NUTRITION AND LIFESTYLE : OPPORTUNITIES FOR CANCER PREVENTION

International Agency For Research On Cancer

The International Agency for Research on Cancer (IARC) was established in 1965 by the World Health Assembly, as an independently financed organization within the framework of the World Health Organization. The headquarters of the Agency are at Lyon, France.

The Agency conducts a programme of research concentrating particularly on the epidemiology of cancer and the study of potential carcinogens in the human environment. Its field studies are supplemented by biological and chemical research carried out in the Agency's laboratories in Lyon, and, through collaborative research agreements, in national research institutions in many countries. The Agency also conducts a programme for the education and training of personnel for cancer research.

The publications of the Agency are intended to contribute to the dissemination of authoritative information on different aspects of cancer research. A complete list is printed at the back of the book. Information about IARC publications and how to order them, is also available via the Internet at: **http://www.iarc.fr/**

This volume is the outcome of the European Conference on Nutrition and Cancer held in Lyon, France on 21–24 June, organized by the International Agency for Research on Cancer, World Health Organization, with the support of the Europe Against Cancer programme of the European Commission.

Cover illustration: The lunch of the Portuguese at Ormuz. Painting of the mid XVIth century. Biblioteca Casanatense, Rome (manuscript 1889)

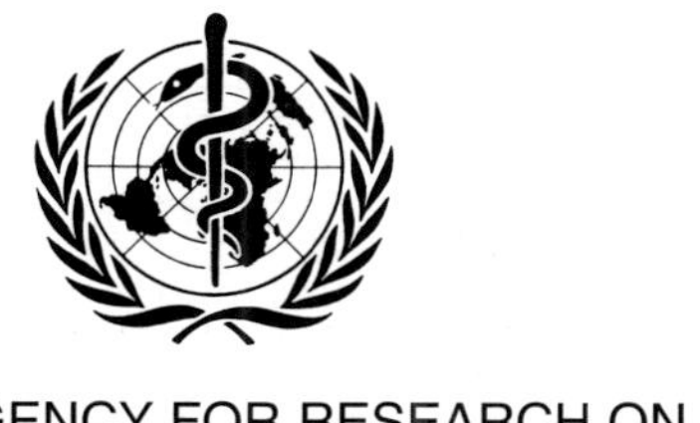

INTERNATIONAL AGENCY FOR RESEARCH ON CANCER

WORLD HEALTH ORGANIZATION

Nutrition and Lifestyle: Opportunities for Cancer Prevention

Edited by

E. Riboli and R. Lambert

IARC Scientific Publications No. 156

International Agency for Research on Cancer
Lyon, France
2002

Published by the International Agency for Research on Cancer,
150 cours Albert Thomas, 69372 Lyon cédex 08, France

Distributed by Oxford University Press, Walton Street, Oxford OX2 6DP, UK (fax: +44 1865 267782) and in the USA by Oxford University Press, 2001 Evans Road, Carey, NC 27513 (fax: +1 919 677 1303). All IARC publications can also be ordered directly from IARC Press (fax: +33 04 72 73 83 02; E-mail: press@iarc.fr).

IARC Library Cataloguing in Publication Data

Nutrition and lifestyle: opportunities for cancer prevention/
editors, E. Riboli, R. Lambert.

(IARC scientific publications; 156)

1. Epidemiology 2. Neoplasms - etiology 3. Nutrition I. Riboli, Elio II. Lambert, René, 1930- III. Title IV. Series

ISBN 92 832 2156 7 (NLM Classification W1)
ISSN 0300-5085

Printed in France

Contents

Chapter 1

Nutrition, past, present and future

Nutrition and cancer: a complex relationship

The search for the links between diet, nutritional and metabolic factors and cancer etiology is an area of research which, over the past two decades has attracted increasing attention both from a scientific and a public health point of view. This growing interest can be explained by exciting scientific developments and their perception by society at large.

The public health relevance is quite evident, due to the universal nature of the factors under study, namely dietary habits, physical activity, and anthropometric, hormonal and metabolic characteristics. Even a weak biological effect on the carcinogenicity process, either causative or preventive, exercised by highly prevalent factors such as the consumption of an unbalanced diet, a sedentary lifestyle and moderate overweight may have a large impact on the cancer burden at the population level. As a consequence, the potential implications of dietary habits and nutritional status for the prevention of cancer and other chronic diseases are progressively being integrated into the public health agenda.

In the 1980s the European Union created the Europe Against Cancer Program, which rapidly identified nutrition as one of the highest priority areas for cancer research and prevention. It was decided to support initiatives on two parallel lines: to formulate, for the first time, European recommendations for cancer prevention that also included nutritional advice, and to promote large, novel epidemiological studies on nutrition and cancer.

Based on the scientific evidence available at that time, the European Code Against Cancer recommended that people consume large amounts of fruit and vegetables, avoid overweight, and moderate their consumption of alcoholic beverages. These recommendations were added to those on the avoidance of well-established risk factors such as tobacco and occupational exposures to carcinogens.

There is, in general, agreement that a diet rich in fruit and vegetables is associated with lower cancer risk, particularly for cancers of the digestive and respiratory tracts. On the other hand, high intake of red and/or processed meats may moderately increase the risk for colorectal cancer and high intake of salt and salt-preserved foods may increase stomach cancer risk.

A major development has been the growing recognition of overweight as a risk factor for cancers of the colon, endometrium, kidney and, in postmenopausal women, of the breast. Lack of physical activity, typical of the sedentary lifestyle of economically developed societies, also seems to increase the risk of colorectal cancer. Several prospective cohort studies have lent strong support for the hypothesis that estrogens and androgens play a prominent role in the etiology of breast cancer. Recent studies have supported new hypotheses on the involvement of hyper-insulinaemia and elevated insulin-like growth factors (IGF) in the pathogenesis of cancers of the prostate, breast and colorectum. Variations in the pattern of estrogens, androgens, IGF and their binding proteins are probably determined by a complex interaction of both nutritional and lifestyle factors as well as inherited genetic susceptibility, as suggested by recent studies on polymorphisms in genes encoding for enzymes that regulate steroid hormone metabolism and hormone receptors.

Thus, the relationship between diet and cancer is much more complex than was previously thought. Research on diet and cancer based solely on simple dietary questionnaire measurements and on a retrospective case–control approach probably has little chance of leading to major breakthroughs in our understanding of this matter. Laboratory investigations on human subjects, within the framework of prospective epidemiological studies are more likely to lead us a step further.

This was the basis of the strategic decision of the International Agency for Research on Cancer (IARC) to give priority to the development of prospective cohort studies on Nutrition and Cancer with repositories of blood samples collected from healthy study subjects. The Europe Against Cancer Program has supported the realization of the European Prospective Investigation into Cancer and Nutrition (EPIC), an unprecedented large prospective study, involving about half a million volunteers in 10 European countries.

Over the past 10–15 years a new generation of large epidemiological prospective cohort studies has also been conducted in North America, Australia and Japan, conceived and designed specifically to investigate the relationship between nutrition and cancer. This book summarizes the results of the European Conference on Nutrition and Cancer that took place at a moment of substantial expansion of research in the field. It offers the opportunity to examine the accumulated scientific evidence on the relationship between nutrition and cancer, with a multidisciplinary and multifactorial approach encompassing epidemiology, nutrition research, endocrinology, carcinogenesis, molecular biology and genetics. All these disciplines contribute to a better understanding of the complex relationship between nutrition and cancer and thereby form the scientific basis for the promotion of effective public health measures.

Elio Riboli
René Lambert
Paul Kleihues

Some methodological issues in nutritional epidemiology

Day N. E.[1], Ferrari P.[2]

[1]University of Cambridge. [2]IARC, Lyon, France.

Introduction

Twenty years ago, it was suggested that dietary factors made a major contribution to the burden of cancer in western populations (Doll & Peto, 1981). Although wide uncertainty over the estimate was acknowledged, a figure of 30% was put on the reduction in cancer incidence potentially achievable through dietary intervention. In the succeeding 20 years, however, progress has been slow in providing the epidemiological evidence to establish conclusively specific diet–disease relationships, as illustrated by the two authoritative reviews that have appeared in recent years (COMA Report, 1998; World Cancer Research Fund, 1997). Much of the earlier data, indicating a substantial role for diet at many cancer sites, consisted of the results of retrospective case–control studies. Many of these results were not later confirmed by the results of prospective cohort studies, which avoid at least some of the potential problems with retrospective studies. An example is given by the relationship of fat consumption to risk of breast cancer. In the 1970s and 1980s, many case–control studies were reported, consistently indicating a smooth increase in risk with increasing fat intake, particularly saturated fat. The results of an overview of the more quantitative of such studies (Howe *et al.*, 1990) are given in Table 1a. They are in striking contrast to the combined results of a number of prospective studies (Hunter *et al.*, 1996), Table 1b, the prospective studies providing no evidence for a relationship. Similar contrasts have been seen, for example, in the relationship between dietary fibre and colorectal cancer (Willett *et al.*, 1990; World Cancer Research Fund, 1997). The methodological problems that could give rise to these conflicting results are well recognized and include:

- The range of variation in diet-associated risk across most populations that have been studied is unlikely to be large, partly reflecting the relative lack of variation in the dietary variables across these populations. With most food constituents, fat and fibre for example, there will not be a nonconsuming subpopulation, as there is with alcohol and tobacco consumption.
- Methods for dietary assessment feasible for use in large epidemiological studies are necessarily rather imprecise.
- Diet may well be modified in the preclinical phase of disease, in the months preceding diagnosis.

To these must be added the problems

Table 1a. Fat consumption and risk of breast cancer: the results of an overview of 12 case–control studies (Howe *et al.*, 1991); odds ratios associated with different quintiles of total fat and saturated fat intake

Quintile of intake	1	2	3	4	5
Total fat[a]	1.0	1.20	1.24	1.24	1.46
Saturated fat[a]	1.0	1.16	1.47	1.36	1.57

[a]Trend test $P<0.0001$ for both.

Table 1b. Fat consumption and risk of breast cancer: the results of an overview of eight cohort studies (Hunter *et al.*, 1996); relative risks associated with different quintiles of total fat and saturated fat intake

Quintile of intake	1	2	3	4	5
Total fat[a]	1.0	1.01	1.12	1.07	1.05
Saturated fat[a]	1.0	1.03	1.04	1.00	1.07

[a]Trend test nonsignificant for both.

typical of retrospective case control studies, namely selection and recall bias, the effects of which are likely to be exacerbated when studying weak effects with imprecise instruments. An elegant study within the Nurses Study demonstrated that these two forms of bias can generate a spurious fat–breast cancer relationship of similar magnitude to that reported by the case–control overview (Giovannucci *et al.*, 1993).

The inference is inescapable that retrospective studies on their own are unlikely to establish conclusively the correct quantitative relationship between diet and cancer. Prospective studies are required. However, it seems surprising that a wide variety of case–control studies, done in different populations with different instruments, each with distinct forms of selection bias, should yield such a consistently false pattern of results. The discrepancy between the case–control and cohort studies may not be entirely the result of errors in the former. The question is whether the dietary instruments used in the moderately large cohort studies which have reported to date are adequate, or whether the negative results reported on fat intake and breast cancer, or fibre intake and colorectal cancer, are artefacts of imprecise measurement and lack of exposure variation in the study population.

The assessment of measurement error

The main dietary instrument used in the majority of cohort studies that have reported results on diet and cancer has been some version of a food frequency questionnaire (FFQ). The precision with which these instruments can quantitatively assess intake of a variety of dietary constituents has customarily been evaluated, in so-called validation studies, by comparison with other record-type instruments (Willett, 1998). Recent work, however, has cast doubt on the validity of such an approach, since there is accumulating evidence that different record-type instruments, whether FFQs, diaries or weighed daily records, have errors which are correlated across individuals (Day *et al.*, 2001; Kipnis *et al.*, 2001; Plummer & Clayton, 1993a, 1993b). This correlation between the errors of the two instruments, which we will call the test instrument (the FFQ) and the calibration instrument, will lead to an underestimation of the error variance of the FFQ, and hence an underestimation of the extent of the regression dilution bias. To avoid this underestimation, one needs a genuinely independent calibration instrument, for example a biochemical or physiological measure, which is closely related to the nutrient intake of interest. For nitrogen and potassium dietary intake, 24-h urinary excretion of nitrogen and potassium have been validated as suitable calibration measures, particularly if a series of such 24-h urine collections are made, since the value of a calibration instrument decreases with increasing error variance.

In a recent paper (Day *et al.*, 2001), both the FFQ and a 7-day diet diary were assessed in relation to the mean of six separate 24-h urinary measures of nitrogen and potassium. These two dietary instruments were evaluated in terms of their error variances (Table 2a), the correlation between the errors in repeated application of the same instrument (Table 2b), the correlation between the errors of different nutrients using the same instrument (Table 2c), and finally the correlation between errors in the same nutrient using the two instruments (Table 2d). The results demonstrate that:

- The error variance of the FFQ is approximately twice that of the 7-day diary for both nutrients, and considerably larger than suggested when using record-type methods as the calibration instrument.
- The errors for both nutrients are substantially correlated between the two instruments. If the 7-day diary had been used to calibrate the FFQ, in the mistaken belief that the two had independent errors, the performance of the FFQ would have been substantially overestimated.
- The correlation between errors in repeat application of both instruments is roughly 0.5, indicating that repeated application of either instrument is not an effective way to reduce regression dilution.
- The correlation between errors in assessment of the two nutrients is high, higher for the FFQ (0.8) than for the 7-day diary (0.7). The estimated correlation between the 'true' intakes of nitrogen and

Table 2a. Performance of a food frequency questionnaire and a 7-day diet diary in assessing intake of nitrogen and potassium, calibrated against six 24-h urine measurements. Variances of the true intake and of the errors of measurement for estimates of N and K intake by the two instruments.

	N (g/day)	K (mmol/day)
True intake	5.1	235
Error of FFQ	14.9	522
Error of 7-day diary	4.8	246

Table 2b. Correlation between errors in repeated measurements with the same instrument.

	N	K
Repeats of FFQ	0.45	0.56
Repeats of 7-day diary	0.52	0.58

Table 2c. Correlation between true intake of N and K and the errors in assessing N and K intake, for the two instruments.

FFQ	0.80
7-day diary	0.70
True intake	0.69

Table 2d. Correlation between the FFQ and 7-day diary in the errors in assessing intake of N and K

	N	K
Correlation between errors	0.27	0.29

potassium is 0.69, i.e. considerably less than the correlation between the errors for the FFQ estimated intakes. The implication of this high level of correlation will be discussed later.

These results indicate that the FFQ that has been used in many of the cohort studies that have reported to date suffers substantially more from regression dilution than had been previously thought. Although the results only apply to nitrogen, and so protein and potassium, they clearly indicate that negative results obtained with this FFQ need to be interpreted cautiously. The disparity between the positive results of the retrospective studies and the negative results of the cohort studies may not be entirely the consequence of excessive bias in the retrospective studies.

Energy adjustment and correlated errors

The discussion in the preceding paragraphs has ignored adjustment for total energy intake. Observational epidemiological studies should mimic the controlled experiment one would ideally have conducted. Dietary experiments would almost always be isocaloric, unless energy itself were the variable of interest, which corresponds, in epidemiological terms, to adjusting for energy consumption (Willett, 1998). The problem is that in using an FFQ as the dietary instrument, energy consumption is poorly estimated. As part of the EPIC Norfolk cohort study, measurement of energy consumption by the FFQ and the 7-day diary was evaluated by comparison with energy expenditure, as measured by 4-day heart rate monitoring – a method validated against doubly labelled water measurements (Wareham *et al.*, 1997). The experiment was conducted in 100 volunteers. Figure 1 displays graphically the relationship between energy expenditure and energy intake assessed by the FFQ and by the 7-day diary. The relationship between energy expenditure and weight is also given. As can be seen, the FFQ estimate of energy intake is only very weakly related to energy expenditure; the 7-day diary estimate is more strongly related. Weight, however, is more strongly related to energy expenditure than either of the dietary estimates of intake. This result indicates that if the aim is to adjust for energy intake, then using weight as a surrogate would be better than using either of the dietary measures. Adjustment for weight is often done, but typically it has only a minimal effect on any diet–disease associations. That is, adjusting for energy *per se*, although indicated biologically, pragmatically has little effect.

Paradoxically, however, adjusting for the FFQ estimate of energy intake can have a substantial effect on FFQ-derived diet–disease associations. The FFQ estimate of energy intake is made up of two components, one reflecting true energy intake, the other comprising the error term. Since, as we have seen, the energy component has little effect, the effect that is seen of adjusting for the FFQ estimate must derive from the error term. One is adjusting for error, and the reason why error adjustment may have a substantial effect is because of the high correlation that can exist between the errors associated with intake of different nutrients, when using the FFQ.

Formally, one would have:

$$\log(\text{relative risk}) = b_1{*}(\text{nutrient1} + \text{error in nutrient1}) + b_2{*}(\text{nutrient2} + \text{error in nutrient2})$$

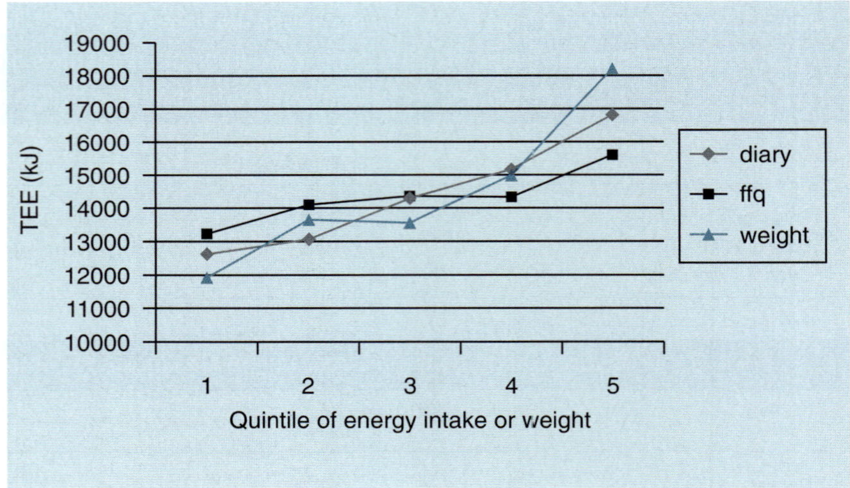

Figure 1
Relationship of total energy expenditure (TEE), as measured by heart rate monitoring, with weight and energy intake assessed by a 7-day food diary (7dd) or a food frequency questionnaire (FFQ).

If the correlation between the error terms dominates, then one might expect to see the estimates of b_1 and b_2 to have opposite signs so that the errors 'cancel'. This would resemble negative confounding and to some extent remove the effect of measurement error. More specifically, if:

1. The true variance of nutrient(i) is $\varsigma_i 2^{**}2$.
2. The error variance of nutrient(i) is $\sigma_i 2^{**}2$.

3. The correlation between the true values of the two nutrients in the population is ρ and the correlation between the two errors is ρ^*. Both correlations are taken to be non-negative.
4. The true value of $b_1 = 1$ and the true value of $b_2 = 0$, i.e. we are considering the situation where only nutrient1 is genuinely associated with disease, and nutrient2 is not a genuine confounder.

When each variable is fitted separately, the univariate estimates of b_1 and b_2 are given by:

b_1 (univ) $= \varsigma_1^2/(\varsigma_1^2 + \sigma_1^2)$, expressing the effect of measurement error, and b_2 (univ) $= \rho\varsigma_1\ \varsigma_2/(\varsigma_2^2 + \sigma_2^2)$, indicating the positive confounding effect of the first nutrients on the second.

When fitting the two variables simultaneously, the bivariate estimates will depend on ρ and ρ^*. Considering first the case of uncorrelated errors, ρ^*0, then we have:

b_1(biv)< b_1(univ)<1
and
0< b_2(biv)< b_2(univ)<1,

In this situation, the effect of measurement error is to spread incorrectly the real exposure disease relationship, which is concentrated on the first nutrient (b_1=1, b_2=0), across both nutrients. If the measurement error for the first nutrient is substantially greater than that for the second, the bivariate regression can suggest that the second nutrient is in fact more strongly related to disease. This phenomenon has been recognized for many years (Tzonou *et al.*, 1986).

Clearly, interpretation of the observed values of the univariate and bivariate regression coefficients requires some knowledge of the error structure.

When ρ^* is not zero, which, as we saw in Table 2, is likely to be the case in nutritional epidemiology, the situation is more complicated. The univariate estimates are unaffected by ρ^*. However, as ρ^* increases, then if the other parameters are held constant, b_1(biv) increases and b_2(biv) decreases. In particular, when:

$$\varsigma_1\sigma_2\rho^* > \varsigma_2\sigma_1\rho$$

we have both

$$0 < b_1(\text{univ}) < b_1(\text{biv})$$

and

$$b_2(\text{biv}) < 0.$$

If we have $\sigma_1\varsigma_1 \sim \sigma_2{}_2$, as is the case in Table 2 and might be approximately true for many pairs of nutrients, then the condition reduces approximately to

$$\rho^* > \rho$$

If the correlation between the errors is greater than the correlation between the true values of the nutrients themselves, as was the case in Table 2 for the FFQ but not the 7-day diary, then:

- An effect resembling negative confounding is induced, and
- The effect of measurement error on the univariate estimate for nutrient1 is partially removed in the bivariate estimate.

Thus, whether adjusting for nutrient2 is helpful, by removing some of the effect of measurement error, or harmful, by introducing spurious positive confounding and hence magnifying the effect of measurement error, depends on the relative values of ρ^* and ρ. These two values are not generally known, and their estimation requires the availability of biomarkers for both nutrient1 and nutrient2.

The implications for adjusting for total energy intake are not straightforward. The intake of most nutrients is likely to be positively correlated with total energy intake. For fat, for example, this correlation might be expected to be high. For a nutrient such as vitamin C, in contrast, the correlation could be only moderate. There is little direct information for most dietary constituents as to the magnitude of the correlation between the errors. Empirically, however, it has been noted that adjusting for estimated energy intake appears to sharpen estimated relative risks. This observation suggests that for the FFQ, the correlation between the errors is greater than the correlation between the true intake of the underlying nutrients. In addition, it appears from Table 2 that the error variances typically dominate the variances of the true intakes. Thus one is led to the conclusion that, when using the FFQ, fitting multivariate dietary models will result in multivariate estimates of relative risk, which in large part reflect the error structure of the underlying variables. If this error structure is not known, then the relationship between the estimated risks and the true underlying risks will be obscure. The estimated risks may be seriously misleading.

Reducing the effect of measurement error

The critical parameters in determining the extent to which measurement error distorts estimated relative risks are the ratios of the error variances to the variances of the true intakes. Even in the multivariate situation, correlation between the errors only enters into the expected values for the regression coefficients through the product

$$\rho^*\sigma_1\sigma_2/\varsigma_1\varsigma_2$$

and its multivariate generalizations.

As the ratios of the error to true variances decrease, so the effect of ρ^* diminishes. There are two ways by which one can decrease these variance ratios. One is by decreasing the error variances themselves, by devising better dietary assessment instruments. From Table 2, it appears that a 7-day diet diary might represent such an improvement. It is currently being employed in EPIC Norfolk (Day *et al.*, 1999) and time will tell whether they provide more accurate estimates of risk than the FFQ, which is also being used. The second approach to reducing the effect of measurement error is to concentrate on ς rather than σ, i.e. to increase the variation of true exposure by choosing more heterogeneous study populations. The range of variation for most dietary factors in the full EPIC cohort is considerably greater than that seen in the majority of single-country cohorts, as in the overview by Hunter *et al.* (1996). Given the error variances associated with the FFQ, even an apparently moderate increase in the observed population variance, i.e. the variance including the error variance, may have a surprisingly large effect. Increasing the observed standard error by 30%, if this increase is entirely due to increased true variance, would change a regression dilution parameter from, for example, 3 to 1.67, or a value of 5 to a value of 1.9. This improvement will only occur if the analysis in the more heterogeneous cohort is not stratified by subcohort in a way that would remove the extra variation. At present in EPIC, the intention is to stratify either by country or by centre. The purpose is to remove centre confounding effects that cannot be removed by known covariates, to reduce the possibility that any observed risks are the result of hidden confounding. An analytic challenge for EPIC is to devise analytic strategies that permit maximum use of the full variation across the cohort, but at the same time minimizing the effect of unobserved confounding factors.

References

COMA Report. (1998) Nutritional aspects of the development of cancer. Report of the Working Group on Diet and Cancer of the Committee on Medical Aspects of Food and Nutrition Policy (COMA). **48**, Norwich, HMSO

Day, N.E.,Oakes S., Luben, R., Khaw, K.T., Bingham, S., Welch, A. & Wareham, N. (1999) EPIC-Norfolk: study design and characteristics of the cohort. *Br. J. Cancer*, **80 (Suppl. 1)**, 95–103

Day, N.E., McKeown, N., Wong, N.Y., Welch, A. & Bingham, S. (2001) Epidemiological assessment of diet: a comparison of a 7-day diary with a food frequency questionnaire using urinary markers of nitrogen, potassium and sodium. *Int. J. Epidemiol.*, **30**, 309–317

Doll, R. & Peto, R. (1981) The causes of cancer. *J. Natl. Cancer Inst.*, **66**, 1191–1308

Giovannucci, E., Stampfer, M.J., Colditz, G.A., Manson, J.E., Rosner, B.A., Longnecker, M., Speizer, F.E. & Willett, W.C. (1993) A comparison of prospective and retrospective assessments of diet in the study of breast cancer. *Am. J. Epidemiol.*, **137**, 502–511

Howe, G.R., Hirohata, T., Hislop, T.G., Iscovich, J.M., Yuan, J.M., Katsouyanni , K., Lubin, F., Marubini, E., Modan, B. & Rohan, T. (1990) Dietary factors and risk of breast cancer: combined analysis of 12 case–control studies. *J. Natl. Cancer Inst.*, **82**, 561–569

Hunter, D.J., Spiegelman, D., Adami, H.O., Beeson, L., van den Brandt, P.A., Folsom, A.R., Fraser, G.E., Goldbohm, R.A., Graham, S. & Howe, G.R. (1996) Cohort studies of fat intake and the risk of breast cancer – a pooled analysis. *N. Engl. J. Med.*, **334**, 356–361

Kipnis, V., Midthune, D., Freedman, L.S., Bingham, S., Schatzkin, A., Subar, A. & Carroll, R.J. (2001) Empirical evidence of correlated biases in dietary assessment instruments and its implications. *Am. J. Epidemiol.*, **153**, 394–403

Plummer, M. & Clayton, D. (1993a) Measurement error in dietary assessment: an investigation using covariance structure models, Part I. *Stat. Med.*, **12**, 925–935

Plummer, M. & Clayton, D. (1993b) Measurement error in dietary assessment: an investigation using covariance structure models, Part II. *Stat. Med.*, **12**, 937–948

Tzonou, A., Kaldor, J., Smith, P.G., Day, N.E. & Trichopoulos, D. (1986) Misclassification in case–control studies with two dichotomous risk factors. *Rev. Epidemiol. Santé Publique*, **34**, 10–17

Wareham, N.J., Hennings, S.J., Prentice, A.M. & Day, N.E. (1997) Feasibility of heart rate monitoring to estimate total level and pattern of energy expenditure in a population-based epidemiological study: the Ely Young Cohort Feasibility Study. *Br. J. Nutr.*, **78**, 889–900

Willett, W.C. (1998) *Nutritional Epidemiology*, 2nd ed., New York, Oxford University Press

Willett, W.C., Stampfer, M.J., Colditz, G.A., Rosner, B.A. & Speizer, F.E. (1990) Relation of meat fat and fibre intake to the risk of colon cancer in a prospective study among women. *N. Engl. J. Med.*, **323**, 1664–1672

World Cancer Research Fund (1997) *Food, Nutrition and the Prevention of Cancer: A Global Perspective.* Washington, D.C., WCRF/American Institute for Cancer Research

A new method for calibration of long-term dietary intake by repeated short-term measurements

Hoffmann K., Kroke A., Klipstein-Grobusch K., Boeing H.
Department of Epidemiology, German Institute of Human Nutrition, Potsdam-Rehbrücke, Germany.

Introduction

Long-term dietary intakes obtained by different food frequency questionnaires (FFQs) are not comparable and cannot be considered as measurements of the same latent exposure variable. This nonconformity is a serious impediment to pool data of the EPIC (European Prospective Investigation into Cancer and Nutrition) study or of other large-scale studies with country-specific FFQs. Nonconformity also occurs as a result of bias specific for groups, i.e. for men and women. To standardize long-term food and nutrient intake, FFQ data should be calibrated by standardized reference measurements such as 24-h recalls based on EPIC-SOFT (Slimani *et al.*, 1999, 2000). A known problem in calibration is that 24-h recalls and other reference assessment tools applied hitherto refer to very short time periods and were not provided to measure long-term habitual dietary intake of individuals. Therefore, a new calibration method was elaborated that firstly estimates the expected distribution of habitual or usual dietary intake from the short-term reference measurements and then standardizes the FFQ data to have a similar distribution.

Method

The proposed method needs one questionnaire measurement and repeated short-term reference measurements for a randomly selected subgroup of study participants. The calibration procedure consists of the following six steps that must be subsequently performed:

1. Transformation of the reference measurements to normality.
2. Average of the transformed reference data for each individual.
3. Shrinkage of the individual means in the transformed scale.
4. Back-transformation of the shrunken individual means to estimate usual intake.
5. Power transformation of the questionnaire data to approximate skewness and kurtosis of the estimated usual intake distribution.
6. Standardization of the power-transformed data to the sample mean and variance of the estimated usual intake distribution.

In the first four steps, the usual intake distribution is estimated by removing the intraindividual variability of the reference measurements. This part of the procedure is similar to a method recently proposed by Nusser *et al.* (1996, 1997) for food consumption surveys. The last two steps define the calibration function. Note that the calibration function is a nonlinear strictly monotone increasing function.

Results

The proposed method was applied to data from the EPIC Potsdam validation study (Kroke *et al.*, 1999). Here, 12 computer-assisted 24-h dietary recall interviews conducted in a 1-year validation study with 134 participants (75 men and 59 women) were used as reference measurements. Because of different FFQ biases, men and women were calibrated separately. The nonlinear calibration method was compared with three linear methods. Besides the most frequently applied linear regression calibration, a so-called additive method with a slope of 1 and a multiplicative method with 0 intercept were included in the comparison. All methods have the property of the arithmetic mean of the calibrated data coinciding with that of estimated usual intake.

In Table 1, the mean, standard deviation, skewness, and kurtosis are given for estimated usual and calibrated

Table 1. Comparison of usual macronutrient intake with intake, obtained by FFQ and calibrated by different methods[a]

	Men (n=75)				Women (n=59)			
Nutrient / method	**AM[b]**	**SD[c]**	**Sk[d]**	**Ku[e]**	**AM[b]**	**S[c]**	**Sk[d]**	**Ku[e]**
Energy (MJ)								
Estimated usual intake[f]	9.71	1.37	0.14	0.39	7.23	1.28	0.37	0.46
Nonlinear calibration	9.71	1.37	0.32	0.29	7.23	1.28	0.48	0.38
Linear calibration	9.71	0.72	0.13	0.06	7.23	0.87	0.65	0.57
Additive calibration	9.71	1.96	0.13	0.06	7.23	1.94	0.65	0.57
Multiplicative calibration	9.71	1.96	0.13	0.06	7.23	1.75	0.65	0.57
Total protein (g)								
Estimated usual intake	82.5	10.1	0.03	0.42	61.6	10.0	–0.16	–0.23
Nonlinear calibration	82.5	10.1	–0.02	0.43	61.6	10.0	–0.16	–0.27
Linear calibration	82.5	4.1	0.15	0.67	61.6	5.7	1.16	1.19
Additive calibration	82.5	17.6	0.15	0.67	61.6	18.2	1.16	1.19
Multiplicative calibration	82.5	17.9	0.15	0.67	61.6	16.9	1.16	1.19
Total fat (g)								
Estimated usual intake	92.6	15.3	–0.25	–0.06	65.0	16.2	0.63	0.96
Nonlinear calibration	92.6	15.3	–0.27	–0.17	65.0	16.2	0.96	0.80
Linear calibration	92.6	8.7	0.22	–0.02	65.0	11.1	0.52	0.08
Additive calibration	92.6	23.6	0.22	–0.02	65.0	20.6	0.52	0.08
Multiplicative calibration	92.6	26.4	0.22	–0.02	65.0	20.4	0.52	0.08
Total carbohydrate (g)								
Estimated usual intake	243.8	48.5	0.40	–0.12	204.3	38.6	0.32	0.20
Nonlinear calibration	243.8	48.5	0.22	0.14	204.3	38.6	0.29	0.23
Linear calibration	243.8	28.2	0.46	0.41	204.3	25.5	0.47	0.45
Additive calibration	243.8	55.8	0.46	0.41	204.3	56.2	0.47	0.45
Multiplicative calibration	243.8	55.5	0.46	0.41	204.3	51.4	0.47	0.45

[a]Data are from a validation study conducted in 1995–1996 as part of the EPIC Potsdam study.
[b]Arithmetic mean.
[c]Standard deviation.
[d]Skewness.
[e]Kurtosis.
[f]The usual intake distribution was estimated on the basis of 12 repeated 24-h recalls.

Table 2. Percentage of men within subjects with total energy intake (MJ/d) below specified threshold values: comparison of calibration methods[a]

Method	Upper limit for individual energy intake (MJ/d)					
	7.5	**8**	**9**	**10**	**11**	**11.5**
Estimated usual intake[b]	10.5	13.5	27.0	44.7	51.6	53.5
Nonlinear calibration	11.4	16.7	28.4	45.2	50.8	53.5
Regression calibration	0	0	18.6	45.9	55.3	55.6
Additive calibration	20.5	27.6	31.4	44.8	49.6	51.7
Multiplicative calibration	20.5	27.6	31.0	43.9	49.6	51.7

[a]Data are from a validation study with 134 participants conducted in 1995–1996 as part of the EPIC Potsdam study.
[b]Usual intake was estimated on the basis of 12 repeated 24-h recalls.

intake of total energy, total protein, total fat and total carbohydrate. Obviously, linear regression calibration is characterized by excessive shrinking of the observed intake distribution. The standard deviation varies between 40% and 70% of that estimated for usual intake. On the other hand, additive and multiplicative calibration result in variances that are too large. However, nonlinearly calibrated data possess the same variability as the estimated usual intake. Moreover, the nonlinear method achieves the best fit of the entire usual intake distribution since after calibration, skewness and kurtosis are close and mean and standard deviation are even equal.

The effect of the calibration methods on the mixture of groups in a pooled data analysis is described in Table 2. Here, the proportion of men in the combined sample of all subjects with energy intake below a threshold is given for specified threshold values. Obviously, the proportions are close for usual and nonlinearly calibrated intake, whereas both genders are more clearly separated by linear regression and excessively mixed by the other two linear methods.

Discussion

In pooled data of linearly calibrated dietary intake, the ranks belonging to one centre or group can markedly deviate from those expected for true habitual intake. This failure of linear calibration can mix up centre and diet effects on a disease and, therefore, cause bias of relative risk estimates in subsequent statistical analyses. The described nonlinear method, however, is aimed at a similarity of ranks of calibrated FFQ intake and estimated usual intake for each centre. Since usual intake is estimated by reference measurements, the reference data supervise the ranking of subjects coming from different centres.

The proposed nonlinear calibration method requires repeated reference measurements. Repetitions are necessary to obtain an estimate of intraindividual variance, which acts as a connecting link between the observed distribution of reference measurements and the usual intake distribution. Without knowledge of intraindividual variation, the shrinkage of the individual means to the grand mean in the normal scale cannot be quantified.

References

Kroke, A., Klipstein-Grobusch, K., Voss, S., Möseneder, J., Thielecke, F., Noack, R. & Boeing, H. (1999) Validation of a self-administered food frequency questionnaire administered in the European Prospective Investigation into Cancer and Nutrition (EPIC) Study: comparison of energy, protein, and macronutrient intakes estimated with the doubly labeled water, urinary nitrogen, and repeated 24-h dietary recall methods. *Am. J. Clin. Nutr.*, **70**, 439–447

Nusser, S.M., Carriquiry, A.L., Dodd, K.W. & Fuller, W.A. (1996) A semiparametric transformation approach to estimating usual daily intake distributions. *Am. Stat. Assoc.*, **91**, 1440–1449

Nusser, S.M., Fuller, W.A. & Guenther, P.M. (1997) Estimating usual dietary intake distributions: adjusting for measurement error and nonnormality in 24-hour food intake data. In: Lyberg, L., Biemer, P., Collins, M., De Leeuw, E., Dippo, C., Schwarz, N. & Trewin, D., eds., *Survey Measurement and Process Quality*, New York, Wiley and Sons, pp. 689–709

Slimani, N., Deharveng, G., Charrondière, R.U., van Kappel, A.L., Ocké, M.C., Welch, A., Lagiou, A., van Liere, M., Agudo, A., Pala, V., Brandstetter, B., Andrén, C., Stripp, C., van Staveren, W.A. & Riboli, E. (1999) Structure of the standardized computerized 24-h diet recall interview used as reference method in the 22 centers participating in the EPIC project. European Prospective Investigation into Cancer and Nutrition. *Comput. Meth. Programs Biomed.*, **53**, 251–266

Slimani, N., Ferrari, P., Ocké, M., Welch, A., Boeing, H., van Liere, M., Pala, V., Amiano, P., Lagiou, A., Mattisson, I., Stripp, C., Engeset, D., Charrondière, R., Buzzard, M., van Staveren, W. & Riboli, E. (2000) Standardization of the 24-hour diet recall calibration method used in the European Prospective into Cancer and Nutrition (EPIC): general concepts and preliminary results. *Eur. J. Clin. Nutr.*, **54**, 900–917

Potential use of the Web to improve dietary habits – the ECP Diet Web-1 Project

Maskens A.

European Cancer Prevention Organisation (ECP) – Brussels, Belgium.

Purpose

Public health authorities, healthcare professionals and scientists do agree that the public should be informed about those aspects of lifestyle, and in particular diet, which can promote better health and quality of life. In the specific case of cancer, and while evidence is not yet sufficient to make very precise recommendations to groups or individuals, careful advice of a global nature can and should be offered.

Among the possible media that can be used for this purpose, the World Wide Web offers a number of advantages over more traditional media. Information posted on a web site is permanently available to the public. It can be updated as new data become available. Different navigation pathways through the site can be offered, so as to meet the requirements of individuals with different backgrounds and interests. Finally, it can be made interactive and also offer links with other, complementary sources of information.

The ECP has therefore undertaken to develop and test a web site dedicated to information on the potential role of diet in the causation and prevention of cancer.

Methods

A multidisciplinary team has been set up to develop the site. It involved scientists, public information experts and web designers. In a stepwise process, the specific requirements and possibilities linked with this information medium were identified and then translated into a first version of the site design, which was then implemented using standard development tools.

Results

The development reached at the end of this first phase of the project can be seen at www.eu-cancer.org.

The site, presented in English, allows readers to access more than 20 specialized documents. A dynamic table, permanently displayed on the left side of the screen, provides access to any of these documents through no more than two or three mouse clicks.

The structure has four layers, the first layer being the home page.

The second layer presents the four main chapter headings as well as their main sections. One chapter is devoted to scientific information on diet and cancer and has three sections: "What do you know about cancer?", "Diet and cancer", and "Current controversies". The second contains the actual recommendations on preventive diets. The third chapter presents the results of recent ECP workshops and meetings related to diet and cancer. The fourth chapter lists web sites that can provide complementary information. It also offers a number of recipes.

The third layer presents a table of the documents available in each of the chapter sections and thus allows easy access to the detailed information. For instance, a mouse click on the section "Recommendations" will display the following list of topics: "Body weight control", "Choice of fat", "More fruits and vegetables", "Eat more fibre-rich food", "Non-alcoholic and low-alcoholic drinks" and "Physical exercise".

The fourth layer comprises web-style documents presenting detailed information on the selected topic. It uses a simple and clear terminology and describes health-promoting approaches in practical terms. It remains cautious about recommendations and always places cancer-specific advice within the broader context of health promotion in general.

While dietary recommendations constitute the central element of the information presented on the web site, the limits of our current knowledge are emphasized and areas of controversy are specifically identified in a special section. Another section lists, under the heading "Myths about cancer", a number of false ideas which are commonly found in the general public.

While the text is primarily intended for the lay public, references and links useful for healthcare professionals (such as links to EU programmes and on-going research) are included.

Conclusion

The web offers a communication platform that can present complex information targeting the general public through the use of dynamic tables and frames, hyperlinks and a rich display. This allows individual users to quickly and easily access the information they wish to find and to browse through the data according to their own level of interest and background knowledge.

In a second phase of this project, we will add interactivity, implement ways to attract visitors, monitor the use of the site, and translate it into additional languages.

Acknowledgements

The work described in this paper is being carried out with the support of the Europe Against Cancer Programme (General Direction, Health and Consumer Protection) of the European Commission.

Comparison of telephone versus face-to-face interviews in the assessment of dietary intake by the 24-hour recall EPIC SOFT programme – the Norwegian calibration study

Brustad M.[1], Skeie G.[1], Braaten T.[1], Slimani N.[2], Lund E.[1]

[1]Institute of Community Medicine, University of Tromsø, Norway. [2]Unit of Nutrition and Cancer, International Agency for Research on Cancer, Lyon, France.

Introduction

The European Prospective Investigation into Cancer and Nutrition (EPIC) is a large multicentre prospective cohort study in 10 European countries (Riboli & Kaaks, 1997). In the EPIC calibration study, single 24-h dietary recalls were collected from a random sample from each country cohort by means of a highly standardized computer program called EPIC SOFT (Slimani *et al.*, 1999). In all countries except Norway the 24-h recalls were accomplished face-to-face. Due to the wide geographical distribution of participants throughout this sparsely populated country, a telephone approach based on the face-to-face method used in the other EPIC centres was designed and implemented for the Norwegian 24-h dietary recall part of the EPIC calibration study. To compare the method of telephone interviews used for the Norwegian 24-h dietary recalls with the face-to-face approach used in the other EPIC countries, another study was undertaken based on an additional random sampling of two groups of women from the Norwegian cohort (Brustad *et al.*, submitted 2001).

The aim of this study was to compare reported food group intakes in grams, total energy, and energy contribution from macronutrients using EPIC SOFT with either a face-to-face or a telephone 24-h recall interview design, similar to the interviews in the Norwegian part of the EPIC calibration study.

Methods and material

Two groups of women living in Tromsø, the major city in northern Norway, were drawn at random from the Norwegian Women and Cancer cohort, NOWAC (Lund & Gram, 1998). One hundred sixty women were invited to a face-to-face interview. There were 111 women who responded positively (crude response rate, 69.4%) and 102 of these were interviewed. For the telephone interview, 180 were invited to participate. One hundred nine women responded positively (crude response rate, 60.6%) and 103 were interviewed.

The EPIC SOFT computer program was used to conduct single 24-h dietary recall interviews, either by telephone or face to face. The face-to-face interviews were performed at the University Hospital of Tromsø in the Department of Clinical Research. For the face-to-face interviews, plates, cups, glasses, and spoons were used for quantification purposes together with the Norwegian food quantification booklet mailed to the participants in the calibration study. The women interviewed by telephone were mainly approached at home, but a few were called at work according to their own choice. The quantification booklet was mailed to the group interviewed by telephone and the interview routines were similar to the telephone recalls in the calibration study. All interviews in both groups were conducted from Monday to Friday. The interviews were conducted by seven interviewers all trained by the nutritionist responsible for the Norwegian part of the EPIC calibration study.

Results

The two randomized groups of women were comparable with respect to age, body mass index, basal metabolic rate, and special diet status. There was no significant difference in the distribution of interview weekdays between the two groups. The number of subjects reporting illness at recall day was significantly different between the two groups (P=0.03) with two and nine subjects in the face-to-face and telephone group, respectively.

No statistically significant differences in reported dietary intakes were found between interviews conducted by telephone and face-to-face interview, except for "egg and egg products" (P<0.01), which was higher in the telephone group (Table 1). For reported intake of "potatoes and tubers" the difference was borderline significant (P=0.052), which indicated a higher reported intake among the face-to-face group than in the telephone group. Thus, reported intake of only 2 out of the 17 food groups differed significantly between women interviewed face to face and by telephone.

As shown in Table 2, the group interviewed by telephone reported a significantly lower energy intake than the face-to-face group (P=0.02). Energy contribution from macronutrients did not differ significantly between groups, except for energy percentage from protein, which was significantly higher in the telephone group (P=0.02).

When assessing energy intake with the Kruscal-Wallis Test using interviewers as the dependent variable, the difference attributed to the interviewers was borderline significant (P=0.056). When the interviewer recording the highest energy intakes was excluded from the analysis, the P values increased from 0.056 to 0.876. The difference in total energy intake between the two groups of women disappeared when the same interviewer was excluded from the analysis (P=0.46).

Conclusion

Telephone versus face-to-face interview design did not influence recalled diet when using the EPIC SOFT program. However, the results of this study

Table 1. Reported intake in grams of food groups as given by the EPIC-SOFT program according to different settings of 24-hour recall interviews

Food groups	Face-to-face n=102 Median (Mean)	Telephone n=103 Median (Mean)	P values[a]
Potatoes and tubers	66.6 (85.9)	39.2 (58.3)	0.05
Vegetables	98.5 (114.6)	126.1 (146.5)	0.06
Legumes	0.0 (0.0)	0.0 (2.3)	0.08
Fruits	124.2 (152.7)	124.2 (138.4)	0.65
Dairy products	209.65 (262.0)	192.7 (247.8)	0.37
Cereals and cereal products	172.9 (188.3)	161.6 (168.4)	0.34
Meat and meat products	72.7 (88.3)	45.0 (77.5)	0.53
Fish and shellfish	0.0 (63.9)	5.0 (71.5)	0.73
Eggs and egg products	0.0 (6.9)	0.0 (16.1)	0.004
Fat	12.9 (16.5)	9.7 (14.0)	0.21
Sugar and confectionery	31.0 (53.8)	21.0 (35.5)	0.14
Cakes	11.0 (43.2)	0.0 (49.7)	0.70
Nonalcoholic beverages	1840 (1901.9)	1712.2 (2017.9)	0.79
Alcoholic beverages	0.0 (64.8)	0.0 (99.4)	0.42
Condiments and sauces	15.0 (40.0)	10.0 (40.1)	0.95
Soups and bouillon	0.0 (29.3)	0.0 (30.5)	0.98
Miscellaneous	0.0 (2.4)	0.0 (0.8)	0.41

[a]Mann-Whitney Test.

Table 2. Intake of total energy and energy contribution from macronutrients[a]

Energy contribution	Face-to-face n=100	Telephone n=94	P values
Total energy (kcal)	1951.0	1768.0	0.02[b]
Energy from fat	35.7%	33.9%	0.07[c]
Energy from protein	15.1%	16.9%	0.02[c]
Energy from carbohydrates	47.9%	46.5%	0.35[c]
Energy from alcohol	1.5%	2.8%	0.28[c]

[a]Subjects reporting illness at recall day were not included in the analysis.
[b]One-way ANOVA.
[c]Mann-Whitney test.

confirm that the 24-h dietary recall method is vulnerable to interviewer effect.

Acknowledgements

The work described in this paper was carried out with support from 'Europe against Cancer' Programme of the European Commission, and the Department of Clinical Research, University Hospital of Tromsø.

References

Lund, E. & Gram, I.T. (1998) Response rate according to title and length of questionnaire. *Scand. J. Soc. Med.*, **26**,154–160

Riboli, E. & Kaaks, R. (1997) The EPIC project: rationale and study design. European prospective investigation into cancer and nutrition. *Int. J. Epidemiol.*, **26** Suppl 1, S6–S14

Slimani, N., Deharveng, G., Charrondière, R.U., van Kappel, A.L., Ocke, M.C., Welch, A., Lagiou, A., van Liere, M., Agudo, A., Pala, V., Brandstetter, B., Andren, C., Stripp, C., van Staveren, W.A. & Riboli, E. (1999) Structure of the standardized computerized 24-h diet recall interview used as reference method in the 22 centers participating in the EPIC project. European prospective investigation into cancer and nutrition. *Comput. Methods Programs Biomed.*, **58**, 251–266

The role of correlated errors in the multivariate analysis of dietary data

Michels K.B.[1,2], Day N.E.[2]
[1]Harvard University, Boston, USA. [2]University of Cambridge, UK.

Background

In epidemiological studies, diet is generally self-reported and thus assessed with error. The degree of error and the correlation of errors may affect the observed association between diet and disease outcomes. Previous authors have attempted to estimate the magnitude of the error. These measurement-error investigations were based on univariate models and therefore did not address the error correlation between foods or nutrients. Multivariate models of diet may introduce correlated errors that make any results difficult to interpret. Since true intake is never known, several assumptions have to be made when estimating the error. Understanding direction and magnitude of the error is essential for interpreting observed associations between diet and disease outcomes in epidemiological studies. The magnitude of measurement error may depend on the dietary assessment instrument and may differ for different foods, food groups, and nutrients.

Methods

We used dietary information obtained from the European Prospective Investigation of Cancer and Nutrition (EPIC) in Norfolk, UK, a prospective population-based study of 30 445 women and men aged 45–74 years in 1993 and residing in Norfolk. Blood samples were obtained from all participants at baseline and 5 years later. For 1962 participants (1049 women and 913 men) of this cohort, we had information on plasma vitamin C and on dietary intake obtained with both

Table 1. Multivariate linear regression model of vitamin C, fibre, fat and total energy intake diet assessed with a 7-day food diary (7DD) and a food frequency questionnaire (FFQ) in relation to plasma vitamin C levels obtained at baseline and 5 years later

Plasma vitamin C	Nutrients	7DD		FFQ	
		β ± SE (β)[a]	*P* value	β ± SE (β)[a]	*P* value
Short-term	Vitamin C	7.1 ± 0.4	<0.0001	5.2 ± 0.5	<0.0001
	Fibre	1.3 ± 0.5	0.004	−0.1 ± 0.6	0.8
	Fat	−1.2 ± 0.8	0.2	−3.9 ± 0.9	<0.0001
	Energy	−0.5 ± 0.9	0.6	1.6 ± 1.0	0.1
Long-term	Vitamin C	4.6 ± 0.6	<0.0001	4.2 ± 0.7	<0.0001
	Fibre	1.8 ± 0.6	0.005	1.2 ± 0.8	0.1
	Fat	0.3 ± 1.2	0.8	−2.8 ± 1.3	0.02
	Energy	−1.5 ± 1.3	0.3	0.1 ± 1.4	0.9

[a]Regression models were adjusted for age, sex, body mass index (BMI), height and current smoking.

a 7-day food diary (7DD) and a food frequency questionnaire (FFQ). We compared the ability of dietary data assessed with a 7DD and an FFQ to predict vitamin C plasma levels in the short and long term using linear regression models. Prediction of vitamin C plasma levels is of interest as a short-term biomarker of vitamin C intake and as an intermediate marker of overall health. Vitamin supplement users were excluded from the analysis.

Results

Univariate linear regression models clearly identified vitamin C intake obtained from both 7DD and FFQ as the most important predictor of short- and long-term plasma vitamin C. In a multivariate model including vitamin C intake, fibre, fat and total energy, the FFQ identified low fat intake as nearly as important as vitamin C intake in predicting short-term as well as long-term vitamin C plasma levels (Table 1).

Conclusions

Univariate models of diet are generally confounded by foods or nutrients not accounted for. Multivariate models are affected by a complex error correlation. The distortion observed in the present data is likely due to correlated measurement errors among foods measured with the same assessment instrument. Energy adjustment did not improve the estimation of the multivariate models. The multivariate error correlation structure is as yet insufficiently understood but has important implications for the analysis of dietary data and the development of dietary pattern models. Any true effect of diet on disease is likely to be moderate to small. Depending on its magnitude, measurement error may well lead to an attenuation of the relative risk that makes the detection of any true association very difficult.

Do cross-check questions improve food frequency questionnaire data?

Nöthlings U., Hoffmann K., Boeing H.

German Institute of Human Nutrition, Department of Epidemiology, Bergholz-Rehbrücke, Germany.

Purpose

The food frequency questionnaire (FFQ) is the primary instrument for collecting information about dietary exposure in epidemiological studies (Willett, 1998). However, the true overall consumption of food groups is often misreported when subjects are asked to report their frequency of intake of a large number of single food items (Haraldsdottir, 1993). An approach to deal with this problem is the use of cross-check questions to correct the total frequency of foods eaten (Calvert *et al.*, 1997). The aim of this study was to calculate correction factors for food groups by means of cross-check questions and to investigate their impact on the accuracy of FFQ data in the EPIC Potsdam Study.

Method

FFQs completed by 134 participants of the EPIC Potsdam validation study (75 men, 59 women) (Kroke *et al.*, 1999) were analysed. Cross-check questions at the end of the FFQ about the average consumption frequency per day, week or month of the food groups fruit, vegetables, bread, meat, sausage, cheese and non-alcoholic beverages were used to calculate the respective correction factors for each individual. Correction factors were calculated by dividing the responses to the cross-check questions by the sum of frequencies from the FFQ for each group of food.

Corrected and not corrected FFQ data were compared to the average of 10–12 24-hour dietary recalls (24-HDR) of each participant, which covered the same period of time as the FFQ. Differences in the daily consumed amounts estimated by the FFQ in comparison to the 24-HDR were calculated. Furthermore, Pearson correlation coefficients adjusted for attenuation due to within-person variability in the 24-HDR (Beaton *et al.*,

Table 1. Deattenuated Pearson correlation coefficients between log-transformed FFQ data (corrected and not corrected) and 24-HDR data

Food Group	Men (n=75)		Women (n=59)	
	FFQ not corrected	FFQ corrected	FFQ not corrected	FFQ corrected
	r deatt	*r* deatt	*r* deatt	*r* deatt
Fruit	0.55	0.65	0.66	0.68
Vegetables	0.45	0.28	0.43	0.27
Bread	0.38	0.52	0.45	0.63
Meat	0.30	0.38	0.53	0.46
Sausage	0.40	0.57	0.33	0.55
Cheese	0.51	0.74	0.61	0.65
Non-alcoholic beverages	0.77	0.80	0.76	0.77

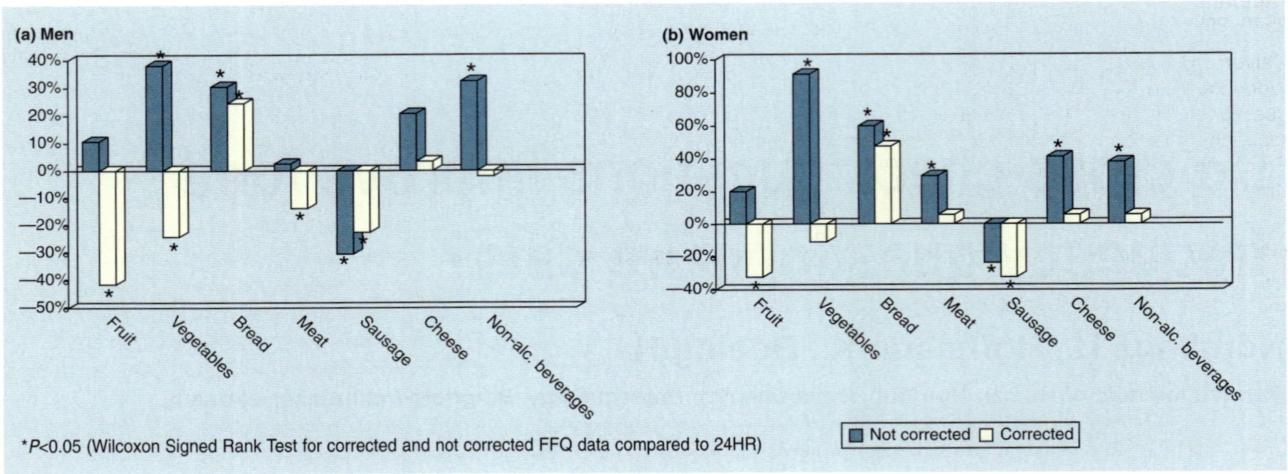

Figure 1
Percent difference of average daily consumption measured by FFQ in comparison to 24-HDR for men **(a)**, *n*=75, and women **(b)**, *n*=59, EPIC Potsdam Validation Study

1979) on logarithmically transformed data were computed. Analysis has been carried out separately for men and women.

Results

Men consumed significantly higher amounts of bread, meat, sausage and cheese than women and women higher amounts of non-alcoholic beverages than men. Consumption of the remaining food groups – vegetables and fruit – showed no significant gender differences (data not shown).

Comparison of crude FFQ data to 24-HDR data indicated significant overreporting for vegetables (39%), bread (31%) and non-alcoholic beverages (33%) in men (Figure 1a). In women, intake of vegetables (91%), bread (60%), meat (29%), cheese (41%) and non-alcoholic beverages (38%) were significantly overestimated (Figure 1b). In contrast, consumption of sausage appeared significantly underreported in both men and women, by 30% and 23%, respectively.

Use of individual correction factors decreased each consumed amount except for sausage in men. After correction, significant underreporting occurred for fruit (–41%), vegetables (–24%), meat (–13%) and sausage (–22%) in men. Bread was still significantly overreported. In women, corrected amounts of fruit (–30%) and sausage (–32%) indicated substantial underreporting. Bread still turned out to be overreported. No relevant differences for cheese and non-alcoholic beverages in both men and women, and additionally, for vegetables and meat in women could be stated.

The use of correction factors improved 11 out of 14 Pearson correlation coefficients (Table 1). The overall percent increase averages 20% in men and 10% in women. Before correction, correlation coefficients ranged from 0.30 for meat to 0.77 for beverages in men and from 0.33 for sausage to 0.76 for non-alcoholic beverages in women. After correction, correlation coefficients increased to values between 0.38 for meat and 0.80 for non-alcoholic beverages in men and from 0.46 for meat to 0.77 for non-alcoholic beverages in women. In contrast to all other food groups, correlation coefficients for vegetables decreased after correction in both genders, from 0.45 to 0.28 and from 0.43 to 0.27 in men and women, respectively.

Conclusion

On the whole, cross-check questions improved the FFQ data. Correction of consumed amounts of food groups was moderate, but all values, except for fruit in both genders, meat in men and sausage in women, were shifted in a profitable way. Cross-check questions also improve the validity of the ranking in reference to 24-HDR data.

In the EPIC Potsdam Study, vegetables seem to be difficult to measure, although overreporting could be reduced by correction, but correlation coefficients with the reference instrument decreased. Thus, a more detailed analysis of reported vegetable consumption in terms of amounts and correlation with 24-HDR is needed.

References

Beaton, G.H., Milner, J., Corey, P., McGuire, V., Cousins, M., Stewart, E., de Ramos, M., Hewitt, D., Grambsch, P.V., Kassim, N. & Little, J.A. (1979) Sources of variance in 24-hour dietary recall data: implications for nutrition study design and interpretation. *Am. J. Clin. Nutr.*, **32**, 2546–2549

Calvert, C., Cade, J., Barrett, J.H. & Woodhouse, A. (1997) Using cross-check questions to address the problem of mis-reporting of specific food groups on Food Frequency Questionnaires. United Kingdom Women's Cohort Study Steering Group. *Eur. J. Clin. Nutr.*, **51**, 708–712

Haraldsdottir, J. (1993) Minimizing error in the field: quality control in dietary surveys. *Eur. J. Clin. Nutr.*, **47**, Suppl 2, S19–S24

Kroke, A., Klipstein-Grobusch, K., Voss, S., Moesenender, J., Thielecke, F., Noack, R. & Boeing, H. (1999) Validation of a self-administered food frequency questionnaire administered in the European Prospective Investigation into Cancer and Nutrition (EPIC) Study: comparison of energy, protein, and macronutrient intakes estimated with the doubly labeled water, urinary nitrogen, and repeated 24-h dietary recall methods. *Am. J. Clin. Nutr.*, **70**, 439–447

Willett, W. (1998) *Nutritional Epidemiology. Monographs in Epidemiology and Biostatistics.* Oxford, United Kingdom, Oxford University Press

Dietscan: a common approach for analysing dietary patterns

Balder H.F.[1], Tan F.[2], Brants H.A.M.[1], Dixon L.B.[3], Virtanen M.[4], Krogh V.[5], Terry P.[6], Pietinen P.[4], Berrino F.[5], Wolk A.[6], Hartman A.[3], Van den Brandt P.A.[2], Goldbohm R.A.[1]

[1]TNO Nutrition and Food Research, Zeist, The Netherlands. [2]Maastricht University, Maastricht, The Netherlands. [3]National Cancer Institute, Bethesda, MD, USA. [4]Finnish National Public Health Institute, Helsinki, Finland. [5]Istituto Nazionale per lo Studio e la Cura dei Tumori, Milano, Italy. [6]Karolinska Institutet, Stockholm, Sweden.

Analysis of dietary patterns is a relatively new approach that identifies combinations of nutrients and foods prevailing in a population (Jacobson & Stanton, 1986; Slattery *et al.*, 1999; Hu *et al.*, 1999). However, a major concern of dietary pattern analysis is the consistency of eating patterns among various populations (Martínez *et al.*, 1998). It remains unclear whether differences in eating patterns observed in previous studies represent true differences in the respective populations, or are simply the result of differences in study methodology. To address this issue, a standardized methodological approach was developed to compare true differences in eating patterns in four different European populations and then to examine the relation between the identified dietary patterns and cancer incidence.

The Dietscan project encompasses four ongoing cohort studies on diet and cancer: the Swedish Mammography Cohort (SMC), The Alpha Tocopherol Beta-Carotene Cancer Prevention Study (ATBC, Finland), the ORmoni e Dieta nella Eziologia dei Tumori (ORDET, Italy) and the Netherlands Cohort Study on diet and cancer (NLCS). Each of these studies was established between 1986 and 1992, with follow-up completed through record linkage of the cohorts with the national or local cancer registries. In all four studies, a semi-quantitative food frequency questionnaire (FFQ) was used, which was validated against dietary records in subsamples of the respective cohorts.

For the food grouping, a priori hypotheses on the association of certain foods and cancer were taken into account. All items from the respective food frequency questionnaires were aggregated into 51 food groups, defined on the basis of the possibly important role in dietary behaviour and their possible relevance to cancer etiology.

Population characteristics of the cohort studies are presented in Table 1. The SMC study and the ORDET study included only women and the ATBC study included only men, whereas the NLCS included both men and women. The participants from the ORDET study were the youngest and the participants from the ATBC study were all current smokers.

The statistical analyses were performed separately for the four cohort studies and separately for men and women. Exploratory factor analysis (EFA) was used to identify dietary patterns (Hatcher, 1994). To assess the impact of arbitrary decisions on the results, sensitivity analyses were carried out with dichotomization of extremely skewed variables, energy adjustment, and EFA options such as the number of factors extracted (2–6) and the type of rotation. On the basis of the scree plot (plot of eigenvalues against the number of factors), four dietary patterns were identified, explaining up to 30% of total variance. The interpretability of the patterns was enhanced by an orthogonal Varimax rotation. Absolute factor loadings larger than 0.35 were considered significant, with a positive loading indicating a positive association with the factor and a negative loading indicating an inverse association. The larger the loading, the greater the contribution of that food group to a specific factor. The first two factors were

Table 1. Study characteristics of the participating cohort studies in the Dietscan project

	ATBC[a]	NLCS[a]	SMC[a]	ORDET[a]
Country	Finland	The Netherlands	Sweden	Italy
Baseline year	1985	1986	1987–1990	1987–1992
Baseline cohort size	27 111	120 852	61 463	9 285
Sex	Men	Men and women	Women	Women
Age range	50–69	55–69	40–74	35–69
FFQ				
Total number of items	276 items	150 items	67 items	107 items
FFQ reference period	12 months	12 months	6 months	12 months
Frequency	Units/times per day/week/month	7 categories (never to 6–7x/week)	8 categories (never/seldom to > 4x/day)	times per week/month
Quantification	Portion size picture booklet (3–5 per item)	Asked in natural or household units (fixed weight per unit)	Age-specific portion sizes	Portion size pictures (less/equal/more than 1–3 pictures)

[a]ATBC, Alpha Tocopherol Beta-Carotene Cancer Prevention Study (Finland); NLCS, Netherlands Cohort Study on Diet and Cancer (Netherlands); SMC, Swedish Mammography Cohort (Sweden); ORDET, ORmoni e Dieta nella Eziologia dei Tumori (Italy)

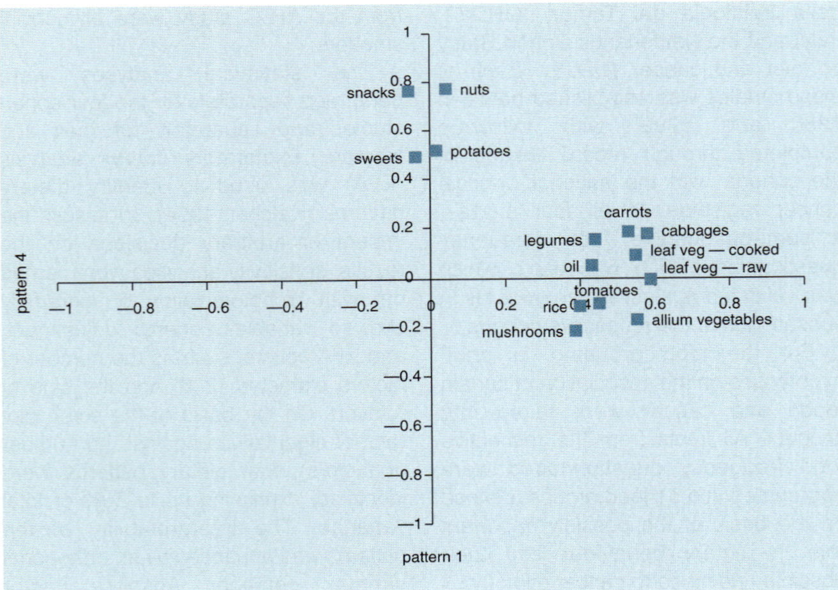

Figure 1
Example of graphical presentation of factor loadings >0.35 on the first and fourth factor in NLCS females

more or less comparable across studies. The first factor had high loadings on raw leaf vegetables and tomatoes and food groups such as dressings, oil, carrots, and cabbages and could therefore be interpreted as a "vegetable" pattern (Figure 1). The second factor had high factor loadings on potatoes, pork, coffee, processed meat and butter and could be labelled as "traditional". In addition to these two comparable factors, various study-specific patterns emerged, such as an "alcohol" pattern (wine, spirits, beer and light beer) and a "fruit" pattern (citrus fruit, fruit juices and berries) in Finland, a "cooked vegetables" (cooked leaf vegetables, cabbages and legumes) pattern in Dutch males and in Italian females, a "snack" pattern (nuts, snacks, potatoes, and sweets) in Dutch females (Figure 1) and a "dairy" pattern (coffee with milk, nonfermented whole milk, nonfermented low fat milk and cakes and cookies) in Italian females. These preliminary findings suggest that some eating patterns are common to the four populations under study, but that other eating patterns are population-specific. In the next step, we will examine the association between the identified patterns and cancer incidence. Of special interest is whether the common eating patterns will show the same associations with cancer risk across the various populations.

References

Hatcher, L. (1994) *A Step-by-Step Approach to Using the SAS System for Factor Analysis and Structural Equation Modeling.* SAS Institute, Cary, NC

Hum, F.B., Rimm, E., Smith-Warner, S.A., Feskanich, D., Stampfer, M.J., Ascherio, A., Sampson, L. & Willett, W.C. (1999) Reproducibility and validity of dietary patterns assessed with a food-frequency questionnaire. *Am. J. Clin. Nutr.*, **69**, 243–249

Jacobson, H.N. & Stanton, J.L. (1986) Pattern analysis in nutrition. *Clin. Nutr.*, **5**, 249–253

Martínez, M.E., Marshall, J.R. & Sechrest, L. (1998) Invited commentary: factor analysis and the search for objectivity. *Am. J. Epidemiol.*, **148**, 17–19

Slattery, M.L., Edwards, S.L., Boucher, K.M., Anderson, K. & Caan, B.J. (1999) Lifestyle and colon cancer: an assessment of factors associated with risk. *Am. J. Epidemiol.*, **150**, 869–877

Demographics and socio-economic differences in adherence to the Mediterranean dietary pattern in Spain

Aller San Juan A.* [6], González C.A.*, * [1], Agudo A.** [1], Argilaga S.** [1], Amiano P.** [2], Barricarte A.* [3], Beguiristain J.M.** [2], Chirlaque M.D.** [4], Dorronsoro M.* [2], Martínez C.* [5], Navarro C.* [4], Quirós J.R.* [6], Rodríguez M.** [5], Tormo M.J.** [4]**

(the EPIC cohort in Spain)

* Principal Investigator, ** Investigator, ***Coordinator of EPIC (in Spain).

[1]Institut Català d'Oncologia, Barcelona. [2]Dirección de Salud de Guipúzcoa, San Sebastián. [3]Departamento de Salud de Navarra, Pamplona. [4]Consejería de Sanidad y Política Social, Murcia. [5]Escuela Andaluza de Salud Pública, Granada. [6]Consejería de Sanidad y Servicios Sociales de Asturias, Oviedo, Spain.

Introduction

Lower social groups usually have a less healthy diet (James, 1997). The aim of this study was to compare social and demographic groups of the Spanish population in their adherence to the Mediterranean dietary pattern (Moreira-Varelas, 1989).

Methods

A cross-sectional study was carried out in three regions of the north and two regions of the south of Spain, in healthy volunteers (15 634 men, 25 812 women) aged 29–69 years, who are members of the EPIC cohort in Spain. The intake of nine groups of food were taken into account to define the pattern of the Mediterranean diet in Spain: vegetables, fruit, legumes, cereals, red meat, fish, olive oil, milk and dairy products, and wine. Two approaches were considered in the analysis: the first was to compare the mean daily intake of each food group and the second was to estimate composite diet scores, using a modified version of the Mediterranean dietary pattern score, developed by Trichopoulou *et al.* (1995) and Olser *et al.* (1997), by educational level and social class of origin. Each component received from 1 to 4 points according to the level of consumption. Quartiles of consumption adjusted for energy were used as cut-off points. Very high consumption (above the 75th percentile) for the groups of fruit, vegetables, fish, legumes, cereals and olive oil, received four points; high consumption (between the 50th and 75th percentile) received 3 points; moderate consumption (between the 25th and 50th percentile) received 2 points and low consumption (under the 25th percentile) received 1 point. Inverse scoring was given for red meat and for milk and dairy products.

For alcohol, the recommendation of having not more than two drinks a day for men, and not more than one drink for women was taken into account. The minimum score (1 point) was given for high consumption of any kind of alcohol (more than 40 g of alcohol a day in men and more than 20 g in women). When the consumption was less than this amount of alcohol, the maximum score (four points) was given for consumption of wine between 1 and 200 mL a day for men and between 1 and 100 mL a day for women. Higher consumption (more than 200 mL of wine in men and more than 100 mL in women), but less than an overall intake of 40 and 30 g of alcohol a

Table 1. Daily mean intake of food group components of the Mediterranean dietary pattern by educational levels in males and females

Food group	Mean intake (g/day)									
	Females					**Males**				
	Primary not completed (*n*=10 146)	Primary (*n*=10 187)	Secondary (*n*=2837)	University (*n*=2445)	*P* value	Primary not completed (*n*=4158)	Primary (*n*=5834)	Secondary (*n*=3240)	University (*n*=2320)	*P* value
Fruit	327.1	322.5	290.0	297.4	0.0001	325.2	320.0	293.5	315.0	0.0007
Vegetables	237.0	243.4	252.8	269.7	0.0001	268.9	270.7	275.4	288.4	0.0001
Fish	51.8	56.1	55.9	56.1	0.0001	74.0	79.3	81.6	77.0	0.0001
Legumes	42.6	41.6	38.9	36.1	0.0001	73.5	72.8	68.2	57.2	0.001
Cereals	201.7	193.1	186.3	185.8	0.0001	298.5	293.6	273.9	253.6	0.0001
Olive oil	18.1	18.9	19.6	20.5	0.0001	23.2	24.2	25.7	24.8	0.0001
Red meat	40.4	49.2	47.4	45.7	0.0002	72.9	80.0	76.9	65.4	0.0001
Milk & dairy products	315.2	318.4	313.2	328.8	0.0001	250.8	260.7	270.9	287.8	0.0001
Wine (in mL)	26.7	38.8	46.4	38.5	0.0001	260.2	267.3	245.1	170.5	0.0001

Table 2. Score of adherence to the Mediterranean dietary pattern by socio-economic group

Socio-economic condition	Number of subjects	Score	
		Mean	**SD**
Highest level of education:			
Primary not finished	14 304	22.57	3.7
Primary finished	16 021	22.29	3.8
Secondary finished	6077	22.5	3.8
University finished	4765	22.57	3.8
		P=0.0851([a])	
Social class of origin:			
I (highest class)	1933	21.98	4.0
II	3516	22.59	3.8
III	13 449	22.58	3.8
IV	6041	22.09	3.7
V (lowest class)	15 957	22.52	3.7
		P=0.0001([a])	

([a]) Adjusted for the other variables (sex, group of age or centre)

day, respectively, received 3 points; no consumption of wine and alcohol received 2 points. Therefore, the potential score ranged from 9 points (minimum adherence to the Mediterranean pattern) to 36 points (maximum adherence to the Mediterranean pattern).

Socioeconomic status was measured by means of the highest completed educational level and by social class of origin. The educational level was classified into four categories from uncompleted primary school to completed university. Social class of origin was indicated by the father's occupation when the subject was 10 years of age. Five categories were used, from class I (professional and executive) to class V (semi-skilled and unskilled manual), following Spanish recommendations for defining social classes from occupational codes (Alvarez-Dardet, 1995).

Results

Lower educational groups eat more fruit, cereals and legumes, and fewer vegetables, olive oil (only in females), and milk and dairy products (only in males) than high educational groups, as shown in Table 1. Given the large number of subjects, even small differences in intake between social groups were statistically significant. Computing a score to assess the overall adherence to the Mediterranean dietary pattern, the differences between food groups are levelled out, and the overall scores show no differences in terms of education levels, although there are slight differences in the social class of origin (Table 2). The adherence score is lower for young subjects (22.01) than for the elderly (22.77) and for females (21.85) than for males (23.53), and slightly higher in the south (23.07) than the north (22.08) of Spain.

Discussion

The scoring approach has a limitation in that all components have the same weight. However, scientific evidence on the effect of the food groups of the Mediterranean pattern is inconsistent. There is strong evidence that the consumption of fruit and vegetables has a protective effect on the risk of cancer and cardiovascular disease. Although there are theoretical reasons in favour of a beneficial effect of a high intake of legumes and cereals, the evidence is considered insufficient. Consequently, the results using the score approach must be considered with caution. In the extrapolation of our results, it should be remembered that they are based on a nonrepresentative sample of the Spanish population. Results suggest that social and geographical differences in adherence to the Mediterranean dietary pattern score are not particularly substantial and show that the pattern in Spain is very uniform, at least in the adult population of the areas included in this study.

Acknowledgement

EPIC is coordinated by the Unit of Nutrition and Cancer of the International Agency for Research on Cancer (IARC) (Agreement AEP/93/02). In Spain it receives financial support from the Europe Against Cancer Programme of the EU (Agreement SOC 99CVF2-034), the Health Research Fund (FIS) of the Spanish Ministry of Health (Exp. 96-0032) and the participating Regional Governments.

References

Alvarez-Dardet, C., Alonso, J., Domingo, A. & Regidor, E. (Grupo de Trabajo de la Sociedad Española de Epidemiología) (1995) Propuesta de un sistema de indicadores para la medición de la clase social. In: Navarro, C., Cabasés, J.M & Tormo, M.A., eds, *La medición de la clase social en Ciencias de la Salud.* Barcelona, SG Editores, pp. 79–83

James, W.P., Nelson, M., Ralph, A. & Leather, S. (1997) Socio-economic determinants of health. The contribution of nutrition to inequalities in health. *BMJ*, **314**, 1545–1549

Moreiras-Varela, O. (1989) The Mediterranean diet in Spain. *Eur. J. Clin. Nutr.*, **43** Suppl. 2, 83–87

Osler, M. & Schroll, M. (1997) Diet and mortality in a cohort of elderly people in a north European community. *Int. J. Epidemiol.*, **26**, 155–159

Trichopoulou, A., Kouris-Blazos, A., Wahlqvist, M.L., Gnardellis, Ch., Lagiou, P., Polychronopoulos, E., Vassilakou, T., Lipworth, L., & Trichopoulos, D. (1995) Diet and overall survival in elderly people. *BMJ*, **311**, 1457–1460

Compliance with the urine marker PABAcheck in cancer epidemiology studies

Runswick S.[1], Slothouber B.[1], Boeing H.[2], Bueno-de-Mesquita H.[2], Clavel F.[2], Key T.[2], Ocke M.[2], Palli D.[2], Trichopoulou A.[2], Tumino R.[2], Slimani N.[2], Riboli E.[2], Powles J.[3], Subar A.[4], Bingham S.[1,2]
(for the EPIC working group on Biomarkers)

[1]Dunn Human Nutrition Unit, Cambridge, UK. [2]EPIC. [3]Institute of Public Health, Cambridge, UK. [4]National Cancer Institute, Bethesda, USA.

Introduction

Because of the well-known difficulty in obtaining accurate dietary information from individuals, the use of biomarker measures as objective measures of food intake have become increasingly common. Useful biomarkers for large-scale epidemiological trials such as EPIC are 24-h urine nitrogen and potassium (Isaksson, 1980; Bingham & Cummings, 1985), the levels of which accurately predict dietary intake and can be used to calibrate and validate the dietary methods used.

The use of analyte measurements from 24-h urines has the drawback that individuals may not always provide complete collections. For this reason the PABAcheck method, which uses PABA (4-aminobenzoic acid) as a marker for the completeness of urine collections has been developed (Bingham & Cummings, 1983).

In this short paper we present information on the degree of compliance with PABA in epidemiological studies. The information was obtained by pooling data from analyses on urine collections from three diet and health calibration studies carried out over the last 5 years, in which a total of approximately 2500 specimens were collected and analysed. These analyses were from the following studies:

1. EPIC (European Prospective Study into Cancer): France, Germany, Greece, Italy, Netherlands, UK. Single 24-h urine collections obtained from 1290 subjects.
2. OPEN (Observing Protein and Energy Nutrition) study: USA. Two non-consecutive 24-h urine collections from 450 subjects.
3. Varna Diet and Stroke Study: Bulgaria. Two non-consecutive 24-h urine collections from 170 subjects.

Methods

Sample collection

Urines were collected in their respective countries according to a common protocol and measurements of urine volume or weight were taken. After thorough mixing, representative aliquots were taken and shipped on dry ice to Cambridge, UK, where they were stored at –20°C until analysis.

Sample analysis

Urines were analysed for total nitrogen using the Kjeldahl technique (Kjeltec 1035/38; Foss UK Ltd, York, UK), for potassium by flame photometry (IL943: Instrumentation Laboratory, Warrington, Cheshire, UK) and for PABA by colorimetry.

The PABAcheck method involves the administration of three 80-mg tablets of PABA at mealtimes concurrently with a 24-h urine collection. If less than 85% (205 mg) of PABA is found in a single 24-h collection it is designated incomplete (Bingham & Cummings, 1983). The average recovery in a group of complete collections is 93% ± 4%. The upper acceptable limit is designated as 110%; readings over this level generally indicate that an interfering drug has been taken.

Correcting up

Because large epidemiological studies are expensive and time-consuming, it is desirable to use as much data as possible. Samples with a PABA recovery of 70%–84% can be used, as it is likely that subjects have taken all three PABA tablets but have not collected all their urine. The level of biomarkers in the urine can therefore be corrected up to the value they would have been if the PABA was the average value of 93% (Johansson *et al.*, 1999). Collections containing less than 70% or more than 110% PABA need to be discarded from further analysis.

Drug interference problem

The main drawback of the PABAcheck method is that the colorimetric method it employs measures aromatic amines generally and is therefore not specific for PABA. Several aromatic amine-containing drugs react to give falsely high PABA recoveries and it is therefore necessary that subjects are instructed not to take drugs or vitamins if possible while undertaking the collection. Paracetamol-based drugs, being structurally similar to PABA, are the most common problem. Aspirin-based drugs do not interfere with the analysis.

HPLC alternative method

An alternative chromatographic method of PABA analysis by HPLC (high-performance liquid chromatography) has been used by some researchers (Jakobsen *et al.*, 1997). This technique has the major advantage of being able to discriminate PABA from other related drugs because of a difference in elution times. The disadvantage of the HPLC method is that it is more costly in terms of time and equipment than the colorimetric method.

Results

HPLC of OPEN samples

For the samples analysed from European countries, the amount of data lost due to high (i.e. over 110%) PABA recovery was small, between 1% and 5% of samples. However, the OPEN study (USA) results yielded a considerably higher proportion of 13% unusable highs. This prompted us to set up the alternative HPLC method described above and the high OPEN samples were re-analysed by this method, resulting in a reduction of the unusable highs to 1%.

Number of usable samples

Out of the total 2574 samples, 1923 (75%) contained 85%–110% PABA. A further 281 samples (11%) contained 70%–84% and were usable after correction. We excluded 317 (12%) because they contained less than 70% PABA and 54 (2%) because they contained more than 110% PABA. EPIC and Bulgarian samples were not analysed by HPLC.

Table 1 shows the percentages of samples for each country designated into four levels of PABA recovery: incomplete, correctable, complete and high. Results for the USA are shown before and after HPLC analysis of highs. In the area with the highest proportion of unusable results, only 10 collections (8%) contained less than 40% PABA while 48 (39%) contained 40%–70% PABA. It is possible that these low apparent recoveries were due to participants' failure to take all three PABA tablets.

Conclusions

Our recent studies in European countries and the USA show that 85%–95% of urines collected in different populations will normally be usable for dietary validation purposes using the described criteria. However, it is important that participants take the PABA tablets.

References

Bingham, S. & Cummings, J.H. (1983) The use of 4-aminobenzoic acid as a marker to

Table 1. Numbers of 24-hour urines classified by four levels of PABA recovery

PABA %	0–69	70–84	85–110	>110	Total % usable PABA results
	Incomplete	**Correctable**	**Complete**	**High**	
Bulgaria	39 (11%)	54 (16%)	234 (69%)	12 (4%)	85%
France	10 (7%)	13 (9%)	113 (82%)	2 (2%)	91%
Germany	7 (4%)	15 (10%)	132 (85%)	1 (1%)	95%
Greece	58 (47%)	38 (31%)	25 (20%)	2 (2%)	51%
Italy	16 (7%)	17 (8%)	180 (84%)	1 (1%)	92%
Netherlands	17 (8%)	14 (7%)	176 (80%)	12 (5%)	87%
UK	34 (8%)	66 (15%)	327 (74%)	14 (3%)	89%
USA	129 (13%)	55 (6%)	639 (68%)	123 (13%)	74%
USA after HPLC of highs	136 (14%)	64 (7%)	736 (78%)	10 (1%)	85%

validate the completeness of 24-h urine collection in man. *Clin. Sci.*, **64**, 629–635

Bingham, S. & Cummings, J.H. (1985) Urine nitrogen as an independent validatory measure of dietary intake. *Am. J. Clin. Nut.*, **42**, 1276–1289

Isaksson, B. (1980) Urinary nitrogen output as a validity test in dietary surveys. *Am. J. Clin. Nutr.*, **33**, 4–6

Jakobsen, J., Ovesen, L., Fagt, S. & Pederson, A.N. (1997) Para-aminobenzoic acid used as a marker for completeness of 24-hour urine: assessment of control limits for a specific HPLC method. *Eur. J. Clin. Nutr.*, **51**, 514–519

Johansson, G., Bingham, S. & Vahter, M. (1999) A method to compensate for incomplete 24-hour urine collections in nutritional epidemiology studies. *Public Health Nutr.*, **2**, 587–591

Differences in calculating fibre intake of a British diet when applying the British, Danish and French food composition tables

Charrondière U.R., Vignat J., Riboli E.

International Agency for Research on Cancer (IARC) WHO, Lyon, France.

Purpose

Fibre is considered as a protecting factor in the risk of developing cardiovascular diseases and cancer, particularly colon cancer. However, due to problems involving its definition and chemical processes, fibre values can differ significantly. Physiologically, fibre is considered as "the indigestible components of the plant cell wall" and can be divided into water-insoluble fibre (cellulose, hemicellulose and lignins) and water-soluble fibre (pectins, gums and mucilages). In food composition tables (FCTs), the definitions adopted for dietary fibre are determined by the analytical methods used (Deharveng *et al.*, 1999):

a. Non-starch polysaccharides (NSP) as measured by the Englyst-type methods do not include lignin, waxes, cutins and resistant starch. They are found only in the British tables.

b. Total dietary fibre (TDF), as measured by the AOAC methods (based on the indigestibility of the components), includes NSP, lignin and resistant starch. It is found in most FCTs.

c. Southgate-type methods, an obsolete colorimetric method, measure NSP, lignins and some starch and are still found in the Greek and British tables.

d. "By difference" total dietary fibre = 100 – (water + protein + fat + ash + available carbohydrate). It includes resistant starch and is rarely used.

e. Crude fibre values, determined by acid hydrolysis, are still cited in some tables even though they are of little or no value for human nutrition.

f. Neutral detergent fibre (NDF) measures insoluble fibre components only (i.e. no water-soluble components) and is therefore not recommended.

The use of these incompatible methods between tables might introduce systematic errors in the dietary fibre intake estimation between countries. Given the importance of having comparable fibre intakes across countries when calculating relative risk, we investigated the magnitude of differences in fibre intake and the impact on the ranking of subjects by applying the dietary fibre values of different FCTs to the same diet.

Material and methods

For 1314 British subjects, the fibre intake was calculated based on reported foods through a single 24-h diet recall (Slimani *et al.*, 1999) collected in the EPIC study (Riboli and Kaaks, 1997). As most fibre is consumed through fruits, vegetables, potatoes, pulses and cereal products, all reported foods of these five food groups were matched to exact or similar foods found in the national FCTs. If the matched foods had a missing fibre value it was replaced by a fibre value of a similar food. No calculations or adjustments were applied to the original fibre values, i.e. a reported cooked food was matched to the corresponding raw food if it was not available in the same or similar cooked form in the national table. The paired *t* test was used to test mean differences between FCTs and the Spearman correlation coefficient served to test overall correlation of values between FCTs.

Results

As shown in Table 1, there are significant differences found between mean dietary fibre intakes when applying the nutrient values as such from three food composition tables to the same diet: 14.4 g for Englyst fibre and 20.5 g for Southgate fibre from the British table and 20.0 g from the French and Danish tables. All tables resulted in significantly different mean intakes ($P<0.0001$), except between the Danish and French tables. Moreover, fibre values are highly correlated between FCTs (r, 0.82–0.94). The dietary fibre intake contribution from different food groups varies between tables even when the total dietary fibre intake is similar. The Englyst method resulted in significantly low fibre intake from fruits and bread, the Southgate method in high fibre intake from bread, the French FCT in a high fibre intake from cereals, and the Danish table in a high fibre intake from vegetables, pulses and pasta/rice. Some of the differences between FCTs can be explained by the real differences between foods, but they can also be accounted for by the differences in analytical methods as well as the values from raw foods for reported cooked and preserved foods. Contrary to the common opinion that Englyst and AOAC dietary fibre values should be comparable for fruits, Englyst values were significantly lower even though lignin and resistant starch levels are low in fruits and cooking does not interfere with nutrient composition as fruits are mainly eaten raw. As expected, Southgate values are similar to AOAC values in most food groups, except for bread, where Southgate values are much higher. The mean dietary fibre intake decreases by up to 25% if foods with missing fibre values are treated as zero values. Even though mean dietary fibre intake differed between tables, the ranking of subjects for dietary fibre intake was not altered.

Conclusions

The dietary fibre intakes calculated with the British, French and Danish FCTs are not comparable and would lead to different calculations of relative risks. However, the ranking of subjects was not altered. The variations in intake stem from random and systematic errors such as different analytical methods and food matching, but also from true differences in the foods between countries, which might be amplified by differences in food intake across countries. Therefore, there is an urgent need for an agreement on one definition for dietary fibre in national food composition tables and for a standardized European food composition table for nutritional research.

References:

Deharveng, G., Charrondière, U.R., Slimani, N., Southgate, D.A.T. & Riboli, E. (1999) Comparison of nutrients in the food composition tables available in the nine European countries participating in EPIC. *Eur. J. Clin Nutr.*, **53**, 60–79

Slimani, N., Deharveng, G., Charrondière, U.R., van Kappel, A.L., Ocke, M.C., Welch, A., Lagiou, A., van Liere, M., Agudo, A., Pala, V., Brandstetter, B., Andren, C., Stripp, C., van Staveren, W.A. & Riboli, E. (1999) Structure of the standardized computerized 24-hour diet recall interview used as reference method in the 22 centers participating in the EPIC project. *Comput. Methods Programs Biomed.*, **58**, 251–266

Riboli, E. & Kaaks, R. (1997) The EPIC project: rationale and study design. *Int. J. Epidemiol.*, **26** (Suppl. 1), S6–S14

Table 1. Dietary fibre intake in grams of 1314 British calibration subjects according to British, Danish and French food composition tables of five food groups (potatoes, vegetables, pulses, fruits, cereals)

	British FCT (Englyst)	British FCT (Southgate)	French FCT (AOAC)	Danish FCT (AOAC)
Mean intake (replace missing values)	14.4[a]	20.5[a]	20.0[a]	20.0[a]
Mean intake (treat missing values = 0)	14.1[a]	18.6[a]	20.0[a]	16.1[a]
Potatoes	1.3	1.5	1.5	1.4
Vegetables	3.4	4.0	4.0	4.3
Pulses	0.6	0.7	0.9	1.8
Fruits and nuts	3.1	4.7	4.4	4.2
Fruits	2.7	4.1	3.9	3.7
Nuts, mixed fruits/nuts, olives	0.4	0.6	0.5	0.5
Cereals	5.9	9.6	9.2	8.3
Flour, pasta, rice, salty biscuits, dough	0.6	1.2	1.1	1.7
Bread	3.4	5.8	4.7	4.7
Crispbread	0.2	0.3	0.1	0.3
Breakfast cereals	1.7	2.3	3.3	1.5

[a]Significant difference for mean intake ($P<0.0001$).

Validity of the Italian EPIC questionnaire to assess past diet

Pasanisi P., Berrino F., Bellati C., Sieri S., Krogh V.
Unit of Epidemiology, INT, Milan, Italy.

Introduction

Within the framework of a European Case Only Study (COS) (Berrino & Bellati, 1999) designed to evaluate the gene–environment interaction in the occurrence of hereditary breast cancer in young women, we were interested in investigating the dietary habits of our participants. Since BRCA1 and BRCA2 genes code for proteins involved in DNA repair mechanisms and in down-regulation of estrogenic action, we hypothesized that mutation carriers may be more sensitive than non-carriers to risk factors (radiation exposure in childhood, oral contraceptives, high glycemic-index food), but also to potential protective factors (dietary anti-oxidants, phytoestrogens, tobacco smoking).

It is critical in a COS to classify patients as to their usual diet in the year before breast cancer diagnosis, which, however, could have occurred from a few months to several years before recruitment.

Several studies on the quality of information on remote diet have been published (Willett, 1990; Pereira & Koifman, 1999); dietary questionnaires on past habits were administered to subjects who had already been investigated on their current diet in the past. Some of these studies showed that the results of the present questionnaires were more correlated to present diet than to the past diet as originally recorded (Willett, 1990).

In COS, questionnaires refer to a period in the past that is clearly defined by a major life event (the year before breast cancer diagnosis). We expect, therefore, that the recall may be easier than just inquiring on the diet many years ago as evaluated in previous studies (Willett, 1990).

We conducted a validation study to use the food frequency questionnaire (FFQ) developed in the EPIC study (Pisani *et al.*, 1997), in the assessment of diet in the year before a major event affecting dietary habits.

Subjects and methods

Subjects

We invited, by phone call and by letter, 194 of the 219 postmenopausal women who participated in two subsequent dietary intervention studies carried out at the Milan National Cancer Institute in 1995 (DIANA 1: 104 healthy women) (Berrino *et al.*, 2001) and in 1997 (DIANA 2: 115 women with previous breast cancer). Twenty-five women were not invited either because they developed metastasis or did not comply with the last follow-up examinations.

In total, 123 women (63%), 53 from the DIANA 1 group and 70 from the DIANA 2 group responded and agreed to participate in the study.

Study design

The women had already completed the Italian EPIC FFQ (FFQ1) at baseline, before the dietary intervention, in January 1995 for the participants in DIANA 1 and in January 1997 for the participants in DIANA 2.

In January 2000, 3–5 years later, they received by mail and were requested to fill in the same self-administered FFQ (FFQ2), enquiring on their usual diet before the intervention study. All questionnaires were returned before January 2001.

EPIC food frequency questionnaire

The Italian EPIC FFQ has been described elsewhere (Pisani *et al.*, 1997).

Statistical methods

The validity of the FFQ2 relative to the reference method FFQ1 was estimated for 37 nutrients and for 55 food groups.

For nutrient intake, validity was assessed by the Pearson correlation moment; mean differences in nutrient intake were tested using the one-way *t* test.

To measure questionnaire reliability, we also computed the intraclass correlation coefficient.

Since the intake of food groups was not normally distributed, non-parametric methods were used in analysis

(Spearman rank order correlation coefficients). We also evaluated correlation separating DIANA 1 and DIANA 2 groups.

Results

Concerning nutrients (Table 1), Pearson correlation coefficients showed values between 0.46 (soluble carbohydrates) and 0.70 (calcium). The mean correlation value was 0.60.

A mean difference significantly different from zero was only observed for vegetable fats, linolenic acid, potassium, vitamin C, folic acid and β-carotene. For all these micronutrients, the FFQ2 tended to give lower estimates than the FFQ1 (Table 1).

Similar correlations were observed computing the intraclass correlation coefficients (mean correlation value

Table 1. Nutrients

Variables	Pearson correlation	*t* test (*P* values)	Intraclass correlation coefficient
Total proteins	0.66	+0.80	0.66
Animal proteins	0.66	+0.72	0.66
Vegetable proteins	0.54	+0.96	0.54
Total fats	0.66	+0.33	0.65
Animal fats	0.61	+0.40	0.61
Vegetable fats	0.65	−0.003	0.61
Total saturated	0.64	+0.96	0.64
Oleic acid	0.62	+0.08	0.59
Total monounsaturated	0.61	+0.10	0.60
Linoleic acid	0.57	+0.14	0.56
Linolenic acid	0.69	−0.05[a]	0.68
Other polyunsaturated	0.51	+0.36	0.51
Total polyunsaturated	0.59	+0.15	0.59
Cholesterol	0.54	+0.44	0.54
Available carbohydrates	0.51	+0.21	0.50
Starch	0.51	+0.20	0.50
Soluble carbohydrates	0.46	+0.45	0.46
Dietary fibre	0.62	+0.29	0.60
Alcohol	0.65	+0.12	0.65
Energy kcal	0.58	+0.59	0.58
Iron	0.62	+0.71	0.62
Calcium	0.70	+0.41	0.69
Sodium	0.60	+0.61	0.59
Potassium	0.64	−0.02[a]	0.63
Phosphorous	0.67	+0.64	0.67
Zinc	0.64	+0.59	0.64
Thiamin	0.62	+0.31	0.61
Riboflavin	0.65	+0.35	0.64
Niacin	0.60	+0.39	0.60
Vitamin C	0.52	−0.03[a]	0.50
Vitamin B6	0.60	+0.66	0.60
Folic acid	0.68	−0.01[a]	0.65
Retinol equivalents	0.63	+0.13	0.61
Retinol	0.60	+0.79	0.60
Beta-carotene	0.56	−0.003[a]	0.49
Vitamin E	0.57	+0.27	0.56
Vitamin D	0.53	+0.92	0.54

[a]Mean difference significantly different from zero ($P<0.05$).

Table 2. Food groups

Variables	Spearman's rho
Fruiting vegetables	0.48
Root vegetables	0.72
Potatoes	0.34
Leafy vegetables (total)	0.52
Leafy vegetables (except cabbages)	0.56
Cabbages	0.20
Mushrooms	0.54
Onion, garlic	0.59
Stalk vegetables	0.59
Mixed salad	0.58
Legumes	0.45
Fruits	0.65
Nuts and seeds	0.43
Milk	0.57
Yogurt	0.61
Cheese	0.62
Pasta	0.56
Rice	0.43
Bread	0.45
Crispbread, rusks	0.42
Salty biscuits	0.34
Pastry	0.52
Red meat (total)	0.48
White meat (total)	0.51
Beef	0.42
Veal	0.44
Pork	0.63
Mutton, lamb	0.74
Chicken, hen	0.53
Processed meat	0.56
Offals	0.66
Fish	0.56
Crustaceans	0.61
Eggs	0.46
Vegetable oils	0.39
Olive oil	0.50
Butter	0.62
Margarines	0.40
Sugar, honey	0.61
Chocolate	0.64
Confectionery	0.60
Ice cream	0.69
Cakes	0.48
Dry cakes	0.63
Fruit or vegetable juices	0.51
Soft drinks	0.49
Coffee	0.70
Tea	0.66
Wine	0.75
Fortified wine	0.54
Beer	0.70
Spirits	0.66
Tomato sauces	0.59
Mayonnaise	0.61
Soups	0.40

0.59), with lower values for those micronutrients in which the mean difference was significantly different from zero (Table 1).

The mean Spearman correlation value was 0.54 for the food group results (Table 2).

Lower correlation coefficients were observed for cabbages (0.20), potatoes (0.34), and for other less important food groups. Values between 0.39 and 0.45 were observed for soups, legumes, beef, veal, margarine, vegetable oil and rice.

Among DIANA 1 women (healthy women), the mean correlation value was 0.71 for nutrients and 0.56 for food groups.

Among DIANA 2 women (breast cancer patients), the mean correlation value was 0.56 for nutrients and 0.55 for food groups.

Conclusion

The correlation was satisfactory for both nutrients and food groups and similar to those reported in previous studies (Willet, 1990; Pereira & Koifman, 1999).

Women overestimated past consumption of some foods that they had been advised to decrease in DIANA studies (e.g. red meat and potatoes) and underestimated some foods they had been advised to increase (e.g. legumes and cabbages).

References

Berrino, F. & Bellati, C. (1999) COS, case only study on breast cancer before the age of 40. Announcement of a new study on gene–environment interaction in breast cancer. *Epid. Prev.*, **23**, 57–58

Berrino, F., Bellati, C., Secreto, G., Camerini, E., Pala, V., Panico, S., Allegro, G. & Kaaks, R. (2001) Reducing bioavailable sex hormones through a comprehensive change in diet: the Diet and Androgens (DIANA) Randomized Trial. *Cancer Epidemiol. Biomarkers Prev.*, **10**, 25–33

Pereira, R.A. & Koifman, S. (1999) Using food frequency questionnaire in past dietary intake assessment. *Rev. Saude Publica*, **33**, 610–621

Pisani, P., Faggiano, F., Krogh, V., Palli, D., Vineis, P. & Berrino, F. (1997) Relative validity and reproducibility of a food frequency dietary questionnaire for use in the Italian EPIC centres. *Int. J. Epidemiol.*, **26**, 152–160

Willett, W. (1990) Recall of remote diet. In: Kelsey, J.L., Marmot, M.G., Stolley, P.D. & Vessey, M.P., eds, *Nutritional Epidemiology*, Oxford, Oxford University Press, pp.148–156

Comparable nutrient intake across countries is only possible through standardization of existing food composition tables

Charrondière U.R., Vignat J., Riboli E.

International Agency for Research on Cancer (IARC) WHO, Lyon, France.

Purpose

Nutritional epidemiological studies, including EPIC, need standardized nutrient and energy intakes across countries to establish correct relationships between nutrient intakes and disease. Errors in nutrient intakes may bias the relation between diet and disease, e.g. shifts in relative risk of disease and in the ranking of subjects in terms of disease risk. Therefore, we investigated the differences in nutrients between food composition tables (FCTs), the impact on nutrient intakes and the need for standardized FCTs.

Material and methods

To compare nutrients, we examined major FCTs in 10 European countries (Denmark, France, Germany, Greece, Great Britain, Italy, The Netherlands, Norway, Spain and Sweden) in terms of definition, analytical methods, modes of expression and units (Deharveng *et al.*, 1999, and unpublished data).

For the investigation of differences in nutrient intake between three FCTs, we calculated the mean intakes for energy, carbohydrates, protein, fat, fibre, and vitamin C for five food groups (fruits, vegetables, potatoes, pulses and cereal products). The calculation was based on reported foods for 1314 British subjects through a single 24-h diet recall collected in the EPIC study. The foods were matched to exact or similar foods found in the national FCT. If the matched foods had a missing value it was replaced by a value of a similar food, except when investigating the impact of missing values on dietary fibre intake. No calculations or adjustments were applied to the original nutrient values, i.e. a reported cooked food was matched to the corresponding raw food if it was not available as such or in a similar form in the national table.

Results

Comparability of FCTs

Despite the existing good quality of national FCTs and international initiatives such as COST ACTION 99 (EUROFOODS), NORFOODS and INFOODS, which have worked over the last 20 years towards standardized analytical methods, definitions and data exchange, a comparison in 1999 between nutrients in existing FCTs in nine European countries concluded that many nutrients give incomparable values, e.g. energy, carbohydrates, fibre, folate, carotenes, and vitamins A and E. (Deharveng *et al.*, 1999). Incomparability of values can be accentuated through differences in national procedures (on calculation, evaluation, or treatment of missing values), the number of foods, food description, and the coverage of foods as consumed (Slimani *et al.*, 2000).

Validity aspects of food intake

Most of the exact concordance between reported foods and those in the table were found in the British table (85%), compared to 58% in the French table and 35% in the Danish table. This can be explained by the fact that the British table contains about 3500 foods, mostly typical British foods and cooked foods. The French table has about 800 raw and cooked foods, whereas the Danish table contains about 800 mainly raw foods. It can be assumed that the more exact the food match is the higher the validity of the nutrient intake is. Another aspect of nutrient intake validity is the treatment of missing values. When replacing the foods that have missing dietary fibre values with similar foods that do have values, the dietary fibre intake increases. The degree of

Table 1. Mean nutrient intake of 1314 British calibration subjects according to British, Danish and French food composition tables of five food groups (potatoes, vegetables, pulses, fruits, cereals)

	British FCT	French FCT	Danish FCT
Energy (kJ)	3063[a]	3206[a]	3736[a]
Protein (g)	22.5	21.6 [a]	22.7
Fat (g)	12.1[a]	11.7[a]	13.0[a]
Carbohydrates (g)	139.6	139.3	168.0[a]
Fibre (g)	14.4[a] (Englyst) 20.5[a] (Southgate)	20.0 (AOAC)	20.0 (AOAC)
Vitamin C (mg)	75.4[a]	86.2[a]	109.0[a]
Potassium (mg)	1521[a]	1576[a]	1452[a]

[a]Significant difference with the two other tables ($P<0.0001$).

Table 2. Differences between national FCTs and ENDB plans to minimize them

	Differences in national FCTs	ENDB objectives
At food level	Between 60 and 11 000 foods, some only in local language Incomparable food classification and description Some FCTs mainly raw foods, others also as consumed Coverage of frequently consumed foods sometimes poor, especially for meat and processed items	Over 1000 foods per country in local language, English and taxonomic names Detailed and common food classification and description Foods are as consumed Coverage of frequently consumed foods sufficient. Nutrient values also from other sources, e.g. food industry, other databases
At nutrient level	Different definitions and analytical methods Different modes of expression and units Missing nutrient values and outdated values exist in most tables	Definitions and analytical methods to be separated into different columns Modes of expression and units to be standardized Missing nutrient values to be calculated or estimated and outdated values to be replaced by better existing data
Documentation of nutrient values	Lacking in most FCTs for: At nutrient level definitions, analytical methods, source of value, e.g. if analysed, calculated, copied Food sampling methods only partly in British FCT Algorithms, coefficients or methods used to calculate missing values are lacking in most FCTs	Documentation provided as far as possible: At nutrient level definitions, analytical methods, and source to evaluate quality and comparability of values Food sampling methods if existing Algorithms, coefficients or methods used to calculate missing values to be listed
At user level of food composition tables	Different treatment of missing values and different calculation procedures, e.g. method and algorithm calculations, retention factors	No missing values to avoid underestimation of nutrient intake Common calculation procedures, algorithms and coefficients

underestimation of nutrient intake depends on the number of missing foods and their importance in the food and nutrient intake. For example, 78 foods with missing dietary fibre values for Southgate fibre led to a 7.8% underestimation of dietary fibre intake; 40 missing values in the Danish table led to a 25.6% underestimation and 32 missing values for Englyst fibre resulted in a 1.5% underestimation, compared with none in the French table, which had no missing fibre values.

Differences in mean nutrient intake

The calculated mean intakes show up to 30–50% differences in nutrient intakes of the same British diet when applying the British, French and Danish FCTs (Table 1). The variation in nutrient intake can be attributed to real differences in the composition of foods between countries but artificial differences due to food matching, analytical methods, definitions of nutrients, percentage of raw foods vs. foods as consumed, and the degree of estimated values of nutrient intake can also contribute to this variation.

Need for a standardized European FCT

As a standardized European FCT seemed necessary, a concept was developed at IARC. The project to build a European Nutrient Database (ENDB) started in 2000 and brings together compilers of FCTs, international studies and industry. As shown in Table 2, the ENDB aims to overcome most of the differences between FCTs by building a database for frequently consumed foods and important nutrients with minimal random and systematic errors. Nutrient values in the ENDB will derive from national FCTs, which will be documented and evaluated according to common criteria, and standardized in terms of definition, analytical method, mode of expression and units. The database will be completed with values from other sources and through common calculation procedures.

Conclusions

The documented, standardized and newly evaluated ENDB with nutrient values from 10 countries will increase the comparability of nutrient intake estimations across countries while minimizing random and systematic measurement errors. However, more chemical analysis of foods and better collaboration with the food industry would increase the precision of data in the future.

References

Deharveng, G., Charrondière, U.R., Slimani, N., Southgate, D.A.T. & Riboli, E. (1999) Comparison of nutrients in the food composition tables available in the nine European countries participating in EPIC. *Eur. J. Clin. Nutr.*, **53**, 60–79

Slimani, N., Charrondière, U.R., van Staveren, W. & Riboli, E. (2000) Standardization of food composition databases for the European Prospective Investigation into Cancer and Nutrition (EPIC): general theoretical concept. *J. Food Comp. Anal.* **13**, 567–584

Do dietary patterns actually vary within the EPIC study?

Slimani N.[1], Fahey M.[1], Welch A.[2], Wirfält E.[3], Stripp C.[4], Bergström E.[5]
(for the EPIC working group on dietary patterns)

[1]Unit of Nutrition and Cancer, IARC, Lyon, France. [2]Dept. of Public Health and Primary Care, Univ. of Cambridge, UK. [3]Dept. of Medicine Malmö, Lund University, Sweden. [4]Inst. of Cancer Epidemiology, Danish Cancer Society, Copenhagen, Denmark. [5]Dept. of Public Health and Clinical Medicine, Epidemiology, Univ. of Umeå, Sweden.

Purpose

The European Prospective Investigation into Cancer and Nutrition (EPIC) is a network of prospective studies involving about 500 000 subjects from 10 Western European countries (France, Italy, Spain, the United Kingdom, Germany, the Netherlands, Greece, Sweden, Denmark and Norway) (Riboli, 2001). The design of the EPIC study was based on the assumption of large heterogeneity in dietary patterns across European study populations. Recent data suggest changes in diet across Europe over the last 30 years, with a trend towards erosion of the differences traditionally existing between European dietary patterns (Hill, 1997). The lack of standardized methodology to assess individual dietary intakes across Europe make it difficult to estimate the actual nature and magnitude of these differences. The aim of this study was to describe the dietary patterns observed among the 10 European countries participating in EPIC, using a common standardized dietary method.

Methods

A single 24-h diet recall was collected from a representative sample of study subjects (*n*=35 955) using standardized software (EPIC-SOFT) (Slimani *et al.*, 2000). In France and Norway, only women were recruited. A health-conscious group from the UK, involving vegans, ovo-lacto vegetarians and fish eaters, was considered separately from a British cohort recruited from the general population. In order to compare 21 main food groups across countries, the country mean intakes were expressed as the percentage of deviation compared to the overall EPIC mean, using multidimensional representations. Mean food consumption (g) for the ith food group, m(i), was first calculated by sex and country for 21 food groups. Secondly, study mean consumption, M(i) was calculated for the same food groups, by sex, as the equally weighted average of the country mean intakes. Finally, in order to express variation in country mean intakes from the overall EPIC mean, the percent deviation relative to the study mean was calculated for each food group, by sex and country, as: $[100\% * m(i)] / M(i)]$. In addition, to take into account the clustering of individuals within centres, a random intercept regression model was used to estimate crude and adjusted country mean intakes and their standard errors (Bryk & Raudenbush, 1991) The patterns of variation among country mean intakes adjusted for age, day of the week, and season were similar to patterns among the crude means, and were not reported.

Results

Italy and Greece have a dietary pattern dominated by plant foods (except potatoes), with lower consumption of animal and processed foods (see Figure 1). The health-conscious group from the UK reported a diet different from the UK general population and closer to Italy and Greece in consumption of vegetables, fruits and legumes. However, apart from some characteristics specific to vegetarian groups (i.e. low consumption of animal products, particularly meat and fish), other patterns more associated with central European or UK dietary habits were also observed in this population (e.g. tea, cakes, margarines and butter). In contrast to Italy and Greece (and the UK health-conscious group), Spain and France have a more

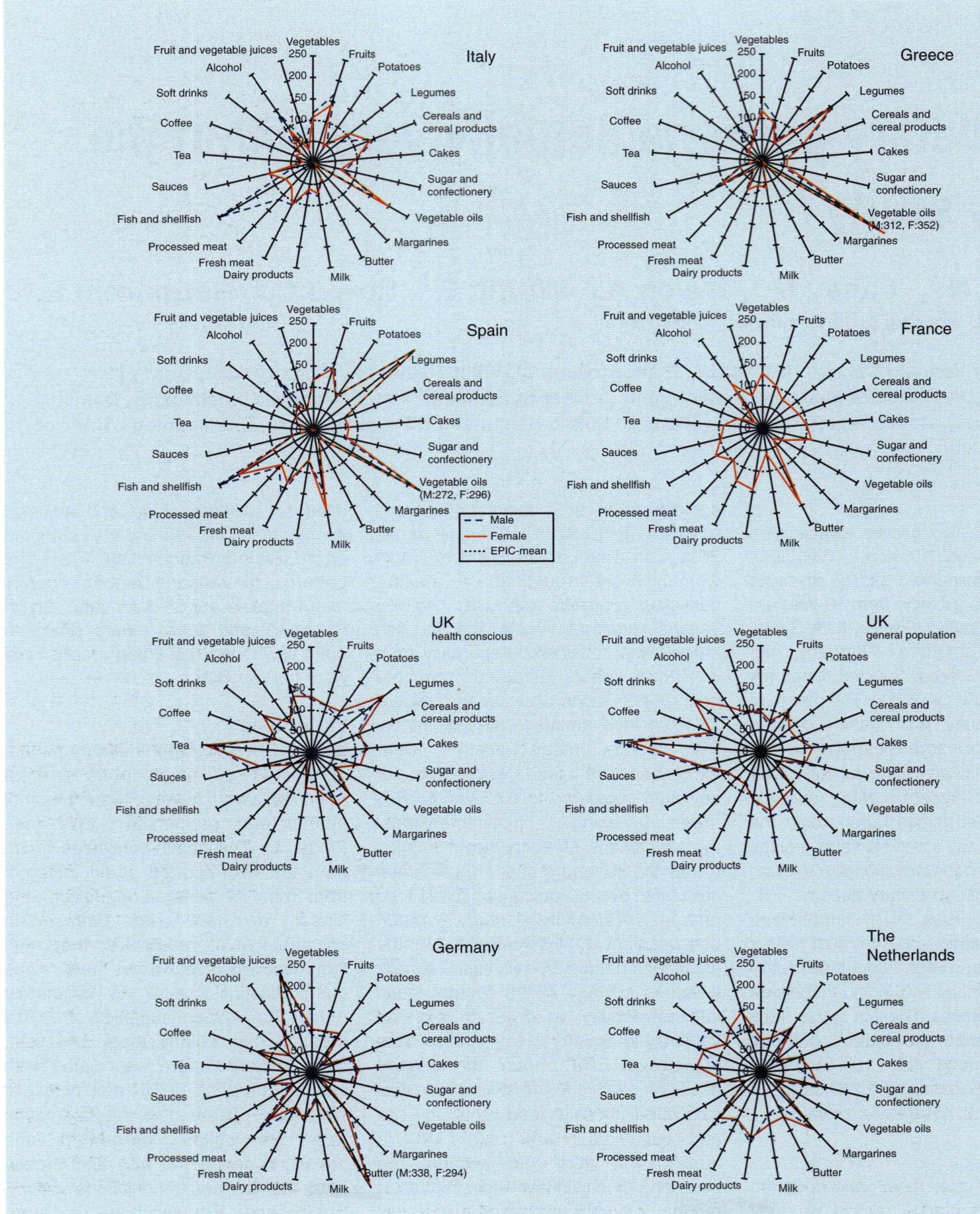
Italy
Greece
Spain
France
UK
health conscious
UK
general population
Germany
The Netherlands
Vegetables
Fruits
Potatoes
Legumes
Cereals and cereal products
Cakes
Sugar and confectionery
Vegetable oils
Margarines
Butter
Milk
Dairy products
Fresh meat
Processed meat
Fish and shellfish
Sauces
Tea
Coffee
Soft drinks
Alcohol
Fruit and vegetable juices
250
200
150
100
50
0
Vegetable oils (M:312, F:352)
Vegetable oils (M:272, F:296)
Butter (M:338, F:294)
Male
Female
EPIC-mean

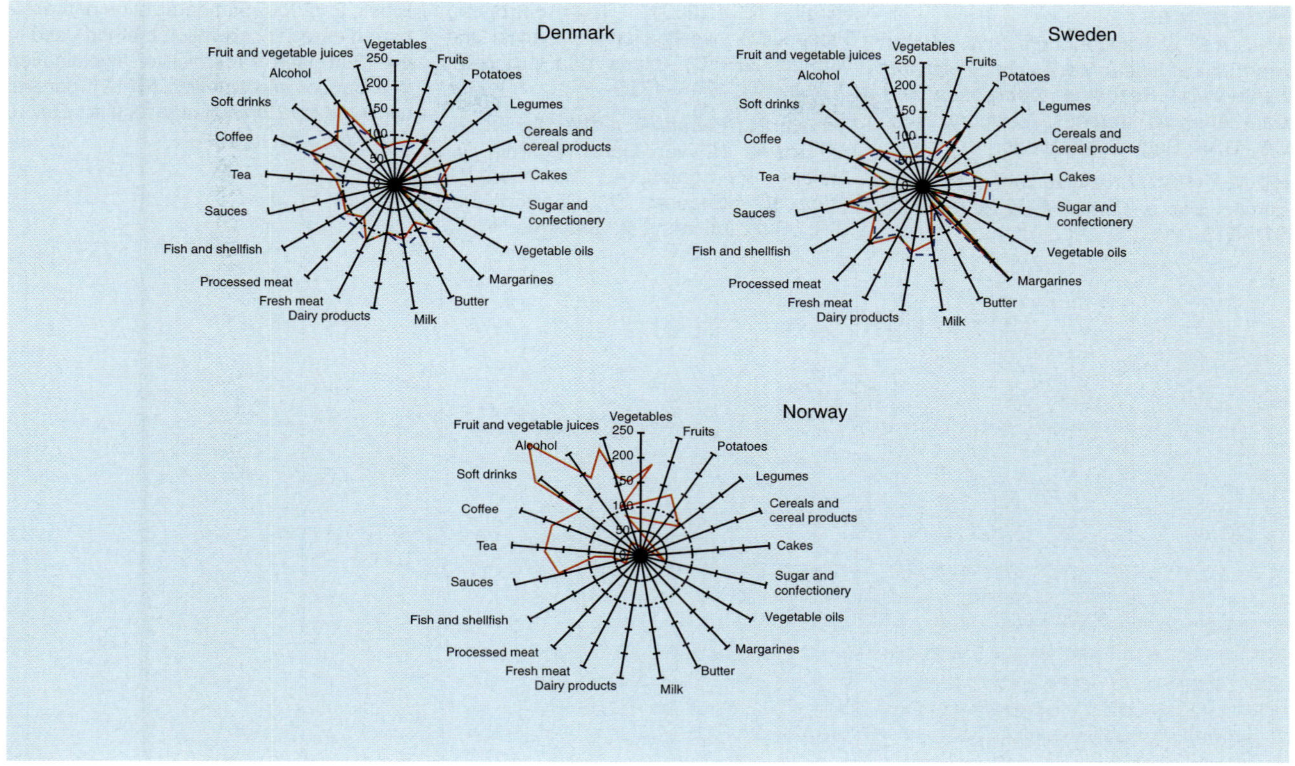

Figure 1
Deviation (%) of the country food group (gr) means from the sex-specific "EPIC" means

heterogeneous dietary pattern. The average Spanish dietary pattern is characterized by high consumption of both plant foods (legumes, vegetable oils, fruits, vegetables) and animal products such as meat (and processed meats), fish, and milk, as well as alcohol. In the French cohort (of women teachers), the dietary pattern is characterized by high consumption of vegetables, but consumption of fruit is near the EPIC mean. Butter appeared as a major characteristic of this diet, followed by other animal products (i.e. dairy products, fresh meats, fish and fish products), sugar products and alcohol.

In contrast, diet in the Nordic countries, The Netherlands, Germany and the UK general population was relatively higher in potatoes and animal, processed and sweetened foods, with a proportion varying across countries. For example, Germany has the highest consumption of butter, processed meat and fruit and vegetable juices, whereas Sweden is characterized by high consumption of margarine, followed by potatoes, processed meat, sauces, coffee, dairy products, sugar products and cakes. Other common characteristics of these countries are that the consumption of vegetables and fruit is at or below the overall EPIC means, and that legumes and vegetable oils do not form a significant part of their diets.

Conclusions

Global dietary patterns vary greatly across EPIC countries. Variation between countries ranged from two to threefold (e.g. for fruits, vegetables, potatoes, cereal and cereal products, milk and dairy products, sugar products) to more than 100-fold differences (margarines and tea), with gender differences particularly for fish, soft drinks, tea, alcohol, legumes, fats and processed meats. The patterns observed in Spain and France, where several centres are involved, suggested large within-country geographical variations that will be investigated further in the future. This large heterogeneity should aid understanding of the relationship between diet and cancer and the formulation of new etiological hypotheses.

References

Bryk, A.S. & Raudenbush, S.W. (1991) *Hierarchical Linear Models for Social and Behavioural Research: Application and Data Analysis Methods*. Newbury Park, CA, USA, Sage Publications

Hill, M.J. (1997) Changing pattern of diet in Europe. *Eur. J. Cancer Prev.*, **6** (Suppl.), S11–S13

Riboli, E. (2001) The European Prospective Investigation into Cancer and Nutrition (EPIC): plans and progress. *J. Nutr.* **131**, 170S–175S

Slimani, N., Ferrari, P., Ocké, M., Welch, A., Boeing, H., van Liere, M., Pala, V., Amiano, P., Lagiou, A., Mattisson, I., Stripp, C., Engeset, D., Charrondière, U.R., Buzzard, M., van Staveren, W. & Riboli, E. (2000) Standardization of the 24-hour diet recall calibration method used in the European Prospective Investigation into Cancer and Nutrition (EPIC): general concepts and preliminary results. *Eur. J. Clin. Nutr.*, **54**, 900–917

Using multiple imputation methods to estimate relative risks in small EPIC lung cancer subsets

Altenburg H.P.[1,2], Agudo A.[1], Berrino F.[1], Boshuizen H.C.[1], Bueno-de-Mesquita H.B.[1], Janzon L.[1], Le Marchand L.[1], Linseisen J.[1,2], Lukanova A.[1], Rasmuson T.[1], Vineis P.[1], Riboli E.[1], Miller A.[1,2]

(for the EPIC working group on lung cancer)

[1]EPIC. [2]German Cancer Research Center, Dept. of Clinical Epidemiology, Heidelberg, Germany.

Purpose

Although most of the relevant variables in the lung cancer subcohort contain only small proportions of missing values, subgroups are possible with higher proportions of missing data. Conventional methods for missing data, such as listwise deletion (as in most statistical software packages) or regression imputation may be sensitive to problems such as:

- Inefficient use of the available information, leading to low power and type II errors.
- Biased estimates of standard errors, leading to incorrect *P* values.
- Biased parameter estimates, due to failure to adjust for selectivity in missing data.

Moreover, listwise deletion of observations is inefficient, because it can dramatically decrease the number of cancer cases in the subgroup. We have similar problems when using methods such as pairwise deletion (available cases), single deterministic imputation, single random imputation or dummy variable adjustment.

More accurate and reliable results can be obtained using maximum likelihood or multiple imputation procedures. In case of data that are missing at random, both methods deliver approximately unbiased as well as efficient parameter estimates and standard errors. Well-developed maximum likelihood methods are *not* available for logistic regression or Cox regression. Therefore the objective of the paper was the use of multiple imputation methods described in Rubin (1987, 1996) or Schafer (1997) to estimate relative risks in subgroups of the lung cancer cohort.

Methods

Multiple imputation inference is performed in three distinct steps:

1. Missing values are represented by a random sample of size five from an appropriate imputation model incorporating random variation. This leads to five complete data sets to be analysed. First of all, one has to choose an appropriate set of variables, e.g. all variables that should be in the intended model, including the dependent variables and other characteristics that may be associated with variables that have missing data. If necessary, one has to transform the variables to achieve approximate normality. Then, running the Expectation-Maximum-Likelihood algorithm provides maximum likelihood estimates of means and the covariance matrix (used as starting values for the imputation process). Next, the actual data augmentation process is run to generate the multiple data sets with imputed values. Finally, the transformed data values have to be transformed back and imputed values of discrete variables have to be rounded.
2. The desired analysis is performed on each of these five data sets using standard software packages, meaning we analyse the data using complete-data methods.

3. The results of the five parameter estimates from each dataset are then combined. We average the parameter estimates across the five samples to obtain a single estimate. The corresponding standard errors are computed by combining the variation within and between the five samples.

The advantage of multiple imputation is that the random error in the imputation process yields approximately unbiased estimates of all parameters. The repeated imputation process gives us good estimates of the standard errors.

Two imputation mechanisms were used:

1. The propensity score and the Markov-Chain-Monte-Carlo (MCMC) mechanism. The propensity score (a nonparametric approach) is the conditional probability of assignment to a particular result given a vector of observed covariables. A propensity score is generated for each variable with missing values, indicating the probability of the observation being missing. The observations are then grouped based on this score and an approximate bootstrap imputation will be applied to each group.

2. The MCMC mechanism (appropriate for arbitrary missing patterns) constructs a Markov chain long enough for the distribution of the elements to stabilize to a common stationary distribution. By repeatedly simulating steps of the chain, it simulates draws from the underlying distribution of the data. The data augmentation process is a Bayesian inference consisting of an imputation step and a posterior step where the information on the unknown parameters is expressed in the form of a posterior distribution. Both steps have to be iterated long enough to get reliable results, thus to reach a stationary distribution and then to simulate an approximately independent draw of the missing values.

Results

Using multiple imputation methods one can find that the coefficient variance estimates can be up to 30% smaller than when using listwise deletion. But the propensity score method can lead to biased (larger) estimates of relative risks, whereas the MCMC method works well.

Conclusion

Use MCMC and include as many variables in the model as necessary. The MCMC method is appropriate for arbitrarily missing data, as is the case in EPIC subcohorts. The relative efficiency varies between 90% and 99% depending on the fraction of missing information on the corresponding parameter.

References

Rubin, D.B. (1987) *Multiple Imputation for Nonresponse in Surveys*. New York, John Wiley & Sons, Inc.

Rubin, D.B. (1996) Multiple imputation after 18+ years. *J. Am. Stat. Asso.*, **91**, 473–489

Schafer, J.L. (1997) *Analysis of Incomplete Multivariate Data*. New York, Chapman and Hall

Socio-economic determinants for participation in the Danish EPIC Diet, Cancer and Health cohort

Olsen A.[1], Tjønneland A.[1], Engholm G.[2], Overvad K.[3]

[1]Danish Cancer Society, Institute of Cancer Epidemiology, Copenhagen, Denmark. [2]Danish Cancer Society, Department of Cancer Prevention and Documentation, Copenhagen, Denmark. [3]Aarhus University, Institute of Epidemiology and Social Medicine, Aarhus, Denmark.

Purpose

To compare socio-economic characteristics among participants and nonparticipants in the Diet, Cancer and Health study.

Background

Participants in population-based cohort studies often differ from the general population with regard to socio-economic characteristics. Although analyses exploring the relation between exposure variables and endpoints are often conducted within the cohort, generalization of results to the background population is still of interest.

Methods

A total of 80 996 men and 79 729 women aged 50–64 years were invited to participate in the study. In all, 27 179 men and 29 785 women (response rate 35%) were recruited. Participants and nonparticipants were compared regarding social, economic and demographic conditions. Information about socio-economic characteristics was obtained from central, administrative registers. A unique 10-digit personal identification number provided by the Central Population Registry (CPR) identified participants and nonparticipants in the registers. All Danish citizens are registered in CPR. Of the invited persons, 158 559 (99%) were found in the registers and were thereby eligible to contribute to the analyses on participation.

Univariate analyses were performed on 20 variables drawn from the registers with participation as the dependent variable. The analyses were stratified according to gender. The variables showing the strongest relation to participation were introduced into a multivariate logistic regression model (proc genmod, SAS). The eight variables chosen for a first introduction in a multivariate analysis were age, education, size of housing, type of housing, years in the workforce, personal income, type of family and social class. In multivariate logistic regression models, each variable is adjusted for the other variables in the model. In this study, the final model was found between models with a subsample of these factors.

Results

Participation was slightly higher among women than among men (37% and 34%, respectively), highest in the youngest age group (50–54 years) and decreasing with increasing age.

In the multivariate logistic regression analyses, the variables showing the strongest explanation of participation differed between men and women. In the analysis performed on females, highest completed education, size of housing, type of housing, years in workforce after 1980 and social class had the strongest effect on participation rate, while the strongest variables in the analysis performed on males were highest completed education, size of housing, years in workforce after 1980, personal income, family type and social class. Results are shown in Tables 1 and 2.

Interpretation

Obvious differences were seen between participants and nonparticipants with regard to socioeconomic variables. In both genders, the variable best discriminating between participants and

Table 1. Variables describing relations between socio-economic situation and participation in a multiple regression model: women

Women (*n*=29 622)	Number of participants	Univariate OR (95% CI)	Multivariate OR (95% CI)
Education			
Basic school	10 004	1.00	1.00
Vocational training	12 011	1.58 (1.52–1.63)	1.29 (1.25–1.34)
Higher education 1–2 years	2269	1.88 (1.77–1.99)	1.38 (1.30–1.48)
Higher education 3–4 years	3268	1.96 (1.86–2.07)	1.32 (1.23–1.41)
Higher education >4 years	1238	1.58 (1.47–1.71)	1.07 (0.98–1.17)
Other	832		
Size of housing			
0–50m^2	345	1.00	1.00
51–100m^2	13 745	1.81 (1.61–2.04)	1.58 (1.39–1.79)
101–150m^2	9930	2.77 (2.46–3.31)	2.01 (1.77–2.28)
151–200m^2	4298	3.27 (2.88–3.71)	2.25 (1.97–2.57)
>200m^2	1304	2.58 (2.19–2.89)	1.90 (1.64–2.29)
Type of housing			
Flat	13 808	1.00	1.00
Single-family house	15 650	1.52 (1.47–1.56)	1.17 (1.13–1.22)
Other	164		
Years in workforce			
<1 year after 1980	3032	1.00	1.00
1–8 years after 1980	6419	1.55 (1.48–1.63)	1.32 (1.23–1.41)
8–15 years after 1980	13 478	2.09 (2.00–2.19)	1.60 (1.48–1.72)
15–16 years after 1980	6693	2.28 (2.16–2.40)	1.59 (1.4–1.72)
Social class			
Highly educated employee	6681	1.00	1.00
Self-employed/family worker	1810	0.69 (0.64–0.74)	0.95 (0.88–1.04)
Other employees	12 256	0.86 (0.83–0.89)	0.96 (0.91–1.02)
Worker (skilled/unskilled)	4857	0.55 (0.52–0.58)	0.73 (0.69–0.77)
Not in workforce	2950	0.38 (0.36–0.40)	0.69 (0.64–0.75)
Other	1068		

OR, odds ratio; CI, confidence interval.

nonparticipants was size of housing, but also a clear difference was seen according to highest completed education and years in workforce. That participants in general had more education and a higher degree of employment than nonparticipants was expected. Various indicators for high social class, e.g. long formal education, was earlier established to have a positive influence on participation (Sonne-Holm *et al.*, 1989; Harlan *et al.*, 1995; Jackson *et al.*, 1996; Lerman & Shemer, 1996). Size of housing is not a regularly used variable and we are not aware of any previous studies considering the effect of size of housing on participation. The effect of size of housing was shown even after adjustment for education, social class and income (except income for women).

Conclusion

Participants differed from nonparticipants according to several factors and it is clear that the participants as a group had a higher socio-economic position compared to nonparticipants. The results from this study are in accordance with findings in other studies and thereby support the assumption that people with lower socio-economic position in general are

Table 2. Variables describing relations between socio-economic situation and participation in a multiple regression model: men

Men (n=26 881)	Number of participants	Univariate OR (95% CI)	Multivariate OR (95% CI)
Education			
Basic school	5705	1.00	1.00
Vocational training	12 333	1.77 (1.71–1.84)	1.45 (1.40–1.51)
Higher education 1–2 years	1477	2.33 (2.17–2.51)	1.67 (1.55–1.81)
Higher education 3–4 years	3303	2.59 (2.46–2.74)	1.63 (1.53–1.73)
Higher education >4 years	2934	1.87 (1.77–1.97)	1.20 (1.12–1.27)
Other	1129		
Size of housing			
0–50m^2	590	1.00	1.00
51–100m^2	9913	1.98 (1.81–2.17)	1.32 (1.20–1.45)
101–150m^2	10 164	3.46 (3.16–3.79)	1.78 (1.61–1.97)
151–200m^2	4782	4.03 (3.66–4.43)	1.98 (1.79–2.21)
>200m^2	1432	2.76 (2.47–3.07)	1.59 (1.41–1.79)
Years in workforce			
<1 year after 1980	1979	1.00	1.00
1–8 years after 1980	2931	1.26 (1.18–1.34)	1.16 (1.08–1.26)
8–15 years after 1980	8462	1.89 (1.78–1.99)	1.45 (1.33–1.58)
15–16 years after 1980	13 509	2.65 (2.51–2.80)	1.66 (1.52–1.82)
Personal income			
1st quartile	4551	1.00	1.00
2nd quartile	6521	1.64 (1.57–1.72)	0.20 (1.14–1.26)
3rd quartile	7575	2.07 (1.98–2.16)	1.26 (1.19–1.32)
4th quartile	8234	2.38 (2.28–2.49)	1.17 (1.11–1.24)
Family type			
Married	19 033	1.00	1.00
Cohabiting	1268	0.71 (0.66–0.76)	0.91 (0.85–0.98)
Single	4159	0.47 (0.45–0.49)	0.74 (0.70–0.77)
Other	2421		
Social class			
Highly educated employee	12 213	1.00	1.00
Self-employed/family worker	2830	0.61 (0.58–0.65)	0.98 (0.91–1.05)
Other employees	3455	0.74 (0.70–0.77)	0.89 (0.84–0.94)
Worker (skilled/unskilled)	7571	0.60 (0.58–0.65)	0.80 (0.77–0.84)
Not in workforce	680	0.21 (0.19–0.22)	0.58 (0.52–0.64)
Other	132		

OR, odds ratio; CI, confidence interval.

underrepresented in epidemiological observational studies.

References

Harlan, W.R., Sandler, SA., Lee, K.L., Lam, L.C. & Mark, D.B. (1995) Importance of baseline functional and socioeconomic factors for participation in cardiac rehabilitation. *Am. J. Cardiol.*, **76**, 36–39

Jackson, R., Chambless, L.E., Yang, K., Byrne, T., Watson, R., Folsom, A., Shahar, E. & Kalsbeek, W. (1996) Differences between respondents and nonrespondents in a multicenter community-based study vary by gender and ethnicity. The Atherosclerosis Risk in Communities (ARIC) Study Investigators. *J. Clin. Epidemiol.*, **49**, 1441–1446

Lerman, Y. & Shemer, J. (1996) Epidemiologic characteristics of participants and nonparticipants in health-promotion programs. *J. Occup. Environ. Med.*, **38**, 535–538

Sonne-Holm, S., Sorensen, T.I., Jensen, G. & Schnohr, P. (1989) Influence of fatness, intelligence, education and sociodemographic factors on response rate in a health survey. *J. Epidemiol. Community Health*, **43**, 369–374

Adjustment for smoking in lung cancer analyses in the EPIC cohort

Boshuizen H.C.[1], Bueno-de-Mesquita H.B.[1], Altenburg H.P., Agudo A., Le Marchand L., Berrino F., Janzon L., Rasmuson T., Vineis P., Lukanova A., Linseisen J., Riboli E., Miller A.

(for the EPIC working group on Lung Cancer)

[1]National Institute for Public Health and the Environment, Bilthoven, The Netherlands.

Introduction

As smoking is strongly related to lung cancer, proper adjustment for smoking is essential in assessing its associations with other factors (Whittemore, 1988). Several methods of adjustment are possible. We will compare the following procedures to adjust for smoking:

1. Number of pack-years;
2. The six-category index: never smoker, former cigarette smoker who stopped more than 10 years ago; former cigarette smoker who stopped less than 10 years ago; currently smoking <15 cigarettes/day; currently smoking 15–24 cigarettes/day; currently smoking ≥ 25 cigarettes/day;other (pipe/cigar/insufficient information);
3. The best fitting model (based on a Schwartz' Bayesian Criterion-type criterion) selected from all available variables on smoking status, intensity and duration, including interaction terms.

Methods

We used the EPIC follow-up data as released by IARC on 25 May 2001, excluding Greece (data not yet complete), prevalent lung cancer cases (*n*=188), those completely lost to follow-up (*n*=534), those with follow-up only in the period when cancer-registry data were judged to be incomplete (*n*=4051) and those with unreliable dietary data (ratio of reported dietary intake to estimated caloric requirement in the 2% most extreme values) (*n*=8157), resulting in a cohort of 441 426 persons of whom 608 developed lung cancer. Of this cohort, 3716 persons were lost to follow-up, roughly half of them because of migration. Dietary data were available on 407 131 persons (499 lung cancer cases). Data were analysed with the Cox proportional hazards model, using age as the time variable and stratification on age at baseline (1-year intervals), gender and region. We studied the effect of different adjustment procedures on the relative risk estimates for quartiles of fruit and vegetable consumption. Results presented are for uncalibrated dietary data. Very similar results were obtained when analyses were repeated with crudely calibrated dietary data, using a multiplication factor which centred the mean of the food frequency questionnaire data in each study centre on the mean of the 24-h recall data from this centre. Dietary data were divided into quartiles, with gender-specific quartile boundaries based on the entire cohort. Quartile boundaries for uncalibrated vegetable consumption were 93, 146 and 227 g/day for men and 124, 191 and 286 g/day for women. For uncalibrated fruit consumption, they were 84, 154 and 273 g/day for men and 131, 226 and 338 g/day for women. All analyses with dietary variables were adjusted for reported total energy intake, height and weight.

Results

The data-driven model (approach 3) contained the following baseline smoking variables: current smoker, former smoker, number of cigarettes currently smoked, duration of smoking and a quadratic term for duration, inhaling (0= not, 1= not deeply, 2= deeply), interaction term between genders and number of cigarettes currently smoked. The data-driven approach yielded the best fitting model, while the pack-years approach fitted the worst. Coefficients for quartiles of vegetable and fruit intake differed between adjustment methods with a

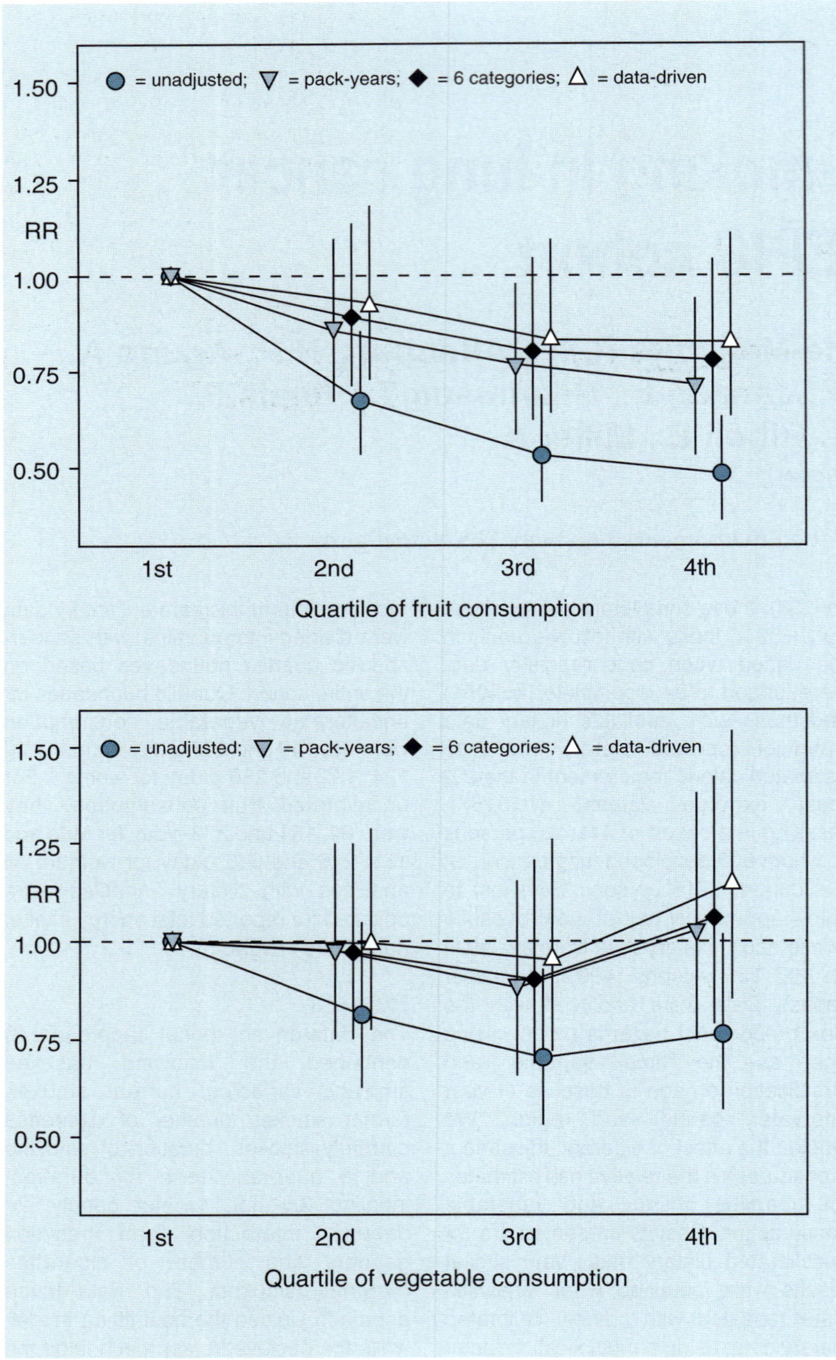

Figure 1
Relative risk of lung cancer from different adjustment procedures by quartile of fruit (above) and vegetable (below) consumption. Reference is the first quartile

magnitude up to the coefficient's standard error (Figure 1). Similar results were obtained when excluding the cases diagnosed within the first 2 years of follow-up from the analysis (Figure 2).

Discussion

As expected, the data-driven approach yields a better-fitting model than a *priori* specified models, and the differences between the crude and the adjusted model are also the largest for this model. It should be remembered that the best model described above relates to lung cancer. For other cancers, the relationship with smoking is likely to be different; thus the best adjustment strategy might also differ. Moreover, the issue of residual confounding by smoking will be less substantial for other cancers, as their association with smoking is weaker to begin with.

Our results suggest that outcomes from models using only pack-years as an adjusting variable may be affected by significant residual confounding compared to data-driven adjustment. However, our analyses do not answer the question of whether residual confounding of smoking is still present in the data-driven model. In principle, residual confounding could still occur as a result of miss-specification of the model or because of important unmeasured aspects of smoking. Although the model was selected from a large set of possible models, this set could have been further extended by including other interaction or polynomial terms, or compounded variables of the basic variables. However, given the large number of models already considered, we feel a considerable improvement in fit and adjustment potential is not to be expected. Residual confounding is more likely to occur due to measurement error present in the smoking data. Information on past smoking behaviour was collected by retrospective recall and thus is prone to some misclassification. Similarly, misclassification could be

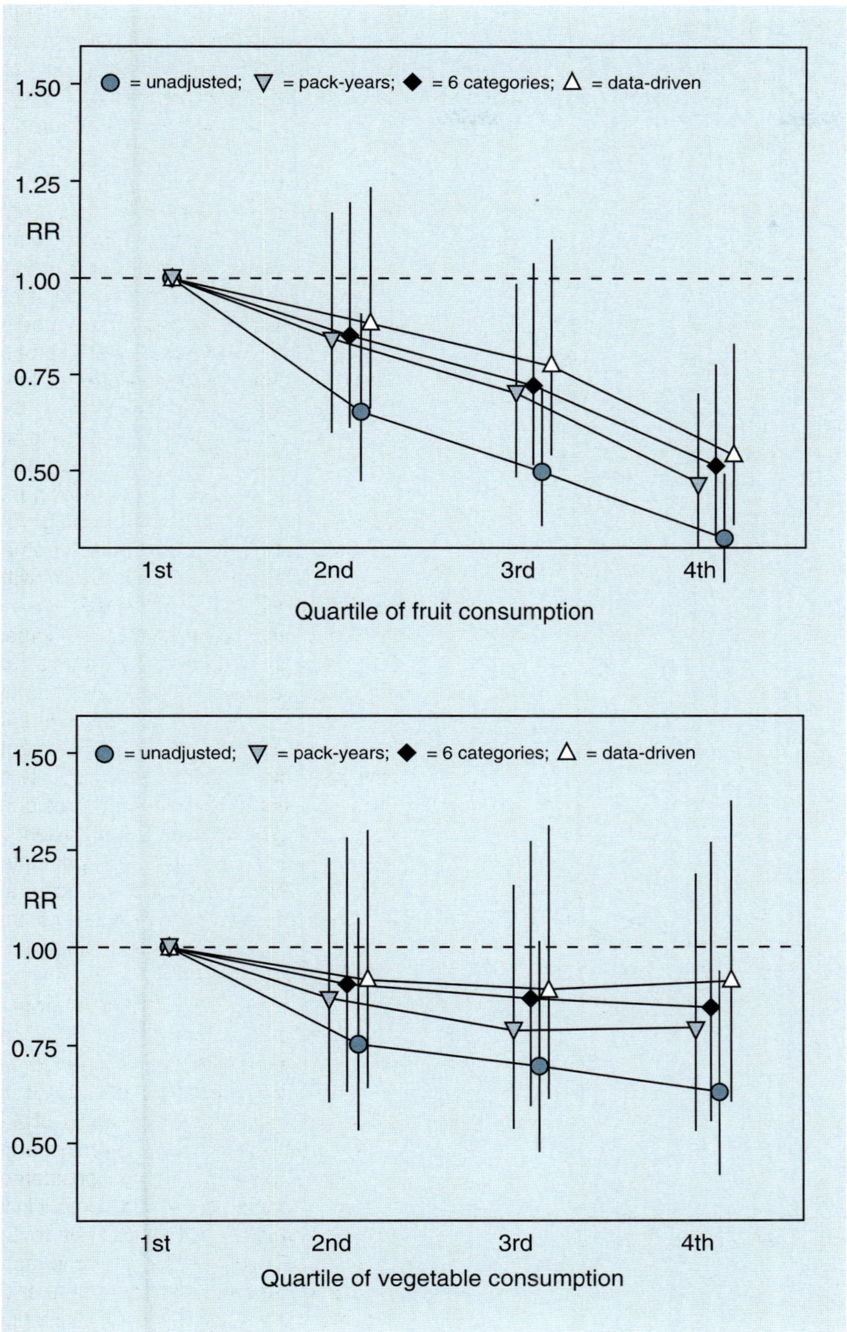

Figure 2
Relative risk of lung cancer from different adjustment procedures by quartile of fruit (above) and vegetable (below) consumption after excluding the first 2 years of follow-up from the analysis. Reference is the first quartile

present because smoking status might have changed during follow-up. Such bias could work in both directions (away or towards unity), depending on the covariance structure of the measurement errors in smoking and dietary data. Simulation studies based on realistic assumptions might shed some light on the possible magnitude of such a bias.

Reference

Whittemore, A.S. (1988) Effect of cigarette smoking in epidemiological studies of lung cancer. *Stat. Med.*, **7**, 223–238

A European case-only study on familial breast cancer

Berrino F., Pasanisi P., Berrino J., Curtosi P., Bellati C.

Epidemiology Unit, National Cancer Institute, Milan, Italy.

Introduction

Heritable breast cancer represents 5%–7% of all breast cancers and about half of these are related to *BRCA* gene mutations. Such mutations confer very high lifetime risks of developing breast cancer (lifetime penetrance, 36%–85%) and ovarian cancer, and most of the cases occur at young ages. The European case-only study (COS) (Berrino & Bellati, 1999) intends to investigate the gene–environment interaction in the occurrence of breast cancer in women before the age of 40.

Several studies have hypothesized that environmental factors may affect the penetrance of *BRCA* genes, including nutritional factors, ionizing radiation, tobacco smoking, reproductive factors, oral contraceptives, and treatment with tamoxifen (Berrino & Bellati, 1999). Nutritional hypotheses refer mainly to the antioxidant effect of fruit and vegetables and to the dietary modulation of sex hormones, insulin-like growth factors and related peptides. These studies suggested that several nutritional and life-style factors are more strongly associated with hereditary than with sporadic breast cancer. If confirmed, these hypotheses would have a great impact on understanding the mechanisms of carcinogenesis and on the perspective of preventing both genetic and sporadic breast cancer.

Subjects and methods

According to the case-only methodology, the frequency of exposure among genetic cases will be compared with the frequency among sporadic cases (Table 1).

If the genetic trait is independent of the exposure under study, the exposure odds ratio measured in a COS study expresses the ratio of the relative risk associated with the exposure among women carrying a *BRCA* gene mutation over the relative risk among women without *BRCA* gene mutations ([(A/E)/(B/F)]/[(C/E)/(D/F)]), i.e. the interaction odds ratio (AD/BC).

Table 1. Frequency of exposure among genetic cases and sporadic cases

	Exposed	Unexposed
Genetic cases	A	B
Sporadic cases	C	D
Source population	E	F

Table 2. Preliminary results of Italian pilot phase: 103 genetic vs 356 sporadic cases

Risk factor	Interaction odds ratio[a]
2+ pregnancies	1.7 (0.7–4.1)
Tobacco	1.0 (0.6–1.6)
Oral contraceptive	0.9 (0.6–1.6)
Radiation exposure	1.6 (0.4–6.2)

[a]Odds ratio adjusted for age and education.

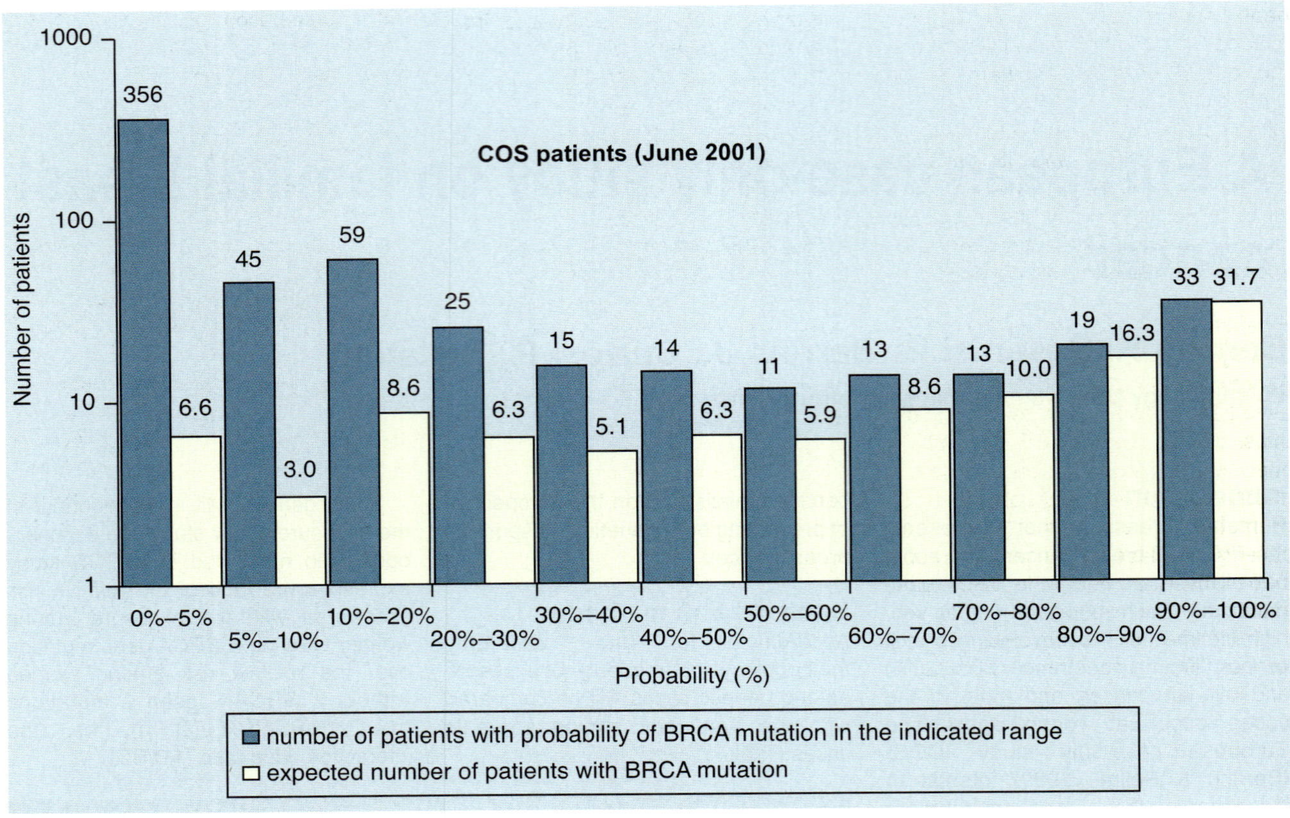

Figure 1
Distribution of 603 COS patients according to their probability of harbouring a deleterious mutation of *BRCA* gene, as established from their family history

In the COS pilot phase carried out in Italy, we have recruited, through the media and general practitioners, 802 Italian women with a breast cancer diagnosis before the age of 40. The participants were requested to fill in a detailed questionnaire on family history (including dates of birth, death and diagnosis of breast and ovarian cancer among first- and second-degree relatives) and on factors under study: dietary habits in the year before breast cancer diagnosis. The study is being expanded to another eight centres in six European countries, with the aim of recruiting 5000 cases.

The major requirement of a case-only study is the unbiased classification of genetic and sporadic cancers. A method (and software) that properly incorporates all information available from each family member has been developed by Parmigiani (Parmigiani *et al.*, 1998). The probability that a given family member is a carrier is obtained from Bayes's theorem, using the mutation prevalence in the population as the prior distribution and the family history as the evidence, taking into account mendelian transmission pathways. The weight of an affected maternal grandmother or aunt for instance, will be higher if the mother also had breast cancer (or if she died when still too young to have breast cancer) than if the mother reached adult or old age without developing the disease. The results of the Parmigiani method are quite sensitive to varying assumptions about the age-specific incidence function of breast and ovarian cancer in mutation carriers and in the general population.

In the COS study, we have improved this method using generation-specific incidence functions estimated from age–period–cohort models (Capocaccia *et al.*, 1990), i.e. a different function for each family member. Cumulative breast cancer risk of a European woman born in the 1950s, in fact, is about three times higher than the risk of her grandmother born at the beginning of the twentieth century. A similar cohort effect has also been shown for mutation carriers (Chang-Claude *et al.*, 1997). Therefore, the output of COS software is the probability that a participant has inherited a *BRCA* gene mutation given her family history and it classifies patients probably affected by hereditable breast cancer (genetic cases) and patients probably affected by sporadic cancer (sporadic cases).

Preliminary results of the pilot study

At present (June 2001), 603 participants have filled in and sent back a complete questionnaire. Using COS software to analyse the information on their family history, the estimated overall proportion of mutation carriers is 17.98%; 103 patients are classified as having greater than 40% probability of carrying a mutation (76% on average) (Fig. 1).

Table 1 shows the frequency of a few relevant exposures in the 103 patients with probability of mutation greater than 40% and in patients with probability of mutation less than 4%, and the corresponding interaction OR (with 95% confidence interval), adjusted for age and education.

The small size of the study does not permit any firm conclusion so far, but suggests that high parity and frequent X-ray exposure in childhood are associated with an increased risk of breast cancer in mutation carriers. Oral contraceptives do not seem to increase the risk and tobacco smoking does not seem to protect.

References

Berrino, F. & Bellati, C. (1999) COS, case only study on breast cancer before the age of 40. Announcement of a new study on gene–environment interaction in breast cancer. *Epid. Prev.*, **23**, 57–58

Brunet, J.S., Ghadirian, P., Rebbeck, T.R., Lerman, C., Garber, J.E., Tonin, P.N., Abrahamson, J., Foulkes, W.D., Daly, M., Wagner-Costalas, J., Godwin, A., Olopade, O.I., Moslehi, R., Liede, A., Futreal, P.A., Weber, B.L., Lenoir, G.M., Lynch, H.T. & Narod, S.A. (1998) Effect of smoking on breast cancer in carriers of mutant *BRCA1* or *BRCA2* genes. *J. Natl. Cancer Inst.*, **90**, 761–766

Capocaccia, R., Verdecchia, A., Micheli, A., Sant, M., Gatta, G. & Berrino, F. (1990) Breast cancer incidence and prevalence estimated from survival and mortality. *Cancer Cause Control.*,**1**, 23–29

Chang-Claude, J., Becher, H., Eby, N., Bastert, G., Wahrendorf, J. & Hamann, U. (1997) Modifying effect of reproductive risk factors on the age at onset of breast cancer for German *BRCA1* mutation carriers. *J. Cancer Res. Clin. Oncol.*, **123**, 272–279

Parmigiani, G., Berry, DA. & Aguilar, O. (1998) Determining carrier probabilities for breast cancer-susceptibility genes *BRCA1* and *BRCA2*. *Am. J. Hum. Genet.*, **62**, 145–158

Follow-up of the ORDET cohort, Lombardy cancer registry, 1987–1997

Tagliabue G.[2], Evangelista A.[1], Tittarelli A.[2], Del Sette D.[1], Contiero P.[2], Crosignani P.[2], Berrino F.[1], Micheli A.[1]

[1]Epidemiology Unit, [2]Lombardy Cancer Registry Unit, Istituto Nazionale per lo Studio e la Cura dei Tumori, Milan, Italy.

Background

The ORDET study (hormones and diet in the etiology of breast tumours) is a prospective cohort study on 10 749 women volunteers, age 35–69 years, recruited in the province of Varese from 1987 to 1992. The aim was to investigate the role of diet and sex hormones in the genesis of breast and other cancers. Several studies on the ORDET cohort have been published (Berrino *et al.*, 1996; Muti *et al.*, 2000; Pala *et al.*, 2001).

Materials and Methods

ORDET cohort

The ORDET cohort overlaps with the EPIC cohort. The 12 079 EPIC volunteers include 7405 women belonging to the ORDET cohort.

At the time of recruitment to ORDET, menstrual and reproductive history and anthropometric measurements were taken, dietary questionnaires were completed and blood and urine were sampled. In addition, all participants received a breast examination by a physician.

Lombardy Cancer Registry

The population of the Varese province, northern Italy, was about 800 000 in the 1991 census. The Lombardy Cancer Registry (LCR) has collected information on all cases of malignant cancer incident in the province since 1976.

Incident cancers

EPILINK, a semiprobabilistic record linkage program, specifically developed by the LCR, was used to link information about the ORDET subjects with other databases, in particular the regional mortality database, the LCR database, and admission and discharge reports from hospitals in the province.

Follow-up

The results of passive follow-up (from mortality, LCR, and hospital discharge files) and active follow-up (searches for clinical information in breast clinics, etc.) were recorded. The expected number of incident cancer cases was calculated from age-, sex- and calendar year-specific incidence rates multiplied by the observed number of person-years at risk (Micheli & Krogh, 1994).

The end of follow-up was determined by death, emigration or last day of follow-up for the present study (31 December 1997).

Results

The average age at recruitment was 48.7 years (SD ± 8.51). Table 1 shows the vital status of the ORDET cohort at 31 December 1997.

Of a total of 480 incident neoplasms, 96.3% were confirmed histologically,

Table 1. ORDET Cohort: vital status at 31 December 1997[a]

VS Code	Description	No. of subjects
1	Alive	10 383
2	Dead	139
7	Emigrated to another region of Italy	185
8	Emigrated to another country	2
9	Unknown	40
	Total	10 749

[a]Median length of follow-up: 7.73 years.

Table 2. ORDET cohort: ratios of observed to expected cases of malignant cancer at 31 December 1997

ICD-9 site	Description	Observed/expected	95% CI
151	Stomach	1.07	0.59–1.55
153	Colon	0.80	0.50–1.10
154	Rectum	0.69	0.26–1.11
157	Pancreas	0.44	0.01–0.87
162	Lung	0.91	0.45–1.37
172	Melanoma	0.96	0.33–1.58
173	Skin	1.03	0.72–1.33
174	Breast	1.34	1.16–1.52
180	Cervix uteri	0.59	0.18–1.01
182	Corpus uteri	0.72	0.40–1.04
183	Ovary	1.01	0.59–1.44
189	Kidney	1.79	0.96–2.61
193	Thyroid	0.75	0.19–1.31
202	Non-Hodgkin lymphoma	1.11	0.62–1.60

whereas 3.3% were confirmed cytologically and only 0.4% were verified by other means (imaging and medical). Breast cancer accounted for 46.2% of the total cancers, followed by cancers of the skin (9.0%), colon (5.6%), ovary (4.6%), and corpus uteri (4.2%).

The ratios of observed to expected cases for each site are shown in Table 2.

Expected cases were calculated from the general population incidence figures for Varese province (1988–1992). It was found that the number of actual cases was greater than the expected number and that this difference did not tend to diminish over the observation period.

Conclusions

The EPILINK software was found to be effective for identifying ORDET participants in other databases and will be useful for further studies in which linking is required and when a unique identification code is not available or not reliable for each subject, or when very large cohorts must be linked.

The high observed/expected ratio found for kidney cancer (Table 2) could depend on the use of the old reference rate while the incidence of kidney cancer is rapidly rising (Chow Wong-Ho *et al.*, 1999), mainly because of the increased use of imaging procedures. In the present cohort, the exceptionally high incidence of kidney cancers relative to those expected could also be due to selection bias, as mainly health-conscious women of high socio-economic status were recruited. Hence the high incidence probably does not apply to the entire population.

The breast cancer cases were significantly in excess of those expected; this might suggest that early diagnosis was a feature of this cohort. However, the ratio of observed to expected cases did not diminish over time (data not shown), suggesting that this did not occur.

Acknowledgements

The ORDET study is financed by the Italian League against Cancer (Milan section) and the Italian Ministry of Health, with a contribution from the Italian National Research Council and the Italian Association for Cancer Research (AIRC). We are indebted to Mrs. Manuela Bellegotti and Mr. Donald C. Ward for technical support.

References

Berrino, F., Muti, P., Micheli, A., Bolelli, G., Krogh, V., Sciajno, R., Pisani, P., Panico, S. & Secreto, G. (1996) Serum sex hormone levels after menopause and subsequent breast cancer. *J. Natl. Cancer Inst.*, **88**, 291–296

Chow, W.H., Devesa, S.S., Warren, J.L. & Fraumeni, J.F. Jr. (1999) Rising incidence of renal cell cancer in the United States *JAMA*, **281**, 1628–1631

Micheli, A. & Krogh, V. (1994) A computer program to calculate expected cases in a dynamic cohort. *Epidemiol. Prev.*, **18**, 164–169

Muti, P., Bradlow, H.L., Micheli, A., Krogh, V., Freudenheim, J.L., Schunemann, H.J., Stanulla, M., Yang, J., Sepkovic, D.W., Trevisan, M. & Berrino, F. (2000) Estrogen metabolism and risk of breast cancer: a prospective study of the 2:16alpha-hydroxyestrone ratio in premenopausal and postmenopausal women. *Epidemiology*, **11**, 635–640

Pala, V., Krogh, V., Muti, P., Chajes, V., Riboli, E., Micheli, A., Saadatian, M., Sieri, S. & Berrino, F. (2001) Erythrocyte membrane fatty acids and subsequent breast cancer: a prospective Italian study. *J. Natl. Cancer. Inst.*, **93**, 1088–1095

The Melbourne Collaborative Cohort Study

Giles G.G., English D.R.

Cancer Epidemiology Centre, Cancer Control Research Institute, Anti-Cancer Council of Victoria, Melbourne, Australia.

Purpose

The principal aim of the Melbourne Collaborative Cohort Study (MCCS) is to improve the prospective investigation of diet and cancer by selecting a study population with an increased range of dietary exposures, by increasing the accuracy of dietary measurements and by collecting blood for the analysis of dietary biomarkers and polymorphisms in the DNA of genes involved in dietary and other metabolic processes. Its second aim is to provide a similar research resource for other common chronic diseases such as heart disease, stroke and type 2 diabetes.

Methods

The MCCS includes both men and women volunteers, aged 40–69 years and recruited from the Melbourne metropolitan area in the early 1990s. In order to recruit a sample with an increased range of dietary exposures, it was decided to deliberately enrich the cohort with migrants to Melbourne from Italy and Greece (Giles 1990).

The baseline questionnaire included questions on personal medical history and family history of common diseases. Smoking and alcohol consumption were asked about in detail and there was a short section on physical activity. Questions were also asked about occupation, household size and composition and social networks and support. A full reproductive history was asked of women. A food frequency questionnaire (FFQ) was developed specifically for the MCCS and was based on 8 days of weighed food records (WFRs) from a sample of 1000 Australian, Italian and Greek men and women. The FFQ food list was selected on the basis of these data, using stepwise regression techniques (Ireland *et al.*, 1994). During recruitment, a random sample of subjects stratified by age, sex, and ethnic group was selected for a calibration study. In the 12 months following attendance, the 256 subjects were asked to complete 2 x 4-day and 2 x 3-day diet diaries and to give blood and 24-h urine samples. A year after their first attendance they were invited to re-attend for repeated measures and blood sampling.

Anthropometric measurements included height, weight, waist and hip circumferences and bio-impedance, the latter using the RJL Systems BIA 101 body composition analyser. Blood pressure measurements were taken using a DINAMAP 1846SX automatic blood pressure monitor.

Blood samples were collected from all subjects in 15-ml lithium-heparin vacutainers. Total plasma cholesterol and glucose were measured immediately using Kodak Ektachem DT60™ desktop analysers. Blood aliquots were placed in a liquid nitrogen inventory and have been maintained at temperatures below –120° C.

A total of 16 962 men and 24 286 women aged between 40 and 69 years were recruited into the cohort between 1990 and 1994. Their age and ethnic breakdowns are given in Table 1. The majority of subjects were Anglo-Celtic (Anglo) and about a quarter were from southern Europe (S. Eur).

Detailed analysis of the dietary data and the calibration study has been, or will be, published elsewhere (Hodge *et al.*, 2000). Figure 1 illustrates some of the differences that we have identified between the ethnic groups in regard to their choice of foods. It is obvious from the figure that the inclusion of southern Europeans has increased the range of intake of foods consumed.

In regard to nondietary risk factors, the inclusion of the southern Europeans in the cohort has also increased variability. This is apparent for obesity-related measures, alcohol consumption, cigarette smoking, physical activity, hypertension, diabetes, cholesterol levels, sex hormone use in women (oral contraceptive and hormone replacement therapy) and family history of cancer. In most instances the levels of these factors appear more adverse for the southern Europeans.

Excluding deaths in the first year of follow-up, 716 deaths were observed between 1991 and 1998 compared with 1664 expected, giving a total standardised mortality ratio (SMR) of

Table 1. Melbourne Collaborative Cohort Study population by sex, ethnic group[a] and age

Age	Men		Women		Total		
	Anglo	S. Eur	Anglo	S. Eur	Anglo	S. Eur	Total
40–49	4103	1028	6305	1568	10 408	2596	13 004
50–59	3578	1713	5798	2420	9376	4133	13 509
60–69	4647	1893	6596	1599	11 243	3492	14 735
Total	12 328	4634	18 699	5587	31 027	10 221	41 248

[a]Anglo, Anglo-Celtic; S. Eur, southern European.

0.43. The SMR for cancer was 0.57, cardiovascular disease 0.32, and other causes 0.34. Cancer incidence data were obtained from record linkage to the Victorian Cancer Registry and the standardized incidence ratio for all cancer was 0.62, breast cancer 0.96, prostate 1.28, bowel 0.59 and lung 0.37.

A case cohort analysis is in progress that includes new cases of cancer of the breast, bowel and prostate, type 2 diabetes and cardiovascular deaths since recruitment until mid 2002. The control subcohort is a random sample of about 5000 individuals. The analysis will use the questionnaire data collected at baseline together with laboratory measurements of selected molecules (fatty acids, carotenoids, hormones) in plasma and polymorphisms in key genes, e.g. in the breast and prostate cancer studies, those involved in the metabolism and action of sex hormones and insulin-like growth factors.

We are currently preparing to conduct another follow-up with repeat physical measures and blood collection. We are investigating ways in which nonfatal, noncancer outcomes might be identified more quickly and accurately than relying on self-report and how best to investigate predictors of disability-free ageing. We are also intending to use the cohort members to perform interventions in regard to smoking, dietary intake and physical activity.

References

Giles, G.G. (1990) The Melbourne Study of Diet and Cancer. *Proc. Nutr. Soc. Aust.*, **15**, 61–68

Hodge, A., Giles, G.G., Patterson, A., Brown, W. & Ireland, P. (2000) The Anti-Cancer Council of Victoria FFQ. Relative validity of nutrient intakes compared with diet diaries in young to middle-aged women in a study of iron supplementation. *Aust. N Z J Public Health*, **24**, 576–583

Ireland, P., Jolley, D. & Giles, G.G. (1994) Development of the Melbourne FFQ: a food frequency questionnaire for use in an Australian prospective study involving an ethnically diverse cohort. *Asia Pac. J. Clin. Nutr.*, **3**, 19–31

Nutrition and cancer prevention in Australia: a national collaboration to promote the evidence

Lee S.[1], Slevin T.[2]

[1]Anti-Cancer Foundation of South Australia, Adelaide, Australia. [2]Cancer Foundation of Western Australia , Perth, Australia.

Introduction

In Australia, the role of diet in cancer prevention has been acknowledged for many years. Only recently, however, have national strategies for the prevention of cancer through diet been documented (The Cancer Council Australia, 2001). The Cancer Council Australia supports collaboration of key agencies to achieve the changes in diet necessary to reduce cancer risk in Australia. Specific strategies to be undertaken, either individually or as a member of relevant committees or bodies, include:

1. Collaboration with the Commonwealth and state health departments, to develop and implement a national public education programme to increase knowledge of the links between cancer and diet, and to change dietary behaviours.
2. Collaboration with state and territory members of The Cancer Council, and other nongovernment health bodies and consumer agencies, to actively advocate for public policy supportive of cancer-preventing diets.
3. Supporting and promoting research into the relationship between nutrition and cancer and how to change diet-related behaviours.

The paper describes recent advances in the implementation of these strategies in Australia.

The National Nutrition and Cancer Working Party

The Cancer Council Australia is the nation's peak nongovernment cancer organization. Its members are the leading state and territory cancer councils. In recent years, a number of member bodies have become actively involved in the area of nutrition and cancer prevention. It was therefore considered timely to establish a more formal alliance.

The Nutrition and Cancer Subcommittee of The Cancer Council Australia's Public Health Committee was formed in February 2001. The group representatives bring together internal expertise from state cancer councils, as well as research experience in nutrition and cancer and substantial experience in conducting public health nutrition programmes. Four areas for action have been identified and are described below:

1. Epidemiology

As new research is published, the nature of the association between diet and cancer causality becomes clearer. It is essential for the working party to remain fully informed on, and guided by, these developments.

2. Evidence on intervention efficacy

For practice to be evidence-based, a sound understanding of the body of evidence on intervention efficacy is essential. The working party will maintain a watching brief on this issue.

3. Cancer Council Programme development

State cancer organizations are currently developing initiatives in the area of nutrition and cancer prevention. The working party will assist in monitoring the progress of programmes currently underway or under development and provide input as to the best investment of resources for programmes developed under the banner of The Cancer Council Australia.

4. Advocacy and lobbying

Many programmes are run, proposed or recommended in the field of nutrition. To ensure efficacy, there is a need for collaboration between organizations. There is also a need to influence government action on the issue of nutrition and cancer, with specific reference to the allocation of resources to conduct meaningful and effective research and interventions. The working party will endeavour to advance these issues.

Nutrition and Cancer Prevention in the 21st Century Workshop

In July 2001, the working party held a national workshop to inform key stakeholders of The Cancer Council Australia's interest in the area of nutrition and cancer prevention. The meeting was held in association with the Strategic Inter-Government Nutrition Alliance (SIGNAL) and attracted over 80 participants from government and nongovernment health organizations, academics, clinicians, industry representatives and researchers.

The meeting sought to update the interested public health community on the current evidence linking nutrition and cancer. Feedback from the workshop was very positive, with a general sense that there is an important place for cancer societies actively involved in the field of promoting healthy nutrition.

Conclusion

The development of the National Nutrition Working Party has been an important step in raising the profile of nutrition and cancer prevention in Australia. Working in collaboration with other relevant organizations will ensure the message remains an essential feature of future national public health nutrition strategies.

Reference

The Cancer Council Australia (2001) *National Cancer Prevention Policy 2001-03.* Canberra, The Cancer Council. Australia

Nutrition and cancer prevention: working together to promote healthy eating

Lee S.

Anti-Cancer Foundation of South Australia, Adelaide, Australia.

The health issue

Evidence shows nutrition to play a major role in cancer prevention. To reduce the risk of cancer through good nutrition, healthy eating patterns must be established at a young age (Child, Adolescent and Family Health Service, 1992), yet it is well documented that children's eating patterns are less than optimal. The 1995 National Nutrition Survey (Australian Bureau of Statistics, 1997) found that a third of children aged 4–11 years had not eaten fruit or fruit products the day before being surveyed, while more than 20% of children under 12 had not eaten vegetables or vegetable products on the day prior to being surveyed. In 1995, the proportion of overweight and obese children and adolescents aged 2–17 years was 21% for boys and 23% for girls. (Australian Institute of Health and Welfare, 2000).

In June 1999, just over 87 000 children attended long-day care, with almost half spending between 10 and 29 hours in care per week (Australian Bureau of Statistics, 1999). For many children, foods eaten while in child care make a significant contribution to their weekly intake. Long-day child care centres can therefore play a crucial role in children's nutrition.

The South Australian Child Care Nutrition Partnership

In an attempt to build on what has already been achieved in South Australia in the area of early childhood nutrition and to minimize duplication, the South Australian Child Care Nutrition Partnership was formed in June 1998; it aims to promote good nutrition for all South Australian children aged 0–5 years in child care. The partnership currently includes representation from the fields of nutrition, dental health, child care, as well as tertiary and vocational education.

Food Matters – a nutrition newsletter for carers of children aged 0–5 years

One of several initiatives of the Partnership is a nutrition newsletter, the need for which was clearly identified. The newsletter is a six-page, two-colour, quarterly publication with a one-page black and white double-sided parent insert. The newsletter contributes to the nutrition education needs of cooks, directors and workers in the early childhood sector, as well as parents and care-givers of preschool-aged children. To date, eight issues of *Food Matters* have been produced.

Evaluation

Self-administered questionnaires and telephone surveys were used to determine the value of the newsletter (n = 116). Results indicate that:

- Over 96% of participants read the newsletter.
- The majority of participants found the newsletter to be relevant or very relevant to their work.
- The majority of participants rated the format of the newsletter, including layout, length and readability, as good or very good.

Benefits of working in partnership

Working in partnership allows the sharing of resources, both human and financial, as well as the sharing of expertise. This shared pool of knowledge and capacity ensures that Food Matters is a credible and sustainable source of consistent nutrition information for carers and families of children aged 0–5 years.

One of the main benefits for individual members of the working party is the opportunity to develop professional networks. These networks can be a valuable resource for other areas of an individual's work. Working closely with people who have different areas of expertise also allows individuals to learn from each other – a simple but effective means of professional development.

For an organization such as the Anti-Cancer Foundation of South Australia, working in partnership is a cost-effective, efficient means of achieving its objectives. It adds to the organization's public profile and, in the case of Food Matters, clearly conveys a commitment to early childhood nutrition.

Conclusions

Cancer prevention nutrition guidelines closely reflect current national dietary guidelines in Australia. Collaboration with organizations that promote these guidelines serves to increase the Anti-Cancer Foundation's capacity for reducing cancer risk. All indications to date suggest Food Matters has been well received as a nutrition resource for carers of children under the age of 5 years. As part of a larger strategy of the South Australian Child Care Nutrition Partnership, it has the potential to positively influence the eating habits of many young South Australians and their families.

Acknowledgements

Thanks go to all members, both past and present, of the Food Matters working group and their respective organizations, for their contributions to the production of this newsletter: Alison Shanks and Jo Meedeniya (Eat Well SA), Julie-Anne McWhinnie and Calli Strongylos (Noarlunga Health Services), Liz Kellett and Caroline Jones (Children's Health Development Foundation), Iris Lindemann and Nadia Cerro (Women's and Children's Hospital), Kathy Simpson and Sue Kleve (Inner Southern Community Health Service), Sue Elliot (TeethSmart SA), Geoff Hayes (Christies Beach Children's Centre).

References

Australian Bureau of Statistics (1997) *National Nutrition Survey Selected Highlights Australia, 1995*, Australian Government Publishing Service, Canberra

Australian Bureau of Statistics (1999) *Child Care, Australia*. Australian Government Publishing Service, Canberra

Australian Institute of Health and Welfare (2000) *Australia's Health 2000: The seventh biennial health report of the Australian Institute of Health and Welfare*, Canberra

Child, Adolescent and Family Health Service (1992) *Health goals and targets for Australian children and youth*. Child, Adolescent and Adolescent and Family Health Service & Department of Community Services and Health, Canberra

Chapter 2

Vegetables, fruit and cereals

Epidemiological studies of cereals, fruit and vegetables

Schatzkin A.

National Cancer Institute. Bethesda, MD, 20814, USA.

The public appears to maintain a healthy dose of scepticism toward diet and cancer research. Even among scientists working in the field, facing continuing inconsistencies in evidence, resolution of key questions has remained elusive.

Nevertheless, there is no dearth of promising, even cherished, hypotheses in this area. And this is hardly new. As Stubs said over 400 years ago. "Doe we not see the poore man that eateth browne bread health fuller, stronger, fayrer complectioned and longer living than the other that fare daintelie every day?" But, as we would all acknowledge now, it's been a rather bad year or two, scientific-evidence-wise, for the long-held fibre hypothesis.

Of course, commercial enterprise has had little compunction against weighing in on these issues. We see claims that breakfast cereals will reduce risk of cancer or that catsup will lower your malignancy risk, and so on. Would that we had the scientific evidence to back up these advertised assertions.

It is not that nutrition and cancer is the only arena of cancer research with inconsistency and uncertainty. There are open questions about certain occupational exposures, low-dose radiation, certain infectious agents. But, there are a number of agents for which the cancer causation evidence is qualitatively greater than that for virtually any nutritional factor. Can we get nutrition to catch up?

As the final bit of introduction to the papers that follow, I would like to indicate some methodological issues to keep in mind when considering both observational and experimental epidemiological studies of cereals and fruits and vegetables in cancer etiology. With respect to observational studies, we need to be cognizant of measurement error (especially the relative risk attenuation that may arise from our use of food frequency questionnaires); inadequate range of intake (in fibre or vegetable studies, for example, does the top quintile really consume an amount that makes for meaningful comparisons); and confounding. On this last issue, unmeasured or unknown confounders are notoriously difficult to rule out. The evidence that may be emerging with respect to hormone replacement therapy and cardiovascular disease – that is, the disparate results from observational epidemiological studies and trials – could turn out to be quite sobering.

With respect to experimental epidemiological studies (trials), we should keep in mind that measurement error may still be operative. That is, misreporting may be affecting the dietary assessments of our intervention participants, thus making the picture rosier. Although trials theoretically can engender a wide range of intake by intervening with dramatically different eating plans, in practice it may be difficult to effect the desired differences in, say, vegetable intake, between intervention and control groups. Finally, trials may not be able to evaluate all relevant aspects of carcinogenesis. Interventions may come too late or not last long enough, for example.

So as we consider the presentations to come, we need to proceed with a certain degree of healthy scepticism and not always believe everything that we read – and write.

Vegetable, fruit and cereal consumption and gastric cancer risk

González C.A.
(for the EPIC working group on gastric cancer)

Department of Epidemiology, Catalan Institute of Oncology, Barcelona, Spain.

Introduction

Incidence and mortality of gastric cancer (GC) is decreasing in the world as well in most European countries but it still represents the fourth most frequent cancer in Europe and the second in the world. Almost 900 000 new cases of gastric cancer in the world and 78 537 new cases in the European Union (EU) have been estimated according to the EUCAN database (Ferlay *et al.*, 2000). Gastric cancer incidence rates vary approximately tenfold in the world and fourfold in the European Union. Portugal, Italy, Spain, Austria and Germany show the highest risk in the EU, while risk is lowest in Denmark, Sweden and France. The 5-year survival of patients affected with GC in the EU is quite low, ranging between 12% in the UK and 28% in Spanish cancer registries. The identification and better control of risk factors represent the most effective way for reducing gastric cancer burden.

Helicobacter pylori infection is an established risk factor of GC (Danesh, 1999). Isolated in 1982, it was recognized as a human carcinogen by IARC in 1994, but the specific mechanisms of action in the complex process of gastric carcinogenesis are not known. *H. pylori* infection is neither a sufficient nor a necessary cause of GC; only a limited correlation exists between the prevalence of infection and the level of risk in a population. In European countries, the prevalence of *H. pylori* infection in adults still ranges from 30% to 70%, but the geographical variation of gastric cancer risk in Europe cannot be completely explained by differences in the prevalence of infection.

On the other hand, only a small fraction of those infected by *Helicobacter* develop GC. In Japan, the country with the highest GC incidence in the world, it has been estimated that 60 million people were infected by *Helicobacter* but only 0.4% had GC (Asaka *et al.*, 1998).

A multifactorial model of carcinogenesis is accepted, according to which different dietary and non-dietary factors, including genetic susceptibility, are involved at different stages in the cancer process. *H. pylori* infection, diet and other environmental factors such as tobacco are thought to play a role in gastric cancer development. However, the interindividual susceptibility differences and the interaction between these environmental and genetic factors have not yet been addressed adequately.

On the other hand, while incidence of gastric cancer is going down in most developed countries, the incidence of gastric cancer of the cardia and adenocarcinoma of the oesophagus is going up (Botterweck *et al.*, 2000). The reason is not well known, although it is possible that cardia and non-cardia gastric cancer cases could be associated, in part, with different risk factors. Combined analyses of nested case–control studies have shown that *H. pylori* infection does not increase the risk of cardia cancer (Helicobacter and Cancer Collaborative Group, 2001).

Scientific evidence up to 1996

International reports (WCRF/AICR, 1997; COMA, 1998) summarized the scientific evidence of the effect of foods and nutrients up to the middle of the last decade. Taking into account the results from epidemiological studies conducted in several European countries, South and North America, Japan and China, the evidence that diets high in vegetables and fruits protect against GC was considered convincing by the WCRF/AICR (1997). Three out of the six previous published cohort studies and 27 of the 32 published case–control studies found a statistically significant protective effect for the intake of one or more vegetable and/or fruit items, or groups, considered collectively or separately. In general, a dose-response pattern was observed, the estimated risk decreasing with increasing vegetable and fruit intake. Evidence was particularly consistent and strong for raw vegetables, citrus fruits and allium vegetables, although the protective effect has been seen for all types of fruits and vegetables. On the contrary, the frequent consumption of pickled or salted vegetables has been associated with a higher cancer risk in most of the studies conducted in Asia.

The evidence that refrigeration protects against GC probably by reducing the need for salt and other preservative methods of foods was also considered convincing. Results on cereal consumption as a group were inconsistent. The observed risk was even increased by cereal intake in many studies, although the consumption of whole grain and brown bread was negatively associated in some studies. The protective effect of vitamin C was considered as probable and the protective effects of carotenoids, allium compounds, whole grain cereals and green tea was considered as possible. It is probable that there was no relationship with nitrate consumption from vegetables, while the evidence on the protective effect of fibre, selenium and garlic was considered insufficient.

It is necessary to emphasize that the evidence on the association between dietary factors and GC in the WCRF/AICR (1997) report was based more on case–control studies than on cohort studies. Relatively few cohort studies, which are supposed to provide the best evidence within nonexperimental studies, had been published at that time. Furthermore, most of these cohort studies included relatively few cases, obtained a poor dietary assessment because of the use of few dietary items in food frequency questionnaires, and suffered from the lack of control of all potentially confounding variables.

The conclusion from the COMA report (1998) in the UK was approximately the same. It was considered that there was moderately consistent evidence of the protective effect of vegetable and fruit consumption. It was stated, however, that confounding by *H. pylori* infection may partly account for these findings, although the working group thought that the strength, consistency and dose-response relationship of the results argue against this hypothesis.

Regarding the most important vitamins and compounds contained in vegetables and fruits, the WCRF/AICR (1997) report considered that vitamin C probably, and carotenoids possibly decrease GC risk, while possibly vitamin E is not associated. The report from the UK concluded that the evidence was strongly consistent for vitamin C, moderately consistent for carotenoids, and inconsistent for vitamin E.

Nevertheless, it was considered in the last decade that approximately 66%–75% of GC risk could be reduced with high intake of fruit and vegetables and low consumption of salted foods (WCRF/AICR, 1997). Other researchers (Steinmetz & Potter, 1991) have estimated that 40%–50% of GC incidence could be prevented by diets high in vegetables and fruit. However, it should be noted that the highest current consumption of vegetables and fruit in Europe is found in Spain and Italy, which are the countries with the highest risk of GC in the EU.

Further evidence in the last 5 years

Further evidence has been published in the last 5 years concerning the protective effect of vegetable and fruit intake, including new evidence on the possibly protective effects of high intake of flavonoids, phytosterols, nonfermented soy products, and cereal fibre. Results from 12 additional case–control studies conducted in Europe, America, and Asia have been published. Eight of them have shown results on vegetables and fruit, and almost all of these studies have supported the protective role of vegetables and fruit (Fig. 1). Six of them presented results on the effect of vitamin C and four found a negative association with its intake. Several have also observed a protective effect of other antioxidants such as alfa-tocopherol and beta-carotene. Within the new and valuable findings, it is important to emphasize the results from the study in Sweden (Ekstrom *et al.*, 2000), which has shown that the protective effects of antioxidants was specially beneficial among subjects who were smokers and/or those infected by *Helicobacter pylori*, in other words, in subjects with a higher risk of gastric cancer. Some of these studies have also shown that the effect of vegetable and fruit intake could be similar for the intestinal and diffuse type of GC (Harrison *et al.*, 1997; Ward *et al.*, 1999; Ekström *et al.*, 2000) and for the cardia and non-cardia subsites (Ekström *et al.*, 2000).

Most of these new case–control studies did not publish results on the effect of cereal intake. Some of the studies carried out in Asian countries observed a positive association with the intake of rice (Mathew *et al.*, 2000) and bread (Ji *et al.*, 1998) while a strong protective effect from consumption of cereal fibre has been observed in Sweden (Terry *et al.*, 2001) for cardia gastric cancer.

Three cohort studies have published further results on vegetable and fruit intake (Fig. 2) but the potential confounding effect of *H. pylori* has not been taken into account. A cohort study in the Netherlands (Botterweck *et al.*, 1998) did not find any association with the consumption of vegetables, fruit, beta-carotene, vitamin C, retinol, nitrate and nitrite. A protective effect was observed only for onions. In this study, more than 120 000 males and females

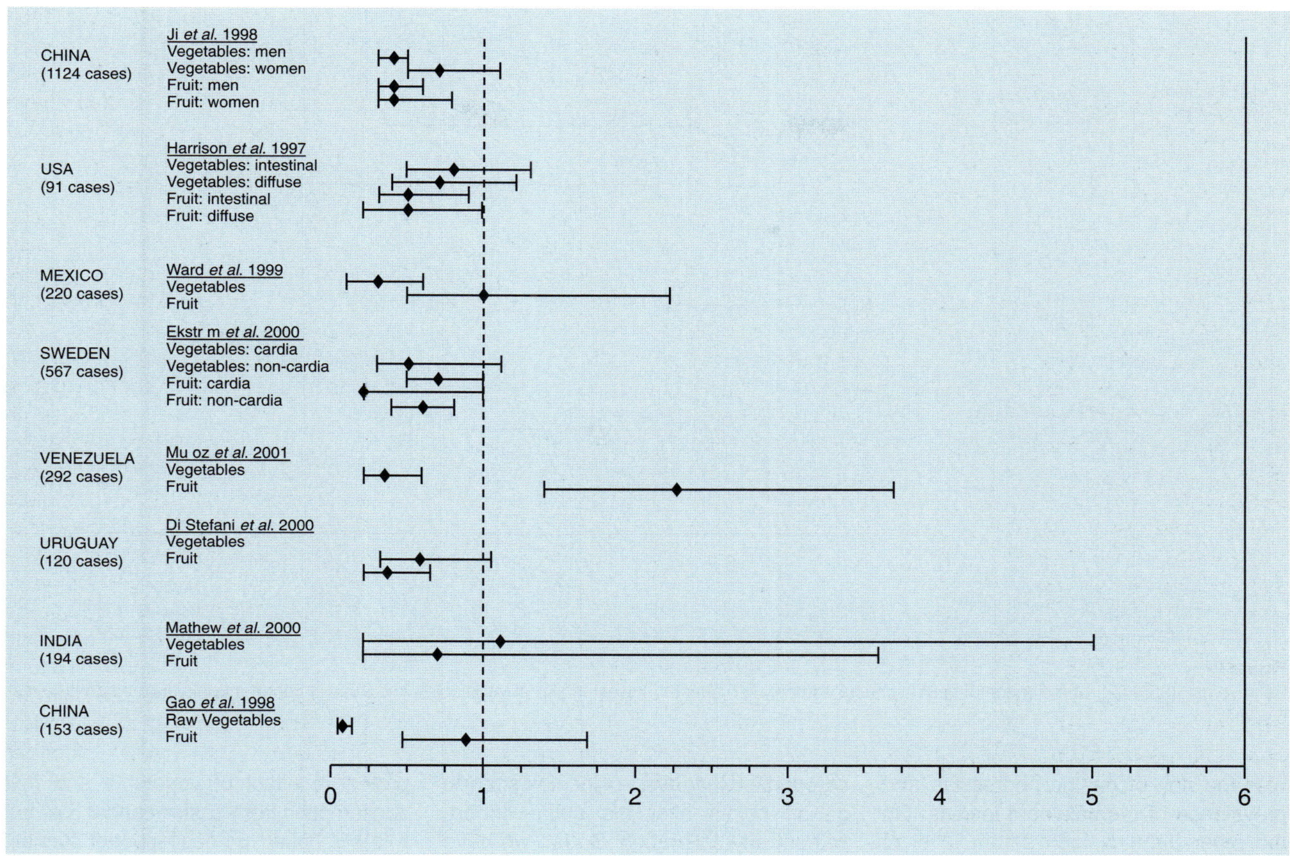

Figure 1
OR (95% CI) for gastric cancer risk comparing highest to lowest intake of vegetables and fruit in case–control studies published in the last 5 years

were included and the analysis was based on 282 GC cases; all recruited subjects were between the ages of 55 and 69. This means that dietary assessment was carried out at a relatively old age, given that the age of the most relevant exposure is probably 20–30 years before the onset of gastric cancer. When the analysis was restricted to the first year of follow-up, this study found a protective effect of the intake of fruit and vegetables for the GC cases diagnosed in this period. The authors have thus suggested that the protective effect observed in case–control studies could be explained by the presence of an information bias in these studies. On the contrary, in a cohort study in Hawaii (Galanis *et al.*, 1998), the association of high consumption of fruit and raw vegetables with reduced risk of GC was statistically significant only for fruit, although the number of cases was low and only 13 food items were included in the questionnaire. Also, a strong protective effect of the consumption of vegetables and fruit was observed in a cohort of twins in Sweden (Terry *et al.*, 1998), but the measure of intake was qualitative, addressing only the relative importance of vegetables and fruit in the diet.

Some additional evidence was recently provided by chemoprevention trials. An intervention study carried out in Colombia (Correa *et al.*, 2000) to assess the effect of supplementation with vitamin C and beta-carotene in volunteers (men and women, mean age 51.1 years) has shown, after 6 years of follow-up, a statistically significant protective effect, that is, an increase in the rate of regression of confirmed histological diagnoses of premalignant lesions in the gastric mucosa (intestinal metaplasia and/or atrophy). In another chemoprevention trial, conducted in Finland (Varis *et al.*, 1998) in male smokers, aged 50–69 years, supplementation with alpha-tocopherol and beta-carotene was not associated

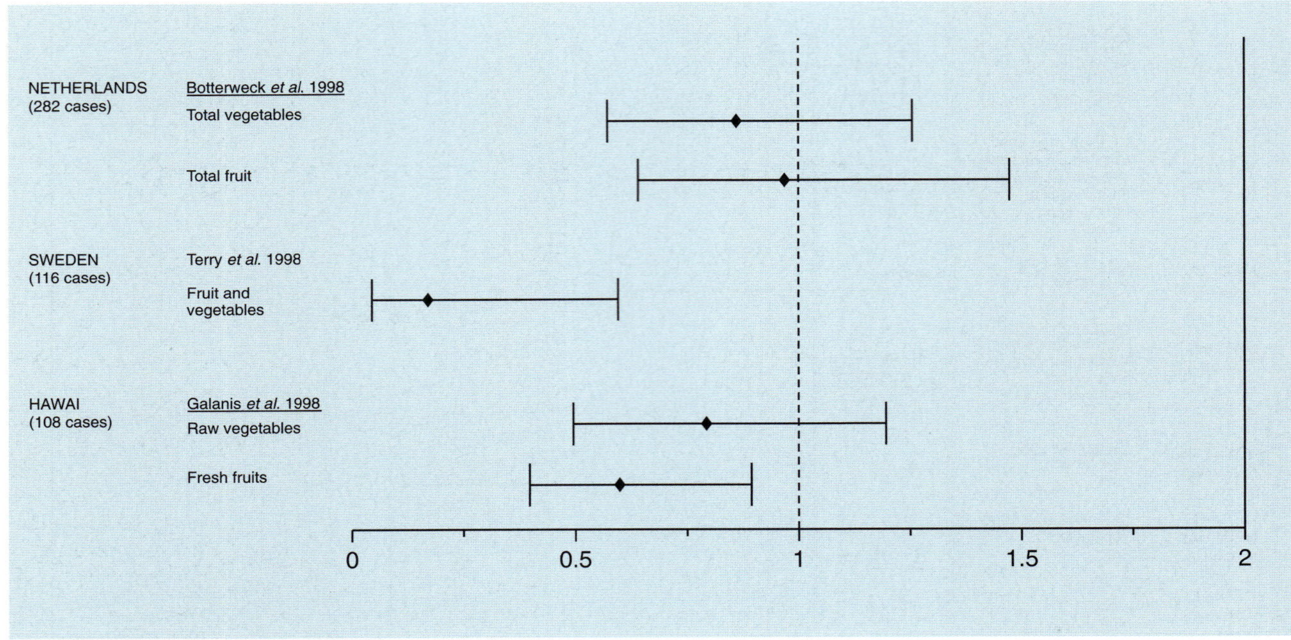

Figure 2
Relative risk (95% CI) for incidence of gastric cancer comparing highest to lowest intake of vegetables and fruits in cohort studies published in the last 5 years

with the risk of gastric neoplasias and prevalence of premalignant lesions. On the other hand, a high serum level of ascorbic acid showed a protective effect in the progression to dysplasia or gastric cancer in an endoscopic follow-up study in China (You *et al.*, 2000).

Very preliminary results from the European Prospective Investigation into Cancer and Nutrition (EPIC) provide data that support the protective effects of fruit intake. In 392 300 subjects included in the cohort, 132 cases of newly diagnosed gastric adenocarcinoma have been identified so far, and are available for preliminary analysis, with a mean of 2.3 years of follow-up. Using Cox regression analysis, age as a time scale variable and length of follow-up as time-dependent covariates, relative risks, stratified by centre and adjusted by total energy, sex, educational level and tobacco smoking, have been estimated. The levels of intake were categorized in tertiles, using sex-specific cut-off points over the entire cohort, without any calibration. So far, we have observed a slight protective effect of total fresh fruit intake and cereals but not of total vegetable intake. Analysing the risk according to the year of diagnosis of the GC cases, the observed protective effect of cereals remains only in cases diagnosed in the first year of follow-up. On the other hand, the protective effect of fruit remains only in cases with 2 or more years of follow-up. These results should be taken with caution because they are based on relatively few cases, with a short follow-up, without adjustment by *H. pylori* infection and with still very heterogeneous identification of cases between centres.

Conclusion

In conclusion, most of the recent epidemiological evidence supports the protective effect of vegetable and fruit consumption from gastric cancer risk, but it is still based on case–control studies. Recall bias is possible in case–control studies and therefore results from well-designed and well-conducted cohort studies are urgently needed. Evidence on whole-grain cereals is still inconclusive. Further research should be addressed to analyse dietary factors separately by cardia and non-cardia gastric cancer. On the other hand, given that vegetable and fruit intake could be specially beneficial among subjects at increased risk of gastric cancer because of a higher level of oxidative damage, such as among smokers and those infected by *H. pylori*, the joint effects of these factors should be assessed. Furthermore, polymorphisms in a wide variety of genes may modify the effect of these exposures. Therefore, in the analysis of GC, it is necessary to consider genetic susceptibility for different risk factors as well.

Gene–environment interaction could explain the high variation in the GC incidence observed in the world. The EUR-GAST project, a nested case–control study within the EPIC cohort, recently funded by the Fifth Framework Programme of the EU, is addressing these aims and we hope that will be valuable in the scientific clarification of the role of these factors.

References

Asaka, M., Kudo, M., Kato, M., Sugiyama, T. & Takeda, H. (1998) Review article: long-term *Helicobacter pylori* infection from gastritis to gastric cancer. *Aliment. Pharmacol. Ther.*, **12**, Suppl 1, 9–15

Botterweck, A.A., van den Brandt, P.A. & Goldbohm, R.A. (1998) A prospective cohort study on vegetable and fruit consumption and stomach cancer risk in the Netherlands. *Am. J. Epidemol.*, **148**, 842–853

Botterweck, A.A., Schouten, L.J., Volovics, A., Dorant, E. & van den Brandt, P.A. (2000) Trends in incidence of adenocarcinoma of the oesophagus and gastric cardia in ten European countries. *Int. J. Epidemiol.*, **29**, 645–654

Correa, P., Fontham, E.T.H., Bravo, J.C., Bravo, L.E., Ruiz, B., Zarama, G., Realpe, J.L., Malcom, G.T., Li, D., Johnson, W.D. & Mera, R. (2000) Chemoprevention of gastric dysplasia: randomized trial of antioxidant supplements and anti-*Helicobacter pylori* therapy. *J. Natl. Cancer Inst.*, **9**, 1881–1887

COMA (Committee on Medical Aspects of Food and Nutrition Policy) (1998) *Nutritional aspects of the development of cancer, Report on Health and Social Subjects No. 48*, The Stationery Office, Norwich, UK

Danesh, J. (1999) Is *Helicobacter pylori* infection a cause of gastric neoplasia? *Cancer Surv. Infec. Human Cancer*, **33**, 263–289

De Stefani, E., Boffetta, P., Ronco, A.L., Brennan, P., Deneo-Pellegrini, H., Carzoglio, J.C. & Mendilaharsu, M. (2000) Plant sterols and risk of stomach cancer: a case–control study in Uruguay. *Nutr. Cancer*, **37**, 140–144

Ekström, A.M., Serafini, M., Nyrén, O., Hansson, L., Ye, W. & Wolk, A. (2000) Dietary antioxidant intake and the risk of cardia cancer and noncardia cancer of the intestinal and diffuse types: a population-based case–control study in Sweden. *Int. J. Cancer*, **87**, 133–140

Ferlay, J., Bray, F., Sankila, R. & Parkin, D.M. (2000) Eucan Database. Cancer Incidence, Mortality and Prevalence in the European Union (1996 estimates). European Network of Cancer registries. International Agency for Research on Cancer (IARC). Version 3.1. Available on the Internet (www-dep.iarc.fr/eucan).

Galanis, D.J., Kolonel, L.N., Lee, J. & Nomura, A. (1998) Intakes of selected foods and beverages and the incidence of gastric cancer among the Japanese residents of Hawaii: a prospective study. *Int. J. Epidemiol.*, **27**, 173–180

Gao, C.M., Takezaki, T., Ding, J.H., Li, M.S. & Tajima, K. (1999) Protective effect of allium vegetables against both oesophageal and stomach cancer: a simultaneous case-referent study of a high-epidemic area in Jiangsu Province, China. *Jpn. J. Cancer Res.*, **90**, 614–621

Harrison, L. E., Zhang, Z., Karpeh, M.S., Sun, M. & Kurtz, R.C. (1997) The role of dietary factors in the intestinal and diffuse histologic subtypes of gastric adenocarcinoma. A case–control study in the U.S. *Cancer*, **80**, 1021–1028

Helicobacter and Cancer Collaborative Group (2001) Gastric cancer and *Helicobacter pylori*: a combined analysis of 12 case control studies nested within prospective cohorts, *Gut*, **49**, 347–353

Ji, B., Chow, W., Yang, G., Zheng, W., Shu, X.O., Jin, F., Gao, R.N., Gao, Y.T. & Fraumeni, J.F. Jr. (1998) Dietary habits and stomach cancer in Shangai, China. *Int. J. Cancer*, **76**, 659–664

Mathew, A., Gangadharan, P., Varghese, C. & Nair, M.K. (2000) Diet and stomach cancer: a case–control study in South India. *Eur. J. Cancer Prev.*, **9**, 89–97

Muñoz, N., Plummer, M., Vivas, J., Moreno, V., De Sanjose, S., Lopez, G. & Oliver, W. (2001) A case–control study of gastric cancer in Venezuela. *Int. J. Cancer*, **93**, 417–423

Steinmetz, K. & Potter, J.D. (1991) Vegetables, fruit, and cancer. I. Epidemiology, *Cancer Causes Control*, **2**, 325–357

Terry, P., Nyrén, O. & Yuen, J. (1998) Protective effect of fruits and vegetables on stomach cancer in a cohort of Swedish twins. *Int. J. Cancer*, **76**, 35–37

Terry, P., Lagergen, J., Ye, W., Wolk, A. & Nyrén, O. (2001) Inverse association between intake of cereal fiber and risk of gastric cardia cancer. *Gastroenterology*, **120**, 387–391

Varis, K., Taylor, P.R., Sipponen, P., Samloff, I.M., Heinonen, O.P., Albanes, D., Harkonen, M., Huttunen, J.K., Laxen, F. & Virtamo, J. (1998) Gastric cancer and premalignant lesions in atrophic gastritis: a controlled trial on the effect of supplementation with alpha-tocopherol and beta-carotene. The Helsinki gastritis study group. *Scand. J. Gastroenterol.*, **33**, 294–300

Ward, M.H. & López-Carrillo, L. (1999) Dietary factors and the risk of gastric cancer in Mexico City. *Am. J. Epidemiol.*, **149**, 925–932

World Cancer Research Fund/American Investigation of Cancer Research (1997) *Food, Nutrition and the Prevention of Cancer: A Global Perspective*, (BANTA Book Group) Menasha, USA

You, W., Zhang, L., Gail, M.H., Chang, Y.S., Liu, W.D., Ma, J.L., Li, J.Y., Jin, M.L., Hu, Y.R., Yang, C.S., Blaser, M.J., Correa, P., Blot, W.J., Fraumeni, J.F. Jr. & Xu, G.W. 2000) Gastric dysplasia and gastric cancer: *Helicobacter pylori*, serum vitamin C and other risk factors. *J. Natl. Cancer Inst.*, **92**, 1607–612

Vegetables and fruits and lung cancer

Miller A.B.
(for the EPIC working group on lung cancer)

Deutsches Krebsforschungszentrum, Im Neuenheimer Feld (DKFZ), Heidelberg, Germany.

Background

In the 1997 report of the World Cancer Research Fund, it was concluded that there was convincing evidence that vegetables and fruits decrease the risk of lung cancer, with the evidence being most abundant and consistent for green vegetables and carrots, as well as for both vegetables and fruits generally. Apart from vegetables and fruits, several micronutrients, vitamins and minerals commonly found in plants have been considered in relation to lung cancer risk. In some studies, the protective effect from fruits and vegetables was attributed to beta-carotene. However, a protective effect of beta-carotene for lung cancer is now considered unlikely because of negative results of trials with beta-carotene supplementation (IARC, 1998).

Since the 1997 report, there have been reports on cohort studies that do not show similar significant associations (Speizer *et al.*, 1999), or an effect of fruit and vegetable intake in women but not in men (Feskanich *et al.*, 2000). Yet a multi-centre case–control study in non-smokers did find a significant effect of increasing vegetable consumption in reducing lung cancer risk (Brennan *et al.*, 2000) and in a European multi-country cohort, fruit intake was inversely related to lung cancer risk in male smokers (Jansen *et al.*, 2001). Part of the difficulty in all studies except in non-smokers could be adequately controlling for potential confounding from tobacco use, while the discrepancies could also be explained by effects of recall bias in the case–control studies and the impact of measurement error in the cohort studies. Therefore, in the preliminary analysis of EPIC data here reported, considerable attention has been paid to controlling for current and past tobacco use, as well as duration of smoking. We also planned to adopt an approach to calibration (Kaaks & Riboli, 1997) to reduce measurement error, but this has so far been judged as unfeasible for these preliminary analyses.

Materials and methods

We analysed a data set which included information on a total cohort of 482 924 subjects; 153 496 (31.8%) were males and 329 428 (68.2%) females. The average follow-up time for the cohort was 4 years. The data set included information on 200 prevalent and 674 incident lung cancer cases, the remaining 482 095 being regarded as lung cancer-free controls (Table 1).

We excluded from the analysis all prevalent cancer cases, the subjects from Malmö and Greece (as there was no dietary data on them in the data base), and the 2% of persons with extreme energy intake/energy requirement ratios.

Table 1. Age distribution of the subjects considered

Age	Controls	Prevalent cases	Incident cases
10–19	240	0	0
20–29	17 908	0	0
30–39	49 849	1	6
40–49	138 478	30	78
50–59	178 776	94	246
60–69	83 225	60	278
70–79	11 981	15	62
80–89	544	0	4
90+	31	0	0

This resulted in an analysed subset of 127 645 male and 289 701 female controls together with 247 males and 245 females with incident lung cancer.

In the analysis we considered the association of lung cancer with smoking and with various food groups (in quartiles and as a continuous, log-transformed variable in units of g/day). The estimation method used was Cox proportional hazard regression, with the dependent variable being age. All analyses were stratified by centre and gender and adjusted for time of follow-up. The food group analyses were also adjusted for smoking. The numbers of cases are at present too low to allow proper control of fruit and vegetable intake in the models relating to individual vegetable subgroups.

The food groups analysed were all vegetables, all fruits, leafy vegetables, fruiting vegetables, root vegetables, cabbages, etc., mushrooms, grain and pod vegetables, onion and garlic, stalk vegetables, mixed salad, mixed vegetables, legumes, cereals, and potatoes and other tubers.

Table 2. Associations with smoking

	Cases	RR
Life-long non-smoker	57	1
Current cigarette smoker		
<15 cig/day	78	6.97
15–24 cig/day	108	13.87
24+ cig/day	60	25.64
Ex-smoker (time since given up)		
<10 years	64	5.18
10+ years	53	1.57
Other (pipe, cigars etc.)	65	3.29
Missing Information	7	1.93
Smoking duration >30 years	304	3.07[a]

[a]After adjustment for smoking behaviour.

Table 3. Hazard ratios for consumption of all vegetables and all fruits

	Quartile	HR	(95% CI)	Continuous	(95% CI)
All vegetables	1	1.00		1.02	(0.87–1.18)
	2	0.82	(0.63–1.06)		
	3	0.80	(0.60–1.05)		
	4	0.96	(0.72–1.28)		
All fruits	1	1.00		0.96	(0.87–1.06)
	2	0.81	(0.63–1.04)		
	3	0.80	(0.62–1.04)		
	4	0.78	(0.58–1.04)		

HR, hazards ratio; CI, confidence interval.

Results

The associations with smoking are shown in Table 2. The effects of smoking on risk of lung cancer were similar in men and women, per amount smoked.

The food groups with no significant association with lung cancer included all vegetables, all fruits, fruiting vegetables, leafy vegetables, onion and garlic, mixed salads, mixed vegetables, cereals and potatoes, and other tubers.

Associations with all vegetables and fruits were the primary hypotheses evaluated; the findings are summarized in Table 3. The other food groups with some evidence of a significant association in at least one quartile were root vegetables, cabbages etc., mushrooms, grain and pod vegetables, stalk vegetables and sprouts, and legumes. The findings for these groups are shown in Table 4.

It is clear that for some of these (root vegetables, cabbages, etc., stalk vegetables and sprouts, and to a lesser extent legumes), there is not a clear reduction in risk with increasing intake. Further, the findings have to be interpreted keeping in mind that no primary hypotheses postulated that individual dietary subgroups (such as consumption of mushrooms) would be protective for lung cancer, even though many statistical tests of significance were applied. Nevertheless, we cannot state that there is no evidence of a possible protective effect of some vegetable subgroups, and further exploration of these possible associations when a larger data set is available (preferably with the inclusion of data from Malmö and Greece) is planned.

It is important to interpret these preliminary findings from EPIC recognizing that the follow-up time was short and the numbers of cases identified so far is relatively small. Although we hope that the dietary data collected on recruitment are representative of the diet these subjects have consumed during the relevant etiological period, we have

Table 4. Hazard ratios for consumption of various vegetable subgroups

	Quartile	HR	(95% CI)	Continuous	(95% CI)
Root vegetables	1	1.00		0.99	(0.92–1.08)
	2	0.87	(0.68–1.12)		
	3	0.70	(0.53–0.93)		
	4	0.87	(0.66–1.15)		
Cabbages, etc.	1	1.00		1.05	(0.96–1.14)
	2	0.85	(0.64–1.12)		
	3	0.69	(0.51–0.94)		
	4	0.92	(0.68–1.25)		
Mushrooms	1	1.00		0.91	(0.83–1.00)
	2	0.80	(0.61–1.04)		
	3	0.78	(0.59–1.04)		
	4	0.64	(0.47–0.89)		
Grain and pod vegetables	1	1.00		0.95	(0.87–1.04)
	2	0.74	(0.56–0.98)		
	3	0.75	(0.56–0.99)		
	4	0.70	(0.51–0.96)		
Stalk vegetables, sprouts	1	1.00		0.98	(0.90–1.08)
	2	0.75	(0.56–0.99)		
	3	0.75	(0.56–1.00)		
	4	0.90	(0.68–1.21)		
Legumes	1	1.00		0.97	(0.89–1.06)
	2	0.74	(0.57–0.98)		
	3	0.83	(0.62–1.10)		
	4	0.71	(0.51–1.00)		

HR, hazards ratio; CI, confidence interval.

to recognize that there have been and there continue to be dietary changes in progress in Europe. It is conceivable that only when it is possible to study cases with a longer period since recruitment (10 or more years) will associations be detectable that truly reflect the impact of the diet at recruitment. Further, with the lack of calibration, and the decision to stratify by centre (albeit with centre-specific cut-off points), much of the heterogeneity in dietary data in EPIC has been submerged. We anticipate that with the solution to these methodological problems, and with adequate correction for measurement error, more reliable data will become available from the very large resource which is EPIC.

In summary, our findings are preliminary, but there was a suggestion of a nonsignificant protective effect for all vegetables or all fruit intake. There was a significant protective effect in some quartiles for some vegetable subgroups, however, including root vegetables, cabbages, mushrooms, grain and pod vegetables, stalk vegetables/sprouts and legumes.

Further analyses of the possible protective effects of vegetables and fruits and the effect on lung cancer risk of consumption of other foods and nutrients are planned when a more complete data set is available.

Acknowledgements

The work described in this paper was carried out with the support of the Europe Against Cancer programme of the European Commission, Deutsches Krebshilfe and Deutsches Krebsforschungszentrum.

References

Brennan, P., Fortes, C., Butler, J., Agudo, A., Benhamou, S., Darby, S., Gerken, M., Jokel, K.H., Kreuzer, M., Mallone, S., Nyberg, F., Pohlabeln, H., Ferro, G. & Boffetta, P. (2000) A multicenter case–control study of diet and lung cancer among non-smokers. *Cancer Causes Control*, **11**, 49–58

Feskanich, D., Ziegler, R.G., Michaud, D.S., Giovannucci, E.L., Speizer, F.E., Willett, W.C. & Colditz, G.A. (2000) Prospective study of fruit and vegetable consumption and risk of lung cancer among men and women. *J. Natl. Cancer Inst.*, **92**, 1812–1823

International Agency for Research on Cancer (1998) *IARC Handbooks of Cancer Prevention (1998), Vol. 2, Carotenoids.* Lyon, International Agency for Research on Cancer

Jansen, M.C.J.F., Bueno-de-Mesquita, H.B., Räsänen, L., Fidanza, F., Nissinen, A.M., Menotti, A., Kok, F.J. & Kromhout, D. (2001) Cohort analysis of fruit and vegetable consumption and lung cancer mortality in European men. *Int. J. Cancer*, **92**, 913–918

Kaaks, R. & Riboli, E. (1997) Validation and calibration of dietary intake measurements in the EPIC project. *Int. J. Epidemiol.*, **26**, Suppl 1, 815–825

Speizer, F.E., Colditz, G.A., Hunter, D.J., Rosner, B. & Hennekens, C. (1999) Prospective study of smoking, antioxidant intake, and lung cancer in middle-aged women (USA). *Cancer Causes Control*, **10**, 475–482

World Cancer Research Fund & American Institute for Cancer Research (1997) *Food, Nutrition and the Prevention of cancer: A Global Perspective*. Washington, D.C.

Plant foods and the risk of colorectal cancer in Europe: preliminary findings

Bueno-de-Mesquita H.B.[1], Ferrari P.[2], Riboli E.[2]
(for the EPIC working group on dietary patterns)

[1]Centre of Chronic Diseases Epidemiology, National Institute for Public Health and the Environment, Bilthoven, Netherlands. [2]Unit of Nutrition and Cancer, International Agency for Research on Cancer, Lyon, France.

Introduction

In the European Union, more than 100 000 men and almost 100 000 women were newly diagnosed with colorectal cancer in 1995 alone. There is roughly a twofold range in the incidence of colorectal cancer across the European Union, with the highest rates in Northwest Europe and the lowest in Finland, Spain and Greece. Outside the EU, high rates for both men and women are found in New Zealand, the USA, Australia, Canada and in Norway, and for men in the Czech Republic and Slovakia. Low rates of colorectal cancer are found in Iceland and Poland. Over the period 1955–1987, there was a rise in the incidence of large bowel cancer in most parts of the world, including Europe, this rise being more marked in men than in women (Coleman *et al.*, 1993). However, in the latter half of this period (1973–1987), several European countries, including Sweden and Denmark, and some urban regions of Switzerland, Poland, and the UK saw a decreased incidence of approximately 10%–20% per 5-year period among those below 65 years of age. In the USA and Canada, clear declines in incidence in all age groups were observed during the period 1973–1987 (Coleman *et al.*, 1993), especially among US whites during the period 1975–1998 (Troisi *et al.*, 1999). Substantial geographic variation in the rates of colorectal cancer, as well as increases and declines in incidence, strongly suggest the existence of preventable lifestyle factors in the etiology of the disease.

In 1997, an international panel of experts concluded: "the evidence that diets high in vegetables decrease the risk of colorectal cancer is convincing" (WCRF, 1997). The same panel also concluded that "no judgement is possible" in the case of fruit and pulses and the risk of colorectal cancer owing to limited and inconsistent data (WCRF, 1997). Reviewing the epidemiology and molecular biology of colorectal cancer in 1999, Potter concluded that "important positive associations exist with family history, meat consumption, smoking and alcohol, whereas important inverse associations exist with vegetables, nonsteroid anti-inflammatory drugs (NSAIDS), hormone replacement therapy (HRT), and physical activity" (Potter, 1999). However, several recent large cohort studies have failed to confirm a protective role for vegetables, fruits or dietary fibre in the occurrence of colorectal cancer. For example, the US Nurses' Health Study "did not support the existence of an important protective effect of dietary fiber against colorectal cancer or adenoma" (Fuchs *et al.*, 1999). In the Health Professionals' Follow-up Study "frequent consumption of fruits and vegetables did not appear to confer protection from colon or rectal cancer" (Michels *et al.*, 2000). Similarly, in a cohort of Finnish men (the ATBC Study), intake of dietary fibre was not associated with risk of colorectal cancer, nor was the consumption of fruits or vegetables (Pietinen *et al.*, 1999). However, evidence recently obtained from two European cohort studies in the Netherlands (Voorrips *et al.*, 2000) and Sweden (Terry, 2001), indicate that subjects with relatively low levels of consumption of vegetables and fruit experience higher risk of colorectal cancer. Epidemiological research has shown that certain types of vegetables may reduce colorectal cancer risk. In his review, Potter identified "the possible importance of green salads for the prevention of rectal cancer and legumes for the prevention of colorectal cancer", and noted that case–control evidence of protection against colon cancer "has been particularly consistent for raw vegetables, green vegetables and cruciferous vegetables" (Potter, 1999).

The European Prospective Investigation into Nutrition and Cancer (EPIC study), co-ordinated by IARC, is a large cohort study designed to examine the association between diet and cancer in nine European countries with substantial variation in the frequency of colorectal cancer (Riboli, 1997; Bueno-de-Mesquita, 1997). Consumption of vegetables and fruit varies greatly across the EPIC study populations (Agudo *et al.*, 2002). Accordingly, we set out to test the hypothesis that intakes of vegetables and fruit, and of certain types of vegetables, are inversely associated with subsequent colorectal cancer risk in the EPIC study.

Subjects and methods

Study population

The EPIC study is a large multicentre prospective cohort study designed to investigate the relation between diet, nutritional, genetic and metabolic characteristics, various lifestyle factors and the risk of cancer. The study, coordinated by the International Agency for Research on Cancer (IARC), is based in 22 collaborating centres in nine European countries (France, Denmark, Germany, Greece, Italy, Netherlands, Spain, Sweden and UK). As such, the study reflects the diversity of dietary habits and cancer risk both between individuals and between populations in Europe. The study was initiated in 1992, and by 1999 about 480 000 subjects with detailed data on diet, lifestyle and anthropometry had been included.

Follow-up was done through cancer registries (Sweden, Denmark, UK, Netherlands, Spain, Italy) or through a combination of methods including health insurance records, cancer and pathology registries, and/or active follow-up (France, Germany, Greece). The end follow-up date was either the date as estimated by the centre itself or the last day of the half-year immediately preceding a notable drop in the incidence of colorectal cancer, whichever was the earlier. Excluding Greece, where follow-up is incomplete, the percentage of subjects lost to follow-up was 1.0%.

By June 2001, after a mean follow-up of 3.3 years in men and 4.4 years in women, a total of 1029 incident cases of colorectal cancer (CRC) were identified. We excluded the data for Malmö and Greece owing to missing dietary information, 745 prevalent cases of CRC, and data for 8379 subjects in the top and bottom 1% of the ratio of energy intake over energy requirement. Cases with prevalent cancer other than CRC were not excluded. This left data for 279 male and 493 female first-incident cases of CRC as well as 122 738 male and 282 929 female non-cases with a mean age of 51.8 (SD 9.9) in men and 50.9 (10.0) in women.

Dietary assessment

Dietary information was collected using a comprehensive food frequency questionnaire (FFQ) covering up to 750 foods and recipes. The FFQ was completed by face-to-face interview in Ragusa, Naples, Spain, and Greece, and by the subjects themselves in all other centres. For this analysis, the main food groups of interest were vegetables and fruit combined, vegetables, fruit, and legumes. Vegetables did not include potatoes and other tubers. Examples of commonly eaten legumes were white beans, haricot beans, chickpeas and lentils. We further evaluated the association with CRC risk in each of five subgroups of vegetables: leafy vegetables excluding cabbages (e.g. lettuce, chicory, green salad, endive); fruiting vegetables (tomato, cucumber, gherkin, french bean, green beans, courgette, sweet pepper); root vegetables (carrots, swedes); cabbages (cauliflower, broccoli, sauerkraut, chinese cabbage, white cabbage); and onions and garlic. Satisfactory grouping of the remaining four vegetable subgroups (mushrooms, grain and pod vegetable, stalk vegetables and sprouts, and mixed salad/mixed vegetables) has not yet been completed.

In order to adjust for possible systematic over- or underestimation in FFQ measurements, a standardized 24-h dietary recall (24-HDR) was collected from 5%–10% subsamples of the EPIC cohort(s) in each country to serve as the reference calibration method. Each calibration sample was designed to be a representative random sample from its EPIC cohort with the age distribution of participants as close as possible to the age distribution of the expected number of incident cancer cases in the first 10 years of follow-up.

Statistical analysis

Subjects were subdivided into sex-specific quintiles of intake of the dietary variables using EPIC-wide cut-off points. To allow for differences in the FFQ between centres, we also calculated calibrated dietary variables. Individual FFQ estimates of food groups of interest were multiplicatively adjusted in order to make the mean of the calibrated FFQ intakes, by centre and sex, equal to the mean intakes given by the 24-HDR. Multiplicative rather than additive adjustment was used to avoid the problem of negative values, to leave zero values unaffected and to influence variation less.

Colorectal cancer incidence rate ratios were calculated using the Cox proportional hazards model, stratified by centre, with attained age as the primary scale variable. We present both sex-adjusted and sex-specific incidence rate ratios adjusted for age at entry, weight and height (sex- and centre-specific tertiles with missing values in a fourth category), intake of energy in 20-tiles, physical activity at work (not working; sedentary; standing; manual; unknown), smoking (never; former with duration less than 22 years; former with duration more than 22 years; current with duration less than 22 years; current with duration more than 22 years; unknown), and alcohol in g/day ethanol (none, 1–10, 11–20, 21–40, 40+ for men and none, 1–5, 6–15,

16–25, 25+ for women). Risk estimates for vegetable intake were adjusted for fruit intake and vice versa. For testing the effect of intake of a subgroup of vegetables over and above the intake of other vegetables, thus keeping other vegetables constant, we adjusted for a factor representing the algebraic difference between the individual intake of vegetables and the individual intake of that subgroup. Partial correlation coefficients by sex and region between subgroups of vegetables and vegetables minus that subgroup were relatively low, i.e. for leafy vegetables 0.39, fruiting vegetables 0.40, root vegetables 0.37, cabbages 0.36, and onion and garlic 0.32. We present *P* values for the Wald χ^2_1 statistic (4 degrees of freedom) for testing the overall significance of the variables used to model quintiles of exposure and *P* values for the χ^2_2 statistic for testing the significance of the trends based on the continuous variable (1 degree of freedom). In additional analyses, 150 male and 213 female incident cases of CRC diagnosed during the first 2 years of follow-up were excluded, leaving 129 male and 280 female cases.

Table 1. Selective characteristics of risk factors of CRC by EPIC-wide quintiles of usual daily consumption of vegetables and fruit (g/d) in 279 male cases with CRC and 122 738 male controls. The EPIC Cohort Study, 1993–1999

	Quintiles of usual consumption of vegetables and fruit in g/d				
	Men				
No. of subjects	24 595	24 596	24 595	24 596	24 595
Mean (quintile ranges)	124 (0–184)	228 (184–273)	324 (273–379)	453 (379–544)	773 (544+)
Age (y)	50.3	51.6	52.3	52.6	52.3
Weight (kg)	81.6	81.8	81.1	80.7	80.7
Height (cm)	175.9	175.8	175.4	174.7	173.2
FFQ mean total energy intake (kcal/d)	2193	2367	2468	2564	2739
Physical activity at work (%)					
Nonworker	21.6	21.7	21.7	22.4	20.0
Sedentary	31.1	37.3	37.0	35.8	34.0
Standing	22.9	19.3	19.4	19.4	22.9
Manual (heavy)	21.5	17.8	18.2	18.9	20.9
Missing	2.9	3.9	3.8	3.5	2.3
Smoking status (%)					
Never	31.9	32.8	33.3	34.0	36.1
Former	30.6	36.4	38.7	39.5	39.4
Current	36.6	30.1	26.8	24.9	23.2
Missing	0.9	0.8	1.2	1.6	1.3
Smoking duration in years					
Never	32.0	32.9	33.4	34.1	36.2
Ever: 0–22	20.4	23.6	24.0	24.5	24.7
Ever: 22 or more	43.1	39.2	37.9	36.3	34.8
Missing	4.5	4.3	4.6	5.0	4.3
FFQ mean ethanol intake (g/d)	21.9	22.5	21.8	21.3	20.8
Nondrinkers (%)	12.8	9.8	10.6	11.9	15.6
1–10 (%)	34.5	29.3	28.1	27.6	27.2
11–20 (%)	17.5	20.9	22.2	22.5	19.3
21–40 (%)	16.2	21.3	21.3	21.1	21.0
40+ (%)	19.4	18.7	17.8	16.9	16.9

Table 2. Selective characteristics of risk factors of CRC by EPIC-wide quintiles of usual daily consumption of vegetables and fruit (g/d) in 493 female cases with CRC and 282 929 female controls. The EPIC Cohort Study, 1993–1999

	Quintiles of usual consumption of vegetables and fruit in g/d				
	Women				
No. of subjects	56 656	56 657	56 656	56 657	56 656
Mean (quintile ranges)	192 (0–268)	326 (268–382)	439 (382–498)	571 (498–658)	873 (658+)
Age (y)	49.6	50.7	51.2	51.6	51.6
Weight (kg)	66.4	65.8	65.2	64.9	65.2
Height (cm)	162.6	162.3	162.0	161.6	161.4
FFQ Mean total energy intake (kcal/d)	1748	1903	1997	2089	2238
Physical activity at work (%)					
Nonworker	31.8	32.7	32.9	33.7	33.7
Sedentary	27.9	26.1	24.1	22.4	20.6
Standing	26.6	28.9	31.5	33.8	36.3
Manual (heavy)	10.3	8.9	7.9	6.7	6.1
Missing	3.4	3.4	3.6	3.4	3.4
Smoking status (%)					
Never	48.4	55.5	59.3	61.8	63.5
Former	21.6	23.2	22.9	22.5	22.7
Current	28.8	19.4	15.5	13.0	11.2
Missing	1.2	1.9	2.4	2.7	2.7
Smoking duration in years					
Never	48.5	55.6	59.4	61.9	63.6
Ever: 0–22	20.3	19.1	17.4	16.8	16.9
Ever: 22 or more	26.6	19.9	16.9	14.4	12.5
Missing	4.6	5.4	6.4	6.9	7.1
FFQ Mean ethanol intake (g/d)	9.8	9.5	9.2	8.7	7.8
Nondrinkers (%)	27.1	25.9	26.7	28.2	32.5
1–5 (%)	26.2	25.1	24.1	23.9	24.4
6–15 (%)	25.1	28.5	29.1	29.2	27.2
16–25 (%)	10.1	10.4	10.4	9.8	8.3
25+ (%)	11.4	10.2	9.7	8.8	7.6

Results

In France, Spain and Italy, usual consumption levels of vegetables and of fruit were higher than in Northern European countries. Usual mean intake of vegetables varied from a low of 70 g per day in men in Umeå, Sweden, to 305 g per day in women in Southern France. Fruit intake ranged from 115 g per day in men from Heidelberg to 486 g per day in men from Central and Southern Italy. We compared selected characteristics across quintiles of usual consumption of the vegetables and fruit combined for men and women separately (Tables 1 and 2). Both men and women with higher reported levels of consumption of vegetables and fruit also reported higher energy intake, while they were slightly older, somewhat lower in weight, and shorter in stature. High vegetable and fruit consumers were less likely to smoke (and if they had smoked to have done so for fewer years) and less likely to be heavy drinkers (defined as 40 or more grams of ethanol per day in men and 16 or more grams per day in women). No clear association between fruit and vegetable consumption and physical activity at work was seen.

Table 3. Multivariate adjusted relative risk estimates[a] of colorectal cancer incidence by quintiles of usual daily consumption of vegetables and/or fruit, and legumes (g/d) in 406 439 subjects: 123 017 men and 283 422 women. The EPIC Cohort Study, 1993–1999

	EPIC-wide quintiles of intake in g/d					*P* values[2]	
	Q1	Q2	Q3	Q4	Q5	Overall effect	For trend; cont.
All vegetables and fruit							
Total no. of cases	168	146	151	159	149		
All	1.00	0.81	0.78[e]	0.79	0.74[e]	0.15	0.45
Without first 2 years of follow-up[c]	1.00	0.63[e]	0.74	0.75	0.72	0.09	0.64
Men[d]	1.00	0.81	0.72	0.70	0.68	0.41	0.80
Without first 2 years of follow-up[c]	1.00	0.41[e]	0.48[e]	0.56	0.53[e]	0.04	0.53
Women[d]	1.00	0.81	0.81	0.83	0.76	0.48	0.40
Without first 2 years of follow-up[c]	1.00	0.76	0.90	0.85	0.81	0.73	0.81
Vegetables							
Total no. of cases	181	144	151	150	147		
All	1.00	0.82	0.84	0.79	0.71[e]	0.14	0.37
Men[d]	1.00	0.82	0.74	0.79	0.60[e]	0.28	0.27
Women[d]	1.00	0.81	0.89	0.78	0.78	0.50	0.78
Fruit							
Total no. of cases	162	129	148	180	154		
All	1.00	0.71[e]	0.76[e]	0.91	0.83	0.03	0.88
Men[d]	1.00	0.66[e]	0.82	1.01	0.79	0.15	0.56
Women[d]	1.00	0.72[e]	0.80[e]	0.93	0.86	0.53	0.46
Legumes							
Total no. of cases	147	141	179	166	140		
All	1.00	1.12	1.29[e]	1.28	1.41[e]	0.15	0.54
Men[d]	1.00	0.82	0.79	0.88	0.95	0.82	0.72
Women[d]	1.00	1.37[e]	1.56[e]	1.53[e]	1.66[e]	0.03	0.35

[a]Hazard ratios stratified by centre and age, and adjusted for (gender), weight, height, smoking (categorical), physical activity at work, intake of energy, intake of ethanol (categorical), and vegetables for fruit and vice versa (categorical).
[b]*P* values of Wald χ^2_1 test for overall effect of variable of interest with 4 DF and of χ^2_2 test for trend using continuous variable with 1 DF.
[c]After excluding cases with colorectal cancer arising during the first 2 years of follow-up, leaving 129 male and 280 female cases of CRC.
[d]Quintile boundaries for all vegetables and fruit in men: 184, 273, 379, 544 and in women 268, 382, 498, 658; for vegetables in men 82, 124, 173, 252 and in women 111, 164, 225, 316; for fruit in men 68, 124, 194, 312 and in women 114, 186, 263, 372; for legumes in men 1, 3, 8, 23 and in women 1, 5, 11, 26.
[e]95% Confidence limits do not include unity.

Comparison with subjects in the lowest quintile of intake, subjects with a higher level of consumption of vegetables and fruit combined had a lower risk of CRC, although there was no clear evidence of a dose–response gradient (Table 3). The same pattern was evident for men and women separately and, in men, was more pronounced when the first 2 years of follow-up were excluded (*P* for overall effect = 0.04). When the quintiles of intake were calculated from calibrated fruit and vegetable intakes, the general pattern of risks remained the same (results not shown). For the consumption of vegetables alone, a weak inverse association with risk was seen, the effect being stronger in men than in women. Excluding the first 2 years of follow-up strengthened the association in men more clearly than in women (results not shown). For the consumption of fruit alone, we also observed a weak inverse association for men and women combined and separately, but with no sign of a dose–response gradient. Excluding the first 2 years of follow-up had only a minor impact on risk (results not shown).

For consumption of legumes, a suggestion of a graded positive association with risk was seen in women but not in men (*P* for overall effect = 0.03 and 0.82, respectively), which remained after excluding the first 2 years of follow-up (results not shown). However, based on calibrated intakes, there were uniformly elevated risks in all categories compared with the lowest quintile of intake (results not shown).

No associations with colorectal cancer risk were seen for any of the subgroups of vegetables, except for the consumption of leafy vegetables. In men only, an overall borderline statistically significant, inverse association was observed (rate ratios 1.00, 0.93, 0.87, 0.84, 0.46; *P* for overall effect = 0.08 and *P* for trend = 0.20), which was only slightly influenced by excluding the first 2 years of follow-up, whereas no effect was seen in women (results not shown). After calibration, however, statistically significant inverse associations with risk were seen for both men and women, with or without excluding the first 2 years of follow-up, but still without any clear dose–response effects (results not shown).

Discussion

Preliminary findings from the EPIC cohort study on dietary risk factors for colorectal cancer showed uniformly reduced risks in all levels of intake of vegetables and fruit combined and in all levels of intake of fruit compared with subjects in the lowest quintile of intake. There was a suggestion of a graded inverse association of risk with the intake of vegetables. For fruiting vegetables, root vegetables, cabbages, and onion plus garlic, no associations were observed, whereas for the consumption of leafy vegetables an inverse association with risk was seen. Conversely, in women, but not in men, the consumption of legumes was positively associated with risk.

The presence of a statistically significant inverse association of risk with an exposure variable after adjustment for the potentially most important confounding factors, in a cohort study that estimates such exposure long enough before the development of the cancer of interest, provides important support for the hypothesis of a causal association. Therefore, we have reason to believe that regular consumption of certain subgroups of vegetables, specifically leafy vegetables, is protective against colorectal cancer. Vegetables are important contributors of dietary fibre/NSP, resistant starch, and other potential anticarcinogenic compounds. In the EPIC calibration study, leafy vegetables accounted for about 5%–20% of total vegetable consumption, with most Mediterranean centres having the highest consumption (Agudo *et al.*, 2002). Leafy vegetables are important sources of several carotenoids, including beta-carotene and lutein, which are known to be strong antioxidants and to have other potentially anticarcinogenic properties.

In comparison to the lowest intake category, the finding of uniformly reduced colorectal cancer risk estimates in all higher levels of intake of vegetables and fruit combined, and of fruit alone, is consistent with results from two European studies in the Netherlands (Voorrips *et al.*, 2000) and Sweden (Terry, 2001), which suggested that subjects at relatively low levels of consumption of vegetables and fruit may experience higher risk of colorectal cancer.

Given that legumes are good sources of dietary fibre/NSP and many vitamins, minerals and other bioactive compounds, the positive relationship with the consumption of legumes in women (but not in men) was unexpected. Residual confounding by other plant foods is an unlikely explanation since the intake of legumes was not strongly related to the consumption of vegetables (partial correlation coefficient by sex and region $r = 0.13$) or fruit ($r = 0.06$). Further, more refined statistical analyses are required before any speculation about specific risk-increasing factors in legumes is justified.

In brief, preliminary findings from EPIC based on an already large number of incident cases of colorectal cancer indicate that a higher consumption of fruit and especially vegetables may protect against the development of colorectal cancer. The lack of a graded inverse association with risk points to the possibility of a threshold level of intake above which no further benefit of increasing consumption of vegetables and fruit can be expected. Of five subgroups of vegetables investigated, preliminary findings clearly show that leafy vegetables may confer the greatest protection against the development of colorectal cancer. More refined analyses, based on a larger number of cases of colorectal cancer and including adjustment for a wider range of potential confounding factors and applying more sophisticated calibration, are essential. Analyses for specific colorectal cancer subsites may also yield further etiological clues.

Acknowledgements

The work described in this paper was carried out with the support of the Europe against Cancer programme of the European Commission.

References

Agudo, A., Slimani, N., Ocke, M.C., Naska, A., Miller, A.B., Kroke, A., Bamia, C., Karalis, D., Vineis, P., Palli, D., Bueno-de-Mesquita, H.D., Peeters, P.H.M., Engeset, D., Hjartäker, A., Navaroo, C., Martinez, C., Wallstom, P., Zhang, J.X., Welch, A., Spencer, E., Stripp, C., Overvad, K., Clavel-Chapelon, F., Casagrande, C. & Riboli, E. (2002) Vegetable and fruit consumption in the EPIC cohorts from ten European countries. *Public Health Nutr.*, (in press)

Bueno-de-Mesquita, H.B. & Gonzalez, C.A. (1997) Main hypotheses on diet and cancer investigated in the EPIC study. *Eur. J. Cancer Prev.*, **6**, 107–117

Coleman, M.P., Esteve, J., Damiecki, P., Arslan, A. & Renard, H., eds. (1993) *Trends in cancer incidence and mortality.* (IARC Scientific Publications No. 121), Lyon, IARC

Fuchs, C.S., Giovannucci, E.L., Colditz, G.A., Hunter, D.J., Stampfer, M.J., Rosner, B., Speizer, F.E. & Willett, W.C. (1999) Dietary fiber and the risk of colorectal cancer and adenoma in women. *N. Eng. J. Med.*, **340**, 169–176

Giovannucci, E., Ascherio, A., Rimm, E.B., Colditz, G.A., Stampfer, M.J. & Willett, W.C. (1995) Physical activity, obesity, and risk for colon cancer and adenoma in men. *Ann. Intern. Med.*, **122**, 327–334

Giovannucci, E. (1999) Tomatoes, tomato-based products, lycopene, and cancer: review of the epidemiologic literature. *J. Natl. Cancer Inst.*, **91**, 317–331

Kaaks, R., Slimani, N. & Riboli, E. (1997) Pilot phase studies on the accuracy of dietary intake measurements in the EPIC project: overall evaluation of results. *Int. J. Epidemiol.*, **26** (Suppl 1), S26–S36

MacFarlane, G.J. & Lowenfels, A.B. (1994) Physical activity and colon cancer. Review. *Eur. J. Cancer Prev.*, **3**, 393–398

Michels, K.B., Giovannucci, E., Joshipura, K.J., Rosner, B.A., Stampfer, M.J., Fuchs, C.S., Colditz, G.A., Speizer, F.E. & Willett, W.C. (2000) Prospective study of fruit and vegetable consumption and incidence of colon and rectal cancers. *J. Natl. Cancer Inst.*, **92**, 1740–1752

Pietinen, P., Malila, N., Virtanen, M., Hartman, T.J., Tangrea, J.A., Albaner, D. & Viramo, J. (1999) Diet and risk of colorectal cancer in a cohort of Finnish men. *Cancer Causes Control*, **10**, 387–396

Potter, J.D. (1996) Nutrition and colorectal cancer. *Cancer Causes Control*, **7**, 127–146

Potter, J.D. (1999) Colorectal cancer: molecules and populations. *J. Natl. Cancer Inst.*, **91**, 916–932

Riboli, E. & Kaaks, R. (1997) The EPIC Project: rationale and study design. *Int. J. Epidemiol.*, **26** (Suppl 1), S6–S14

Riboli, E., Hunt, K., Slimani, N., Hémon, B., Ferrari, P., Norat, T., Fahey, G.C., Casagrande, C., Vignat, J., Overvad, K., Tjønneland, A., Clavel-Chapelon, F., Wahrendorf, J., Boeing, H., Trichopoulos, D., Trichopoulou, A., Vineis, P., Palli, D., Bueno-de-Mesquita, H.B., Peeters, P.H.M., Lund, E., Engeset, D. A., González, C.A., Barricarte, A., Berglund, G., Hallmans, G., Day, N. Key, T., Kaaks, R. & Saracci, R. (2002) The EPIC Project: rationale and study design. *Public Health Nutr.* (in press)

Slattery, M.L., Edwards, S.L., Ma, K.N., Friedman, G.D. & Potter, J.D. (1997) Physical activity and colon cancer: a public health perspective. *Ann. Epidemiol.*, **7**, 137–145

Terry, P., Giovannucci, E., Michels, K.B., Bergkvist, L., Hansen, H., Holmberg, L. & Wolk, A. (2001) Fruit, vegetables, dietary fiber, and risk of colorectal cancer. *J. Natl. Cancer Inst.*, **7**, 525–533

Troisi, R.J., Freedman, A.N. & Devesa, S.S. (1999) Incidence of colorectal carcinoma in the U.S. An update of trends by gender, race, age, subsite, and stage, 1975–1994. *Cancer*, **85**, 1670–1676

Voorrips, L.E., Goldbaum, R.A., van Poppel, G., Sturmas, F., Hermus, R.J. & van den Brandt, P.A. (2000) Vegetable and fruit consumption and risks of colon and rectal cancer in a prospective cohort study: The Netherlands Cohort Study on Diet and Cancer. *Am. J. Epidemiol.*, **152**, 1081–1092

Willett, W.C. & Trichopoulos, D. (1996) Summary of the evidence: nutrition and cancer. *Cancer Causes Control*, **7**, 178–180

World Cancer Research Fund (1997) *Diet, Nutrition, and the Prevention of Cancer: A Global Perspective.* Washington, D.C., WCRF/American Institute of Cancer Research

Carbohydrate consumption in 10 European countries

McTaggart A.[1], Wirfält E.[2], Pala V.[3]
(EPIC working group on dietary patterns)

[1]Department of Public Health and Primary Care, University of Cambridge, UK. [2]Dept of Community Medicine, Lund University, Malmö, Sweden. [3]Dept of Epidemiology, National Cancer Institute, Milan, Italy.

Purpose

To look at the main sources and types of carbohydrate consumed within the 10 countries making up the EPIC (European Prospective Investigation in Cancer) population, as a means of studying dietary patterns and diet-related chronic disease. The focus here is to look particularly at the consumption of staple foods and sucrose.

Methods

A computerized 24-h recall interview program (EPIC-SOFT) was developed for use in this large multicentre study, as a calibration method for standardization of interviews between the 27 EPIC centres. Intake was estimated from EPIC-SOFT data for a subsample of the EPIC subjects, in 35 955 men and women (13 031 men from 19 study centres and 22 924 women from 27 centres) in 10 countries within Europe. The potential major contributors of carbohydrate in the diet were identified and 17 food groups were looked at for their relative contributions to the diet for each centre and country in terms of the mean weight of each food group consumed and the proportion of consumers.

Results

Results are shown in Fig. 1 and 2. The main sources of complex carbohydrate and starchy foods for all centres and countries were bread, potatoes, and pasta and rice. For most countries, bread and potatoes formed the main staple foods, except for Italy, which consumed 3–4 times more pasta than all other countries. For most countries, more than 90% of the sample consumed bread with the highest intake in Denmark. The exception was Umeä, Sweden where crispbread was also consumed by a high proportion of the sample. Consumption of potatoes was less common, but there was a trend to higher consumption in northern countries and less in Greece, Italy and Spain. Vegetables and legumes also contributed to carbohydrate intake and were consumed in all countries by more than 80% of the sample with a general trend towards lower consumption in more northern countries. The UK, Sweden, Denmark and Norway were the main consumers of breakfast cereals but they appeared in a small proportion of peoples' diets. Fruit also contributed to carbohydrate intake and showed more female consumers, with a definite increase in the Mediterranean countries.

The consumption of more refined carbohydrates and foods containing sucrose was generally low. The more southern countries, France, Italy and Spain consumed less sucrose in the form of cake, sweet biscuits, sugar, confectionery and soft drinks than the northern countries, Sweden, Denmark, Norway, the UK, Germany and the Netherlands. There were similar patterns of consumption for men and women for most foods except cake and sweet biscuits, for which women consumed more in six out of eight countries.

Conclusions

The data reflects the traditional habits of countries arising from their geography and patterns of agriculture, with high intakes of pasta in Italy, bread in Denmark, crispbread in Sweden, the greater use of potatoes in northern countries and higher intakes of fruit and vegetables in the southern climates. This confirms the established idea that food selection in Mediterranean countries traditionally differs from that in other European countries. Data on consumption of different types of carbohydrate and the variations in levels of consumption within Europe may play a part in determining cancer incidence.

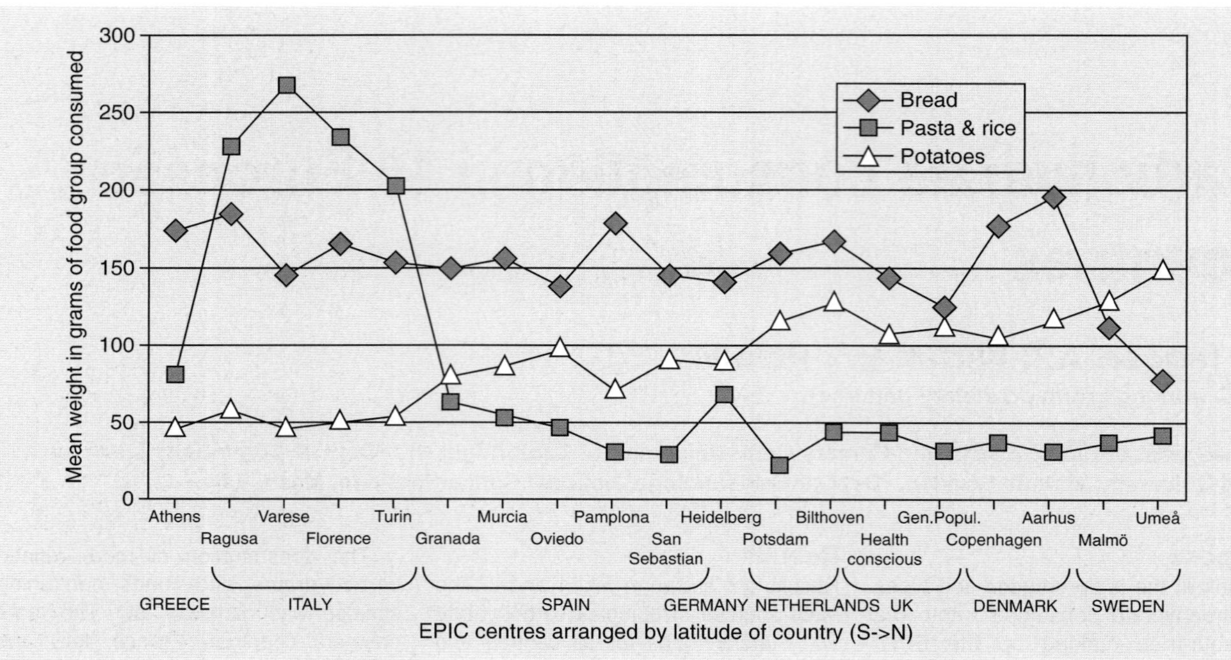

Figure 1
Average intake for men of staple foods within EPIC centres

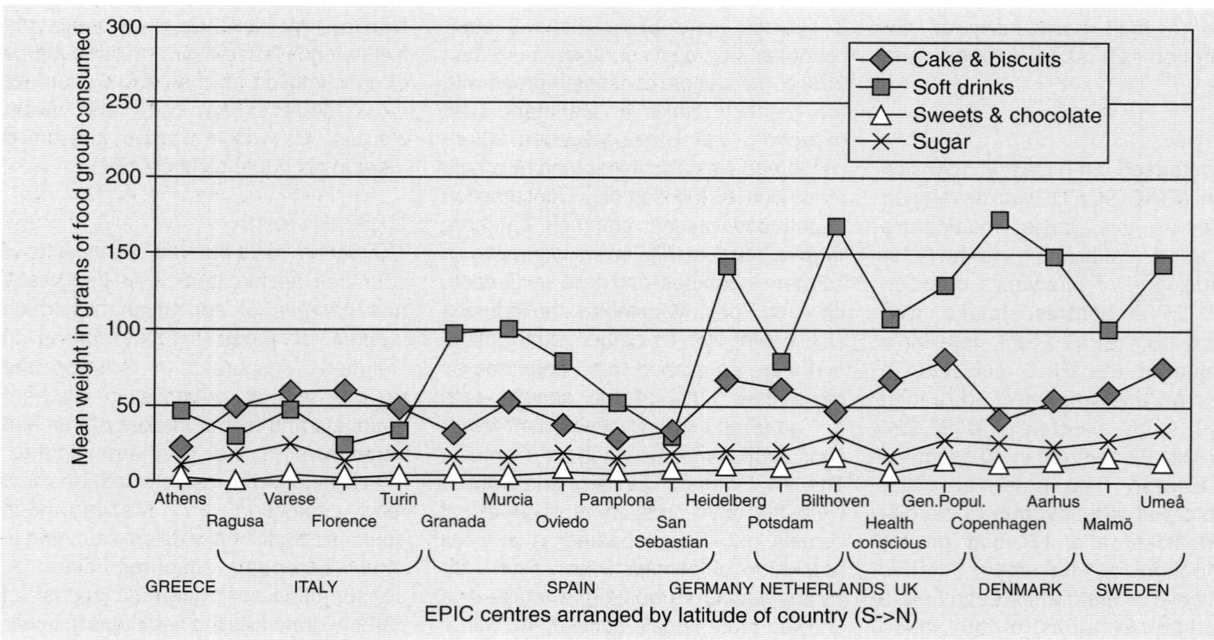

Figure 2
Average intake for men of food groups supplying sucrose within EPIC centres

Vegetable and fruit consumption in the EPIC cohorts from 10 European countries

Agudo A.[1], Slimani N.[2], Ocké M.C.[3], Naska A.[4]
(for the EPIC working group on dietary patterns)

[1]Department of Epidemiology, Catalan Institute of Oncology (ICO), 08907 L'Hospitalet, Barcelona, Spain. [2]International Agency for Research on Cancer, 69372 Lyon cedex 08, France. [3]National Institute for Public Health and the Environment, 3720 BA Bilthoven, The Netherlands. [4]University of Athens Medical School, Athens 11572, Greece.

Epidemiological data strongly support a protective effect of increased vegetable and fruit consumption against epithelial cancers from the respiratory and digestive tract, as well as cardiovascular disease. The differences in consumption patterns between regions as well as within populations need to be considered to improve knowledge on nutrition and the health effects of dietary factors. The present report assesses the vegetable and fruit consumption in adult populations from 10 European countries.

Methods

A calibration study was carried out within the EPIC project, a large prospective study involving 519 978 subjects in 10 European countries. The calibration population was a random sample from each cohort according to the number and age–sex distribution of expected cancer cases. After exclusions, 35 955 individuals (13 031 men and 22 924 women) from 27 centres were included in the present analysis. Information on dietary intake was gathered by means of a computerized 24-h diet recall interview (Slimani *et al.*, 1999). Each reported food was described and quantified according to common rules.

Data from the following subgroups of vegetables are presented separately: leafy vegetables, fruiting vegetables, root vegetables, cabbage, and onion and garlic. Separate results are presented for citrus fruits and fruits other than citrus (including fresh, dried and canned). Intake of other subgroups was collected as well, but no separate results are provided. Potatoes, legumes, fruit juices and tomato sauces were considered in different groups in our classification system. Although they are foods of plant origin they were excluded from this report.

Adjusted means and standard errors were estimated for each centre separately for men and women using weighted regression. A model was fitted using the variable of interest as the dependent variable and centre and age as covariates; weights were calculated for all subjects in each particular season and weekday combination, as the ratio between the expected frequency under ideal conditions and the actual frequency. The adjusted means reported correspond to populations with balanced distribution over seasons and between weekend and weekdays, with a mean age of 57 years for men and 55 years for women.

Results

Regarding consumption of vegetables among men (Table 1) there was a clear south-north gradient of total consumption, with a ratio of 2.6 between Greece and Umeå, the highest and lowest adjusted means. An exception to this pattern is the health-conscious group in the UK, with a high proportion of vegetarians. Among women (Table 2), the highest consumption was observed in the south of France and the lowest in the north of Spain (Asturias), with a ratio of 2.5. There was also a south-north pattern, although some centres in Italy and Spain had low intake. A different picture arises regarding vegetable subgroups. Fruiting vegetables are the most consumed, accounting for about half of total intake in many centres. Leafy vegetables, root vegetables and cabbages have similar proportions of overall consumption (10%–15%), but they show different patterns: Mediterranean countries have a high

Table 1. Consumption of vegetables by subgroups, men[a]

Country and centre	*n*	Total veg.	Leafy veg.	Fruiting veg.	Root veg.	Cabbage	Onion, garlic
Italy							
Florence	271	212.8	28.5	106.8	10.8	17.0	4.4
Varese	328	204.9	34.3	80.6	14.8	15.6	10.6
Ragusa	168	179.5	35.3	78.3	2.3	11.1	14.6
Turin	677	246.1	43.7	114.2	12.6	19.1	14.3
Spain							
Asturias	386	150.2	22.5	68.3	7.7	15.6	21.7
Granada	214	221.6	31.1	145.0	8.0	2.0	25.7
Murcia	243	266.8	29.3	164.4	11.7	15.6	34.7
Navarra	444	246.9	89.2	103.5	6.8	7.1	18.4
San Sebastian	490	234.0	45.8	111.9	13.2	12.3	30.7
United Kingdom							
General population	404	160.8	6.6	53.7	27.5	31.2	9.7
Health conscious	114	225.4	14.2	76.5	25.3	35.7	17.8
The Netherlands							
Bilthoven	1024	136.7	27.7	41.6	10.3	27.1	12.6
Greece							
Greece	1312	269.7	30.1	178.6	8.6	13.6	28.6
Germany							
Heidelberg	1033	169.5	20.8	69.2	18.1	21.6	7.6
Potsdam	1235	151.3	7.7	71.0	14.7	25.8	7.7
Sweden							
Malmö	1421	120.3	7.7	56.3	19.2	14.7	8.3
Umeå	1344	103.4	9.7	47.2	17.4	10.7	8.8
Denmark							
Aarhus	567	134.1	8.9	46.8	21.5	17.7	16.2
Copenhagen	1356	147.4	11.1	56.6	20.6	17.5	13.6

[a]Mean adjusted by age, season and day of week.

consumption of leafy vegetables, Scandinavian countries and the UK have the highest intake of root vegetables, and the UK, the Netherlands and Germany are the highest consumers of cabbage.

Regarding fruits (Tables 3 and 4), the ratio between highest and lowest consumers was 3.7 among men and 2.7 in women, comparing Murcia and Ragusa, respectively, to Malmö. The highest consumption of citrus fruits was observed in Spanish centres while the Italian centres lead the intake of non-citrus fruits. The apple is the most consumed fruit in all countries, accounting for approximately 25% of total intake. In addition to apples, the most consumed fruits in countries with high consumption (Italy and Spain) are oranges and pears, while bananas and oranges take the second and third place in Northern countries.

Discussion

The large variability across centres at the subgroup level is one of the most interesting findings of our study. The different geographical patterns must be kept in mind when interpreting results from both descriptive and etiological studies. The principal limitation of 24-h diet recall is that it does not provide a reliable estimate of an individual's intake because of day-to-day variations (Bingham & Nelson, 1991). However, since it is less prone to recall errors than questionnaires, which refer to usual diet, it is particularly suited to assessing group means. Nevertheless, since we did not study representative population samples, the results shown here should not be considered as being representative at the country level.

Table 2. Consumption of vegetables by subgroups, women[a]

Country and centre	*n*	Total veg.	Leafy veg.	Fruiting veg.	Root veg.	Cabbage	Onion, garlic
France							
North-east	2009	215.1	40.9	91.8	30.6	15.8	7.7
North-west	622	208.7	40.6	81.4	33.2	11.8	6.5
South	1396	218.0	45.5	93.8	25.2	17.2	5.1
South coast	612	260.9	51.7	127.1	23.4	13.3	11.0
Italy							
Florence	785	197.2	24.3	91.6	11.4	12.9	9.6
Varese	794	160.0	30.6	72.5	10.7	7.9	6.6
Ragusa	138	138.3	30.8	54.8	3.0	11.7	11.0
Turin	392	233.8	36.8	116.5	14.7	16.0	12.6
Naples	403	173.7	19.3	88.4	9.1	22.4	5.9
Spain							
Asturias	324	103.3	17.8	42.5	6.1	11.3	14.1
Granada	300	216.0	24.9	148.2	8.9	5.0	20.9
Murcia	304	253.3	30.2	142.1	11.9	15.0	44.4
Navarra	271	196.1	63.6	88.3	5.8	11.6	11.0
San Sebastian	244	212.7	32.9	101.1	15.5	14.0	23.6
United Kingdom							
General population	571	163.7	8.6	65.3	25.3	30.0	8.4
Health conscious	197	220.1	20.6	82.8	23.0	34.0	12.7
The Netherlands							
Bilthoven	1086	128.3	22.0	40.6	11.7	26.0	11.0
Utrecht	1874	131.7	23.9	47.4	11.7	24.4	8.5
Greece							
Greece	1374	207.0	28.6	126.8	9.6	12.2	19.4
Germany					20.2	24.7	6.3
Heidelberg	1087	165.4	22.0	66.7	19.3	23.8	7.0
Potsdam	1063	167.0	11.2	80.8	21.2	25.7	5.6
Sweden							
Malmö	1711	130.5	11.7	65.6	17.2	13.7	6.7
Umeå	1574	122.5	10.1	55.0	22.6	16.1	7.8
Denmark							
Aarhus	510	149.2	10.9	55.8	30.7	19.1	11.3
Copenhagen	1485	149.8	10.2	60.0	25.1	19.4	10.3
Norway							
South and east	1136	130.7	9.2	40.5	34.0	23.3	5.6
North and west	662	118.3	4.2	32.1	40.9	22.6	5.0

[a]Mean adjusted by age, season and day of week.

Consumption of vegetables in our study was slightly higher than estimates based on national dietary surveys (Roos *et al.*, 2000) in several countries, except in women from Norway and the Netherlands. A similar pattern was observed for fruit intake, although our estimates are lower for men in Sweden and women in Norway. Except for Greece and Norway (fruits only), we also found estimates for vegetable and fruit intake slightly higher than those from household budget surveys (both genders combined) from Germany, Greece, Norway, Spain and the UK (Naska *et al.*, 2000).

Table 3. Consumption of fruits by subgroups, men[a]

Country and centre	*n*	Total fruits	Citrus fruits	Other fruits[b]
Italy				
Florence	271	396.1	58.0	326.2
Varese	328	348.2	73.3	264.3
Ragusa	168	447.6	76.2	361.8
Turin	677	421.5	59.4	356.5
Spain				
Asturias	386	340.7	49.5	282.4
Granada	214	360.4	86.7	260.8
Murcia	243	453.6	151.3	277.8
Navarra	444	317.4	89.4	217.3
San Sebastian	490	386.1	92.1	279.4
United Kingdom				
General population	404	148.7	21.2	116.5
Health conscious	114	264.2	53.5	183.6
The Netherlands				
Bilthoven	1024	167.8	39.6	114.1
Greece				
Greece	1312	273.0	51.1	207.5
Germany				
Heidelberg	1033	175.1	24.2	142.2
Potsdam	1235	239.3	31.0	194.6
Sweden				
Malmö	1421	121.5	22.4	94.0
Umeå	1344	121.9	27.9	90.8
Denmark				
Aarhus	567	178.1	27.6	145.2
Copenhagen	1356	142.3	18.0	117.4

[a]Mean adjusted by age, season and day of week. Standard errors of adjusted means reported, as well as crude means and SE are available on request to authors.
[b]Other fruits includes fresh fruits other than citrus, as well as dried and canned fruits, but not including nuts and seeds, olives, mixed, and unclassified fruits.

References

Bingham, S.A. & Nelson, M. (1991) Assessment of food composition and nutrient intake. In: Margetts, B.M. & Nelson, M., eds. *Design Concepts in Nutritional Epidemiology*, Oxford, Oxford University Press, pp. 153–191

Naska, A., Vasdekis, V.G., Trichopoulou, A., Friel, S., Leonhauser, I.U., Moreiras, O., Nelson, M., Remaut, A.M., Schmitt, A., Sekula, W., Trygg, K.U. & Zajkas, G. (2000) Fruit and vegetable availability among ten European countries: how does it compare with the 'five-a-day' recommendation? *Br. J. Nutr.*, **84**, 549–556

Roos, G., Johansson, L., Kasmel, A., Kumbiené, J. & Prättälä, R. (2000) Disparities in vegetable and fruit consumption: European cases from the north to the south. *Public Health Nutr.*, **4**, 35–43

Slimani, N., Deharveng, G., Charrondière, R.U., van Kappel, A.L., Ocke, M.C., Welch, A., Lagiou, A., van Liere, M., Agudo, A., Pala, V., Brandstetter, B., Andren, C., Stripp, C., van Staveren, W.A. & Riboli, E. (1999) Structure of the standardized computerised 24-h diet recall interview used as reference method in the 22 centers participating in the EPIC project. *Comput. Methods Programs Biomed.*, **58**, 251–266

Table 4. Consumption of fruits by subgroups, women[a]

Country and centre	*n*	Total fruits	Citrus fruits	Other fruits[b]
France				
North-east	2009	248.0	41.8	193.0
North-west	622	247.9	45.1	191.3
South	1396	257.7	35.0	207.5
South coast	612	249.3	39.1	196.4
Italy				
Florence	785	328.1	54.3	263.5
Varese	794	335.0	66.0	259.6
Ragusa	138	399.9	63.8	332.7
Turin	392	361.1	60.8	294.3
Naples	403	292.7	71.1	214.2
Spain				
Asturias	324	336.4	58.0	267.4
Granada	300	353.3	101.0	244.7
Murcia	304	378.9	116.8	247.2
Navarra	271	332.4	98.7	225.9
San Sebastian	244	372.8	78.4	283.6
United Kingdom				
General population	571	171.7	28.2	134.3
Health conscious	197	274.1	35.5	215.9
The Netherlands				
Bilthoven	1086	169.8	37.1	123.9
Utrecht	1874	213.5	49.9	152.7
Greece				
Greece	1374	241.9	45.1	188.3
Germany				
Heidelberg	1087	212.7	26.0	173.8
Potsdam	1063	259.9	38.4	210.5
Sweden				
Malmö	1711	151.0	30.0	116.4
Umeå	1574	159.4	38.9	117.4
Denmark				
Aarhus	510	231.2	37.2	188.6
Copenhagen	1485	181.4	31.0	142.1
Norway				
South and east	1136	173.7	32.5	135.9
North and west	662	162.7	28.7	129.2

[a]Mean adjusted by age, season and day of week. Standard errors of adjusted means reported, as well as crude means and SE are available on request to authors.
[b]Other fruits includes fresh fruits other than citrus, as well as dried and canned fruits, but not including nuts and seeds, olives, mixed, and unclassified fruits.

Consumption of soy products in 10 European countries

Keinan Boker L.[1], Peeters P.H.M.[1], Mulligan A.A.[2], Navarro C.[3], Slimani N.[4]
(for the EPIC working group on dietary patterns, sub-group on soy consumption)

[1]Julius Center for General Practice and Patient Oriented Research, Utrecht, The Netherlands. [2]University of Cambridge, Cambridge, UK. [3]Regional Health Council, Murcia, Spain. [4]IARC, Lyon, France.

Background

Soy products may have a protective role against certain chronic diseases, including hormone-related cancers (Adlercreutz & Mazur, 1997). Most studies have been conducted among populations with frequent and relatively high soy intake. Data regarding soy product intake in Western societies is limited. In light of the possible beneficiary consumption of soy, the aim of this study was to describe the distribution of soy product intake in 10 European countries (Denmark, France, Germany, Greece, Italy, Norway, Spain, Sweden, The Netherlands, UK) by using a standardized reference dietary method.

Methods

A 24-h dietary recall (24-HDR) interview was conducted among a sample (5%–12%) of all EPIC cohorts (calibration study, *n*=35 955) (Slimani *et al.*, 2000). All relevant soy items were subdivided by similarity into seven subgroups (beans and sprouts, dairy products, grain products, meat substitutes, pastes and spreads, traditional foods and nonspecific foods). Results were presented separately for males and females. Distributions of seven soy subgroups were described across countries. Crude and age-adjusted means of consumption were computed per soy subgroup across countries and expressed in g/day. Adjusted means were weighted according to weekday and season of dietary recall interview. Further adjustment for energy intake did not change results substantially (less than 5% change).

Results

In total, 195 men and 486 women reported consumption of soy products in their 24-h recall dietary interviews. Table 1 describes the number of total participants, the number of subjects reporting soy consumption in their 24-HDR interviews, and the soy subgroup most frequently consumed, per country and gender. Although reporting soy consumption was generally low, the highest percentages of soy intake report were observed in the UK, due to inclusion of a subgroup which habitually avoids intake of meat (fish eaters, vegetarians and vegans), and in The Netherlands (4.2–8.3%). The lowest percentages of soy intake reports were observed in Spain, Greece, Sweden and Norway (0.2–0.8%). In Mediterranean countries such as France, Spain, Italy and Greece, the soy products mostly consumed were dairy products, grain products and beans and sprouts. In mid-European countries such as The Netherlands and Germany, the soy products most consumed were beans and sprouts. Intake patterns in the Nordic countries were not clear; soy meat substitutes were mostly consumed in Denmark and soy grain and dairy products in Sweden and Norway. In the UK, soy dairy products were most often consumed.

Table 2 presents crude and adjusted means of intake for selected soy subgroups across countries. In general, the subgroup of soy dairy products was consumed by both genders in the highest quantities (males: 1.19, SE, 0.18; females: 1.94, SE, 0.18 g/day). The subgroup of soy grain products was consumed by males in the lowest quantities (0.05, SE, 0.03 g/day) and the subgroup of soy pastes, by females (0.02, SE, 0.01 g/day). Among 681 participants reporting consumption of soy products in their 24-HDR, soy dairy products were consumed in the highest quantities (62.56, SE, 8.60 and 32.82, SE, 2.90 g/day for males and females, respectively), soy grain products were

Table 1. Distribution of soy product consumption among the calibration study population – men and women

Country – gender (*n*)	Number of individuals reporting soy consumption (% of total)	Soy subgroup mostly consumed (% of consumption events)
France		
M (0)	NA	–
F (4639)	150 (3.2)	Soy dairy products
Italy		
M (1444)	24 (1.7)	Soy grain products/soy beans and sprouts
F (2512)	52 (2.1)	Soy grain products
Spain		
M (1777)	7 (0.4)	Soy beans and sprouts
F (1443)	6 (0.4)	Soy beans and sprouts
UK		
M (518)	43 (8.3)	Soy dairy products
F (768)	58 (7.6)	Soy dairy products
The Netherlands		
M (1024)	61 (6.0)	Soy beans and sprouts
F (2960)	124 (4.2)	Soy beans and sprouts
Greece		
M (1312)	5 (0.4)	Soy meat substitutes
F (1374)	11 (0.8)	Soy dairy products
Germany		
M (2268)	33 (1.5)	Soy beans and sprouts
F (2150)	37 (1.7)	Soy beans and sprouts
Sweden		
M (2765)	10 (0.4)	Soy grain products
F (3285)	23 (0.7)	Soy dairy products
Denmark		
M (1923)	12 (0.6)	Soy meat substitutes
F (1995)	21 (1.1)	Soy meat substitutes
Norway		
M (0)	NA	–
F (1798)	4 (0.2)	Soy dairy products
Total		
M (13 031)	195 (1.5)	Soy dairy products
F (22 924)	486 (2.1)	Soy dairy products
Total (M+F) (35 955)	681 (1.9)	Soy dairy products

M, male; F, female; NA, non-applicable.

consumed in the lowest quantities among males (2.78, SE, 1.44 g/day) and soy pastes, among females (0.31, SE, 0.09 g/day) (Table 2).

Conclusions

Soy product consumption is rather low in Western Europe. As no standardization of soy or phytoestrogen content for each soy item across countries was available in the calibration study, we were unable to calculate a total mean of soy or isoflavone intake and had to use the intake means of the seven soy subgroups as a proxy to total soy intake. However, when applying values of isoflavones for specific soy products as published in the literature (USDA Iowa University Database, 1999) to our population's means of the intake of soy subgroups, estimates of isoflavone consumption are in agreement with previously published data concerning consumption of phytoestrogens in Western populations (Horn-Ross *et al.*, 2000; De Kleijn *et al.*, 2001). Low as it is, the soy intake in the calibration study population might be underestimated, as soy protein has been long utilized in food systems and exposure to unsuspected and hidden sources of soy is generally unaccounted for.

Not only are intake quantities of soy products among Western subjects substantially lower than Asian subjects, but sources of soy foods also differ; while Japanese, Chinese and Korean subjects mostly consume traditional soy foods such as tofu in variant forms, Western populations mostly consume soy milk and dairy products.

This study is the first one to describe consumption of soy products in Western Europe. Its population is derived from a variety of geographical and cultural regions. However, the study population is not, in itself, a representative sample on the national level. In addition, lack of data concerning soy and isoflavone content of each relevant soy item has limited our ability to directly estimate soy – and isoflavone – intake in the study population. As soy intake is currently studied worldwide with regard to its possible associations with many chronic diseases, improvement of the information on soy intake in Europe is of great importance.

Table 2. Adjusted means (standard errors)[a] of selected soy products consumption. Means of consumption in g/day

Country	$n1$; $n2$[b]	Soy beans and sprouts		Soy dairy products		Soy meat substitutes		Soy traditional foods	
		Males	Females	Males	Females	Males	Females	Males	Females
France	0; 4639	NA	0.41 (0.10)	NA	4.23 (0.55)	NA	0.16 (0.07)	NA	0.02 (0.02)
Italy	1444; 2512	0.1 (0.03)	0.12 (0.04)	0.72 (0.35)	1.13 (0.34)	0.23 (0.21)	0.08 (0.06)	0.05 (0.04)	–
Spain	1777; 1443	0.02 (0.01)	0.05 (0.03)	0.81 (0.43)	0.10 (0.10)	–	–	–	–
UK	518; 768	–	–	22.62 (3.77)	24.66 (3.74)	2.71 (0.86)	1.03 (0.38)	1.26 (0.55)	1.15 (0.39)
The Netherlands	1024; 2960	0.70 (0.12)	0.66 (0.14)	0.71 (0.53)	1.31 (0.55)	0.71 (0.26)	0.56 (0.13)	0.52 (0.32)	0.33 (0.11)
Greece	1312; 1374	–	–	–	0.79 (0.49)	0.89 (0.63)	0.17 (0.17)	–	–
Germany	2268; 2150	0.28 (0.06)	0.35 (0.07)	0.28 (0.27)	0.15 (0.11)	–	<0.01 (<0.01)	0.09 (0.07)	0.11 (0.06)
Sweden	2765; 3285	–	0.05 (0.04)	0.03 (0.03)	0.25 (0.09)	0.11 (0.08)	0.08 (0.05)	–	–
Denmark	1923; 1995	0.01 (0.01)	0.03 (0.02)	0.14 (0.14)	0.49 (0.36)	0.18 (0.07)	0.17 (0.05)	–	–
Norway	0; 1798	NA	0.12 (0.09)	NA	0.30 (0.30)	NA	0.07 (0.07)	NA	–
Total	13 031; 22 924	0.11 (0.01)	0.22 (0.03)	1.19 (0.18)	1.94 (0.18)	0.28 (0.06)	0.18 (0.03)	0.11 (0.03)	0.10 (0.02)
Reports of soy consumption	195; 486	5.87 (0.64)	3.69 (0.47)	62.56 (8.60)	32.82 (2.90)	14.62 (3.06)	3.05 (0.46)	5.76 (1.80)	1.61 (0.34)

[a]Means are adjusted for age and weighted by day and season of recall.
[b]$n1$; $n2$, number of males; number of females.
NA, Non-applicable.

References

Adlercreutz, H. & Mazur, W. (1997) Phyto-oestrogens and Western diseases. *Ann. Med.*, **29**, 95–120

De Kleijn, M.J.J., van der Schouw, Y.T., Wilson, P.W.F., Adlercreutz, H., Mazur, W., Grobbee, D.E. & Jacques, P.F. (2001) Intake of dietary phytoestrogens is low in postmenopausal women in the United States: the Framingham study (1–4). *J. Nutr.*, **131**, 1826–1832

Horn-Ross, P.L., Lee, M., John, E.M. & Koo, J. (2000) Sources of phytoestrogen exposure among non-Asian women in California, USA. *Cancer Causes Control*, **11**, 299–302

Slimani, N., Ferrari, P., Ocke, M., Welch, A., Boeing, H., Liere, M., Pala, V., Amiano, P., Lagiou, A., Mattison, J., Stripp, C., Engeset, D., Charrondière, R., Buzzard, M., Staveren, W. & Riboli, E. (2000) Standardisation of the 24-hour diet recall calibration method used in the European Prospective Investigation into Cancer and Nutrition (EPIC): general concepts and preliminary results. *Eur. J. Clin. Nutr.*, **54**, 900–917

USDA Iowa State University Database on the Isoflavone Content of Foods – 1999 (1999), www.nalusda.gov/fnic/foodcomp/Data/isoflav/isfl_tbl.pdf

Consumption of soy products among European consumers of a health-conscious diet

Keinan Boker L.[1], Peeters P.H.M.[1], Mulligan A.A.[2], Navarro C.[3], Slimani N.[4]
(for the EPIC working group on dietary patterns, sub-group on soy consumption)

[1]Julius Center for General Practice and Patient Oriented Research, Utrecht, The Netherlands. [2]University of Cambridge, Cambridge, UK. [3]Regional Health Council, Murcia, Spain. [4]IARC, Lyon, France.

Background

Soy products may have a protective role against certain chronic diseases, including hormone-related cancers (Adlercreutz & Mazur, 1997). Soy product intake among Western societies is lower than in Asian populations. It is hypothesized that Western subjects consuming a meat-free diet also consume higher quantities of soy products. The aim of the study was to describe the distribution of soy product intake in European consumers of a health-conscious diet (meat-free diet) by using a standardized reference dietary method.

Methods

A 24-h dietary recall (24-HDR) interview was conducted among a sample (5%–12%) of all EPIC cohorts (calibration study, *n*=35 955) (Slimani *et al.*, 2000). All relevant soy items were subdivided by similarity into seven subgroups (beans and sprouts, dairy products, grain products, meat substitutes, pastes and spreads, traditional foods and nonspecific foods). Self-reported habitual consumers of a meat-free fish-based diet, as well as vegetarians and vegans, were identified through the 24-HDR questionnaires and subsequently defined as consumers of a health-conscious diet. Results were presented separately for males and females. In order to define them with regard to demographic, anthropometric and nutritional factors, we compared consumers of a health-conscious diet to the other participants by means of the unpaired *t* test. We computed crude and age-adjusted means of soy product consumption among consumers of a health-conscious diet and compared these results (by the unpaired *t* test) to means of consumption among the rest of the cohort. Adjusted means were weighted by weekday and season of dietary recall interview. Further adjustment for energy intake did not change results substantially (less than 5% change).

Results

In total, 412 consumers of a health-conscious diet were identified: 136 (33.0%) males and 276 (67.0%) females. Most of the consumers of a health-conscious diet (*n*=235, 57.0%) were in the UK, as they were deliberately oversampled in the Oxford arm of EPIC.

Table 1 presents a comparison of selected demographic, anthropometric and nutritional factors between consumers and non-consumers of a health-conscious diet. Consumers of a health-conscious diet, both males and females, seem to be significantly younger, taller, lighter, more educated and less often current smokers than the others. They consume significantly less energy from protein and fat sources and more energy from carbohydrate sources, have significantly higher daily intake of fruit, vegetables, legumes and cereals and significantly lower daily intake of dairy products and eggs.

Table 2 presents the adjusted means of consumption of seven soy subgroups among consumers of a health-conscious diet as compared to non-consumers. Dairy products were most frequently consumed among consumers and non-consumers of a health-conscious diet (both genders). Of all soy subgroups, dairy products were consumed in highest quantities among consumers of a health-conscious diet (approximately 106.50 and 70.80 g/day for males and females, respectively), as well as among non-consumers of a health-conscious diet (approximately 0.34 and 1.21 g/day for males and females, respectively). Compared to non-consumers, consumers of a health-conscious diet

Table 1. Characteristics of consumers of a health-conscious diet

Variable	Males			Females		
	Consumers of a health-conscious diet (*n*=136)	Non-consumers of a health-conscious diet (*n*=12 895)	*P* value	Consumers of a health-conscious diet (*n*=276)	Non-consumers of a health-conscious diet (*n*=22 648)	*P* value
Current smokers (%)	13.4	27.9	0.00	8.1	18.5	0.00
Academic education (%)	49.3	21.4	0.00	41.7	20.9	0.00
Mean age in years (SD)	54.6 (7.4)	56.8 (8.0)	0.00	52.9 (8.2)	55.3 (8.0)	0.00
Mean height in cm (SD)	177.1 (7.1)	174.2 (7.4)	0.00	164.2 (6.2)	162.3 (6.6)	0.00
Mean weight in kg (SD)	73.4 (9.9)	81.8 (11.8)	0.00	62.6 (10.4)	67.0 (11.7)	0.00
Mean energy intake in kcal/day (SD)	2216.0 (762.7)	2533.3 (872.0)	0.00	1881.8 (679.1)	1874.7 (637.2)	0.73
% of daily energy from carbohydrates	52.2	42.2	0.00	51.2	45.2	0.00
% of daily energy from protein	11.8	14.7	0.00	12.2	15.5	0.00
% of daily energy from fat	34.2	37.1	0.00	34.7	36.4	0.00
Mean intake of fruit in g/day (SD)	282.3 (264.1)	220.4 (251.6)	0.00	284.5 (240.6)	226.4 (215.2)	0.00
Mean intake of vegetables in g/day (SD)	249.9 (200.4)	169.5 (162.1)	0.00	235.4 (172.9)	167.9 (149.2)	0.00
Mean intake of legumes in g/day (SD)	34.0 (108.7)	14.5 (57.4)	0.00	15.3 (46.1)	7.1 (34.1)	0.00
Mean intake of dairy products in g/day (SD)	196.8 (264.7)	298.6 (289.1)	0.00	244.5 (307.3)	289.1 (241.6)	0.02
Mean intake of eggs and egg products in g/day (SD)	7.3 (21.4)	17.4 (35.7)	0.00	5.4 (16.0)	13.7 (29.0)	0.00
Mean intake of cereals in g/day (SD)	283.6 (203.0)	246.8 (172.7)	0.01	199.9 (139.2)	170.3 (118.6)	0.00

Table 2. Comparison of soy product consumption between consumers and non-consumers of a health-conscious diet[a]

Soy subgroup	Males			Females		
	Consumers of a health-conscious diet (*n*=136)	Non-consumers of a health-conscious diet (*n*=12 895)	*P* value	Consumers of a health-conscious diet (*n*=276)	Non-consumers of a health-conscious diet (*n*=22 648)	*P* value
Beans and sprouts	–	0.11 (0.01)	–	0.67 (0.38)	0.21 (0.03)	0.28
Dairy products (milk, drink, cheese, yoghurt, dessert, ice-cream)	106.50 (16.18)	0.34 (0.10)	0.00	70.80 (10.70)	1.21 (0.14)	0.00
Grain products (bread, pasta, flour, flakes)	0.01 (0.01)	0.05 (0.03)	0.86	0.19 (0.20)	0.10 (0.02)	0.73
Meat substitutes (hamburger, frankfurter, schnitzel, balls)	12.17 (3.83)	0.18 (0.05)	0.00	5.47 (1.55)	0.12 (0.02)	0.00
Soy pastes and spreads	1.46 (0.92)	0.08 (0.04)	0.14	0.31 (0.17)	0.02 (0.01)	0.09
Traditional foods (tofu, tempeh, miso)	7.75 (2.86)	0.05 (0.03)	0.00	3.30 (1.07)	0.06 (0.02)	0.00
Nonspecific	15.92 (5.55)	<0.01 (0.01)	0.00	8.46 (2.79)	<0.01 (<0.01)	0.00

[a]Means of consumption are age-adjusted and weighted according to weekday and season of 24-HDR interview, expressed in g/day (SE).

consume significantly higher amounts (between 18- to 313- and 2- to 58-fold higher, for males and females, respectively) of almost all soy subgroups.

Conclusions

Subjects who habitually avoid consumption of meat, i.e. consumers of a health-conscious diet, are significantly different from the rest of the cohort with regard to certain anthropometric, nutritional and dietary factors. Some of these findings were previously reported for Western vegetarians and vegans (Key *et al.*, 1999; Appleby *et al.*, 1999). Their soy product consumption is much higher as compared to non-consumers of a health-conscious diet. When estimating the isoflavone intake of consumers of a health-conscious diet according to published data regarding phytoestrogen content in certain food items (USDA Iowa University Database, 1999), intake levels among them are comparable to levels of intake in traditional Asian diets.

Therefore, the higher consumption of soy products may possibly indicate one sort of a healthier habitual diet. In addition, consumers of a health-conscious diet may serve as a reference group in the EPIC study when testing hypotheses in future analytical studies.

References

Adlercreutz, H. & Mazur, W. (1997) Phyto-oestrogens and Western diseases. *Ann. Med.*, **29**, 95–120

Appleby, P.N., Thorogood, M., Mann, J.I. & Key, T.J.A. (1999) The Oxford vegetarian study: an overview. *Am. J. Clin. Nutr.*, **70** (Suppl), 525S–531S

Key, T.J., Davey, G.K. & Appleby, P.N. (1999) Health benefits of a vegetarian diet. *Proc. Nutr. Soc.*, **58**, 271–275.

Slimani, N., Ferrari, P., Ocke, M., Welch, A., Boeing, H., Liere, M., Pala, V., Amiano, P., Lagiou, A., Mattison, J., Stripp, C., Engeset, D., Charrondière, R., Buzzard, M., Staveren, W. & Riboli, E. (2000) Standardisation of the 24-hour diet recall calibration method used in the European Prospective Investigation into Cancer and Nutrition (EPIC): general concepts and preliminary results. *Eur. J. Clin. Nutr.*, **54**, 900–917

USDA Iowa State University Database on the Isoflavone Content of Foods – 1999 (1999), www.nalusda.gov/fnic/foodcomp/Data/isoflav/isfl_tbl.pdf

Dietary and lifestyle characteristics of meat-eaters, fish-eaters, vegetarians and vegans

Davey G., Allen N., Appleby P., Spencer E., Verkasalo P., Knox K., Postans J., Tipper S., Hobson C., Key T.
(the Oxford EPIC cohort)

Imperial Cancer Research Fund, Cancer Epidemiology Unit, University of Oxford, Oxford, OX2 6HE, UK.

Introduction

EPIC Oxford is a cohort of 57 500 men and women. A unique feature of the cohort was the UK-wide targeted recruitment of vegetarians and health-conscious individuals, designed to maximize dietary heterogeneity.

Methods

Principally, two methods of recruitment to the Oxford cohort were used. Firstly, nurse recruitment: an invitation to attend the subject's General Practitioner's surgery for interview with a nurse and completion of a diet and lifestyle questionnaire (age range, 40–70). Secondly, postal recruitment: the distribution of the diet and lifestyle questionnaire to members of diet-interest groups (e.g. the Vegetarian Society of the UK), their families and friends (age range, 20–97).

The baseline questionnaire consists of a food frequency questionnaire (FFQ) (Bingham *et al.*, 1994, 1995) and questions on health and lifestyle. Mean nutrient intakes were estimated from the FFQ data, using standard portion sizes derived largely from the Ministry of Agriculture Fisheries and Food (1993) and nutrient contents from the fifth edition of McCance and Widdowson's The Composition of Foods (Holland *et al.*, 1991) and its supplements. Additionally, responses to four simple questions (Do you eat meat? Do you eat fish? Do you eat dairy products? Do you eat eggs?) enabled one of four diet groups to be assigned to each subject: meat-eaters (those that eat meat), fish-eaters (those that do not eat meat but do eat fish), vegetarians (those that do not eat meat or fish but do eat dairy products and/or eggs) and vegans (those that eat no animal products). Results presented are adjusted for age where appropriate (10-year age groups).

Results

Median ages for 13 213 men were 52, 43, 39, 36 years and for 44 239 women were 49, 40, 36, 33 years for the meat, fish, vegetarian and vegan diet groups, respectively.

Body mass index (BMI)

Mean BMI was 24.2 kg/m^2 for men and 23.6 kg/m^2 for women (Table 1).

Figure 1 shows BMI by diet group and 10-year age group (20–29, 30–39 ... 70–79, 80+). The highest mean BMI for both men and women at each age group was for meat-eaters, whereas the lowest was for vegans, with fish-eaters and vegetarians demonstrating similar BMI at intermediate values.

Lifestyle factors

Activity at work was assessed according to the type of current or most recent job, whether a sedentary occupation (e.g. office work), a standing occupation (e.g. shop assistant) or a manual/heavy manual occupation (e.g. construction worker). Overall, 57% of men and 51% of women reported sitting occupations; 18% of men and 9% of women reported manual occupations. Of the four diet groups, more vegans reported manual work than the other diet groups (men 20% and women 11%) (Table 1).

The health-conscious character of the cohort was reflected in the high numbers that had never smoked (53% of men and 61% of women). There were relatively small differences in smoking habits between the diet groups, though current smoking was most prevalent in meat-eaters (11% for both men and women).

Dietary patterns

Consumption of dairy products was higher in meat-eaters than in both fish-eaters and vegetarians. Consumption of fruit and vegetables (excluding potatoes) was highest in vegans and lowest in meat-eaters (Table 1).

Patterns of nutrient intake across the diet-groups were generally the same for men and women. Percentage energy from fat was lower for vegan men and women compared with the other diet groups. Percentage energy from alcohol was also lowest in vegans, although the differences between the diet groups were small.

Daily intake of fibre, carotene, folate and vitamin C was considerably higher in vegans than in meat-eaters, with fish-eaters and vegetarians taking intermediate values.

Conclusions

Striking differences in both lifestyle and dietary factors are shown between meat-eaters and vegans, with fish-eaters and vegetarians usually taking intermediate values. In particular, vegans have substantially lower BMI and substantially higher fruit, vegetable, fibre, carotene, folate, and vitamin C intake than meat-eaters.

References

Bingham, S.A., Gill, C., Welch, A., Day, K., Cassidy, A., Khaw, K.T., Sneyd, M.J., Key, T.J.A., Roe, L. & Day, N.E. (1994) Comparison of dietary assessment methods in nutritional epidemiology: weighed records vs 24 h recalls, food-frequency questionnaires and estimated-diet records. *Br. J. Nutr.*, **72**, 619–643

Bingham, S.A., Cassidy, A., Cole, T.J., Welch, A., Runswick, S.A., Black, A.E., Thurnham, D., Bates, C., Khaw, K.T., Key, T.J.A. & Day, N.E. (1995) Validation of weighed records and other methods of dietary assessment using the 24-h urine nitrogen technique and other biological markers. *Br. J. Nutr.*, **73**, 531–550

Holland, B., Welch, A.A., Unwin, I.D., Buss, D.H., Paul, A.A. & Southgate, D.A.T. (1991) *McCance and Widdowson's The Composition of Foods*, 5th ed. Cambridge, Royal Society of Chemistry

Ministry of Agriculture Fisheries and Food. (1993) *Food Portion Sizes*, 2nd ed. London, HMSO

Table 1. Body mass index, lifestyle factors, food and nutrient intake by diet group

	Men			
	Meat eaters	**Fish eaters**	**Vegetarians**	**Vegans**
Number of subjects	7073	1533	3813	794
Body mass index[a]	24.9	23.5	23.5	22.5
Activity at work[b] (%)				
Sitting	57.2	57.1	57.4	54.3
Standing	24.8	26.7	26.9	25.3
Manual	18.0	16.2	15.7	20.4
Smoking[b] (%)				
Never	50.1	53.7	56.7	53.4
Ex	39.1	35.6	35.7	40.6
Current	10.8	8.5	7.7	6.0
Dairy products (g/day)	450.9	381.5	372.4	0.0
Fruit (g/day)	304.0	353.6	347.1	462.0
Vegetables, excl. potatoes (g/day)	227.9	280.0	279.3	319.3
% energy from fat	32.0	31.1	31.1	28.2
% energy from alcohol	5.2	5.2	4.7	3.9
Fibre (g/day)	18.9	22.5	23.0	27.5
Carotene (mg/day)	2.9	3.3	3.3	4.0
Folate (µg/day)	333.4	363.9	370.1	428.5
Vitamin C (mg/day)	120.0	132.8	131.7	154.3

	Women			
	Meat eaters	**Fish eaters**	**Vegetarians**	**Vegans**
Number of subjects	23 379	7014	12 494	1352
Body mass index[a]	24.3	22.8	22.7	21.9
Activity at work[b] (%)				
Sitting	51.0	52.7	52.0	47.0
Standing	40.7	39.0	39.7	42.2
Manual	8.3	8.3	8.3	10.9
Smoking[b] (%)				
Never	61.6	58.9	62.6	59.0
Ex	27.4	33.0	30.3	32.8
Current	11.0	8.1	7.1	8.1
Dairy products (g/day)	423.1	376.3	359.7	0.0
Fruit (g/day)	362.9	401.7	389.2	486.9
Vegetables, excl. potatoes (g/day)	263.3	306.0	302.8	362.9
% energy from fat	31.6	30.8	30.4	27.9
% energy from alcohol	2.9	3.2	3.0	2.6
Fibre (g/day)	19.2	21.8	22.0	26.7
Carotene (mg/day)	3.2	3.6	3.5	4.3
Folate (µg/day)	325.4	348.9	352.7	415.7
Vitamin C (mg/day)	139.1	148.5	148.1	170.6

[a]kg/m^2, adjusted by 10-year age group.
[b]Adjusted by 10-year age group.
[c]Non-starch polysaccharides.

Consumption of wild vegetables in the EPIC cohort of Ragusa (Sicily)

Tumino R.[1], Frasca G.[1], Giurdanella M.C.[1], Lauria C.[1], Krogh V.[2]
(The Ragusa EPIC cohort)

[1]Cancer Registry, Azienda Ospedaliera "Civile, M.P. Arezzo", Ragusa, Italy. [2]Epidemiology Unit, National Cancer Institute, Milan, Italy.

The consumption of edible vegetables which grow naturally in the countryside has been a poorly investigated aspect of the Mediterranean diet, despite some evidence of beneficial effects related to their antioxidant content (Trichopoulou *et al.*, 2000). The European Prospective Investigation into Cancer and Nutrition (EPIC) has given us an opportunity to explore the intake of wild greens within the cohort.

In the food frequency questionnaire (FFQ) used in the Ragusa (Sicily) collaborating centre for the EPIC project, we investigated the consumption of the following vegetables: Greek mustard (Italian name, senapa canuta; colloquial name, lassini; Latin name, *sinapis incana*), black mustard (Italian name, senapa; colloquial name, sanapu; Latin name, *sinapis nigra*), white wall rocket (Italian name, ramolaccio; colloquial name, rariceddi; Latin name, *diplotaxis eracoides*), wild radish (Italian name, ruchetta selvatica; colloquial name, sinacciuola; Latin name, *raphanus raphanistrum*), wild chicory (Italian name, cicoria; colloquial name, cicuoria; Latin name, *cichorium intybus L.*), borage (Italian name, borragine; colloquial name, vurrania; Latin name, *borrago officinalis*) and purselane (Italian name, portulaca; colloquial name, purciddana; Latin name, *portulaca oleracea*). With the exception of purselane, which is eaten either cooked or raw, all of the others are traditionally eaten cooked (boiled) according to their seasonal availability in late winter, early spring and autumn.

The basic descriptive statistics (Tables 1 and 2) of 6185 food frequency questionnaires (males, 2921; females, 3264) show that in the Ragusa EPIC cohort, only 13.1% of men and 15.7% of women never eat such vegetables, whereas 28.3% of males and 25.5% of females consume them 1–2 times a month, and 14.9% of men and 13.5% of women eat them more frequently. There is a significant positive trend of consumption with age only in men (P=0.0001). Among the consumers, the mean daily intake was 9.1 g in males and 7.2 g in females; the medians were 5.0 g and 4.3 g, respectively. Of the total cooked leafy vegetables plus cabbage daily intake (30.4 g in men and 29.6 g in women), wild greens account for 30.0% in men and 24.2% in women. In both sexes, their consumption is positively associated (P<0.0001) with the consumption of cabbage, leafy and root vegetables, fruiting vegetables, legumes, mushrooms and olive oil (data not shown).

These results suggest that, in the context of a relatively low intake of cooked leafy vegetables and cabbage, consumption of wild greens is surprisingly high. Further, despite the stereotype of an old-fashioned dietary habit and the expectation that only old people eat wild greens, in the Ragusa EPIC cohort, a relatively high percentage of young men (aged 35–44) consumed wild greens twice a month; in women, similar proportions of younger and older (aged 55–69) subjects reported consumption twice a month or more. In Ragusa, these vegetables are eaten with a generous amount of olive oil, like in Greece, another Mediterranean country where wild greens are common. The combination of vegetables and olive oil seems to be a healthy nutritional habit, as reported by Trichopoulou *et al.*, 1998. In contrast to the traditional Greek diet, in which wild greens are eaten both cooked (fried pies) and raw (Trichopoulou *et al.*, 2000), in Ragusa these foods are eaten only cooked (except purselane). Another difference with the Greek diet is the number of edible wild greens, which in

Table 1. Frequency of intake of wild greens in the EPIC cohort of Ragusa by age group: men

Frequency	Age group			Total
Times per month	35–44	45–54	55–69	35–69
Never	177 (16.4%)	146 (11.9%)	60 (9.6%)	383 (13.1%)
Up to 1	446 (41.8%)	565 (46.2%)	266 (42.5%)	1277 (43.7%)
Up to 2	302 (28.1%)	334 (27.3%)	190 (30.4%)	826 (28.3%)
More	143 (13.7%)	178 (14.6%)	109 (17.5%)	426 (14.9%)
Total	1073 (100.0%)	1223 (100.0%)	625 (100.0%)	2921 (100.0%)

Pearson χ^2 on 6 d.f = 24.6799, *P*=0.0001.

Table 2. Frequency of intake of wild greens in the EPIC cohort of Ragusa by age group: women

Frequency	Age group			Total
Times per month	35–44	45–54	55–69	35–69
Never	278 (17.1%)	161 (14.1%)	72 (14.3%)	511 (15.6%)
Up to 1	690 (42.6%)	482 (42.2%)	217 (43.3%)	1482 (45.4%)
Up to 2	446 (27.5%)	337 (29.5%)	143 (28.6%)	835 (25.5%)
More	207 (12.8%)	162 (14.2%)	69 (13.8%)	436 (13.5%)
Total	1621(100.0%)	1142 (100.0%)	501 (100.0%)	3264 (100.0%)

Pearson χ^2 on 6 d.f = 6.7124, *P*=0.3481.

Greece surpasses 150 (Trichopoulou *et al.*, 2000), whereas in Ragusa this is restricted to the above-mentioned seven foods and a very few others; the most commonly eaten are Greek mustard, black mustard, wild radish and wild chicory. All except wild chicory belong to the Cruciferae family. Since this group of vegetables is reported to be rich in certain glucosinolates, which seem to have anticarcinogenic properties (Stoewsand, 1995), it is reasonable to speculate that wild mustard greens might also contain similar compounds. Unfortunately, official food tables do not report nutrient content for these vegetables, with the exception of chicory (cichorium intybus) and probably wild radish (Salvini *et al.*, 1998), if we assume the wild counterparts are equivalent to the cultivated ones. Nevertheless, according to the website www.hoptechno.com/nightcrew/sante7000, reporting information on over 7000 foods from the U.S. Department of Agriculture (USDA) Human Nutrition Information Service, the contents of carotene, vitamin C and vitamin E in mustard greens is much higher than that of cabbage. To our knowledge, nothing is known about the chemical composition of the wild greens eaten in Ragusa and, therefore, about their putative effect in nutritional anticarcinogenesis and carcinogenesis; but it should be mentioned that one of these vegetables, purselane (*Portulaca oleracea*), was used in the DIANA randomized trial in which the authors showed the effect of a dietary intervention on the bioavailability of serum sex hormones, the latter being a risk factor for postmenopausal breast cancer (Berrino *et al.*, 2001).

Acknowledgements

Gioacchino Gurrieri, Micologist, AUSL 7 Ragusa (Italy)
Foto studio Fr.lli Tidona Ragusa (Italy)

References

Berrino, F., Bellati, C., Secreto, G., Camerini, E., Pala, V., Panico, S., Allegro, G. & Kaaks, R. (2001) Reducing bioavailable sex hormones through a comprehensive change in diet: the diet and androgens (DIANA) randomized trial. *Cancer Epidemiol. Biomarkers Prev.*, **10**, 25–33

Salvini, S., Parpinel, M., Gnangarella, P., Maisonneuve, P. & Turrini, A. (1998) *Banca Dati di Composizione Degli Alimenti per Studi Epidemiologici in Italia.* Istituto Europeo di Oncologia, Milano

Stoewsand, G.S. (1995) Bioactive organosulfur phytochemicals in Brassica oleracea vegetables – a review. *Food Chem. Toxic.*, **33**, 537–543

Trichopoulou, A., Lagiou, P. & Papas, A. (1998) Mediterranean diet: are antioxidants central to its benefits? In Papas, A., ed. *Antioxidant Status, Diet, Nutrition and Health.* CRC Press, Boca Raton Fla, USA , pp. 107–116

Trichopoulou, A., Vasilopoulou, E., Holman, P., Chamalides, C., Foufa, E., Kaloudis, T.R., Kromhout, D., Miskaki, P., Petrochilou, I., Poulima, E., Stafilakis, K. & Theophilou, D. (2000) Nutritional composition and flavonoid content of edible wild greens and green pies: a potential rich source of antioxidant nutrients in the Mediterranean diet. *Food Chem.*, **70**, 319–323

Plasma vitamin C, cancer mortality and incidence in men and women: a prospective study

Luben R., Khaw K.T., Welch A., Bingham S., Wareham N., Oakes S., Day N.E.
(The Norfolk EPIC cohort)

Dept. of Public Health and Primary Care, University of Cambridge, UK.

Introduction

A number of prospective studies have suggested that a high dietary intake of antioxidants may be protective against cancer, but findings have not been consistent and trial results to date have not been conclusive.

Vitamin C plays a role in many biological processes including free radical scavenging, collagen and hormone synthesis, haemostasis, and protection of lipid membranes, which might plausibly affect chronic disease risk. However, only some prospective studies have reported a significant inverse relationship between vitamin C and cancer and even those that reported such an effect vary over the level of vitamin C which may be important and the potential magnitude of the relationship.

We present data from a prospective population study examining the relationship between plasma vitamin C and subsequent all-cause mortality, cancer mortality and cancer incidence in men and women.

Methods

We examined the relationship between plasma vitamin C measured in 8860 men and 10 636 women aged 45–79 years in the EPIC Norfolk cohort and subsequent all-cause mortality, cancer mortality (to January 2001) and cancer incidence (to December 1999). We excluded subjects who reported a history of heart attack, stroke or any cancer.

Participants attended a clinic where blood was taken by venepuncture into citrate bottles and stabilized in a standardized volume of metaphosphoric acid stored at –70°C. Plasma vitamin C concentration was estimated using a fluorometric assay within 1 week of sampling. At the clinic visit, all participants were asked to complete a 7-day diet diary prospectively. Because of the labour-intensive requirements for analysis of diet diaries, only a sample of diaries have been coded and analysed to date for average daily nutrient and food intake.

All participants have been flagged for death certification at the Office for National Statistics in the United Kingdom. Death certificates were coded according to the International Classification of Disease (ICD) 9th revision. Cancer incidence in Norfolk was obtained by linkage to the East Anglian Cancer Registry and coded using the ICD 10th revision. Cancer mortality was defined as those who had ICD9 140–239 as underlying cause on the death certificate and cancer incidence as ICD10 C00–C97, excluding C44 non-melanoma skin cancer.

Results

Table 1 presents age-adjusted relative risks for all-cause mortality, cancer mortality and cancer incidence by sex-specific quintile of plasma vitamin C in men and women who had no history of cardiovascular disease or cancer at the baseline survey. In both men and women, there is a significant trend across quintiles of plasma vitamin C for all-cause mortality. In men, there is a significant trend for cancer mortality and cancer incidence but this is not seen in women.

Site-specific cancer incidence and cancer mortality in the EPIC Norfolk cohort is shown in Table 2. Lung cancer accounts for 41.9% of mortality and 16.1% of the incidence in men but only 20.4% and 6.3%, respectively, in women.

Table 1. Age-adjusted relative risks for all-cause mortality and cancer mortality and cancer incidence by vitamin C quintile for men and women

	Plasma vitamin C quintile					Trend	
	1	2	3	4	5	χ^2	*P*
Men	*n*=1787	*n*=1791	*n*=1761	*n*=1727	*n*=1794		
Plasma vitamin C mg/dl mean (SD)	20.8 (7.1)	38.1 (3.5)	48.1 (2.6)	56.8 (2.6)	72.6 (11.5)		<0.001
All-cause mortality (*n*=327)	1.00	0.69	0.62	0.47	0.54	17.22	<0.001
Cancer mortality (*n*=138)	1.00	0.71	0.59	0.66	0.52	5.86	0.016
Cancer incidence (*n*=507)	1.00	0.82	0.76	0.66	0.70	9.92	0.002
Women	*n*=2099	*n*=2046	*n*=2297	*n*=2158	*n*=2036		
Plasma vitamin C mg/dl mean (SD)	30.3 (10.1)	49.5 (3.1)	59.1 (2.6)	67.8 (2.6)	85.1 (13.7)		<0.001
All-cause mortality (*n*=218)	1.00	0.84	0.66	0.59	0.54	11.36	<0.001
Cancer mortality (*n*=108)	1.00	1.12	0.70	0.60	0.82	2.34	0.127
Cancer incidence (*n*=447	1.00	0.85	0.90	0.96	0.87	0.26	0.612

Table 2. Cancer incidence (to December 1999) and cancer mortality (to January 2001) in EPIC Norfolk men and women with no history of heart disease, stroke or cancer at baseline

		Lung	Ovarian	Breast	Prostate	Stomach	Colorectal	Other	All
Men	Incidence	31 (16.1%)	–	–	75 (38.9%)	10 (5.2%)	55 (28.5%)	22 (11.4%)	193
	Mortality	26 (41.9%)	–	–	11 (17.7%)	6 (9.7%)	13 (21.0%)	6 (9.7%)	62
Women	Incidence	13 (6.3%)	17 (8.2%)	112 (54.1%)	–	2 (1.0%)	44 (21.3%)	19 (9.2%)	207
	Mortality	10 (20.4%)	10 (20.4%)	12 (24.5%)	–	1 (2.0%)	13 (26.5%)	3 (6.1%)	49

Conclusions

Increased plasma vitamin C concentration is associated with a reduced risk of all-cause mortality in both men and women and is associated with a reduced risk of cancer mortality and cancer incidence in men.

How vegetables are eaten in Italy EPIC centres: still setting a good example?

Pala V.[1], Berrino F.[1], Vineis P.[2], Palli D.[3], Celentano E.[4], Tumino R.[5], Krogh V.[1]
(the Italian EPIC cohort)

[1]Epidemiology Unit, National Cancer Institute, Milan, Italy. [2]University of Turin, Turin, Italy. [3]Cancer Study and Prevention Centre, Florence, Italy. [4]Pascale Institute, Naples, Italy. [5]Cancer Registry, Azienda Ospedaliera "Civile M.P. Arezzo", Ragusa, Italy.

Background and purpose

Westernization of diet and the increased variety of food available for purchase have moved Italians away from the Mediterranean diet defined as the "dietary pattern of people living in southern Italy in the 1960s" (Iacoviello, 2001, personal communication). People buy greater quantities of food but it is not clear that the overall nutritional value of foods consumed has improved. To investigate these issues, we assessed the consumption of fruit and vegetables using the detailed information gathered in the 24-h dietary recall interview of the EPIC calibration study (Slimani *et al.*, 2000). We compared metropolitan areas (Turin, Florence, Naples) with smaller towns and surrounding rural areas (Varese, Ragusa) and also the northern centres (Turin, Varese, Florence) with the southern cities (Naples, Ragusa).

Vegetable intake was also related to socioeconomic variables, an index of the variety of the diet, and the age class of participants.

Methods

The cohort studied was a sample (~10%) of the Italian EPIC cohort examined on total diet in the 24 h up to interview using the EPIC-SOFT computer program. Mean food intakes (g/ m^2 per day) were calculated from individual consumption divided by body surface area (BSA) to take account of anthropometric variation. BSA was calculated from height (H) and weight (W) using the Du Bois formula:

$$BSA = 0.007184 \times (H)^{0.725} \times (W)^{0.425}$$

Analysis of covariance in combination with weighting procedures to take account of the nonuniform distribution of interviews over the seasons were used to calculate weighted mean consumption. The variables used for adjustment are listed in the notes to Table 1. Statistical analysis employed Stata Statistical Software, version 7.0 (Stata Corp.).

Results

Town versus country, north versus south

Comparison between Italian EPIC centres was in terms of mean weighted daily vegetable intake divided by BSA. In general, women tended to eat more vegetables than men. Both sexes ate more vegetables in big towns (Turin, Florence) than provincial towns (Ragusa, Varese): consumption ranged from 142 g/m^2 per day for women in Turin to 88 and 90 g/m^2 per day for men in Varese and Ragusa, respectively. When only raw fresh items were considered, again the cities (Turin, Florence) consumed more than the provincial centres. Furthermore, women in the north consumed more raw fresh vegetables by BSA than women in the south, with intakes ranging from 32 g/m^2 per day (Turin) and 28 g/m^2 per day (Florence) to 19 g/m^2 per day (Ragusa, Naples).

Occupation and vegetable intake

Table 1 shows how fresh vegetable intake varies with occupation. Farmers and shopkeepers of both sexes ate the least vegetables; teachers, white collar workers (men) and people in professions (particularly women) ate the most. Adjusting for energy intake did not change these rankings (data not shown).

Education and eating greens

Table 1 shows how fresh vegetable intake varies with education. Few years of schooling corresponded to low vegetable intake in both sexes;

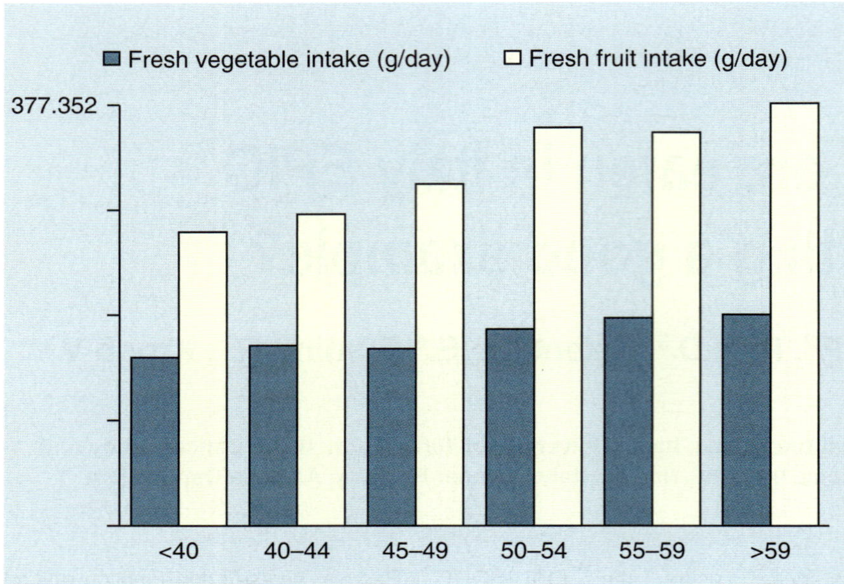

Figure 1
Daily fruit and vegetable intake by age class

Table 1. Daily fresh vegetable intake by socio-economic variables

	Males		Females	
	Mean (g)	± SE (g)	Mean (g)	± SE (g)
Present job				
Farmer	126.8	59	147.6	76
Shopkeeper	161.3	18	144.3	15
Unemployed & housewife	170.7	57	175	6
White-collar & teacher	191.5	6	176.2	6
Professional	183.9	13	199.8	21
Unskilled worker	182.6	12	168.7	10
Skilled worker	178.9	7	180.1	10
Education[b]				
None	104.5	49	132.6	29
Primary school	159.8	9	172.8	6
Junior high school	170.3	9	175.7	6
Technical high school	171.0	9	199.7	10
High school	168.1	8	174.5	7
Junior college	80.8	35	238.4	20
University degree	180.5	14	191.5	11

[a]Adjusted for age, EPIC centre and weighted for season.
[b]Adjusted for energy intake, age, EPIC centre and weighted for season.

conversely, highly educated women were the greatest consumers of vegetables.

Variety in diet

People with higher energy-adjusted vegetable intake also ate a greater variety of foods. As a descriptor of diet variety, we used the number of different food items consumed daily. Consumers of up to 20 different food items ate 147 g/day (men) or 154 g/day (women) of vegetables; consumers of 20–40 different items ate 154 g/day (men) and 184 g/day (women) of vegetables; consumers of more than 40 different foods ate 171 g/day (men) and 217 g/day (women) of vegetables.

Age and fruit and vegetable consumption

Figure 1 shows fruit and vegetable intake by age. Consumption increased with age. We were unable to determine whether this was mainly an age–cohort effect (people born earlier, e.g. before World War II, might cling to traditional eating habits) or to an ageing effect (switch to more digestible/easily masticated foods with advancing age). We suspect a strong cohort effect that is partly enhanced by an ageing effect. Subsequent studies might distinguish these.

Conclusions

The eating habits revealed by this unrepresentative but highly detailed survey suggest that the poor but healthy food consumption pattern of our (Italian) grandparents is fast disappearing. The health-food extremist was not observed in Italy but differences in eating habits between town and country, the educated and less educated, suggest an effect of health consciousness and knowledge of the possible health effects of different foods on eating.

In contrast, people with lower incomes and less education from economically disadvantaged or rural areas are probably abandoning the traditional diet: they are more likely to eat a less varied diet characterized in particular by lower vegetable intake. Information access and nutritional education might be important in promoting healthier eating among these less advantaged groups.

Acknowledgements

The EPIC study is financed by the Europe Against Cancer Program, the Italian Ministry of Health and the Italian Association for Cancer Research (AIRC). We are indebted to D.C. Ward for help with the English.

References

Slimani, N., Ferrari, P., Ocke, M., Welch, A., Boeing, H., Liere, M., Pala, V., Amiano, P., Lagiou, A., Mattison, J., Stripp, C., Engeset, D., Charrondière, R., Buzzard, M., Staveren, W. & Riboli, E. (2000) Standardisation of the 24-hour diet recall calibration method used in the European Prospective Investigation into Cancer and Nutrition (EPIC): general concepts and preliminary results. *Eur. J. Clin. Nutr.*, **54**, 900–917

Fruit and vegetable consumption and risk of cancer of the digestive tract: meta-analysis of published case–control and cohort studies

Norat T., Riboli E.

Unit of Nutrition and Cancer, International Agency for Research on Cancer, Lyon, France.

It is widely considered that diets rich in fruits and vegetables might decrease the risk for some cancers, particularly those of the alimentary and respiratory tracts (WCRF/AICR, 1997). The possible cancer preventive effect of vegetables and fruits is explained by different mechanisms. Potentially anticarcinogenic agents found in fruits and vegetables include carotenoids, vitamins C and E, dietary fiber, selenium, glucosinolates and indoles, isothiocyanates, flavonoids, phenols, protease inhibitors, and plant sterols (Steinmetz & Potter, 1996).

Purpose

To summarize the epidemiological evidence on the association between vegetable and fruit intake and cancers of the digestive tract. To estimate the proportion of cancers preventable by current fruit and vegetable consumption levels and the possible reduction in cancer incidence that may follow a hypothetical increase in fruit and vegetable consumption.

Methods

Criteria for inclusion of studies: case–control or cohort studies on total vegetable or total fruit consumption and oesophageal, gastric or colorectal cancer risk were included in the meta-analysis if they provided the information necessary for the statistical analysis, were published in English between 1973 and 2000 and were referenced in the Medline database.

Statistical methods: in this meta-analysis, two overall effect-size statistics were estimated: 1) the average of the logarithm of the observed relative risks (estimated as the odds ratio in most of the studies) associated with the highest versus the lowest level of consumption, as reported in the articles, and 2) the pooled coefficient b in the

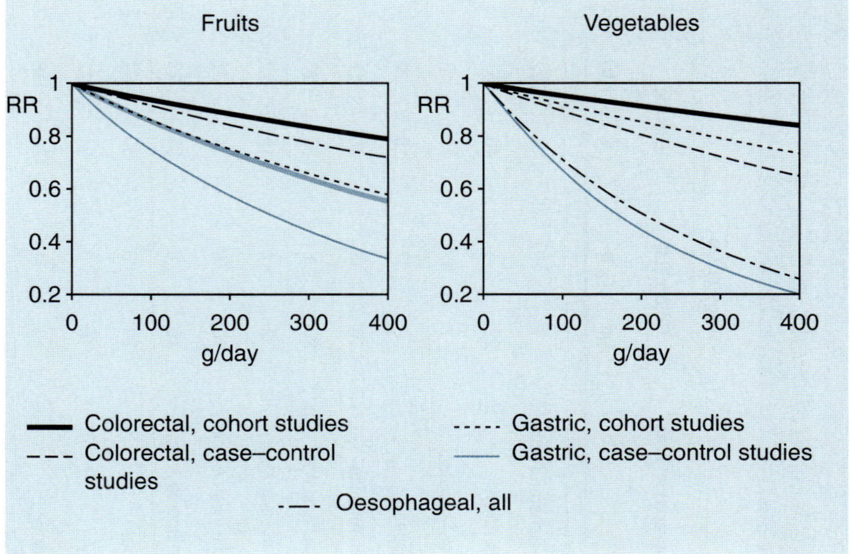

Figure 1
Dose–response relationship between fruit and vegetable consumption and risk of cancers

Table 1. Preventable proportion (%) of cancer risk by current fruit and vegetables consumption and preventable proportion by increasing consumption up to 350 g/day when lower

Geographical area	Vegetables						Fruits					
	Colorectal		Gastric		Oesophageal		Colorectal		Gastric		Oesophageal	
	a	b	a	b	a	b	a	b	a	b	a	b
Sub-Saharan Africa	7	19	14	22	5	20	12	8	45	20	37	22
North Africa	22	6	40	31	16	28	9	11	34	31	27	28
Central America	7	19	15	16	5	14	16	6	53	16	45	14
Caribbean	9	17	18	21	7	19	13	8	46	21	38	19
South America	10	16	20	17	7	15	15	6	52	17	43	15
Middle East Asia	20	8	36	26	15	23	10	10	40	26	33	23
Low income Asia	8	18	12	27	4	24	10	9	39	27	32	24
Middle income Asia	18	9	34	31	13	28	9	11	34	31	28	28
High income Asia	19	8	35	23	14	21	12	8	43	23	36	21
China	29	3	50	34	22	30	8	12	32	34	26	30
India	18	9	34	22	13	26	9	10	36	29	29	26
Oceania	15	11	28	18	11	16	14	7	50	18	42	16
Southern Europe	24	5	43	19	18	27	13	7	47	19	29	27
North-Central Europe	15	11	28	24	11	30	11	8	42	24	26	30
Eastern Europe	18	9	34	28	13	25	10	10	38	28	31	25
North America	18	9	32	21	13	19	13	8	46	21	39	19
Australia, New Zealand	14	12	29	30	12	27	9	11	35	30	29	27
Ex-USSR Asia	8	18	17	50	6	43	3	17	15	50	12	43

[a]By current consumption.
[b]Up to 350 g/day.

dose–response model lnRR=bX using the Greenland and Longnecker method (1992). When consumption was expressed as frequency, it was multiplied by "mean portion sizes" published in previous studies. When consumption was expressed qualitatively, the mean and variance derived from published studies were applied to the distribution of the study population. The preventable proportion was estimated as proposed by Miettinen (1974). The pooled slope b was used to estimate relative risks associated with quartiles of consumption of fruit or vegetables in different populations, using non-consumption as the reference category. As estimates of the prevalence of fruit or vegetable consumption by geographical area, per caput intakes provided in Food Balance Sheets (FAO) were used, corrected for overestimation with data published from national dietary surveys (FAO, 1994).

Conclusions

- The pooled analysis of all studies indicates that high intake of vegetables was associated with a significantly decreased risk of gastric and colorectal cancer, and with a nonsignificantly decreased risk of oesophageal cancer (Fig. 1).
- The average association with vegetables in case–control studies was significant for the three cancer sites. The meta-analysis of the cohort studies did not find an association between vegetable consumption and the risk of oesophageal and colorectal cancer. However, the protective effect of vegetables for stomach cancer was statistically significant over the cohort studies examined.
- Fruit consumption is significantly associated with a reduction in cancer risk for the oesophagus and the stomach. The association with colorectal cancer risk is, over these studies, not significant.
- Both case–control and cohort studies reported an overall significant protection of fruits against stomach cancer. Cohort studies did not find a significant reduction in oesophageal cancer as a result of high fruit intake.
- The protective effect estimated by pooling case–control studies is stronger than the effect estimated from cohort studies. These results could be caused by recall bias in case–control studies. The association could have been underestimated by cohort studies by an error effect in the measurement of intake. Nevertheless, the average relative risks from both case–control and cohort studies were always lower than 1, supportive of a moderate protective effect of vegetables and fruits against oesophageal and colorectal cancer, and a higher protective effect for gastric cancer.
- Worldwide, increasing vegetable consumption could potentially prevent up to 50% of gastric cancer and up to 29% of colorectal cancer. Increasing fruit consumption could potentially prevent up to 45% of cases of oesophageal cancer and 50% of gastric cancer cases (Table 1).
- In European countries, the population preventable fraction by increasing vegetable consumption is 28% for gastric cancer and 18% for colorectal cancer. The population preventable fraction by increasing fruit consumption is 30% for gastric cancer and 30% for oesophageal cancer.
- The figures of preventable fractions presented above should be interpreted cautiously. A causal relationship between fruit and vegetable consumption with cancer risk has been assumed. Interaction between fruit and vegetable consumption and between the consumption of these foods and other lifestyle factors could not be taken into account. It is unlikely that any major cancer preventive effect can be achieved in practice by varying only one of these risk factors, but our results indicate that there is a substantial potential for preventing cancer through diet.

References

Food and Agriculture Organization of the United Nations, Statistical Division. (1994) *Compendium of Food Consumption Statistics from Household Surveys in Developing Countries, Vol. 1: Asia, Vol. 2: Africa, Latin America and Oceania*, Food and Agriculture Organization of the United Nations, Rome

Greenland, S. & Longnecker, M.P. (1992) Methods for trend estimation from summarized dose–response data, with applications to meta-analysis. *Am. J. Epidemiol.*, **135**, 1301–1309

Miettinen, O.S. (1974) Proportion of disease caused or prevented by a given exposure, trait or intervention. *Am. J. Epidemiol.*, **99**, 325–332

Steinmetz, K.A. & Potter, J.D. (1996) Vegetables, fruit, and cancer prevention: a review. *J. Am. Diet. Assoc.* **96**, 1027–1039

World Cancer Research Fund/American Institute for Cancer Research (1997) *Food, Nutrition and the Prevention of Cancer: A Global Perspective.* WCRF/AICR, Washington, DC

Subregional variations of dietary consumption and incidences of cancers in southern France

Siari S.[1], Scali J.[1], Richard A.[1], Tretarre B.[2], Daurès J.P.[2], Padilla M.[3], Grosclaude P.[4], Gerber M.[1]

[1]Groupe d'Epidémiologie Métabolique, INSERM-CRLC, 34298 Montpellier cedex 5. [2]Registre des tumeurs de l'Hérault, 34298 Montpellier. [3]CIHEAM-IAM, 3191 Route de Mende, 34033 Montpellier. [4]Registre des cancers du Tarn, 81000 Albi, France.

Objective

This study describes the variations of dietary intake and incidences of cancers in five socioeconomic zones in southern France: Greater Montpellier (1), Bassin de Thau (2), Bitterrois (3), Haut-Cantons (4) Tarn (5), in the context of the Mediterranean diet.

Method

Nutritional assessment was obtained by a validated food frequency questionnaire (FFQ) (Bonifacj *et al.*, 1997; Daurès *et al.*, 2000) for 922 subjects (aged 34–76) in five subregions characterized by socio-economic variables such as income, population density, employment, number of shopping centres, fast-food restaurants and women's activity.

We included food and cancer incidences as quantitative variables and the five socio-economic subregions as individuals in a principal component analysis (PCA) to reveal the association between quantitative variables (food intake and cancer incidence columns of the matrix) and individuals (the five subregion lines of the matrix) and to interpret simultaneously the contributions of variables and individuals. Because incidences are aggregated values for each of the five subregions, individuals' nutrition data were reaggregated for each of the five subregions and introduced as the median value of the individual's data. This analysis is illustrated in Fig. 1 and 2 for 454 men and 468 women, respectively.

Results

In Fig. 1 and 2, the radius of the circle represents the values of the contributions of the variables to the plane defined by axes 1 and 2 (the closer to the circle, the higher the coefficient; threshold: 0.50).

The individuals are represented along the two dimensions that define the plane of the circle. Three different dietary patterns can be seen in both sexes:

- A Mediterranean type dietary pattern, with typical foods such as olive oil, fish and seafood, olives and herbs;
- a rich diet characteristic of the French southwest region with a high intake of processed meat, foie gras and wine, but also fruits and vegetables;
- a fast-food diet characterized by a high intake of fast food (various sandwiches, hamburgers and pizza), cheeses, meat and dried fruit.

A Mediterranean diet and a fast-food diet were found to be on opposite ends of the spectrum (all cancer sites, prostate and lung cancer incidences in men and all cancer sites, cervix, lung, breast and stomach cancer incidences in women) and were associated with the fast-food dietary pattern and hence not associated with the Mediterranean diet pattern.

High intakes of fresh and cooked vegetables are opposite stomach cancer in both sexes, whereas colon–rectum cancer incidence appears associated with the rich diet, especially wine and alcohol intake in men (Fig. 1), despite the association with a high intake of fruit and vegetables. In women, a close association was observed between cheese and stomach, breast and cervix cancer incidences (Fig. 2). For each figure, the two axes define the plane of the circle with location of the variables (food intake, cancer incidence) in its plane (close association, opposition). The length of the radius illustrates the value of the contribution coefficient of

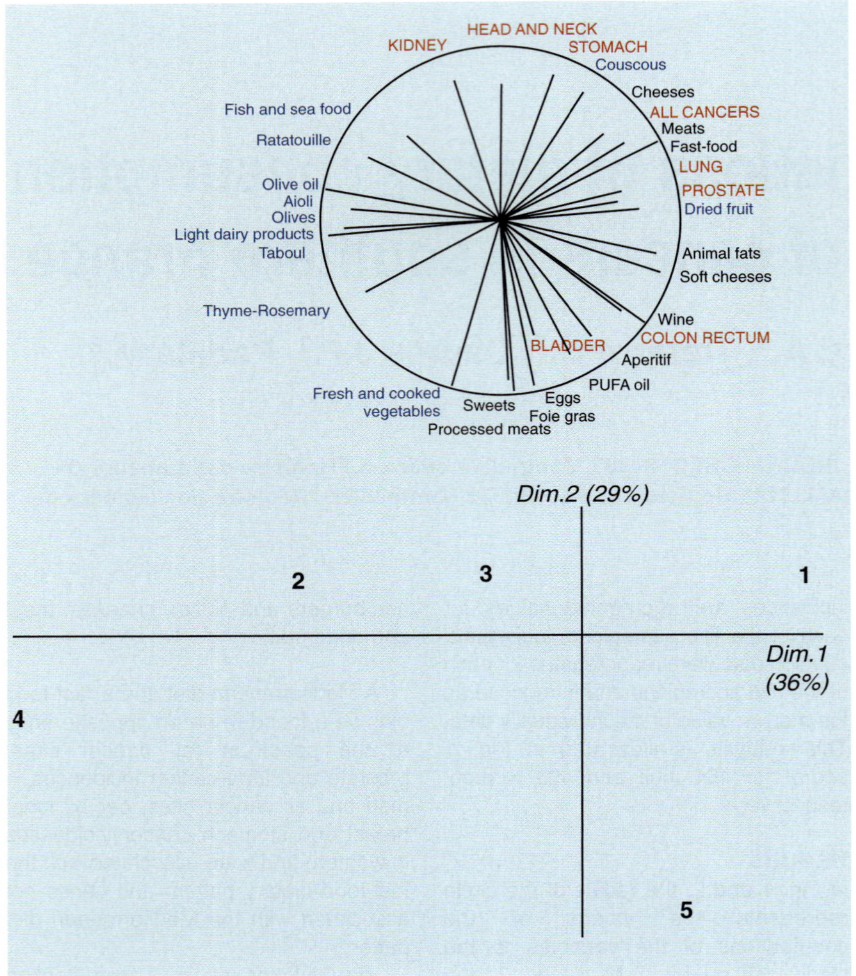

Figure 1
Principal component analysis of cancer incidences and nutritional data in men

the variables in relation to the plane.

Individuals (subregions) are characterized by the coordinate that situates each region in relation to each axis. Subregions 1, 4 and 5 are clearly dissociated along the two axes in both sexes. When they are projected on this representation, regions 4 (rural area in keeping with traditional dietary pattern) and 2 (coastal area in keeping with traditional dietary pattern) are clearly projected onto the Mediterranean diet pattern. Region 5 (the southwest subregion) is related to its typical dietary pattern. Bladder cancer in men shows a weak association with the dietary pattern of region 5, but this risk may be confounded by occupational risk in this region (use of solvents in the leather industry). Region 1 (the city of Montpellier and the suburbs) is projected on the fast-food pattern. Region 3, which contains a medium-sized city in a wine-producing area with an intermediary diet pattern (loss of Mediterranean or traditional pattern, influence of urbanization), shows a high incidence of kidney cancer in both sexes, and head and neck cancers in men, without any clear association with an identified food pattern.

For both sexes, PCA has displayed a fast-food profile, associated with a strong incidence of cancers within Greater Montpellier and a Mediterranean food profile, associated with low incidences of cancer in the rural area of Haut-Cantons.

Therefore, the urban way of life and its food components seem to be associated with risk of cancer.

References

Bonifacj, C., Gerber, M., Scali, J. & Daurès, J.P. (1997) Comparison of dietary assessment methods in Southern French population. Use of weighed records, estimated-diet records and food-frequency questionnaire. *Eur. J. Clin. Nutr.*, **51**, 217–231

Daurès, J.P., Gerber, M., Scali, J., Astre, C., Bonifacj, C. & Kaaks, R. (2000) Validation of a food frequency questionnaire using multiple day records and biochemical markers: application of the methods of triads. *J. Epidemiol. Biostat.*, **5**, 109–115

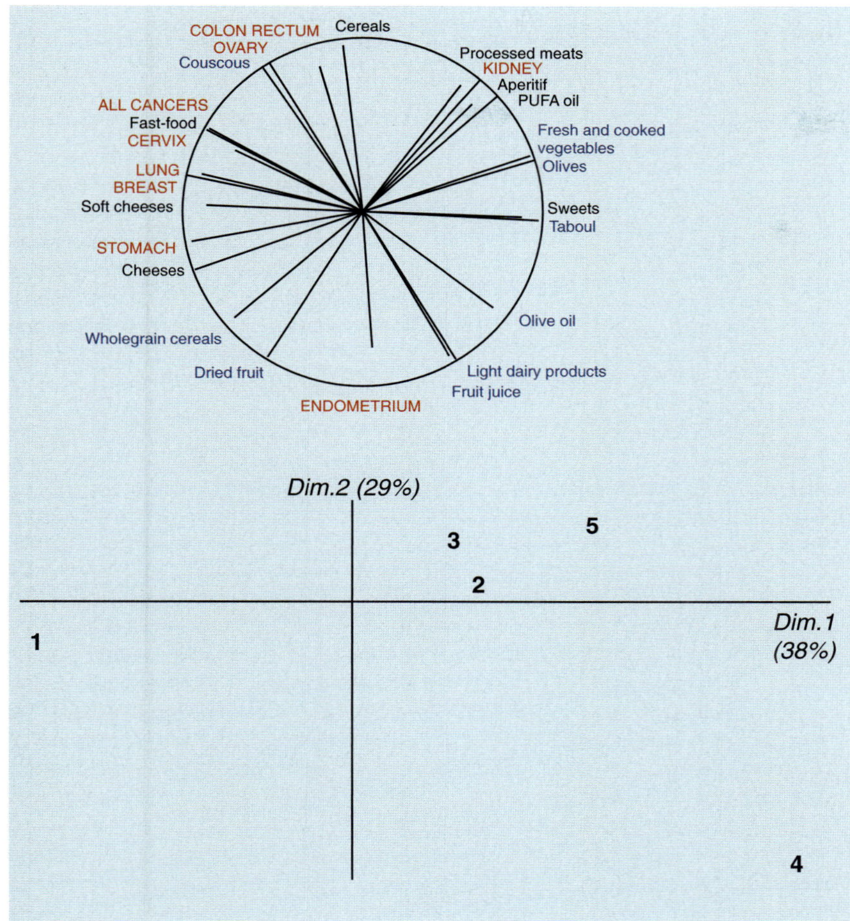

Figure 2
Principal component analysis of cancer incidences and nutritional data in women

Mortality and fresh fruit consumption

Appleby P.N.[1], Key T.J.[1], Burr M.L.[2], Thorogood M.[3]

[1]Cancer Research UK Epidemiology Unit, University of Oxford, Gibson Building, The Radcliffe Infirmary, Oxford, OX2 6HE, UK. [2]Centre for Applied Public Health Medicine, Temple of Peace and Health, Cathays Park, Cardiff, CF1 3NW, UK. [3]Department of Public Health and Policy, London School of Hygiene and Tropical Medicine, Keppel Street, London, WC1E 7HT, UK.

Introduction

It has been estimated that diets containing substantial and varied amounts of fruits and vegetables could prevent at least 20% of all cases of cancer (World Cancer Research Fund, 1997). A recent analysis of data from the EPIC Norfolk cohort found an inverse association between plasma vitamin C (of which fruits and vegetables are the major dietary source) and mortality from all causes of death, cardiovascular disease, and ischaemic heart disease, and from cancer in men only (Khaw *et al.*, 2001). To estimate the benefits that might arise from a greater consumption of these foods, we examined mortality with respect to fresh fruit intake in the Health Food Shoppers Study. The analysis reported here updates previous analyses of mortality data from this study after follow-up to 1980 (Burr & Sweetnam, 1982), 1985 (Burr & Butland, 1988) and 1995 (Key *et al.*, 1996).

Study population

The Health Food Shoppers study is a prospective study of nearly 11 000 health-conscious British subjects who completed a simple diet and lifestyle questionnaire between 1973 and 1979 (Burr & Sweetnam, 1982). Subjects were followed up to 31 December 1997. Those who died were coded for underlying cause of death using the 9th revision of the International Classification of Diseases (ICD-9). We analysed mortality up to age 90 among subjects aged 16–89 years at recruitment who provided information on fresh fruit intake and smoking habits and had no prior cancer registration, except for non-melanoma skin cancer (ICD-9 173). Cox regression analysis was used to estimate death rate ratios for subjects consuming fresh fruit daily compared with less frequent consumers for each of 13 major causes of death, including several cancers, adjusted for age, sex and smoking. Subset analyses examined mortality in men, women, and non-smokers, and mortality further adjusted for four other dietary factors.

Results

Most subjects (77%) reported eating fresh fruit daily. Daily consumers of fresh fruit were more likely to be female (63% versus 50%), less likely to smoke (16% versus 31%), and were generally older (median age at recruitment 47 versus 44) than less frequent consumers. There were 2529 deaths before age 90 in more than 213 000 person-years of observation. Compared with less frequent consumers, subjects consuming fresh fruit daily had lower mortality for all of the causes of death examined. Death rate ratios were significantly below 1 for all causes of death combined, all malignant neoplasms, lung cancer, circulatory diseases, ischaemic heart disease, and respiratory disease (Table 1). The results were similar among non-smokers, but the benefits of daily fresh fruit consumption appeared to be greater among women than among men (Table 1). In no instances were death rates significantly higher among daily consumers of fresh fruit.

Subjects were also classified according to their consumption of wholemeal bread, nuts or dried fruit, raw vegetable salads, and bran cereals. For each of these foods, especially wholemeal bread, daily consumers usually had lower mortality than less frequent consumers (results not shown). We calculated death rate ratios for mortality up to age 90 for daily consumers of each of these foods, plus fresh fruit, adjusted for age, sex and smoking and for each other food (Table 2). Death rate ratios for daily consumers of fresh fruit compared with less frequent consumers remained significantly below 1 for all causes of death combined, all malignant

Table 1. Mortality by fresh fruit consumption[a, b, c]

Cause of death (ICD-9 codes)	All subjects (*n*=10741)	Men (*n*=4325)	Women (*n*=6416)	Non-smokers (*n*=8675)
All causes of death	612 vs 1917	326 vs 834	286 vs 1083	427 vs 1628
(1–999)	0.81 (0.74–0.89)[e]	0.90 (0.79–1.03)	0.72 (0.63–0.82)[e]	0.81 (0.73–0.90)[e]
All malignant neoplasms	172 vs 508	96 vs 188	76 vs 320	110 vs 433
(140–208)	0.79 (0.66–0.95)[d]	0.72 (0.56–0.93[d]	0.88 (0.68–1.13)	0.86 (0.70–1.07)
Stomach cancer	9 vs 31	3 vs 14	6 vs 17	5 vs 27
(151)	0.88 (0.41–1.88)	1.73 (0.49–6.16)	0.52 (0.20–1.34)	1.12 (0.43–2.93)
Colorectal cancer	22 vs 78	13 vs 27	9 vs 51	18 vs 68
(153–154)	0.88 (0.54–1.43)	0.67 (0.34–1.32)	1.13 (0.55–2.32)	0.81 (0.48–1.37)
Pancreas cancer	10 vs 29	7 vs 10	3 vs 19	7 vs 24
(157)	0.74 (0.35–1.55)	0.50 (0.18–1.34)	1.22 (0.36–4.14)	0.72 (0.31–1.68)
Lung cancer	35 vs 46	26 vs 25	9 vs 21	10 vs 27
(162)	0.53 (0.33–0.85)[e]	0.47 (0.27–0.84)[d]	0.62 (0.28–1.38)	0.65 (0.31–1.35)
Female breast cancer	–	–	20 vs 70	16 vs 63
(174)			0.77 (0.46–1.27)	0.79 (0.45–1.37)
Prostate cancer	–	13 vs 28	–	6 vs 27
(185)	–	0.66 (0.34–1.29)	–	1.18 (0.49–2.85)
Circulatory diseases	282 vs 920	156 vs 435	126 vs 485	204 vs 777
(390–459)	0.83 (0.73–0.96)[e]	0.95 (0.79–1.14)	0.70 (0.58–0.86)[e]	0.80 (0.69–0.94)[e]
Ischaemic heart disease	161 vs 444	95 vs 252	66 vs 192	121 vs 363
(410–414)	0.74 (0.61–0.89)[e]	0.89 (0.70–1.14)	0.52 (0.39–0.70)[e]	0.67 (0.54–0.82)[e]
Cerebrovascular disease	78 vs 278	37 vs 105	41 vs 173	56 vs 247
(430–438)	0.83 (0.64–1.07)	0.89 (0.61–1.31)	0.78 (0.55–1.09)	0.87 (0.65–1.17)
Respiratory disease	74 vs 215	41 vs 92	33 vs 123	51 vs 190
(460–519)	0.71 (0.54–0.93)[d]	0.75 (0.52–1.10)	0.66 (0.45–0.98)[d]	0.77 (0.56–1.05)
All other causes	84 vs 274	33 vs 119	51 vs 155	62 vs 228
(1–139, 210–389, 520–999)	0.85 (0.66–1.09)	1.37 (0.92–2.03)	0.57 (0.41–0.79)[e]	0.77 (0.58–1.02)

[a]Table shows numbers of deaths among subjects eating fresh fruit less than daily (first number) versus those eating fresh fruit daily.
[b]Death rate ratios with their 95% confidence interval for daily consumers compared with less frequent consumers, adjusted for age at recruitment and, where applicable, sex and smoking.
[c]Age at recruitment categories: <40, 40–44, 45–49, 50–54, 55–59, 60–64, 65–69, 70–74, 75–79, 80–84, 85–89; smoking categories: non-smoker, light smoker (<15 or unknown number of cigarettes per day, or other tobacco user), heavy smoker (15 or more cigarettes per day).
[d]$P<0.05$.
[e]$P<0.01$.

neoplasms, lung cancer, ischaemic heart disease, and respiratory disease. In contrast, of the other foods only wholemeal bread consumption showed significant differences in mortality between daily consumers and less frequent consumers.

Conclusions

Daily consumption of fresh fruit can make a significant contribution to cutting death rates from a wide variety of causes, including cancer. The fact that the results for fresh fruit stand out in comparison with those for other foods generally associated with a healthy diet suggests that fruit consumption is not simply acting as a marker for other diet or lifestyle factors and that the benefits are probably real.

Table 2. Mortality by consumption of various foods[a]

Cause of death (ICD-9 codes)	Fresh fruit	Wholemeal bread	Nuts/dried fruit	Raw vegetable salads	Bran cereals
All causes of death (1–999)	0.83 (0.75–0.91)[c]	0.89 (0.82–0.98)[b]	1.00 (0.92–1.10)	0.98 (0.90–1.07)	1.02 (0.94–1.12)
All malignant neoplasms (140–208)	0.78 (0.65–0.95)[b]	1.01 (0.85–1.20)	0.98 (0.83–1.17)	1.03 (0.87–1.23)	0.93 (0.78–1.11)
Stomach cancer (151)	1.01 (0.45–2.25)	0.84 (0.42–1.67)	0.53 (0.26–1.12)	1.19 (0.60–2.38)	0.77 (0.36–1.65)
Colorectal cancer (153–154)	0.93 (0.55–1.56)	1.21 (0.76–1.93)	0.83 (0.52–1.30)	0.93 (0.60–1.46)	1.14 (0.73–1.77)
Pancreas cancer (157)	0.83 (0.38–1.80)	0.86 (0.43–1.73)	0.79 (0.38–1.66)	0.82 (0.40–1.71)	1.10 (0.54–2.26)
Lung cancer (162)	0.52 (0.32–0.86)[b]	1.08 (0.67–1.76)	0.85 (0.48–1.49)	1.03 (0.60–1.76)	0.90 (0.52–1.58)
Female breast cancer (174)	0.66 (0.38–1.14)	1.22 (0.75–1.97)	1.32 (0.82–2.12)	1.29 (0.81–2.07)	0.63 (0.37–1.07)
Prostate cancer (185)	0.73 (0.35–1.50)	1.24 (0.59–2.57)	1.06 (0.52–2.14)	0.60 (0.29–1.25)	0.52 (0.23–1.18)
Circulatory diseases (390–459)	0.89 (0.77–1.03)	0.86 (0.76–0.98)[b]	0.94 (0.83–1.07)	0.94 (0.83–1.07)	1.04 (0.92–1.18)
Ischaemic heart disease (410–414)	0.80 (0.66–0.98)[b]	0.86 (0.72–1.03)	0.95 (0.79–1.14)	0.85 (0.71–1.02)	1.13 (0.94–1.35)
Cerebrovascular disease (430–438)	0.85 (0.64–1.12)	0.89 (0.70–1.13)	0.92 (0.73–1.17)	1.11 (0.88–1.41)	0.92 (0.73–1.17)
Respiratory disease (460–519)	0.73 (0.54–0.98)[b]	0.88 (0.67–1.14)	1.14 (0.87–1.48)	0.84 (0.64–1.10)	1.13 (0.88–1.47)
All other causes (1–139, 210–389, 520–999)	0.81 (0.62–1.06)	0.79 (0.63–1.00)	1.14 (0.90–1.44)	1.18 (0.93–1.49)	1.06 (0.84–1.34)

[a]Table shows death rate ratios with their 95% confidence interval for daily consumers compared with less frequent consumers of each food, adjusted for age at recruitment, sex where applicable, smoking, and each other food. Age at recruitment and smoking categories as Table 1.
[b]$P<0.05$.
[c]$P<0.01$.

References

Burr, M.L. & Butland, B.K. (1988) Heart disease in British vegetarians. *Am. J. Clin. Nutr.*, **48**, 830–832

Burr, M.L. & Sweetnam, P.M. (1982) Vegetarianism, dietary fibre, and mortality. *Am. J. Clin. Nutr.*, **36**, 873–877

Key, T.J., Thorogood, M., Appleby, P.N. & Burr, M.L. (1996) Dietary habits and mortality in 11 000 vegetarians and health conscious people: results of a 17-year follow-up. *Br. Med. J.*, **313**, 775–779

Khaw, K.-T., Bingham, S., Welch, A., Luben, R., Wareham, N., Oakes, S. & Day, N. (2001) Relation between plasma ascorbic acid and mortality in men and women in EPIC-Norfolk prospective study: a prospective population study. *Lancet*, **357**, 657–663

World Cancer Research Fund (1997) *Food Nutrition and the Prevention of Cancer: A Global Perspective.* WCRF/American Institute for Cancer Research, Washington, D.C.

Validation study of soya intake and plasma isoflavone levels among British women

Verkasalo P.K.[1], Appleby P.N.[1], Allen N.E.[1], Davey G.K.[1], Spencer E.A.[1], Postans J.[1], Adlercreutz H.[2], Key T.J.[1]

[1]Cancer Epidemiology Unit, Imperial Cancer Research Fund, University of Oxford, UK. [2]Institute for Preventative Medicine, Nutrition and Cancer, Helsinki, Finland.

Introduction

Soya products contain high levels of the isoflavones, genistein, daidzein and their glycosides, which have been identified as possible protective factors against hormone-dependent cancer. Ecological comparisons have shown rates of breast and prostate cancer to be lower in Asian populations, where soya bean consumption is high, than in Western countries where soya bean consumption is low (Adlercreutz and Mazur, 1997). However, little is known about the consumption of soya products in Western countries and whether soya intake is an accurate marker of serum isoflavone levels in these populations. The aim of this study was to examine the relationship between soya intake estimated from food frequency questionnaires (FFQ) and food diaries with serum isoflavone concentrations, among 80 women with a wide range of soya intakes.

Material and Methods

Cross-sectional data were taken from 80 women, aged between 20 and 39 years, who were participants in the Oxford arm of the European Prospective Investigation into Cancer and Nutrition (EPIC). All subjects completed a questionnaire containing questions of age, anthropometry, smoking and other lifestyle factors as well as a detailed semi-quantitative food frequency questionnaire (FFQ). This included two questions relating to the type and amount of milk consumed most often and a third question relating to the frequency of consumption of solid soya foods (such as tofu, soya meat, textured vegetable protein and vegeburgers) during the previous year. The study population of 80 women was selected to give a wide range of soya intakes as reported in the FFQ, and divided into four groups of 20 women each: Group I consumed no soya milk and no solid soya products; Group II consumed no soya milk but regularly consumed solid soya products (at least 5–6 times per week); Group III consumed some soya milk (142 ml per day) and some solid soya products (at most once per week); Group IV consumed a high amount of soya milk (284 ml or more per day) and a high amount of solid soya products (at least 2–4 times per week). Estimated intakes of daidzein and genistein were calculated from the FFQ and the food diary according to values provided by the United States Department of Agriculture (USDA, 1999). A 30-ml non-fasting blood sample was taken at the time of recruitment and plasma concentrations of daidzein and genistein were measured by time-resolved fluoroimmunoassay (Wang *et al.*, 2000).

Results

Reported soya intakes varied more than 100-fold between the four intake groups and plasma isoflavone concentrations increased with increasing soya. Women who consumed the most soya milk and solid soya products (Group IV) had mean plasma isoflavone levels of 378 and 525 nmol/l for genistein and daidzein, respectively (Figure 1). This is comparable to that of Asian populations who are known to consume large amounts of soya.

Soya intake as measured by the FFQ and the food diary correlated well with plasma isoflavone concentrations. Spearman correlation coefficients between soya intakes based on the food diary and serum daidzein and genistein concentrations were high (0.78–0.80 for total soya, 0.74–0.77 for soya milk and 0.66–0.69 for solid soya products). Of the FFQ-based estimates, high correlations were observed for total soya (0.78 for both isoflavones) and soya milk intake (0.72 for both

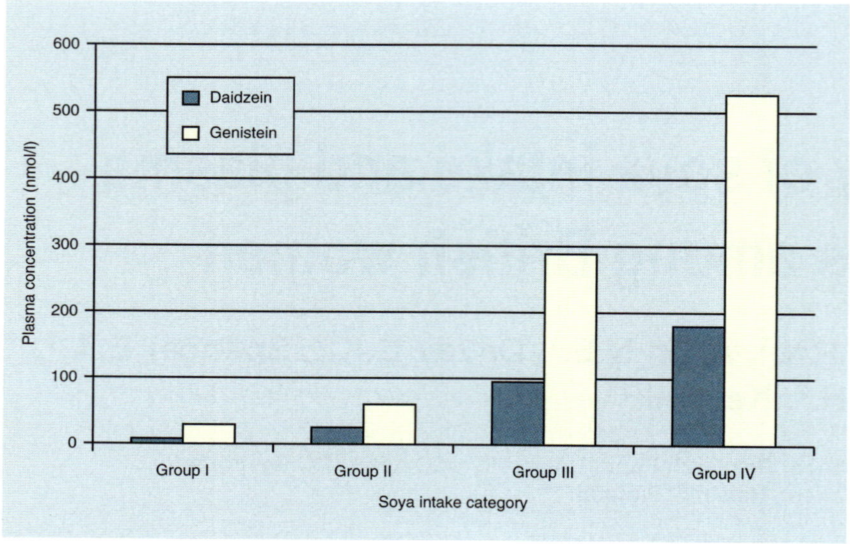

Figure 1
Geometric mean concentrations of plasma daidzein and genistein in 80 premenopausal women by soya intake group

Group I, no soya intake; Group II, no soya milk and soya foods 5–6 times per week; Group III, 142 ml per day soya milk and soya foods once a week or less; Group IV: 284+ ml per day soya milk and soya foods 2–4 times per week.

isoflavones), but the correlations for solid soya product intake were low (0.24–0.28). Compared to information provided by the food diary, the FFQ had a tendency to overestimate low intakes of solid soya foods and underestimate high intakes of solid soya.

Discussion

British women with high intakes of soya have plasma isoflavones that are comparable with Asian women on a traditional diet, which has recently been reported to provide about 30 mg of isoflavones per day (Chen *et al.*, 1999; Arai *et al.*, 2000). The plasma isoflavone concentrations in British women who eat little or no soya were comparable to other Western populations (Adlercreutz and Mazur, 1997). Both the FFQ and the food diary provide estimates for soya intake that correlate well with plasma isoflavone levels. The diary performed somewhat better, but for many purposes, the questions related to soya milk consumption on the FFQ will provide reasonably valid estimates of isoflavone consumption in this population.

References

Adlercreutz, H. & Mazur, W. (1997) Phyto-oestrogens and Western diseases. *Ann. Med.*, **29**, 95–120

Arai, Y., Watanabe, S., Kimira, M., Shimoi, K., Mochizuki, R. & Kinae, N. (2000) Dietary intakes of flavonols, flavones and isoflavones by Japanese women and the inverse correlation between quercetin intake and plasma LDL cholesterol concentration. *J. Nutr.*, **130**, 2243–2250

Chen, Z., Zheng, W., Custer, L.J., Dai, Q., Shu, X.O., Jin, F. & Franke, A.A. (1999) Usual dietary consumption of soy foods and its correlation with the excretion rate of isoflavonoids in overnight urine samples among Chinese women in Shanghai. *Nutr. Cancer*, **33**, 82–87

USDA (1999) *USDA-Iowa State University Database on Isoflavone Content of Foods.* release 12. http://www.nal.usda.gov/fnic/foodcomp/Data/isoflav/isoflav.html. accessed 06/2000

Wang, G.J., Lapcik, O., Hampl, R., Uehara, M., Al-Maharik, N., Stumpf, K., Mikola, H., Wahala, K. & Adlercreutz, H. (2000) Time-resolved fluoroimmunoassay of plasma daidzein and genistein. *Steroids*, **65**, 339–348

Fruit and vegetable intake and chronic disease risk in Portugal

Reis M.F.[1], Oliveira L.[1], Pereirinha A.[2], Pereira Miguel J.M.[2]

[1]Food Safety and Nutrition Centre, INSA, Lisbon, Portugal. [2]Institute of Preventive Medicine, Faculty of Medicine, Lisbon, Portugal.

Introduction

High intake of fruits and vegetables has been associated with decreased risk of chronic disease, namely cardiovascular disease (CVD) and cancer. This beneficial effect on health may be related to fruit- and vegetable-component antioxidant capacity and to their participation in homocysteine metabolism. Total plasma homocysteine (tHcy) is an accepted independent marker for atherosclerotic cardiovascular risk and a moderate rise in tHcy level (≥ 15 μmol/l) has been described to result in a 1.5- to 3-fold higher risk for coronary and cerebral events. A moderate rise in tHcy seems to be associated with unbalanced eating habits leading to a decrease in vitamin B_{12}, B_6 and folate blood levels. These dietary factors are involved in methionine/homocysteine metabolism and recent studies have demonstrated the influence of dietary patterns on tHcy plasma levels. Oxidative DNA damage has been implicated in several diseases, including cancer, and 8-hydroxy-deoxyguanosine (8-OHdG) is generally regarded as a reliable indicator of such damage. The antioxidant activity of fruit and vegetable components, vitamins C and E and possibly carotenoids, has been associated with protection against oxidative stress. Although high carotenoid blood levels have been related to a decreased risk of cancer and CVD, supplementation trials with carotenoids did not confirm this relationship. However, carotenoid concentration in blood has been proved to correlate directly with fruit and vegetable intake and can be used as markers of consumption.

CVD is the main cause of death in Portugal (40%) followed by cancer (20%). Little is known about the actual fruit and vegetable consumption and the related essential nutrient intake by the Portuguese population and its potential effects in chronic disease risk in our country.

Purpose

The general aim of this study is to contribute to the characterization of the Portuguese population regarding fruit and vegetable consumption and its potential effects on morbidity and mortality indexes associated with chronic disease.

The specific objectives of this project are:

1) to determine carotenoid serum levels in well-known Portuguese population groups and to relate these levels to the estimate of fruit and vegetable consumption obtained by a semi-quantitative food frequency questionnaire;

2) to determine tHcy, folate and vitamin B_{12} and B_6 plasma levels in the same population groups and to relate tHcy blood levels with the determined vitamin and carotenoid levels;

3) to determine vitamin C and E plasma levels and 8-OHdG in the same individuals and to relate these with both tHcy blood levels and the conventional CVD risk factors.

Methods

Population groups and sampling procedure

Participants will be adult well-informed volunteer (≤ 55 years) patients at the Santa Maria Hospital or the National Institute of Health services in Lisbon. Two samples will be considered for the case–control study: the control sample will comprise individuals from the target population without vascular or alimentary disease; the case sample will comprise patients suffering from recent acute myocardial infarction.

Evaluation instruments

A questionnaire tested for this sample type will be used. The questionnaire includes general socio-demographic questions and specific questions on clinical history, food intake, smoking and physical activity habits, psychosocial aspects and anthropometric data.

Analytical methods

Analysis of tHcy, 8-OHdG, vitamins C, B_6, E and carotenoids will be performed by HPLC validated methods with different final detection methods (ultraviolet, diode array detector, fluorometric, electrochemical). Folates and vitamin B_{12} will be analysed using microbiological methods.

Data analysis

The data obtained will be coded and validated and a database will be created. Statistical analysis will be performed with appropriate models using SPSS and Epi-info software.

Expected results

- Characterization of Portuguese population groups regarding fruit and vegetable intake as well as several related nutrient blood levels.
- Evaluation of CVD risk and the relation between classic CVD risk factors and tHcy blood levels in these groups.
- Evaluation of the association of fruit and vegetable intake with myocardial infarction.

References

Appel, L.J., Miller E.R. III, Jee, S.H., Stolzenberg-Solomon, R., Lin, P-H., Erlinger, T., Nadeau, M.R. & Selhub, J. (2000) Effect of dietary patterns on serum homocysteine. *Circulation*, **102**, 852–857

Broekmans, W.M., Klopping-Ketelaars, I.A., Schuurman, C.R., Verhagen, H., van den Berg, H., Kok, F.J. & van Poppel, G. (2000) Fruits and vegetables increase plasma carotenoids and vitamins and decrease homocysteine in humans. *J. Nutr.*, **130**, 1578–1583

Collins, A.R., Olmedilla, B., Southon, S., Granado, F. & Duthie, S. J. (1998) Serum carotenoids and oxidative DNA damage in human lymphocytes. *Carcinogenesis*, **19**, 2159–1262

Eichholzer, M., Luthy, J., Gutzwiller, F. & Stahelin, H. B. (2001) The role of folate, antioxidant vitamins and other constituents in fruit and vegetables in the prevention of cardiovascular disease: the epidemiological evidence. *Int. J. Vitam. Nutr. Res.*, **71**, 5–17

Olmedilla, B., Granado, F., Southon, S., Wright, A.J., Blanco, I., Gil-Martinez, E., Berg, H., Corridan, B., Roussel, A.M., Chopra, M. & Thurnham, D.I. (2000) Serum concentrations of carotenoids and vitamins A, E, and C in control subjects from five European countries. *Br. J. Nutr.*, **85**, 227–238

Fruit and vegetable consumption and colorectal cancer incidence

Michels K.B., Giovannucci E., Joshipura K.J., Rosner B.A., Stampfer M.J., Fuchs C.S., Colditz G.A., Speizer F.E., Willett W.C.
Harvard University, Boston, MA, USA.

Background

Frequent consumption of fruits and vegetables has been associated with a reduced risk of colorectal cancer in many observational studies, most of which were retrospective case–control studies. Fruits and vegetables could confer protection through anticarcinogenic components such as antioxidants, folic acid, flavonoids, organosulfides, isothiocyanates, and protease inhibitors as well as fermentable fiber. The purpose of this study was to examine the relation between repeatedly assessed fruit and vegetable consumption and subsequent incidence of colon and rectal cancer among women and men.

Methods

We prospectively investigated the association of fruit and vegetable consumption with the incidence of colon and rectal cancers in two large cohorts: the Nurses' Health Study (data from 88 764 female registered nurses) and the Health Professionals Follow-up Study (data from 47 328 male health professionals). The incidence of newly diagnosed cancer of the colon and rectum was confirmed by review of medical records and pathology reports and ascertained up to 1996 in both cohorts. Diet was assessed and cumulatively updated in 1980, 1984, 1986, and 1990 among women and in 1986 and 1990 among men, using a detailed food frequency questionnaire (FFQ). We created food groups of fruit and vegetable consumption and subgroups of fruits and vegetables including citrus fruit, fruits and vegetables rich in vitamin C, green leafy vegetables, cruciferous vegetables, potatoes, and legumes. Consumption of fruits and vegetables was grouped into five frequency categories. In addition, relative risk estimates for an increase in intake by one serving per day were obtained using daily consumption as a continuous variable. Analyses were adjusted for age, family history of colorectal cancer, history of sigmoidoscopy, height, body mass index, physical activity, regular aspirin use, pack-years of smoking, vitamin supplement use, alcohol consumption, total caloric intake, red meat consumption, and (among women) menopausal status and post-menopausal hormone use.

Results

With a follow-up including 1 743 539 person-years and 937 cases of colon cancer, we found little association with fruit and vegetable intake. A difference in fruit and vegetable consumption of one additional serving per day was associated with a covariate-adjusted relative risk (RR) of 1.02 (95% confidence interval [CI], 0.99–1.05). A difference in vegetable consumption of one additional serving per day was associated with a RR of 1.03 (CI, 0.99–1.08). These associations were similar for women and men. A difference in fruit consumption of one additional serving per day was associated with a RR of 0.96 (95% CI, 0.89–1.03) among women and 1.08 (CI, 1.00–1.16) among men. For rectal cancer (244 cases), the respective estimate for fruit and vegetable consumption was 1.00 (CI, 0.94–1.06). None of the subgroups of fruits and vegetables emerged as an important predictor of colon or rectal cancer in women and men.

Conclusions

In these two longitudinal studies of women and men with repeated diet assessment over time, we found no overall association between fruit and vegetable consumption and colon or rectal cancer incidence. Further, we did not find evidence of any appreciable benefit from any of the specific subgroups of fruits and vegetables considered, including citrus fruit, fruits and vegetables rich in vitamin C, green leafy vegetables, cruciferous vegetables, potatoes, and legumes. As the assessment of diet is inevitably affected by measurement error, this has to be considered in interpreting the observed results. The use of cumulatively updated dietary data, however, should have reduced at least random within-person measurement error. A careful evaluation of previous studies revealed that often only one food or food group emerged as inversely related to colon or rectal cancer.

In summary, although frequent consumption of fruits and vegetables may have beneficial effects on some chronic diseases, these data do not support an important protective effect against colorectal cancer.

References

Michels, K.B., Giovannucci, E., Joshipura, K.J., Rosner, B.A., Stampfer, M.J., Fuchs, C.S., Colditz, G.A., Speizer, F.E. & Willett, W.C. (2000) A prospective study of fruit and vegetable consumption and colorectal cancer incidence. *J. Natl. Cancer Inst.*, **92**, 1740–1752

Diet and the risk of cancers of the lung, oral cavity and pharynx, and larynx: a population-based case–control study in north-east Italy

Pisa F.E.[1], **Barbone F.**[1, 2]

[1]Cattedra di Igiene, DPMSC, University of Udine, Italy. [2]Dept. Epidemiology and Intl. Health, Univ. of Alabama at Birmingham, Birmingham, AL, USA.

The province of Udine, north-east Italy, has among the highest mortality rates in Italy for cancers of the lung (ICD-IX 162), oral cavity and pharynx (ICD-IX 140–149) and larynx (ICD-IX 161) (Bidoli *et al.*, 1999). The role of diet on the risk of these cancers has reached sound international evidence (WCRF/AIRC, 1997) and is confirmed in hospital-based studies in north-east Italy. Using a population-based case–control design, we studied the role of diet on the risk of cancers of the lung, oral cavity and pharynx, and larynx in three health districts of the province. Among residents in the three health districts, we identified all histologically confirmed cases diagnosed from 1 March to 31 December 1996. Using a validated food frequency questionnaire, we interviewed 111 cases of cancer of the lung, 58 of the oral cavity and pharynx and 43 of the larynx as well as 247 population controls matched by sex, year of birth, and health district of residence. Year of birth- sex- and dose of smoking-adjusted odds ratios (OR) and 95% confidence intervals (95% CI) were calculated by unconditional logistic regression. Other variables did not modify the results and were excluded from the final model.

As expected, cigarette smoking was strongly associated with these cancers (Table 1). An association was also found between alcohol consumption and cancers of the lung (drinkers of 30.5 and more drinks/week versus abstainers, OR, 2.0, 95% CI, 0.6–6.4), oral cavity and pharynx (OR, 4.0, 95% CI, 0.9–18.9) and larynx (OR, 1.6, 95% CI, 0.3–9.8). Decreased risk was associated with frequent consumption of vegetables and fruits (Table 3). Frequent consumption of meat and processed meat was associated with an increased risk (Table 2).

Although the most relevant risk factors are tobacco smoking and alcohol drinking, efforts to prevent cancers of the lung, oral cavity and pharynx, larynx in the province of Udine should also focus on diet.

References

Bidoli, E., Franceschi, S., Redivo, A., Simon, G., Piffer, S., Zanier, L. & Simonato, L. (1999) *Atlas of Cancer Mortality in Northeastern Regions and Provinces and in Italy, 1990–1994.* Centro di Riferimento Oncologico, Aviano, Italy

World Cancer Research Fund/American Institute for Cancer Research (1997) *Food, Nutrition and the Prevention of Cancer: A Global Perspective.* WCRF/AICR, Washington, DC

Franceschi, S., Bidoli, E., Baron, A.E., Barra, S., Talamini, R., Serraino, D. & La Vecchia, C. (1991) Nutrition and cancer of the oral cavity and pharynx in North-east Italy. *Int. J. Cancer*, **47**, 20–25

Table 1. Odds ratio and 95% confidence interval for cancer of the lung, oral cavity and pharynx, and larynx according to cigarette smoking and alcohol drinking

	Cases												Controls	
	Lung				Oral cavity + pharynx				Larynx					
	n	%	OR[b]	95% CI	*n*	%	OR[b]	95% CI	*n*	%	OR[b]	95% CI	*n*	%
Smoking status														
Never smoker[a]	8	7	1.0	–	5	9	1.0	–	1	2	1.0	–	86	35
Ex-smoker	38	34	4.3	1.8–10.3	24	41	6.0	2.1–17.3	22	51	20.6	2.6–159.7	101	41
Current smoker	65	59	12.9	5.5–29.9	29	50	9.6	3.4–27.1	20	46	27.5	3.5–214.2	60	24
Dose of smoking, packs per year														
Never smoker[a]	8	7	1.0	–	5	9	1.0	–	1	2	1.0	–	86	35
<45	46	41	5.3	2.3–12.5	31	53	6.0	2.2–16.9	21	49	17.1	2.2–132.4	118	48
45–89	36	32	20.8	7.8–55.3	15	26	15.8	4.8–51.9	16	37	62.1	7.4–520.5	28	11
90+	21	19	22.9	7.8–66.8	7	12	14.2	3.7–55.4	5	12	34.7	3.6–335.8	15	6
Total drinks/week														
Abstainer[a]	9	8	1.0	–	3	5	1.0	–	3	7	1.0	–	23	9
1–5.5	8	7	0.5	0.2–1.9	6	10	1.2	0.2–6.2	1	2	0.1	0.0–1.0	39	16
6–13.5	14	13	1.1	0.3–3.6	6	10	1.2	0.2–6.1	1	2	–	–	43	17
14–20.5	19	17	1.2	0.4–3.8	11	19	1.8	0.4–8.1	5	12	0.5	0.1–3.2	49	20
21–30	21	19	1.3	0.4–4.2	8	14	2.3	0.4–12.0	14	33	2.7	0.4–17.7	46	19
30.5+	40	36	2.0	0.6–6.4	23	40	4.0	0.9–18.9	19	44	1.6	0.3–9.8	46	19

[a]Reference category.
[b]Odds ratio (OR) adjusted for year of birth and sex.
CI, confidence interval.

Table 2. Odds ratio and 95%CI for cancer of the lung, oral cavity and pharynx, and larynx according to the intake[a] of selected foods

	Cases												Controls	
	Lung				Oral cavity and pharynx				Larynx					
	n	%	OR[c]	95% CI	*n*	%	OR[c]	95% CI	*n*	%	OR[c]	95% CI	*n*	%
Green salad														
≤ 1[b]	12	11	1.0	–	12	21	1.0	–	6	14	1.0	–	23	9
2–3	18	16	1.5	0.6–4.1	10	17	0.7	0.2–2.2	8	19	1.9	0.5–7.2	25	10
4–6	34	31	1.3	0.5–3.2	16	28	0.6	0.2–1.5	10	23	1.1	0.3–3.8	50	20
7+	47	42	0.7	0.3–1.6	20	34	0.3	0.1–0.7	19	44	0.9	0.3–3.0	148	60
Apples														
≤ 1[b]	21	19	1.0	–	17	29	1.0	–	12	28	1.0	–	31	13
2–3	27	24	1.2	0.5–2.7	11	19	0.6	0.2–1.6	11	26	0.9	0.3–2.7	33	13
4–6	27	24	0.7	0.3–1.6	11	19	0.3	0.1–0.7	6	14	0.3	0.1–0.8	66	27
7+	36	32	0.5	0.3–1.1	19	33	0.3	0.2–0.8	14	33	0.4	0.2–1.1	116	47
Tomatoes														
≤ 1[b]	15	13	1.0	–	19	33	1.0	–	14	33	1.0	–	35	14
2–3	44	40	1.9	0.9–4.3	17	29	0.5	0.2–1.2	8	19	0.4	0.1–1.1	63	26
4–6	30	27	1.1	0.5–2.5	8	14	0.2	0.1–0.4	8	19	0.3	0.1–0.9	87	35
7+	22	20	1.2	0.5–2.9	14	24	0.4	0.1–1.0	13	30	0.7	0.2–1.7	61	25
Citrus fruits														
≤ 1[b]	15	14	1.0	–	15	26	1.0	–	14	33	1.0	–	47	19
1–3	52	47	2.8	1.3–6.0	21	36	1.1	0.5–2.5	15	35	0.8	0.3–2.2	61	25
4–6	22	20	1.0	0.5–2.4	13	22	0.5	0.2–1.1	7	16	0.3	0.1–1.0	79	32
7+	21	19	1.3	0.6–3.0	9	15	0.4	0.1–1.1	7	16	0.4	0.1–1.2	59	24
Carrots														
≤ 1[b]	38	34	1.0	–	18	31	1.0	–	15	35	1.0	–	55	22
1	24	22	0.8	0.4–1.7	13	22	1.0	0.4–2.3	12	28	1.0	0.4–2.7	50	20
2–3	34	31	0.8	0.4–1.6	17	29	0.8	0.3–1.8	9	21	0.6	0.2–1.7	77	31
4+	15	14	0.5	0.2–1.0	10	17	0.6	0.2–1.5	7	17	0.7	0.2–1.9	63	26
Meat														
≤ 1[b]	14	13	1.0	–	9	15	1.0	–	6	14	1.0	–	61	25
2–3	53	48	1.8	0.9–3.7	27	47	1.5	0.6–3.5	24	56	1.7	0.6–4.8	123	50
4+	44	40	2.4	1.1–5.1	22	38	2.0	0.8–5.1	13	30	1.4	0.5–4.4	62	25
Processed meat														
≤ 1[b]	12	11	1.0	–	6	10	1.0	–	6	14	1.0	–	46	19
1	17	15	1.2	0.5–3.0	9	15	1.0	0.3–3.2	7	16	0.6	0.2–2.0	56	23
2–3	57	51	2.4	1.1–5.2	26	45	2.0	0.7–5.4	17	39	1.0	0.3–3.0	98	40
4+	25	22	2.1	0.8–5.1	17	29	2.1	0.7–6.6	13	30	1.4	0.4–4.5	46	19

[a]Servings per week.
[b]Reference category.
[c]Adjusted for year of birth, sex and dose of smoking.
OR, odds ratio; CI, confidence interval.

Dietary factors and epithelial cell exfoliation in the human colon

Bailey N., Bandaletova T., Loktionov A., Cross A.J., Bingham S.
MRC Dunn Human Nutrition Unit, Hills Road, Cambridge CB2 2XY, UK.

Introduction

Diet is a major factor in colon cancer risk with nutrients influencing either the development or the prevention of tumours. A typical Western diet high in meat, fat and calories but low in vegetables and fibre may contribute to the risk of colon cancer development (WCRF 1997). Abnormal renewal of the gastrointestinal tract epithelium is also associated with a disposition to this disease (Eastwood, 1995) but the relationship between proliferation, differentiation and exfoliation is poorly understood. In this study we used a noninvasive immunomagnetic technique to isolate exfoliated colonocytes from human stool samples. Eleven healthy non-smoking male volunteers participated in three different dietary periods, one high in meat, one low in meat and one void of meat, to study the relationship between diet and colonic cell turnover.

Materials and methods

Study design

Eleven healthy non-smoking males were recruited for the study which followed a random crossover design with three 15-day dietary periods: low red meat 60 g/day (LM), high red meat 420 g/day (HM) and vegetarian diet providing the same amount of protein as the high red meat diet, but from non-meat sources of protein (VEG). Diets were isoenergetic and contained the same amount of fat.

Isolation of exfoliated colonocytes

Fresh cooled faecal samples were washed with ice-cold dispersing solution (pH 7.4) and sieved. Addition of 40 µl Immunomagnetic beads was followed by a 30-min incubation at 4°C. Bead-cell complexes were magnetically isolated by passing the wash through a column attached to a strong magnetic field. Labelled cells remained in the column and were washed with PBS before removal from the magnet and the cells then gently eluted by means of a plunger.

Cytological analysis

Prepared hematoxylin stained smears were analysed using direct cell counting in 40 microscope fields. Squamous epithelial cells were ignored and only single or clusters of colonocytes that were characteristically distinguishable were included.

Immunocytochemistry

Exfoliated cells were further characterized using immunostaining for epithelium-specific cytokeratin 5/8 C50.

Results

Exfoliated colonocytes were successfully isolated from all subjects though not necessarily during each dietary period. Figure 1 shows exfoliated colonocytes positively stained for cytokeratin C50. There was a variation in cell number recovery from sample to sample in each volunteer and between individual volunteers. Figure 2 presents results of the assessment of mean exfoliated cell numbers expressed as cell numbers per gram of stool from volunteers from each dietary period. There were no significant differences by analysis of variance according to diet and mean values (±SE) were as follows: VEG, 0.350 ± 0.363; LRM, 0.252 ± 0.218; HRM, 0.202 ± 0.306, $P>0.05$.

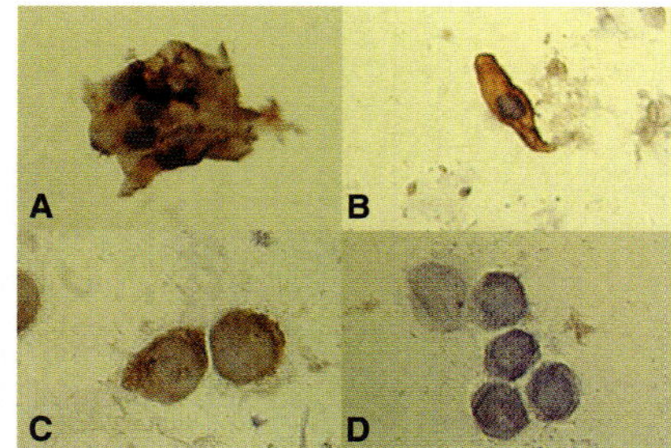

Figure 1
Exfoliated colonocytes stained with cytokeratin 5/8 C50 (A, B). (C) shows the human colon carcinoma cell line stained with cytokeratin 5/8 C50 HT-29 as a positive control and (D) shows the cell line with secondary antibody replaced with PBS as a negative control

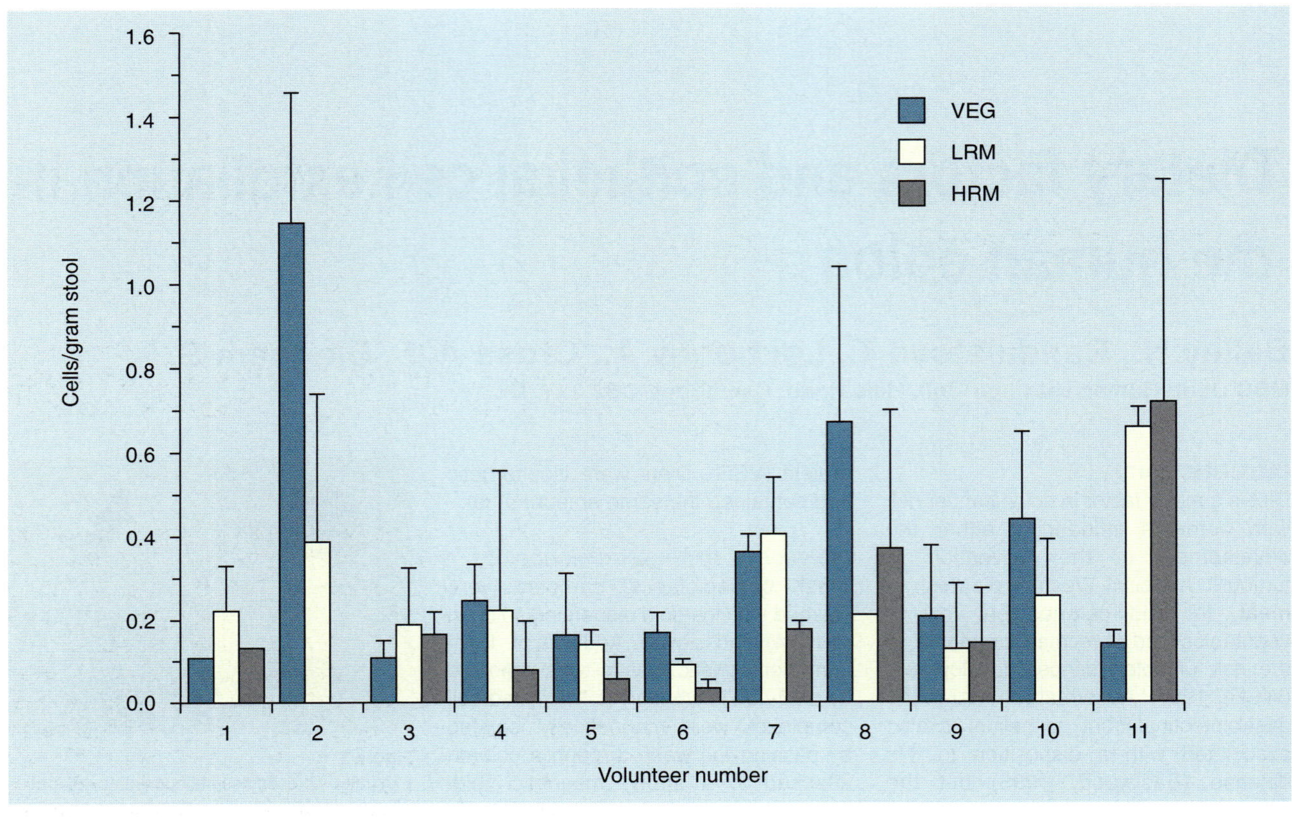

Figure 2
Mean exfoliated cell numbers per gram of stool for each volunteer over the three different dietary periods

Discussion

The direct contact between food residues and the large bowel mucosa plays an important role in the development of colon cancer with cellular turnover being directly associated with colon tumour development (Owen 2001). Because the colonic epithelium undergoes such a rapid renewal, culminating in exfoliation of differentiated colonocytes into the gut lumen, it can be seen as a viable source of material for biomarker analysis (Iyengar *et al.*, 1991). In this study we have been able to reliably isolate exfoliated cells from stool samples as predicted. This material is potentially useful for biomarker analysis. Cells were shown to be derived from the gut epithelium by staining with cytokeratin C50, a marker of epithelial origin. The considerable variation in the number of exfoliated cells between different subjects can possibly be explained by individual traits such as transit time, gut flora, and stool composition. Although cells were successfully isolated and characterized by immunocytochemistry, there were no obvious effects from diet, because no significant difference in exfoliation was observed between the three different dietary periods.

References

Eastwood, G.L. (1995) A review of gastrointestinal epithelial renewal and its relevance to the development of adenocarcinomas of the gastrointestinal tract. *J. Clin. Gastroenterol.*, **21**, Suppl 1, S1–S11

Iyengar, V., Albaugh, G.P., Lohani, A. & Nair, P.P. (1991) Human stools as a source of viable colonic epithelial cells. *FASEB J.*, **5**, 2856–2859

Owen, R.W. (2001) Biomarkers in colorectal cancer. In: Miller, A.B., Bartsch, H., Boffetta, P., Dragsted, L. & Vainio, H. *Biomarkers in Cancer Chemoprevention* (IARC Scientific Publications No. 154), Lyon, IARC, pp. 101–111

World Cancer Research Fund (1997) *Food, Nutrition and the Prevention of Cancer*, American Institute for Cancer Research, Washington D.C.

Chapter 3

Alcoholic beverages

Alcoholic beverages and smoking

Franceschi S.

International Agency for Research on Cancer, 150, Cours Albert Thomas, 69372 Lyon Cédex 08, France.

Tobacco smoking and alcohol drinking stand out, in the epidemiological scenario, as the two risk factors for which the association with cancer is the strongest and most consistent. In addition to the strong effect of these two carcinogens or, better, carcinogenic cocktails, reasons include the relatively good validity of intake measurement and the generally prolonged duration of smoking and drinking habits.

Still, many aspects of smoking and drinking await further elucidation. With respect to cigarette smoking, for instance, the difference between modern filtered low-tar, low-nicotine cigarettes and older types with respect to cancer risk is far from clear. The inaccuracy of current estimates of tar content on cigarette packets only complicates the issue.

For alcohol drinking, aside from the very marked associations with cancer of the oral cavity, pharynx, oesophagus and larynx, weaker associations with cancers of the stomach, colon and rectum, liver, cervix uteri, and breast are more puzzling (Bagnardi *et al.*, 2001). For some cancer sites (e.g., liver, cervix), the important issue is confirming the role of alcohol in the absence of well-established additional causes (e.g., hepatitis B and C viruses and human papilloma virus). It seems unlikely, however, that the moderate, but consistent, association observed between alcohol and cancer of the breast is strongly confounded by the effect of known risk factors (e.g. menstrual and reproductive factors).

The metabolic effects of alcohol drinking and smoking are also new research priorities. It remains unclear, for instance, why, despite the apparent caloric density of alcohol, body weight, adipose tissue, and lean body mass are reduced among drinkers, or are not as great as expected (Hellerstedt *et al.*, 1990; Franceschi *et al.*, 2001). Also, smokers do tend to be consistently thinner (and former smokers fatter) than lifetime non-smokers (Franceschi *et al.*, 2001). Understanding the mechanism(s) of weight control among smokers is also an important question from a prevention viewpoint. The fear of weight gain, in a period when a real epidemic of obesity is taking place in developed as well as developing countries, should not be left to interfere with people's determination to stop smoking.

References

Bagnardi, V., Blangiardo, M., La Vecchia, C. & Corrao, G. (2001) A meta-analysis of alcohol drinking and cancer risk. *Br. J. Cancer*, **85**, 1700–1705

Franceschi, S., Levi, F., Conti, E., Talamini, R., Negri, E., Dal Maso, L., Boyle, P., Decarli, A. & La Vecchia, C. (1999) Energy intake and dietary pattern in cancer of the oral cavity and pharynx. *Cancer Causes Control*, **10**, 439–444

Franceschi, S., Dal Maso, L., Levi, F., Conti, E., Talamini, R. & La Vecchia, C. (2001) Leanness as early marker of cancer of the oral cavity and pharynx. *Ann. Oncol.*, **12**, 331–336

Hellerstedt, W.L., Jeffery, R.W. & Murray, D.M. (1990) The association between alcohol intake and adiposity in the general population. *Am. J. Epidemiol.*, **132**, 594–610

Alcohol and risk of cancer of the upper gastrointestinal tract: first analysis of the EPIC data

Boeing H.
(for the EPIC working group on dietary patterns)

German Institute of Human Nutrition, Dept of Epidemiology, Bergholz- Rehbrücke, Germany.

Introduction

About 390 000 new cancer cases of the oral cavity and oropharynx are seen worldwide today as well as about 412 000 new cases of oesophageal cancer. This is approximately 8% of the total cancer incidence (Ferlay *et al.*, 2001).

Cancer of the oral cavity and oropharynx is particularly high in Melanesia, South-Central Asia, South Africa and Europe. The highest incidence of oral cancer is seen in some areas of France (up to 55/100 000 males) (Blot *et al.*, 1996). This is about 20 times the number being found in low-incidence areas. The incidence of cancer at this site has increased in some Western European countries in the past. This trend, however, has not been observed in many other countries. The male-to-female ratio is about 2 for cancer of the mouth and about 4 for cancer of the oropharynx (Ferlay *et al.*, 2001). A well-established risk factor for oral cancer is tobacco smoking, showing a relative risk of about 6–10 for smokers versus non-smokers (Blot *et al.* 1996). A similar magnitude of relative risk was also seen for those drinking more then 30 g alcohol per day, although most studies did not support the idea that both factors act in a supra-multiplicative fashion (Jensen *et al.*, 1996). Nonetheless, the majority of cancer cases can be attributed to the risk factors of tobacco smoking and alcohol drinking. Other risk factors pertain to diet: often, cancer cases reported lower intake of vegetable and fruit in the past than their healthy counterparts. Thus, it is thought that vegetable and fruit intake reduces the risk of occurrence of cancer at this site. It is currently not clear which of the many substances in vegetables and fruit are responsible for the observed reduction in risk.

High incidences of oesophageal cancer can be found in eastern and southern Africa, North-Central China, Central Asia and South America. The male-to-female ratio is about 2 (Ferlay *et al.*, 2001). In Europe, the highest incidence of this cancer site, with 26.5/100 000, is found in Calvados, France, among males (Munoz & Day, 1996). Other high-incidence areas of Europe report 9–12 new oesophageal cancer cases per 100 000 (age-standardized) per year. The low-incidence areas of Europe show fewer than three new cancer cases per 100 000 per year. The secular trend of oesophageal cancer has been more or less stable in Europe over time over the past years. Important epidemiological etiological research into this type of cancer, particularly with regard to the risk factors prevailing in the high-risk regions in Europe, was conducted by scientists of the International Agency of Research into Cancer (IARC) in the early 1970s. The first studies pointed to a particular kind of spirit, calvados, as a major etiological cause of cancer at this site in the Calvados region. Subsequent studies linked all kinds of alcohol with the occurrence of this disease (Tuyns *et al.*, 1979). Heavy drinking (>120 g alcohol/day) showed a dramatic increase in risk (RR, 50–100) compared with moderate drinking (<40 g alcohol/day). In this study, tobacco smoking was the next important factor, showing a relative risk of 5–10 for heavy smoking. The joint relative risk of alcohol drinking and tobacco smoking follows the multiplicative model, as for cancer of the oral cavity and pharynx. A diet with nutritional deficits, particularly in micronutrients such as vitamin A and C, beta-carotene, riboflavin and zinc, were often linked with this cancer (Munoz & Day, 1996). Such a diet is usually characterized by a high intake of staple foods and a low intake of vegetables and fruit.

Most of the oesophageal cancers are squamous cell carcinomas. Adenocarcinomas of the oesophagus seem to be increasing over time in some European regions covered by cancer registries but not in all regions (Botterweek *et al.*, 2000). Particularly for adenocarcinomas appearing in the lower part of the oesophagus, overweight and a high waist circumference are important risk factors in addition to alcohol drinking and tobacco smoking, probably due to an increased reflux from the stomach because of abdominal pressure (IARC, 2001).

In the first analysis of the EPIC Study, we looked at the influence of alcohol, tobacco smoking, and fruit and vegetable intake on risk for cancers of the upper gastrointestinal tract in total. Due to the small numbers available for this analysis, we concentrated on overall effects and did not perform subtype analyses.

Methods

The recruitment procedures and the geographical distribution of the EPIC study population is described in detail elsewhere (Riboli & Kaaks, 1997). The total number of available EPIC study subjects without Norway was 482 924 persons. In this analysis, the study centres in Greece (*n*=28 572) and Malmö (*n*=28 098) were not considered because dietary information had not yet been approved. Further exclusion criteria were prevalent cancers of the upper gastrointestinal tract (*n*=81), extreme diet defined as the lowest and highest 1% of the ratio of energy to estimated basal metabolic rate (*n*=8388), and missing follow-up information (*n*=33). The study population from which the incident cases were identified counted 417 752 subjects.

Case identification occurred by active and passive follow-up depending on the situation in the individual centres. The original number of incident cases (ICD-O C00.0–C10.9., C13.0–C13.9 and C15.0–C15.9) in this study population were 146. This number includes cancers of the above-mentioned sites, identified as neoplasms, squamous cell carcinoma and adenocarcinomas. Due to missing values in some of the variables being used in the statistical model, the actual number of cases for this analysis was reduced to 124. These cases occurred in the following sites: oral cavity, *n*=42; oro-/hypopharynx, *n*=14; and oesophagus, *n*=68. Also, control subjects with missing information (*n*=30 484) were excluded from analysis, leaving 124 cases and 387 268 non-cases for final analysis.

Relative risk was derived by using the proportional hazard model (SAS PHREG). Age at first diagnosis of the cancer or age at censoring date formed the dependent variable. As censoring date, age at the date of the last active follow-up information or at the date a cancer registry was considered complete was taken. Follow-up time was included as the independent variable in the statistical model. Further independent variables included mean alcohol consumption at age 20, 30, 40 and at baseline examination. Each study participant gave detailed information about his or her consumption of alcoholic beverages at the specific ages. The mean alcohol consumption at these ages was categorized into four levels (no alcohol consumption, >0–30 g/d, >30–60 g/d, >60 g/d), and also tobacco smoking (never smoking, ex-smoking, 1–20 cigarettes per day, and >20 cigarettes per day). Other variables were calibrated vegetable and fruit consumption (first tertile ≤ 287 g/d, second tertile >287–456 g/d, and third tertile >456 g/d), sex, BMI (continuous variable), energy intake (coded into deciles) and education (none, primary/technical school, secondary school/university). All independent variables were used in one model and, thus, the estimated relative risks were adjusted to each other. Interaction between tobacco smoking and alcohol drinking were also calculated using all other independent variables as confounders.

Results

The centres of the UK contributed the greatest number of cases (*n*=40), followed by Denmark (*n*=39), Germany (*n*=14), Italy (*n*=12), Spain (*n*=7), the Netherlands (*n*=6), and Sweden (*n*=6). In EPIC France, including only women, no case of this cancer site has yet been identified. The mean age of cases in each country were 60 years of age or older; the mean age of the non-cases was between 53 and 55 years in most countries and up to 59 years in Denmark and France. Mean alcohol consumption at different ages of more than 60 g/day was found to be related with a relative risk (RR) of 9 (Table 1). A significant elevated risk was also found for the alcohol category 30–60 g/d (RR=3.17). Smoking was also a risk factor. Compared to never smoking, current smoking showed a relative risk of 2.7 for 1–20 cigarettes, and of 9.0 for more than 20 cigarettes per day (Table 2). The joint effect of alcohol drinking and tobacco smoking was analysed in a separate model in which the first nonsignificant categories were collapsed. There was a relative risk of about 50 for heavy drinking and smoking, indicating that the joined exposure of heavy drinking and smoking followed the multiplicative model (Table 3). In this analysis, vegetable and fruit consumption was linked with reduced risk adjusted for other risk factors. Compared to the consumption in the first tertile, the

Table 1. Alcohol drinking and risk of cancer of the upper GI tract – first analysis of the EPIC Study

Mean lifelong alcohol consumption	Cases/non-cases	Hazard rate ratio (95% CI)[a]
No alcohol	4/31 638	1
>0–30 g/day	83/322 564	1.21 (0.43–3.40)
>30–60 g/day	20/24 934	3.17 (1.00–10.05)
>60 g/day	17/8008	9.22 (2.75–30.93)

[a]Adjusted for follow-up time, sex, education, BMI, vegetable and fruit consumption, tobacco smoking, energy intake.

Table 2. Tobacco smoking and risk of cancer of the upper GI tract – first analysis of the EPIC Study

Tobacco smoking	Cases/non-cases	Hazard rate ratio (95% CI)[a]
Never smoker	26/199 028	1
Ex-smoker	43/107 974	1.52 (0.91–2.54)
1–20 cigarettes/day	34/67 488	2.74 (1.57–4.78)
>20 cigarettes/day	21/12 654	9.02 (4.64–17.56)

[a]Adjusted for follow-up time, sex, education, BMI, vegetable and fruit consumption, alcohol consumption, energy intake.

Table 3. Joint effect of alcohol drinking and tobacco smoking on risk of cancer of the upper GI tract – first analysis of the EPIC Study

	Tobacco smoking Hazard rate ratio[a] (95% CI)/no. of cases		
Alcohol drinking	non-smoker	1–20 cigarettes	>20 cigarettes
0–30 g/day	1/58	2.0 (1.2–3.5)/22	6.8 (3.0–15.5)/7
>30–60 g/day	2.6 (1.1–6.0)/7	5.1 (2.1–12.7)/6	20.7 (8.7–49.0)/7
>60 g/day	6.9 (2.3–20.7)/4	22.0 (8.3–58.1)/6	48.7 (20.0–118.9)/7

[a]Adjusted for follow-up time, sex, education, BMI, vegetable and fruit consumption, energy intake.

relative risk was reduced by about one-third for the second tertile and by about half for the third tertile (Table 4).

Discussion

Alcohol drinking and tobacco smoking showed a high relative risk for the cancers of the upper gastrointestinal tract compared to non-drinking and non-smoking. In this analysis, both variables seem to exhibit a similar increase in risk, taking the more extreme lifestyle habits in the EPIC population into account. About 8000 subjects were identified in the EPIC Study among the controls drinking more than 60 g alcohol per day and about 12 500 smoking more than 20 cigarettes per day. The category with the highest number of subjects among the non-cases were never smoking, comprising 199 028 subjects, and among the alcohol categories, moderate alcohol consumption of up to 30 g, with 322 564 subjects. Thus, the observed higher relative risk estimates in connection with alcohol drinking and tobacco smoking do not relate to the majority of the EPIC population. However, heavy smoking and drinking often coincide and taking the EU population as a whole, such lifestyle habits nevertheless will exist in a considerable number of subjects.

Tobacco smoking and alcohol drinking probably follow the multiplicative model. Thus subjects who smoke and are heavy consumers of alcohol experience a relative risk of about 50 compared to non-smoking and no- to moderate-alcohol-drinking subjects. We observed crude rates of 235 per 100 000 for cancer in the upper gastrointestinal tract in the heavy smoking and alcohol-drinking population in EPIC and 33 per 100 000 in the non-smoking and no- to moderate-alcohol-drinking population. With respect to prevention, none of the two factors have obvious preferences in terms of prevalence and effect size for the studied cancer sites in the EPIC population.

The finding that vegetable and fruit consumption reduces the risk of cancer at these sites is a good signal that initiatives to increase the consumption of this type of food, as is currently being done in the "5-a-Day-Campaigns" of the different EU countries, may be effective in reducing cancer risk. The observed risk-reducing effect of vegetables and fruit might be particularly important for cancer of the upper gastrointestinal tract since the majority of cases appeared in countries of Western, Central and Northern Europe. These countries

Table 4. Vegetable and fruit intake and risk of cancer of the upper GI tract – first analysis of the EPIC Study

Vegetable and fruit consumption[a]	Cases/non-cases	Hazard rate ratio (95% CI)[b]
1st tertile (≤ 287 g/day)	71/129 666	1
2nd tertile (>287 to 456 g/day)	31/129 072	0.64 (0.41–0.99)
3rd tertile (>456 g/day)	22/128 406	0.55 (0.32–0.95)

[a]FFQ mean of a centre calibrated against 24-h recalls.
[b]Adjusted for follow-up time, sex, education, BMI, tobacco smoking, alcohol consumption, energy intake.

traditionally have a low intake of vegetables and fruit (Agudo *et al.*, 2002).

It will be premature to draw further and definite conclusions from this first analysis. The results show that disease occurrence within the EPIC population is following a pattern similar to that of other study populations regarding alcohol intake and upper gastrointestinal tract cancers. In the future, more detailed analyses are needed, in particular for the different cancer sites and histological types being combined in this analysis. A forthcoming analysis will also certainly specify the effect of specific alcoholic beverages and other risk factors including diet.

Acknowledgement

Many thanks to Naomi Allen from Oxford who reviewed the manuscript.

References

Agudo, A., Slimani, N., Ocké, M., Naska, A., Miller, A., Kroke, A., Karalis, D., Vineis, P., Palli, D., Bueno-de-Mesquita, H.B., Peeters, P.H.M., Hjartäker, A., Engeset, D., Navarro, C., Martinez, C., Wallström, P., Zhang, J.-X., Welch, A., Key, T., Stripp, C., Overvad, K., Clavel, F., Casagrande, C. & Riboli, E. (2002) Vegetables and fruit consumption in the EPIC cohorts from ten European countries. *Public Health Nutr.* (in press)

Blot, W.J., McLaughlin, J.K., Devesa, S.S. & Fraumeni, J.F. (1996) Cancers of the oral cavity and pharynx. In: Schottenfeld, D. & Fraumeni, J.F. Jr., eds. *Cancer Epidemiology and Prevention*, 2nd ed., pp 666–680

Botterweek, A.A., Schouten, L.J., Volovics, A., Dorant, E. & van den Brandt, P.A. (2000) Trends in incidence of adenocarcinoma of the oesophagus and gastric cardia in ten European countries. *Int. J. Epidemiol.*, **29**, 645–654

Ferlay, J., Bray, F., Pisani, P. & Parkin, D.M. (2001) *GLOBOCAN 2000: Cancer Incidence, Mortality and Prevalence Worldwide*, Version 1.0. (IARC CancerBase No. 5), Lyon, IARC Press

International Agency for Research on Cancer (2002) *The Role of Weight Control and Physical Activity in Cancer Prevention* (IARC Handbook of Cancer Prevention No. 6), Lyon, IARC

Jensen, O.M., Paine, S.L., McMichael, A.J. & Ewerts, M. (1996) Alcohol. In: Schottenfeld, D. & Fraumeni, J.F. Jr., eds, *Cancer Epidemiology and Prevention*, 2nd ed., pp 290–318

Munoz, N. & Day, N.E. (1996) Esophageal Cancer. In: Schottenfeld, D. & Fraumeni, J.F. Jr., eds, *Cancer Epidemiology and Prevention*, 2nd ed., pp 681–706

Riboli, E. & Kaaks, R. (1997) The EPIC Project: rationale and study design. European Prospective Investigation into Cancer and Nutrition. *Int. J. Epidemiol.*, **26**, Suppl 1, S6–S14

Tuyns, A.J., Pequignot, G. & Abbattucci, J.S. (1979) Oesophageal cancer and alcohol consumption: importance of type of beverage. *Int. J. Cancer*, **23**, 443–447

Alcohol consumption and breast cancer risk. Preliminary results of the EPIC cohort

Clavel-Chapelon F.[1], Thiebaut A.[1], Berrino F.[2]
(for the EPIC working group on Diet and Breast Cancer)

[1]E3N-EPIC Group, INSERM, Institut Gustave-Roussy, 94805, Villejuif, France. [2]National Cancer Institute, Milan, Italy.

Introduction

The relationship between alcohol and breast cancer is a major public health problem in Western countries where alcohol drinking is frequent and breast cancer is common.

Epidemiological studies suggest a link between alcohol consumption and breast cancer, though the evidence has been considered as probable and unconvincing by a panel of experts (World Cancer Research Fund, 1997). A recent meta-analysis on the published data found a relative risk of 1.10 (1.06–1.14) for a consumption of 12 g of alcohol per day versus nondrinking (Curtis Ellison *et al.*, 2001). In a pooled analysis of six large prospective studies, a statistically significant linear increase in breast cancer incidence with increasing alcohol consumption was found (Smith Warner *et al.*, 1998). The pooled multivariate relative risk suggested an increase close to 10% (RR, 1.09, 1.04–1.13) for an increment of 10 g/day of ethanol. This last dataset was characterized by very high percentages of nondrinkers, ranking from 22.5% to 55.3%, and by Anglo-Saxon dietary and alcohol consumption patterns, with four studies out of six being from North America, one from Sweden and one from the Netherlands.

The European Prospective Investigation into Cancer and Nutrition (EPIC), a multi-centre prospective cohort study investigating the relation between diet and cancer, offers the opportunity to analyse heterogeneous drinking habits across Europe. We report here preliminary results on the relationship between alcohol and breast cancer from a large sample of European women participating in this study.

Material and methods

The EPIC multi-centre cohort study was set up in 1992 in 10 Western European countries: France, Italy, Spain, UK, Germany, The Netherlands, Greece, Sweden, Denmark and Norway (Riboli & Kaaks, 1997). The total study population comprises men and women. Only women, i.e. 329 428 subjects, were considered in this paper.

Data on diet, anthropometry and lifestyle factors as well as blood samples were collected from each study subject. Information on usual dietary intakes was collected using a semi-quantitative food frequency questionnaire or a dietary history (Spain, France) developed in each of the participating countries. The dietary questionnaires have been either self-administered or administered by an interviewer (Spain, Greece). All used photographs of different portion sizes of food items and commonly known units of portions. Their validity and reliability were tested. The reference method was 12 monthly 24-h recalls covering 1 calendar year. Two centers (Sweden and UK) used multiple food records as the reference method (Margetts & Pietinen, 1997). In these studies, correlation coefficients between the mean consumption, as reported in the dietary questionnaire, and the average of the 24-h recalls, ranked, among females, from 0.71 (France) to 0.91 (Germany) (Kaaks *et al.*, 1997).

Greece, Norway and the Malmö centre of Sweden are not considered in this analysis, because the dietary data had not been completely checked out.

Participants are followed with cancer registries in all countries except France, Germany and Greece, where follow-up is active, by the means of follow-up questionnaires. Follow-up time was between return of the dietary questionnaire and 2001. The mean duration of follow-up was 4.3 years.

For this analysis, we considered all EPIC centres with available data on diet and follow-up, with no previous breast cancer at enrolment and with an acceptable ratio of energy intake over energy requirement (in comparison to energy requirements computed as 1.55 times the basal metabolic rate; bottom and top 1% were excluded). The relationship between alcohol and breast cancer was investigated on 279 231 women. Of these, a total of 2758 breast cancer cases were reported by cancer registries or by the participants.

To take into account potential confounders simultaneously, proportional hazard models were used (Cox, 1972), with age as the time scale. Results were not calibrated, but stratified on centre. RRs were adjusted for energy intake (continuous), body mass index (continuous), follow-up time (<1, 1–2 or 3+ years), educational level (4 categories), smoking habits (non-smokers, current and ex-smokers) and reproductive factors. Non-consumers were taken as the reference category. We calculated 95% confidence intervals for all relative risks.

Results

The distribution of participants by EPIC centre and the description of their alcohol drinking habits is shown in Table 1. Overall, 14.0% of women never drink alcohol beverages. Drinking is common in Denmark, Germany and the UK, with less than 5% nondrinkers. Among drinkers, the average consumption was 10.4 g of ethanol per day (SD, 12.8). Daily ethanol consumption among drinkers was high in Denmark and France. It was low in Spain, the UK and Sweden.

Wine and beer were the major contributors to ethanol intake.

Overall, 21.0% of women were not wine consumers and 45.7% never drank beer.

The relationship between alcohol drinking and breast cancer risk was studied (Table 2). We first analysed the relationship between reproductive factors and breast cancer. As expected, the risk increased with decreasing age at menarche and increasing age at first full-term pregnancy. It decreased as the number of children increased. The risk increased with the educational level. No significant association was observed with smoking status. Compared to nondrinkers, the RR of drinkers was equal to 1.01 (95% CI, 0.91–1.14). A modest increase in risk with increasing ethanol intake (*P*<0.07) was observed, equal to 3% (RR, 1.03; 0.99–1.06) per 10 g per day ethanol intake. As compared to nondrinkers, the relative risk of drinkers moderately increased up to 1.16 (0.95–1.42) for women who drank 30–40 g of ethanol per day and decreased thereafter, to 1.07 (0.86–1.32) in the highest category of consumption.

Similar results were observed among postmenopausal women. The test for trend was significant (*P*<0.02) with an increase of 5% (RR, 1.05; 1.01–1.09) per 10 g per day ethanol intake. The RR for the intermediate category of consumption was equal to 1.39 (1.06–1.82) and that of the highest category (40+ g/d ethanol) was 1.29 (0.96–1.74).

We also specifically considered wine and beer consumption, with a separate category for non-ethanol drinkers (Table 2). The risks associated with consumption of wine were all close to unity. Relative risks modestly increased with increasing beer consumption.

Table 1. Description of drinking habits by country

		Ethanol			Wine			Beer		
Country	**No. of study participants**	**% Non-consumers**	**Mean[a] (g/d)**	**SD**	**% Non-consumers**	**Mean[a] (mL/d)**	**SD**	**% Non-consumers**	**Mean[a] (mL/d)**	**SD**
France	68 931	12.5	12.9	14.5	23.1	120.5	140.1	66.4	63.4	119.6
Italy	31 299	22.2	10.9	12.8	31.8	114.5	129.0	50.2	36.7	85.4
Spain	25 189	51.7	9.4	11.3	63.4	96.2	113.3	79.9	122.4	155.9
UK	55 920	4.6	7.7	9.6	6.2	53.8	81.5	18.6	47.9	114.2
The Netherlands	26 528	16.8	10.4	12.8	28.2	59.2	88.3	70.0	70.6	152.7
Germany	29 234	4.2	10.0	12.5	5.8	80.0	117.4	31.0	77.5	158.1
Sweden	12 913	10.3	2.3	2.6	21.4	12.3	16.6	18.1	41.3	56.2
Denmark	29 217	2.7	14.1	15.0	4.8	93.0	120.1	19.1	106.7	184.6
Total	279 231	14.0	10.4	12.8	21.0	84.2	116.6	45.7	65.4	135.4

[a]Among consumers.

Table 2. Multivariate relative risks[a] of breast cancer according to alcohol consumption. EPIC study 1992–2001

	All women		Postmenopausal women	
Alcohol intake	**No. of cases**	**Multivariate RR**	**No. of cases**	**Multivariate RR**
Ethanol (g/d)				
0	421	1.00	215	1.00
>0	2713	1.01 (0.91–1.14)	1429	0.89 (0.76–1.05)
0–10	1630	0.97 (0.86–1.10)	862	1.09 (0.93–1.29)
10–20	528	0.94 (0.82–1.09)	273	1.09 (0.90–1.33)
20–30	272	1.05 (0.89–1.24)	141	1.21 (0.96–1.52)
30–40	150	1.16 (0.95–1.42)	82	1.39 (1.06–1.82)
40+	133	1.07 (0.86–1.32)	71	1.29 (0.96–1.74)
Trend[b]		1.03 (0.99–1.06) P<0.07%		1.05 (1.01–1.09) P<0.02%
Wine (glasses/d)				
No ethanol	421	0.98 (0.83–1.15)	215	0.87 (0.69–1.09)
No wine	272	1.00	141	1.00
0–1	1732	0.94 (0.82–1.09)	910	0.94 (0.78–1.14)
1–2	373	0.94 (0.80–1.11)	194	0.98 (0.77–1.23)
2–3	207	0.96 (0.79–1.16)	117	1.04 (0.80–1.36)
3+	129	1.03 (0.82–1.28)	67	1.16 (0.85–1.58)
Trend[c]		1.01 (0.98–1.05) NS		1.04 (0.99–1.09) P<0.1
Beer (glasses/d)				
No ethanol	421	1.04 (0.92–1.18)	215	0.94 (0.79–1.11)
No beer	1296	1.00	712	1.00
0–1	1323	1.03 (0.94–1.13)	662	1.04 (0.91–1.18)
1–2	67	1.30 (0.99–1.69)	41	1.48 (1.05–2.10)
2+	27	1.44 (0.97–2.13)	14	1.56 (0.91–2.68)
Trend[c]		1.09 (1.00–1.20) P<0.06%		1.10 (0.98–1.25) NS

[a]Adjusted for energy intake, BMI, follow-up time, educational level, smoking habits, age at menarche, age at first full-term pregnancy and parity; RRs on wine (beer) also adjusted for beer (wine) consumption.
[b]Per 10 g/d ethanol intake.
[c]Continuous variable expressed in glasses.

Discussion

The results of the present study provide support for an increase to a limited magnitude in breast cancer risk with ethanol intake and with wine or beer consumption. The associations were similar in the subgroup of postmenopausal women.

The fact that our population originates from several countries throughout Europe increased the heterogeneity of the drinking habits with, across centres, percentages of nondrinkers ranking from 2.7 to 51.7, and among drinkers, mean quantities consumed varying from 2.3 to 14.1 g/d. However, the level of consumption in our data was not sufficient to allow the study of very high categories of consumption.

The length of follow-up, equal to 4.3 years on average, varied from 2.3 in Denmark to 6.9 in France. Due to the relatively short time lag between recording the dietary data and breast

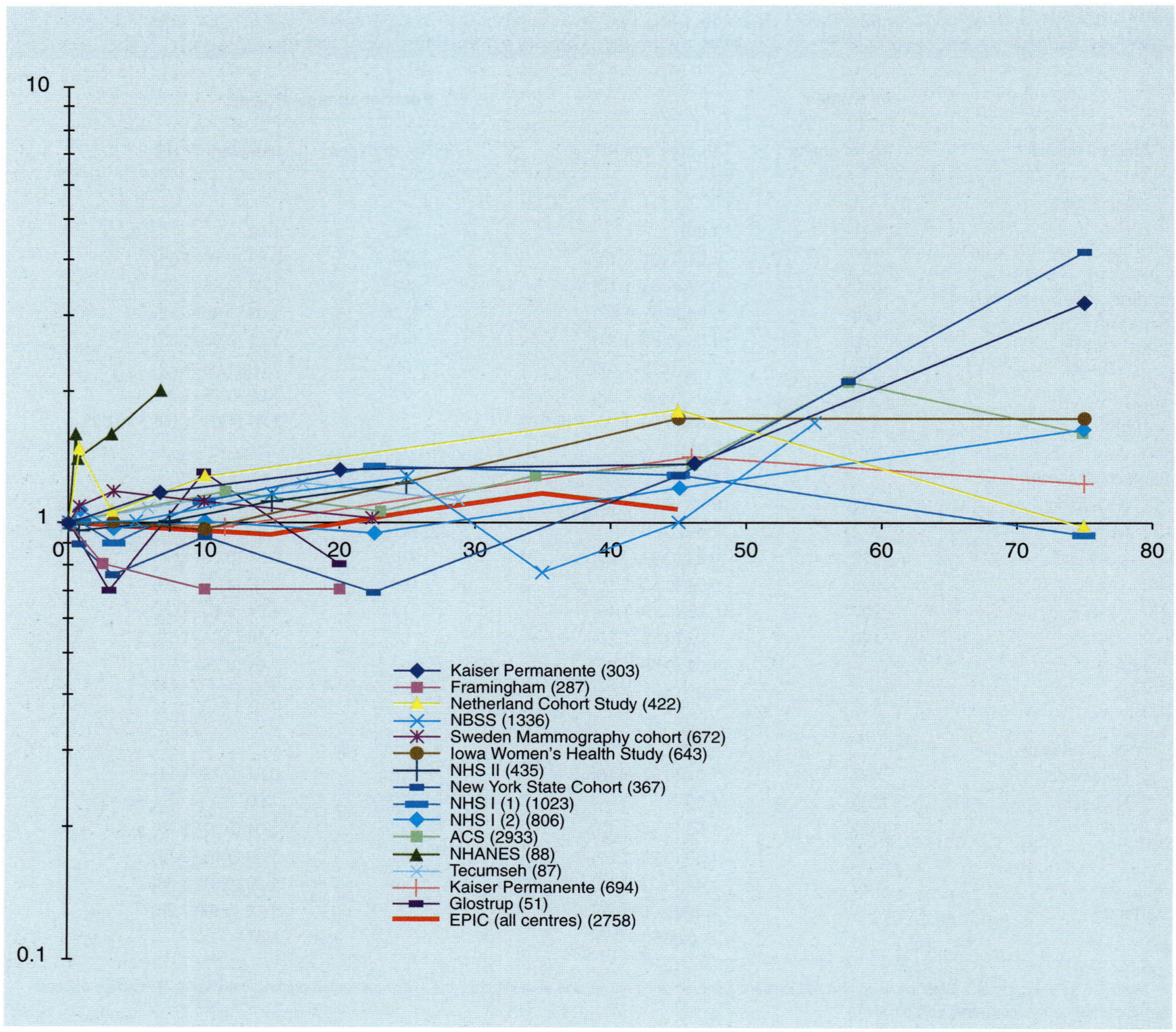

Figure 1
Ethanol intake and risk of breast cancer. Results from cohort studies (no. of breast cancer cases)

cancer occurrence, and to an insufficient number of cases for analysis after exclusion of the cases occurring in the first 2 years of follow-up, a bias due to the influence of preclinical disease on alcohol consumption cannot be excluded. Results are only presented on the subgroup of women who were postmenopausal at inclusion, since the information on occurrence of menopause during the follow-up was not available.

In the validation studies, alcohol was accurately reported. Moreover, the prospective nature of our data makes a recall bias unlikely.

Because we controlled for known breast cancer risk factors, our results are unlikely to be explained by confounding.

The relationship between alcohol consumption and breast cancer risk has been addressed in several epidemiological studies. A number of meta-analyses have also been published (Curtis Ellison *et al.*, 2001; Longnecker *et al.*, 1988; Longnecker, 1994; Howe *et al.*, 1991). However, most considered only a selection of studies. We examined results from all existing cohort studies, together with the EPIC results and pooled them in Fig. 1. The number of cases in these studies varies, from less than 100 in the Glostrup, Tecumseh and NHANES studies to almost 3000 in the study of the American Cancer Society and in the EPIC cohort. For each study, the multivariate RRs corresponding to different levels of ethanol intake were plotted on a logarithmic scale. Results originate from the original publication (Hiatt & Bawol, 1984; Schatzkin *et al.*, 1987; Garfinkel *et al.*, 1988; Hiatt *et al.*, 1988; Simon *et al.*, 1991; Pernille Hoyer *et al.*, 1992; Zhang *et al.*, 1999b; Garland *et al.*, 1999; Rohan *et al.*, 2000a) or, for comparison purposes, from those reported in the paper by Smith-Warner (Willett *et al.*, 1987; Graham *et al.*, 1992; Gapstur *et al.*, 1992; van den Brandt *et al.*, 1995; Holmberg *et al.*, 1995). A trend of increasing risk with increased consumption is obvious among existing data, up to a daily amount of 45 g of ethanol. A higher intake leads to heterogeneous results with eight studies having reported on consumers of 50 and over grams of ethanol daily. As compared to the existing literature, EPIC results are much closer to unity.

Data from animal and epidemiological studies have been recently reviewed (Singletary & Gapstur, 2001). Animal models of breast cancer, although not entirely consistent, provide support for an enhancing action of ethanol on mammary carcinogenesis. Several pathways have been put forward from animal studies and from cell culture experiments, such as increased circulating estrogens and androgens, enhancement of mammary gland susceptibility to carcinogenesis, increased mammary carcinogen DNA damage and greater potential for invasiveness of breast cancer cells (Singletary, 1997). Epidemiological studies have raised plausible biological mechanisms. Alcohol was reported to be associated with increased breast area occupied by mammographically dense tissue (Vachon, 2000). Of interest is a recent report that mammographic density is positively associated with plasma IGF-1 levels and inversely with plasma IGFBP-3 (Byrne, 2000). The interrelationship between plasma IGF-1, IGFPB-3, alcohol and mammographic density warrants evaluation.

The impact of alcohol on hormonal status provides another plausible explanation. In premenopausal women (in some instances, only among oral contraceptive users), alcohol intake has been associated with higher levels of various estrogens and androgens, and with modifications of the menstrual cycle pattern, leading to an increase in blood hormone levels. In postmenopausal women, an interaction with estrogen replacement therapy use has been put forward (Ginsburg *et al.*, 1996), with increased estradiol levels among alcohol consumers as compared to abstainers, an effect possibly explained by an altered clearance of estradiol in these women. Among postmenopausal women not using hormone replacement therapies (HRT), heterogeneous findings were reported.

An interaction with dietary components was also suggested. As folate is involved in DNA synthesis and methylation, its role in reducing breast cancer risk, particularly among women with high alcohol consumption, was studied. In three cohort studies, the highest RR of drinkers was consistently found among women with the lowest folate consumption as compared to those with the highest (Zhang *et al.*, 1999a; Rohan *et al.*, 2000b; Sellers *et al.*, 2000).

In the EPIC study, a weaker association was observed between alcohol and breast cancer as compared to the bulk of the literature. More investigations on the EPIC data are needed to determine whether this is due to a possible interaction with some nutrients in diet, with HRT use, with the specific content of the HRTs or with patterns of drinking across countries.

The preliminary nature of this analysis should be acknowledged. As soon as possible, consideration will be given to confounding factors and effect modification, in particular in relation to hormone use and nutrient intake.

References

Byrne, C., Colditz, G.A., Willett, W.C., Speizer, F.E., Pollack, M. & Hankinson, S.E. (2000) Plasma insulin-like growth factor (IGF)I, IGF-binding protein 3, and mammographic density. *Cancer Res.*, **60**, 3744–3748

Cox, D.R. (1972) Regression models and life tables (with discussion). *J. R. Stat. Soc. B.* **34**, 187–220

Curtis Ellison, R., Zhang, Y., McLennan, C.E. & Rothman, K.J. (2001) Exploring the relation of alcohol consumption and risk of breast cancer. *Am. J. Epidemiol.*, **154**, 740–747

Gapstur, S.M., Potter, J.D., Sellers, T.A. & Folsom, A.R. (1992) Increased risk of breast cancer with alcohol consumption in postmenopausal women. *Am. J. Epidemiol.*, **136**, 1221–1231

Garfinkel, L., Boffetta, P. & Stellman, S.D. (1988) Alcohol and breast cancer: a cohort study. *Prev. Med.*, **17**, 686–693

Garland, M., Hunter, D.J., Colditz, G.A., Spiegelman, D.L., Manson, J.E., Stampfer, M.J. & Willett, W.C. (1999) Alcohol consumption in relation to breast cancer risk in a cohort of United States women 25–42 years of age. *Cancer Epidemiol. Biomarkers Prev.*, **8**, 1017–1021

Ginsburg, E.S., Mello, N.K., Mendelson, J.H., Barberi, R.L., Teoh, S.K., Rothman, M., Gao, X. & Sholar, J.W. (1996) Effects of alcohol ingestion on estrogens in postmenopausal women. *J.A.M.A.*, **276**, 1747–1751

Graham, S., Zielezny, M., Marshall, J., Priore, R., Freudenheim, J., Brasure, J., Haughey, B., Nasca, P. & Zdeb, M. (1992) Diet in the epidemiology of postmenopausal breast cancer in the New York State cohort. *Am. J. Epidemiol.*, **136**, 1327–1337

Hiatt, R.A. & Bawol, R.D. (1988) Alcoholic beverage consumption and breast cancer incidence. *Am. J. Epidemiol.*, **120**, 676–683

Hiatt, R.A., Klatsky, A.L. & Armstrong, M.A. (1988) Alcohol consumption and the risk of breast cancer in a Prepaid Health Plan. *Cancer Res.*, **48**, 2284–2287

Holmberg, L., Baron, J.A., Byers, T., Wolk, A., Ohlander, E.M., Zack, M. & Adami, H.O. (1995) Alcohol intake and breast cancer risk: effect of exposure from 15 years of age. *Cancer Epidemiol. Biomarkers Prev.*, **4**, 843–847

Howe, G., Rohan, T., DeCarli, A., Iscovich, J., Kaldor, J., Katsouyanni, K., Marubini, E., Miller, A., Riboli, E. & Toniolo, P. (1991) The association between alcohol and breast cancer risk: evidence from the combined analysis of six dietary case–control studies. *Int. J. Cancer*, **47**, 707–710

Hoyer, A. & Engholm G. (1992) Serum lipids and breast cancer risk: a cohort study of 5207 Danish women. *Cancer Causes Control*, **3**, 403–408

Kaaks, R., Slimani, N. & Riboli, E. (1997) Pilot phase studies on the accuracy of dietary intake measurements in the EPIC project: overall evaluation of results. *Int. J. Epidemiol.*, **26**, S26–S36

Longnecker, M., Verlin, J., Orza, M. & Chalmers, T. (1988) A meta-analysis of alcohol consumption in relation to risk of breast cancer. *J.A.M.A.*, **260**, 652–656

Longnecker, M. (1994) Alcoholic beverage consumption in relation to risk of breast cancer: meta-analysis and review. *Cancer Causes Control*, **5**, 73–82

Margetts, B.M. & Pietinen, P. (1997) European Prospective Investigation into Cancer and Nutrition: validity studies on dietary assessment methods. *Int. J. Epidemiol.*, **26**, S1–S5

Riboli, E. & Kaaks, R. (1997) The EPIC Project: rationale and study design. European Prospective Investigation into Cancer and Nutrition. *Int. J. Epidemiol.*, **26**, S6–S14

Rohan, T.E., Jain, M., Howe, G.R. & Miller, A.B. (2000) Alcohol consumption and risk of breast cancer. *Cancer Causes Control*, **11**, 239–247

Rohan, T.E., Jain, M.G., Howe, G.R. & Miller, A.B. (2000) Dietary folate consumption and breast cancer risk. *J. Natl. Cancer Inst.*, **92**, 266–269

Schatzkin, A., Jones, D.Y., Hoover, R.N., Taylor, P.R., Brinton, L.A., Ziegler, R.G., Harvey, E.B., Carter, C.L., Licitra, L.M. & Dufour, M.C. (1987) Alcohol consumption and breast cancer in the epidemiologic follow-up study of the first National Health and Nutrition Examination Survey. *N. Engl. J. Med.*, **316**, 1169–1173

Sellers, T.A., Kushi, L.H., Cerhan, J.R., Vierkant, R.A., Gapstur, S.M., Vachon, C.M., Olson, J.E., Therneau, T.M. & Folsom, A.R. (2000) Dietary folate intake, alcohol, and risk of breast cancer in a prospective study of postmenopausal women. *Epidemiology*, **12**, 420–428

Simon, M.S., Carman, W., Wolfe, R. & Schottenfeld, D. (1991) Alcohol consumption and the risk of breast cancer: a report from the Tecumseh community health study. *J. Clin. Epidemiol.*, **44**, 755–761

Singletary, K. (1997) Ethanol and experimental breast cancer: a review. *Alcohol Clin. Exp. Res.*, **21**, 334–339

Singletary, K.W. & Gapstur, S.M. (2001) Alcohol and breast cancer. *J.A.M.A.*, **286**, 2143–2151

Smith-Warner, S.A., Spiegelman, D., Yaun, S.S., van den Brandt, P.A., Folsom, A.R., Goldbohm, R.A., Graham, S., Holmberg, L., Howe, G.R., Marshall, J.R., Miller, A.B., Potter, J.D., Speizer, F.E., Willett, W.C., Wolk, A. & Hunter, D.J. (1998) Alcohol and breast cancer in women: a pooled analysis of cohort studies. *J.A.M.A.*, **279**, 535–540

Vachon, C., Kushi, L., Cerhan, J., Kuni, C. & Sellers, T. (2000) Association of diet and mammographic breast density in the Minnesota Breast Cancer Family Cohort. *Cancer Epidemiol. Biomarkers Prev.*, **4**, 727–733

Van den Brandt, P.A., Goldbohm, R.A. & van 't Veer, P. (1995) Alcohol and breast cancer: results from The Netherlands Cohort Study. *Am. J. Epidemiol.*, **141**, 907–915

Willett, W.C., Stampfer, M.J., Colditz, G.A., Rosner, B.A., Hennekens, C.H. & Speizer, F.E. (1987) Moderate alcohol consumption and the risk of breast cancer. *N. Engl. J. Med.*, **316**, 1174–1180

World Cancer Research Fund (1997) *Food, Nutrition and the Prevention of Cancer: A Global Perspective.* Washington, D.C., American Institute for Cancer Research, pp. 261–269

Zhang, S., Hunter, D.J., Hankinson, S.E., Giovannucci, E.L., Rosner, B.A., Colditz, G.A., Speizer, F.E. & Willett, W.C. (1999a) A prospective study of folate intake and the risk of breast cancer. *J.A.M.A.*, **281**, 1632–1637

Zhang, Y., Kreger, B.E., Dorgan, J.F., Splansky, G.L., Cupples, L.A. & Ellison, R.C. (1999b) Alcohol consumption and risk of breast cancer: the Framingham Study revisited. *Am. J. Epidemiol.*, **149**, 93–101

Smoking and diet quality in teenage girls: are they related?

Baer Wilson D., Nietert P.J.

The Center for Healthcare Research, The Medical University of South Carolina, Charleston, South Carolina.

Objective

To explore the associations of smoking with measures of diet quality among white, black and Hispanic teenage girls in grades 9–12.

Introduction

Tobacco use is one of the most problematic public health issues of modern times and is associated with 87% of lung cancer deaths. According to Cooper *et al.* (1999) and the World Cancer Research Project (1997), antioxidant vitamins found in fruits and vegetables have been identified as helping to minimize lung cancer risk. Further, there is evidence that vitamin C, vitamin E and carotenoids play a crucial role in mediating the oxidant damage delivered by tobacco smoke.

Data from the Youth Risk Behavior Survey (YRBS), reported from the Center for Disease Control (2000), show that adolescent girls in grades 9–12 have surpassed smoking rates of males, with 34.9% of females currently smoking. Tomeo *et al.* (1999) and Austin & Gortmaker (2001) report that female smokers are also likely to be dieting, thus potentially compromising their intake of cancer-protective antioxidants from fruits and vegetables, beginning at a young age.

Little data exists about the effect of smoking on diet quality in female teens, particularly in various racial/ethnic groups. It is important that we understand dietary implications of smoking in various racial/ethnic groups so that we may adequately tailor cancer prevention interventions. This study was designed to examine how smoking is related to diet quality among white, black and Hispanic teenage girls in grades 9–12.

Methods

The study sample included white (n=2797), black (n=2196) and Hispanic (n=2052) girls in grades 9–12 who responded to the 1999 Youth Risk Behavior Survey (YRBS). The main study outcome was diet quality as measured by consumption of fruit, fruit juice, milk, (at least one serving/day in the last 7 days) and vegetables (at least one serving of either salad, carrots, or other vegetables at least 4–6 times in the last week). The independent variable was smoking status ($\geq$ 1 cigarette/day on any days smoked in the last 30 days) with covariates being age, depression, body image perception, body mass index (BMI), dieting behaviour, exercise habits and vomiting/use of laxatives to control weight.

Statistical analyses were performed to test bivariate associations between smoking and each of the study variables using chi-square and paired t tests. Logistic regression models were developed to test for a significant association between smoking and fruit, fruit juice, milk, and vegetable consumption. All analyses were stratified by ethnic/cultural group. Dose–response relationships were explored for all statistically significant associations between smoking (using a graduated smoking variable (<1, 1–5, >6 cigarettes in the last 30 days) and the dependent diet quality variables for white, black and Hispanic teenage girls. All models were adjusted for covariates. SUDAAN software was used to account for the complex sampling design of the survey.

Results

In the total sample, smokers tended to be older (P<0.001), were more likely to view themselves as overweight (P=0.058), more likely to have dieted in the past 30 days (P=0.058), more likely to have vomited or used laxatives to control weight (P<0.01) and less likely to have eaten salad, carrots, or other vegetables in the past 7 days (P<0.01) than non-smokers. Using logistic regression analyses with adjusted figures, among white girls, smoking was associated with significantly decreased

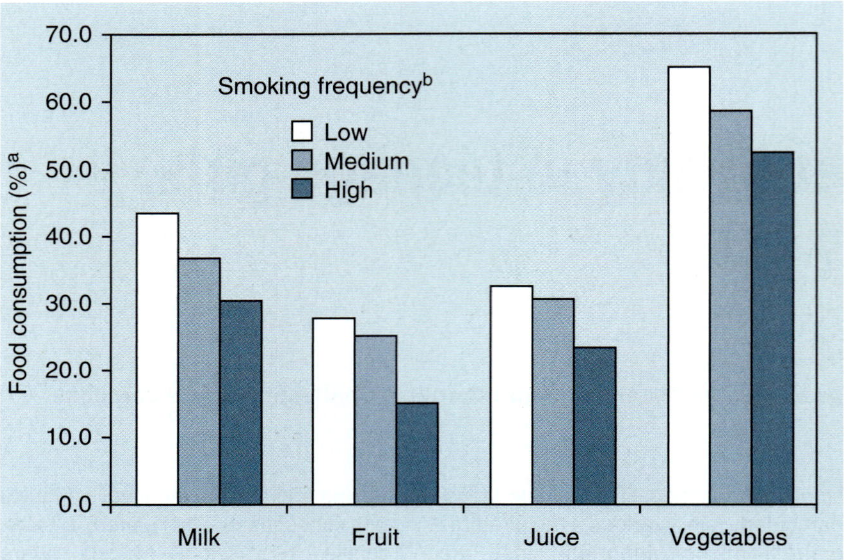

Figure 1
Dose–response effect of smoking on food consumption in white teenage girls
[a]Fruit, juice, milk consumption defined ->1 serving/day in the past week, vegetables ≥ 4-6 servings in past week
[b]Smoking low 0–<1 cigarette, med 1–5 cigarettes, high ≥ 5 cigarettes/day in last 30 days

odds of consuming milk 0.74 (95% CI, 0.56–0.98), fruit 0.70 (95% CI, 0.54–0.92), fruit juice 0.74 (95% CI, 0.56–0.98), and salads, carrots or other vegetables 0.75 (95% CI, 0.63–0.89), than non-smokers. Among Hispanic girls who smoked, only fruit juice was associated with significantly decreased odds of consumption 0.59 (95% CI, 0.56–0.98) compared with non-smokers. Black teenage girls who smoked appeared to consume higher levels of the foods studied than non-smokers; however, the effects were not statistically significant. For each of the significant smoking and food variables, a significant dose–response relationship was detected. Figure 1 depicts this effect among white smokers.

Conclusions

These results are consistent with the hypothesis that white teenage girls who smoke are less likely to consume the foods studied, when compared with girls who do not smoke, because of dieting behaviour. However, these associations were not consistent across ethnic/cultural groups. While Hispanic female adolescent smoking/diet quality behaviours demonstrate some similarities to white girls, black female teen smokers consumed higher levels of fruit, fruit juice, vegetables and milk than did non-smokers. This supports results reported by Headen *et al.* (1991) indicating that black teens initiate smoking for different reasons than do white teens.

Implications

This is one of the first studies to report on the association of smoking with diet quality in teenage girls across ethnic/cultural lines in the U.S. The results showing a dose–response effect among white teenage girls, and for one food variable in Hispanic girls, indicate that smokers are compromising cancer protective nutrients found in fruits and vegetables. This may compound their risk of developing lung cancer over a lifetime, compared to smoking alone.

The strong differences by race indicate the need for tailoring interventions accordingly, given that both smoking and diet/body size are influenced by cultural norms. These study results underscore the need for educating health care providers and school clinics to rigorously emphasize the need to eat multiple servings of fruits, vegetables, and dairy foods according to recommendations, along with smoking cessation counseling for teenage girls who smoke. Further study is needed to understand the intricacies of these behaviours, particularly in black and Hispanic populations.

References

Austin, S.B. & Gortmaker, S.L. (2001) Dieting and smoking initiation in early adolescent girls and boys: a prospective study. *Am. J. Public Health*, **3**, 446–450

Center for Disease Control. (2000) Trends in cigarette smoking among high school students, United States, 1991–1999. MMWR Weekly Report, *JAMA*, **284**, 1507–1508

Cooper, D.A., Eldridge, A.L., & Peters, J.C. (1999) Dietary carotenoids and lung cancer: a review of recent research. *Nutr. Rev.* 133–145

Headen, S.W., Bauman, K.E., Deane, G.D. & Koch, G.G. (1991) Are the correlates of cigarette smoking initiation different for black and white adolescents? *Am. J. Public Health*, **81**, 854–857

Tomeo, C.A., Field, A.E., Berkey, C.S., Colditz, G.A. & Frazier, A.L. (1999) Weight concerns, weight control behaviors and smoking initiation. *Pediatrics*, **104**, 918–924

World Cancer Research Fund, American Institute for Cancer Research. (1997) *Food Nutrients and the Prevention of Cancer: A Global Perspective.* Washington, D.C., American Institute for Cancer Research.

Alcohol consumption and oxidative damage

Bianchini F.[1], Boeing H.[2], Vineis P.[3], Elmstahl S.[4], Martinez-Garcia C.[5], van Kappel A.L.[1], Ohshima H.[1], Riboli E.[1], Kaaks R.[1]

[1]IARC, Lyon, France. [2]Deutsches Institut für Ernährungsforschung, Potsdam, Germany. [3]Servizio di Epidemiologia dei Tumori, Torino, Italy. [4]Malmö University Hospital, Malmö, Sweden. [5]Granada Cancer Registry, Granada, Spain.

Introduction

Oxidative damage to macromolecules has been implicated in the etiology of cancer and other age-related diseases. Several studies have shown that dietary factors, including fat, vegetables and antioxidants, can have a modulator effect on markers of oxidative damage (Bianchini *et al.*, 2000; Djuric *et al.*, 1991; Duthie *et al.*, 1996; Verhagen *et al.*, 1995). In the present study, we show the relationship between habitual alcohol consumption and lymphocyte levels of 8-hydroxy-2'-deoxyguanosine (8-oxodGuo), a commonly used marker of oxidative damage to DNA, in a cross-sectional study within the European Prospective Investigation into Cancer and Nutrition (EPIC).

Methods

Premenopausal women, aged 45–50, were selected in Potsdam (Germany), Turin (Italy), Malmö (Sweden) and Granada (Spain). Information on alcohol consumption in different beverages was obtained by previously validated food frequency questionnaires and assuming 11 vol% alcohol in wine, 16 vol% in fortified wines, 4 vol% in beer and cider, and 40 vol% in spirits and brandy. 8-oxodGuo was measured in lymphocytes, obtained from a fasting blood sample immediately after the blood draw, using HPLC with electrochemical detection (Bianchini *et al.*, 2000).

Results

Levels of 8-oxodGuo ranged from 0.36 to 6.23 8-oxodGuo x 10^{-6} deoxyguanosines (dG), confirming the high inter-individual variation already observed in previous studies. Mean values differed significantly ($P<0.03$) between Granada and the other centres (Table 1).

Consumption levels of total alcohol were significantly different between the four centres (Table 1). Mean total alcohol intake (drinkers and non-drinkers) was highest in Turin (13.1 mL alcohol/day) and lowest in Granada (1mL alcohol/day), where only 12 out of 28 women reported drinking alcohol. Centres also differed in the consumption levels of specific

Table 1. Lymphocyte levels of 8-oxodGuo x 10^{-6}dG and daily consumption (mL) of alcohol in different alcoholic beverages in Potsdam, Turin, Malmö and Granada (means ± SD)

Variable	Potsdam (*n*=27)	Turin (*n*=36)	Malmö (*n*=24)	Granada (*n*=28)
8-OxodGuo	1.72±1.45[a]	1.50±1.12[a]	1.59±1.02[a]	2.30±0.78[b]
Total alcohol	9.9±9.4[a]	13.1±15.7[a]	9.7±11[a]	1.0±2[b]
Wine	6.7±9.1[a,b]	11.4±15.2[a]	4.5±6.3[b,c]	0.6±1.5[c]
Fortified wines	0.05±0.06[b]	0.2±0.3[a]	–	–
Beer, cider	3.0±4.9[a]	0.7±1.2[b]	4.0±4.6[a]	0.4±1.2[b]
Spirits, brandy	0.2±0.6[b]	0.7±1.4[a,b]	1.2±3.3[a]	–

[a, b, c, d]For the same variable, only mean values with different alphabetical letters are statistically different (i.e. consumption of spirits and brandy in Turin was not significantly different from Potsdam and Malmö, while consumption in Potsdam was significantly different from Malmö).

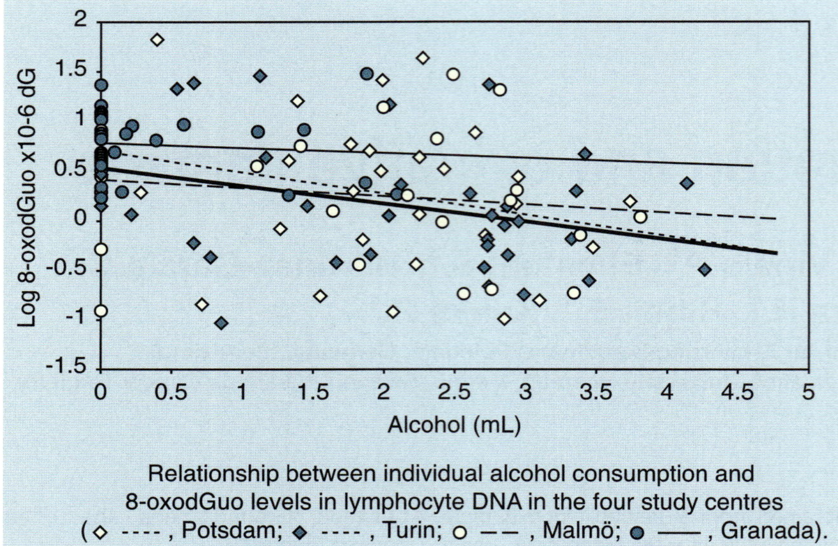

Figure 1
Relationship between individual alcohol consumption and 8-oxodGuo levels in lymphocyte DNA in the four study centres

beverages. For example, in Turin wine represented 87% of total alcohol consumed, while in Potsdam and Malmö 30%–40% of total alcohol consumption derived from beer.

At the individual level, a negative relationship between 8-oxodGuo and total alcohol consumption was observed in Potsdam (*r*= –0.22), Turin (*r*= –0.25) and Malmö (*r*= –0.24) (Figure 1). In addition, on a group level, mean alcohol intakes and mean 8-oxodGuo levels were inversely correlated (*r*= 0.98).

The data were also analysed by generalized linear regression models (GLM) with 8-oxodGuo levels (log-transformed values) as a dependent variable and "centre", storage time and total alcohol consumption as predictor variables (Bianchini *et al.*, 2001). Additional variables included the Quetelet index, total fruit and vegetable consumption, plasma total carotenoids, α- and γ-tocopherol. The variable "study centre" showed a significant effect on 8-oxodGuo levels (*P* = 0.001), explaining 13% of variation. This effect diminished when the variable "alcohol intake" was introduced in the model. Alcohol itself explained approximately 4% of the variation and was negatively correlated with 8-oxodGuo levels (*P* = 0.02), while total plasma carotenoids and tocopherol showed a positive correlation (*P* = 0.03), thus confirming our previous findings (Bianchini *et al.*, 2000).

Considering different types of beverages, 8-oxodGuo levels were inversely correlated with consumption of wine in Turin (*r*= –0.23) and Malmö (*r*= –0.27), with consumption of fortified wines in Turin (*r*= –0.23), with consumption of beer in Potsdam (*r*= –0.46) and Granada (*r*= –0.37), and with consumption of spirits and brandy in Potsdam (*r*= –0.25).

Discussion

Our results show a negative relationship between levels of alcohol intake and lymphocyte levels of 8-oxodGuo across the four study populations. The mechanisms responsible for such associations are not clear. The associations appear to be independent of beverage type, thus suggesting an independent effect of alcohol itself, although the involvement of other components, such as flavonoids, cannot be excluded. Our results persisted after controlling for possible confounding effects of total fruit and vegetable consumption and plasma carotenoid levels. However, confounding from possible unidentified factors is still possible and could be assessed only by randomized intervention trials, where subjects are given different amounts and types of alcoholic beverages for various periods of time.

References

Bianchini, F., Elmstahl, S., Martinez-Garcia, C., van Kappel, A.L., Douki, T., Cadet, J., Ohshima, H., Riboli, E. & Kaaks, R. (2000) Oxidative DNA damage in human lymphocytes: correlations with plasma levels of alpha-tocopherol and carotenoids. *Carcinogenesis*, **21**, 321–324

Bianchini, F., Jaeckel, A., Vineis, P., Martinez-Garcia, C., Elmstahl, S., van Kappel, A.L., Boeing, H., Ohshima, H., Riboli, E. & Kaaks, R. (2001) Inverse correlation between alcohol consumption and lymphocyte levels of 8-hydroxy-deoxyguanosine in humans. *Carcinogenesis*, **22**, 885–890

Djuric, Z., Heilbrun, L.K., Reading, B.A., Boomer, A., Valeriote, F.A. & Martino, S. (1991) Effects of a low-fat diet on levels of oxidative damage to DNA to human peripheral nucleated blood cells. *J. Natl. Cancer Inst.*, **83**, 766–769

Duthie, S.J., Ma, A., Ross, M.A. & Collins, A.R. (1996) Antioxidant supplementation decreases oxidative DNA damage in human lymphocytes. *Cancer Res.*, **56**, 1291–1295

Verhagen, H., Poulsen, H.E., Loft, S., van Poppel, G., Willems, M.I. & van Bladeren, P.J. (1995) Reduction of oxidative DNA damage in humans by Brussels sprouts. *Carcinogenesis*, **16**, 969–970

Effect of smoking on the association between alcohol consumption and cancer mortality among middle-aged Japanese men: JPHC Study Cohort I

Hara M., Sasaki S., Tsugane S.
(for the JPHC Study Group)

Epidemiology and Biostatistics Division, National Cancer Center Research Institute East, Chiba, Japan.

Introduction

Many epidemiological studies have consistently shown heavy alcohol consumption to be a risk factor for alcohol-related cancer, especially cancer of the mouth, pharynx, larynx, oesophagus, and liver. Studies on the combined effects of alcohol and smoking on these cancers have indicated that the risk rose with increasing alcohol consumption regardless of smoking status, and that heavy drinking is a cancer risk factor even in never smokers (IARC, 1988). However, few studies have investigated the combined effects of alcohol and smoking on other than alcohol-related cancers. We earlier reported that the risk of alcohol on cancer mortality was modified by smoking status (Tsugane *et al.*, 1999). The purpose of this investigation was to examine the interaction by cancer type (alcohol-related cancer versus other cancers) using extended follow-up data.

Methods

A population-based prospective study was conducted in the Japan Public Health Center prospective study on cancer and cardiovascular disease (JPHC Study). From 1990 through 1999, 19 227 men aged 40–59 years who reported their alcohol intake and did not have serious diseases at baseline were followed. Weekly ethanol intake was calculated by combining the amount of ethanol per day and frequency per week. The validity of alcohol intake as measured by Spearman's correlation with 7-day dietary records repeated 4 times was 0.79 among 94 subsamples. We calculated the crude mortality rate per 100 000 person-years for each cause. Cox's proportional hazard model was used to compare mortality according to the weekly dose of ethanol ingested.

Results

We documented 928 deaths, 381 of which were due to cancer, including 62 alcohol-related cancers (3 mouth cancers, 2 pharynx cancers, 3 larynx cancers, 21 oesophagus cancers and 33 liver cancers). As expected, the risk for alcohol-related cancers was closely associated with alcohol consumption. However, alcohol consumption was also associated with the risk of other cancer deaths; the relative risk (RR) among the heaviest drinkers (ethanol intake >450 g/week) compared with occasional drinkers was significantly high after adjustment for possible confounders (Table 1). Table 2 illustrates how smoking status influences the relation between alcohol drinking and mortality from alcohol-related and other cancers. The risk of alcohol-related cancers was closely associated with alcohol consumption regardless of smoking status and a linear trend in RRs was found among current smokers. For cancer mortality except for alcohol-related cancer, the RRs of non-smokers did not increase, while the RRs of smokers increased in a dose-dependent manner.

Table 1. Number of deaths, death rate per 100 000 person-years and relative risks for death by cause and alcohol intake categories in 19 227 men, Japan, 1990–1999

	Nondrinker	Occasional drinker	Weekly ethanol intake (g/week)				*P* for trend[d]
			1–150	151–300	301–450	>450	
Mortality from alcohol-related cancers[a]							
No. of deaths (*n*=62)	11	3	7	16	15	10	
Person-years	38 473	20 388	32 821	36 888	28 477	29 515	
Death rate per 100 000 person-years	28.6	14.7	21.3	43.4	52.7	33.9	
Multivariate RR[b]	1.71	1.00	1.02	2.52	3.25	1.88	0.14
95%CI	(0.46–6.38)		(0.24–4.29)	(0.71–8.95)	(0.90–11.76)	(0.48–7.34)	
Multivariate RR[c]	1.65	1.00	0.99	4.24	4.72	3.12	0.06
95%CI	(0.32–8.63)		(0.16–5.95)	(0.94–19.10)	(1.01–21.94)	(0.63–15.37)	
Mortality from cancers other than alcohol-related							
No. of deaths (*n*=319)	73	25	40	53	57	71	
Person-years	38 473	20 388	32 821	36 888	28 477	29 515	
Death rate per 100 000 person-years	189.7	122.6	121.9	143.7	200.2	240.6	
Multivariate RR[b]	1.28	1.00	0.99	1.12	1.47	1.85	0.01
95%CI	(0.78–2.10)		(0.59–1.67)	(0.68–1.85)	(0.89–2.45)	(1.13–3.02)	
Multivariate RR[c]	1.27	1.00	0.91	1.03	1.40	1.71	0.02
95%CI	(0.77–2.12)		(0.53–1.57)	(0.61–1.73)	(0.83–2.37)	(1.03–2.84)	

[a]Alcohol-related cancer: mouth, pharynx, larynx, oesophagus, and liver.
[b]RR, relative risk, adjusted for age in 1990 (40–44, 45–49, 50–54, 55–59), area (Iwate, Akita, Nagano, Okinawa), flushing response (yes, no), and cigarette smoking (never, past, 1–19/day, 20–29/day, 30/day+).
[c]RR further adjusted for educational background (junior high school, high school, college or more), sports participation (<1 day/month, 1–3 days/month, >1 day/week), and four categories of selected dietary habits (yellow vegetables, fruits, fish, miso soup, pickled vegetables).
[d]*P* for trend was tested for linear hypothesis about the regression coefficient among drinkers.
CI, confidence intervals.

Discussion

We considered that there might be some difference in the way in which alcohol-related cancer develops compared to other cancers. The most interesting finding in this study is that an elevated risk of cancer mortality (excluding alcohol-related cancer due to heavy drinking) was limited in current smokers. We assumed that elevated microsomal cytochrome P450 (CYP) and microsomal enzyme activity might play important roles. Chronic ethanol consumption reportedly enhanced the activation of procarcinogens and mutagens in the rat (Seitz *et al.*, 1981). For example, CYP2E1 is naturally inducible by ethanol, acetaldehyde, and smoking, and is involved in the metabolic activation of various N-nitrosamines, including the potent tobacco-specific carcinogen. Activated nitrosamines have been related to development of many common human

Table 2. Number of deaths, death rate per 100 000 person-years and relative risks for death by cause and alcohol intake categories in 14 901 men, Japan, 1990–1999

	Nondrinker	Occasional drinker	Weekly ethanol intake (g/week)				*P* for trend[d]
			1–150	151–300	301–450	>450	
Mortality from alcohol-related cancers[a]							
Non-smokers[b]							
No. of deaths	3	1	1	1	2	3	
Multivariate RR[c]	1.69	1.00	2.13	3.39	7.04	3.22	0.57
95%CI	(0.17–16.42)		(0.22–20.85)	(0.37–31.13)	(0.79–63.12)	(0.28–37.14)	
Current smokers							
No. of deaths	5	2	3	12	9	7	
Multivariate RR[c]	1.56	1.00	0.60	4.79	4.23	2.59	0.15
95%CI	(0.16–15.11)		(0.04–9.63)	(0.60–38.21)	(0.51–35.20)	(0.29–23.0)	
Mortality from cancers other than alcohol-related							
Non-smokers[b]							
No. of deaths	18	12	13	10	2	5	
Multivariate RR[c]	1.34	1.00	0.58	0.62	0.76	0.65	0.56
95%CI	(0.73–2.44)		(0.29–1.18)	(0.30–1.27)	(0.36–1.61)	(0.29–1.45)	
Current smokers							
No. of deaths	31	8	22	34	42	57	
Multivariate RR[c]	1.86	1.00	1.50	2.10	2.73	3.61	<0.01
95%CI	(0.81–4.24)		(0.62–3.67)	(0.92–4.80)	(1.20–6.22)	(1.62–8.07)	

[a]Alcohol-related cancer includes mouth, pharynx, larynx, oesophagus, and liver.
[b]Non-smokers are limited to never smokers.
[c]RR, relative risk, adjusted for age in 1990 (40–44,45–49,50–54,55–59), area (Iwate, Akita, Nagano, Okinawa), educational background (junior high school, high school, college or more), medication (none, any), past history of hypertension (no, yes), sports participation (< 1 day/month, 1–3 days/month, ≥ 1 day/week), and four categories of selected dietary habits (yellow vegetables, fruits, fish, miso soup, pickled vegetables). For current smokers, further adjusted for numbers of cigarettes smoked (1–19/day, 20–29/day, 30+/day)
[d]*P* for trend was tested for linear hypothesis about the regression coefficient among drinkers.
CI, confidence intervals.

cancers, including lung cancer (Bandera *et al.*, 2001). We suspected that CYP2E1 in current smokers might be induced by an increase in weekly ethanol intake and might activate nitrosamine from tobacco smoking. One explanation that the risk of cancer mortality (except for alcohol-related cancer due to heavy drinking) was not increased in never-smokers might be the lack of apparent carcinogens activated by CYP2E1.

To explain why no apparent increase in the risk of alcohol-related cancer was seen among the heaviest drinkers and why an increased risk was observed among non-drinkers, we then considered the influence of abstainers among former heavy drinkers. In our study, a high percentage of alcohol-related cancer was due to hepatocellular carcinoma (HCC), and almost all HCC in Japan is developed through infection by the hepatitis C virus (HCV) or liver cirrhosis (LC). Some heavy drinkers might have stopped or restricted alcohol drinking due to liver dysfunction before the survey and were categorized as non-drinkers or light-to-moderate drinkers, respectively.

In conclusion, the risks of cancer mortality due to alcohol drinking might be modified by smoking status and they are different between alcohol-related cancer and other cancers. We found that the RRs of even non-alcohol-related cancers increased with the increase in weekly ethanol consumption by current smokers. Alcohol might activate tobacco-derived procarcinogen, resulting in a higher cancer risk.

Acknowledgement

This work was supported by grants for Cancer Research and for the Second-Term Comprehensive Ten-Year Strategy for Cancer Control from the Ministry of Health, Labor and Welfare of Japan.

References

Bandera, E.V., Freudenheim, J.L. & Vena, J.E. (2001) Alcohol consumption and lung cancer: a review of the epidemiologic evidence. *Cancer Epidemiol. Biomarkers Prev.*, **10**, 813–821

International Agency for Research on Cancer (1988) IARC *Monographs on Evaluation of Carcinogenic Risks to Humans. Alcohol drinking*, Vol. 44, Lyon

Seitz, H.K., Garro, A.J. & Lieber, C.S. (1981) Enhanced pulmonary and intestinal activation of procarcinogens and mutagens after chronic ethanol consumption in the rat. *Eur. J. Clin. Invest.*, **11**, 33–38

Tsugane, S., Fahey, M.T., Sasaki, S. & Baba, S. (1999) Alcohol consumption and all-cause and cancer mortality among middle-aged Japanese men: seven-year follow-up of the JPHC study Cohort I. Japan Public Health Center. *Am. J. Epidemiol.*, **150**, 1201–1207

Trends in self-reported past alcohol intake from 1950 to 1995 observed in eight European countries participating in the European Investigation into Cancer and Nutrition (EPIC) project

Klipstein-Grobusch K.[1], Slimani N.[2], Krogh V.[3], Boeing H.[1]
(for the EPIC working group on dietary patterns)

[1]German Institute of Human Nutrition, Department of Epidemiology, Potsdam-Rehbrücke, Germany. [2]IARC, Unit of Nutrition and Cancer, Lyon, France. [3]Instituto Nazionale di Tumori, Milano, Italy.

Introduction

Alcohol intake has been studied intensively as a risk factor for chronic diseases. Studies on trends in alcohol intake showed that alcohol consumption and beverage consumption preference are unlikely to be constant over time. Dose–response relationships between alcohol use and risk assessment might be distorted when current intake is assessed instead of life-time use (Lemmens, 1998). In the cohorts contributing to the European Prospective Investigation into Cancer and Nutrition (EPIC) project (Riboli & Kaaks, 1997), data on recalled consumption of alcoholic beverages in the past were obtained. The aim of the present investigation was to describe trends of self-reported past consumption of alcoholic beverages and alcohol intake from 1950 to 1995 within EPIC.

Methods

Subjects for the present analysis came from 21 EPIC study centres in eight European countries. Numbers of subjects in each study centre and country are given in Table 1. Subjects younger than 35 years and older than 75 years were excluded from analysis as well as those with missing alcohol consumption data.

Consumption of glasses of alcoholic beverages per week expressed as beer/cider, wine, sweet liquor/distilled spirits was estimated retrospectively for age 20, 30, and 40 years by self-administered life-style questionnaires phrased similarly in study centres.

Daily consumption of alcohol intake (g/day) for the time periods 1950–1975, 1960–1985 and 1970–1995 was calculated based on average glass volume and alcohol content for each type of alcoholic beverage. This information was derived for each study centre from 36 900 computerized 24-h dietary recall interviews collected in the EPIC calibration substudy using a standardized computerized system (EPIC-SOFT) common across countries (Slimani *et al.*, 2000). The participants' date of birth was used to calculate calendar time when participants were 20, 30, or 40 years old and to construct corresponding time periods: information on alcohol consumption at age 20 corresponds to information on alcohol consumption during the time period 1950–1975, information at age 30 to the time period 1960–1985, and information at age 40 to the time period 1970–1995. Because of the wide age range (35–75 years) of study participants and the availability of information on consumption of alcoholic beverages at a

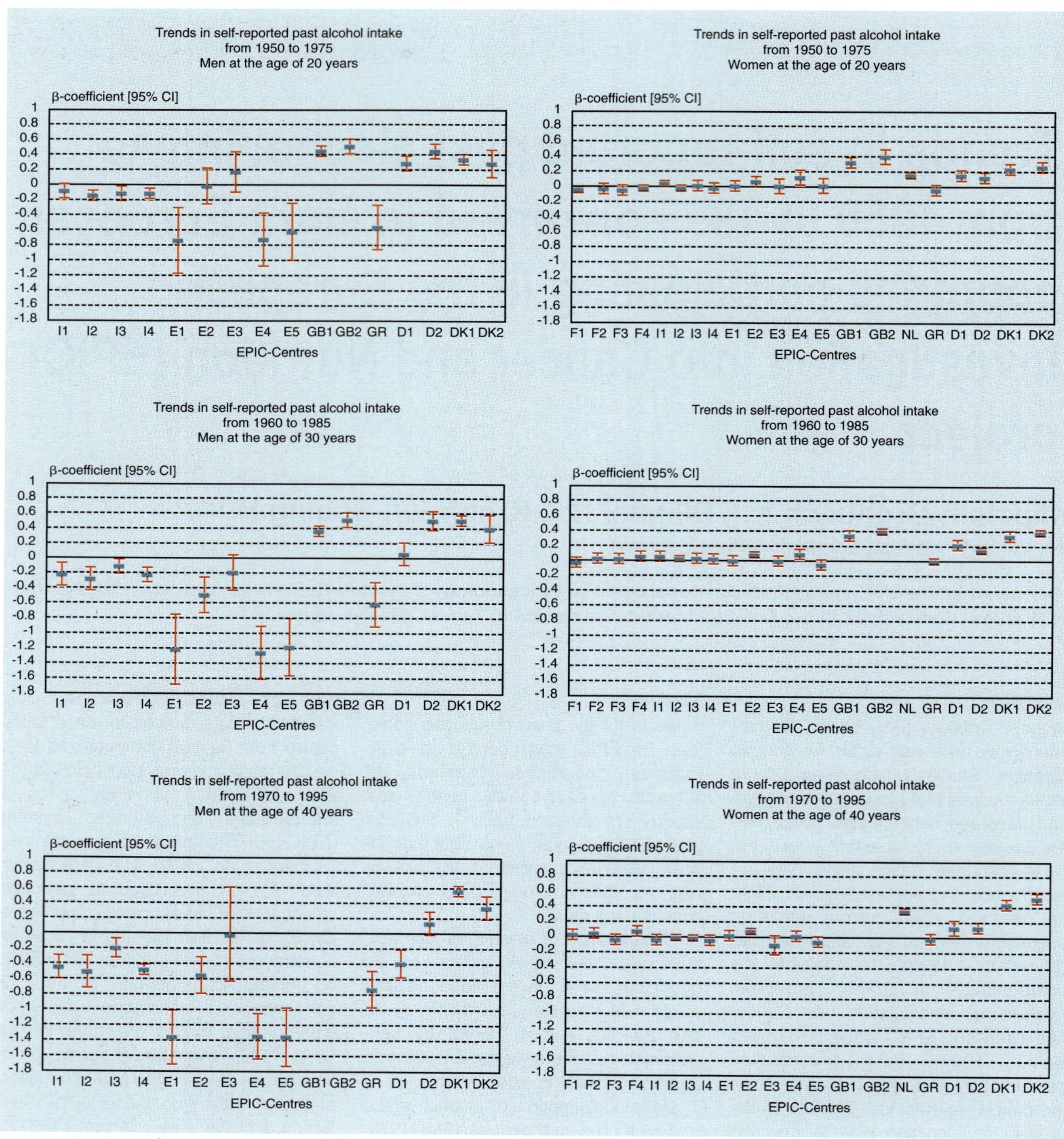
Trends in self-reported past alcohol intake
from 1950 to 1975
Men at the age of 20 years
β-coefficient [95% CI]
I1 I2 I3 I4 E1 E2 E3 E4 E5 GB1 GB2 GR D1 D2 DK1 DK2
EPIC-Centres
Trends in self-reported past alcohol intake
from 1950 to 1975
Women at the age of 20 years
β-coefficient [95% CI]
F1 F2 F3 F4 I1 I2 I3 I4 E1 E2 E3 E4 E5 GB1 GB2 NL GR D1 D2 DK1 DK2
EPIC-Centres
Trends in self-reported past alcohol intake
from 1960 to 1985
Men at the age of 30 years
β-coefficient [95% CI]
I1 I2 I3 I4 E1 E2 E3 E4 E5 GB1 GB2 GR D1 D2 DK1 DK2
EPIC-Centres
Trends in self-reported past alcohol intake
from 1960 to 1985
Women at the age of 30 years
β-coefficient [95% CI]
F1 F2 F3 F4 I1 I2 I3 I4 E1 E2 E3 E4 E5 GB1 GB2 NL GR D1 D2 DK1 DK2
EPIC-Centres
Trends in self-reported past alcohol intake
from 1970 to 1995
Men at the age of 40 years
β-coefficient [95% CI]
I1 I2 I3 I4 E1 E2 E3 E4 E5 GB1 GB2 GR D1 D2 DK1 DK2
EPIC-Centres
Trends in self-reported past alcohol intake
from 1970 to 1995
Women at the age of 40 years
β-coefficient [95% CI]
F1 F2 F3 F4 I1 I2 I3 I4 E1 E2 E3 E4 E5 GB1 GB2 NL GR D1 D2 DK1 DK2
EPIC-Centres

Figure 1

given age (20, 30, and 40 years) we were able to calculate the average consumption of alcoholic beverages (glasses/week) and alcohol intake (g/day) for the three above-mentioned time periods. The percentage of alcohol abstainers, i.e. study participants not reporting any consumption of alcoholic beverages, was determined and contribution of alcoholic beverages to total alcohol intake was calculated. Regression analysis was conducted to assess trends in past alcoholic beverage and alcohol intake with time for the cohorts in the study centres for the three time periods. All analyses were performed separately for men and women.

Results

For self-reported beer/cider consumption, a positive trend was generally observed for all time periods, i.e. 1950–1975, 1960–1985, and 1970–1995 for most of the study centres. Trends in beer/cider consumption were considerably less pronounced for women than for men.

Trends in wine consumption differed according to geographical location: for men in southern European study centres, a negative trend in wine consumption was observed for all time periods, whereas for men of middle/northern European study centres, a positive trend was observed. The level of initial wine consumption was considerably higher in southern compared to middle/northern European study centres. Similar, although less pronounced trends were observed for women.

Trends for self-reported alcohol intake are depicted in Figure 1. The graphs describe the yearly increase/decrease of alcohol intake expressed as a β-coefficient (95% confidence interval) of the linear regression over the time periods of interest. Because wine consumption was the major contributor to total alcohol intake for both men (with the exception of middle/northern European EPIC centres) and women, time trends for alcohol intake showed a similar geographical pattern as for wine consumption.

Table 1. Number and origin of study participants[a]

EPIC cohort	Country	Abbreviation	Women (*n*)	Men (*n*)
North-east of France	France	F1	32 235	–
North-west of France	France	F2	11 405	–
South of France	France	F3	17 978	–
South coast of France	France	F4	9615	–
Florence	Italy	I1	9963	3458
Varese	Italy	I2	9491	2551
Ragusa	Italy	I3	3263	2929
Turin	Italy	I4	4263	5655
Oviedo	Spain	E1	5448	3084
Granada	Spain	E2	6076	1795
Murcia	Spain	E3	5830	2684
Pamplona	Spain	E4	4057	3785
San Sebastian	Spain	E5	4259	4158
UK general population	U.K.	GB1	14 447	12 370
UK health-conscious population	U.K.	GB2	43 440	13 010
Utrecht	The Netherlands	NL	17 234	–
Greece	Greece	GR	16 432	11 522
Heidelberg	Germany	D1	13 616	11 927
Potsdam	Germany	D2	16 636	10 895
Aarhus	Denmark	DK1	8696	8413
Copenhagen	Denmark	DK2	20 865	18 579
Total			275 249	116 815

[a]Number of subjects consuming beer, wine or liquor at the age of 20 years.

Generally, men reported higher alcohol intakes than women; the average male/female ratio for self-reported past alcohol intake was 5.8 (range, 2.4–16.2) for 1950–1975, 5.2 (range, 2.1–15.5) for 1960–1985, and 5.2 (range, 2.1–14.1) for 1970–1995. For most study centres, however, it was below 5 with moderate changes, mostly slight decreases with time.

More women than men reported no alcohol consumption: figures for male alcohol abstainers were 11.7% for 1950–1975, 6.8% for 1960–1985, and 5.3% for 1970–1995 and were 46.5%, 29.4%, and 22.9% for female alcohol abstainers, respectively. For most cohorts, a considerable decrease in the percentage of alcohol abstainers with time was observed.

Conclusion

Trends in alcoholic beverage consumption, alcohol intake, and changes in the percentage of alcohol abstainers over time, i.e. for the time periods 1950–1975, 1960–1985, and 1970–1995 differed for both sexes and within the 21 EPIC centres. More women refrained from alcohol consumption than men and generally, over time, the percentage of alcohol abstainers for most EPIC centres decreased considerably. The different trends in alcohol intake suggest that information depicting life-long history of alcohol intake should be included in analyses of the relation between alcohol and chronic diseases, particularly in multicenter studies such as EPIC.

References

Lemmens, P.H. (1998) Measuring lifetime drinking histories. *Alcohol Clin. Exp. Res.*, **22**, 29S–36S

Riboli, E. & Kaaks, R. (1997) The EPIC Project: rationale and study design. European Prospective Investigation into Cancer and Nutrition. *Int. J. Epidemiol.*, **26**, S6–S14

Slimani, N., Ferrari, P., Ocké, M., Welch, A., Boeing, H., Liere, M., Pala, V., Amiano, P., Lagiou, A., Mattisson, I., Stripp, C., Engeset, D., Charrondière, R., Buzzard, M., Staveren, W. & Riboli, E. (2000) Standardization of the 24-hour diet recall calibration method used in the European prospective investigation into cancer and nutrition (EPIC): general concepts and preliminary results. *Eur. J. Clin. Nutr.*, **54**, 900–917

Alcohol consumption in EPIC cohorts from ten European countries

Sieri S.[1], Agudo A.[2], Kesse E.[3], Klipstein-Grobusch K.[4], San-José B.[5], Welch A.A.[6], Krogh V.[1]
(for the EPIC working group on dietary patterns)

[1]Epidemiology Unit, National Cancer Institute, Milan, Italy. [2]Catalan Institute of Oncology, Barcelona, Spain. [3]Institut Gustave Roussy, Villejuif, France. [4]Department of Epidemiology, German Institute of Human Nutrition, Postdam-Rehbrücke, Germany. [5]University of Athens, Athens, Greece. [6]University of Cambridge, Institute of Public Health, Strangeways, Research Laboratory, Cambridge, UK.

Alcohol may have contrasting effects on health. Moderate intake has been related to reduced risk of coronary heart disease by increasing high-density lipoproteins (HDL) and lowering low-density lipoproteins (LDL), total cholesterol and clotting factors. Conversely, alcohol consumption is reported to increase the risk of cerebrovascular disease and of cancers of the oral cavity, larynx, oesophagus and liver (IARC, 1988). The overall effect on health may be related to the types of alcoholic beverage consumed and drinking patterns (Fillmore *et al.*, 1998).

The purpose of this study was to compare the quantities of alcohol and types of alcoholic beverage consumed in the 27 centres, from ten European countries participating in the EPIC study, which differ in terms of drinking patterns and frequency of alcohol-related diseases.

Methods

Twenty-four-hour dietary recalls were collected in a standardized way using EPIC-SOFT (Slimani *et al.*, 2000) from a sample of 35 955 members of the EPIC cohort (13 301 men, 22 824 women, age 21–79).

Adjusted means of consumption of alcoholic beverages and total alcohol were calculated using a mixture approach to take into account the uneven distribution, among centres, of the interviews by day of week and season, and of the possible confounding effect of age. Individual alcohol consumption was calculated as the sum of ethanol content of all alcoholic beverages consumed.

Results

The types of the alcoholic beverage and quantity of alcohol consumed differed between sexes and centres, as shown in Tables 1 and 2.

Among men, wine consumption was highest in Varese and Turin (northern Italy) and San Sebastian (Spain) and lowest in Umeå (Sweden). Beer was mainly consumed in the German, Dutch and Danish centres. Consumption of spirits was high in the Spanish centres and the UK general population, and low in Italy (Table 1).

Among women, wine consumption was lower than men in the Mediterranean centres of Spain, Greece and Italy. Female wine consumption was highest in the Danish centres and lowest in Granada (Spain). Beer consumption was also lower in women than men; but was particularly high in Murcia (Spain) and Denmark and low in the Mediterranean countries. In general, women consumed very low quantities of spirits (Table 2).

Total alcohol intake, among men, was high in the northern Spanish centres of San Sebastian and Navarra and low in Umeå (Sweden) and southern Italy (Ragusa). Among women, the highest alcohol consumption was observed in Danish centres and the lowest in Mediterranean centres.

Thus, women consumed much less total alcohol than men in the Mediterranean countries, whereas differences between men and women in terms of total alcohol consumption were less marked in central and northern

Table 1. Adjusted[a] means of total ethanol and alcoholic beverage intake (g/day) among men in the 19 EPIC centres

	n	Wine		Beer, cider		Spirits		Total ethanol	
		Mean ± SE		Mean ± SE		Mean ± SE		Mean ± SE	
Italy									
Florence	271	202.4	13.5	12.3	27.6	2.9	1.9	20.8	2.0
Varese	328	305.0	12.3	32.3	25.0	5.7	1.7	31.9	1.8
Ragusa	168	141.5	17.2	12.5	35.0	0.8	2.4	14.0	2.5
Turin	677	294.1	8.6	31.2	17.5	3.8	1.2	30.0	1.2
Spain									
Asturias	386	228.7	11.3	138.1	23.1	11.2	1.6	35.6	1.6
Granada	214	146.2	15.2	126.9	31.0	8.6	2.1	24.5	2.2
Murcia	243	155.0	14.3	214.8	29.1	11.8	2.0	28.2	2.1
Navarra	444	260.5	10.5	49.4	21.5	14.6	1.5	38.1	1.5
San Sebastian	490	293.8	10.1	91.8	20.7	9.6	1.4	41.4	1.5
United Kingdom									
UK general population	404	87.9	11.1	229.4	22.6	11.9	1.5	21.5	1.6
UK health conscious	114	58.3	20.8	218.1	42.5	1.8	2.9	16.5	3.0
The Netherlands									
Bilthoven	1024	60.6	7.2	347.4	14.7	10.1	1.0	23.6	1.0
Greece									
	1312	119.0	6.3	85.3	12.7	5.5	0.9	19.7	0.9
Germany									
Heidelberg	1033	123.1	7.0	396.9	14.2	3.3	1.0	29.5	1.0
Potsdam	1235	50.5	6.3	407.9	12.9	5.5	0.9	23.4	0.9
Sweden									
Malmö	1421	47.1	6.2	234.9	12.7	10.7	0.9	15.9	0.9
Umeå	1344	28.0	6.1	177.0	12.4	6.5	0.8	10.2	0.9
Denmark									
Aarhus	567	154.5	9.3	344.8	19.1	10.2	1.3	33.7	1.3
Copenhagen	1356	193.9	6.0	350.0	12.3	8.0	0.8	37.2	0.9

[a]Adjusted by age and weighted for weekday and season.

Europe. These findings are consistent with those of a previous study on alcohol consumption in the European Community, which found a marked difference in the frequency of wine consumption between men and women in southern countries (Hupkens *et al.*, 1993).

In our study, the main source of alcohol consumed by men in the Mediterranean centres was wine; in the German, Dutch, Swedish and UK centres, it was beer. For women, the main source of alcohol was wine in all centres except Murcia.

It was also evident that European centres differed in terms of patterns of alcohol consumption (with or without

Table 2. Adjusted[a] means of total ethanol and alcoholic beverage intake among women in the 27 EPIC centres

	n	Wine Mean ± SE		Beer, cider Mean ± SE		Spirits Mean ± SE		Total ethanol Mean ± SE	
France									
North-east	2009	102.2	3.3	27.3	3.2	1.9	0.4	12.5	0.4
North-west	622	103.7	5.8	20.0	5.7	2.0	0.6	12.6	0.7
South	1396	94.1	3.9	13.2	3.8	2.1	0.4	10.6	0.5
South coast	612	101.2	5.9	11.9	5.8	1.2	0.7	11.6	0.7
Italy									
Florence	785	71.0	5.2	10.3	5.1	0.5	0.6	7.6	0.6
Varese	794	67.1	5.2	9.3	5.0	0.7	0.6	7.1	0.6
Ragusa	138	34.7	12.4	5.6	12.1	0.0	1.4	3.7	1.5
Turin	392	102.9	7.3	9.7	7.2	0.7	0.8	10.7	0.9
Naples	403	72.8	7.2	7.0	7.1	0.2	0.8	7.6	0.9
Spain									
Asturias	324	42.8	8.1	29.4	7.9	0.4	0.9	6.7	1.0
Granada	300	17.7	8.4	26.0	8.2	0.1	0.9	3.5	1.0
Murcia	304	29.4	8.3	114.6	8.2	1.1	0.9	7.4	1.0
Navarra	271	33.1	8.8	4.4	8.6	0.2	1.0	4.2	1.0
San Sebastian	244	64.2	9.3	10.2	9.1	0.8	1.0	7.8	1.1
United Kingdom									
UK general population	571	91.5	6.1	20.3	6.0	7.4	0.7	12.9	0.7
UK health conscious	197	61.7	10.4	21.1	10.1	4.5	1.2	8.6	1.2
The Netherlands									
Bilthoven	1086	59.8	4.5	49.1	4.4	2.4	0.5	10.3	0.5
Utrecht	1874	71.2	3.4	17.4	3.3	3.3	0.4	11.9	0.4
Greece									
	1374	21.5	3.9	24.7	3.8	1.1	0.4	3.4	0.5
Germany									
Heidelberg	1087	99.5	4.5	70.4	4.4	1.0	0.5	13.3	0.5
Potsdam	1063	58.8	4.5	43.6	4.4	1.0	0.5	8.4	0.5
Sweden									
Malmö	1711	53.7	3.6	79.5	3.5	2.1	0.4	8.6	0.4
Umeå	1574	32.5	3.7	58.3	3.6	1.5	0.4	5.6	0.4
Denmark									
Aarhus	510	120.1	6.4	98.7	6.3	4.4	0.7	18.5	0.8
Copenhagen	1485	146.6	3.8	90.4	3.7	4.7	0.4	20.9	0.4
Norway									
South-east	1136	55.0	4.4	43.2	4.3	2.8	0.5	8.2	0.5
North-west	662	50.6	5.7	27.4	5.6	1.7	0.6	7.1	0.7

[a]Adjusted by age and weighted for weekday and season.

meals and weekend versus weekday). Alcohol was mainly drunk during meals in Italian centres, by both sexes; whereas alcohol consumption out of mealtimes was higher in most other centres.

For both sexes, alcohol consumption was higher at weekends, particularly in the Swedish centres and among Norwegian women. However, in most Spanish centres (both sexes) and the Norwegian north-west centre (women), the proportion of alcohol consumed outside of mealtimes increased during weekends.

Conclusions

The most commonly consumed alcoholic beverages were wine by southern European men and beer by men in other countries. In the overwhelming majority of centres, women preferred wine. No clear geographic patterns were discerned for spirits consumption. Increased weekend drinking seems to be a characteristic of northern Europe, while alcohol consumption is generally restricted to mealtimes in Mediterranean countries. Thus we have found that detailed patterns of alcohol consumption vary markedly with geography among the European centres participating in EPIC. Naturally our data refer to restricted regions, and should not be taken as indicative of means patterns of consumption at the country level. These findings will form a useful basis for future prospective studies on alcohol-related diseases.

References

IARC (1988) *IARC Monographs on the Evaluation of Carcinogenic Risks to Humans,* Vol. 44, *Alcohol drinking,* Lyon, IARC

Fillmore, K.M., Golding, J.M., Graves, K.L., Kniep, S., Leino, E.V., Romelsjo, A., Shoemaker, C., Ager, C.R., Allebeck, P. & Ferrer, H.P. (1998) Alcohol consumption and mortality. I. Characteristics of drinking groups. *Addiction*, **93**, 183–203

Hupkens, C.L., Knibbe, R.A. & Drop, M.J. (1993) Alcohol consumption in the European community: uniformity and diversity in drinking patterns. *Addiction*, **88**, 1391–1404

Slimani, N., Ferrari, P., Ocké, M., Welch, A., Boeing, H., Liere, M., Pala, V., Amiano, P., Lagiou, A., Mattisson, I., Stripp, C., Engeset, D., Charrondière, R., Buzzard, M., Staveren, W. & Riboli, E. (2000) Standardization of the 24-hour diet recall calibration method used in the European prospective investigation into cancer and nutrition (EPIC): general concepts and preliminary results. *Eur. J. Clin. Nutr.*, **54**, 900–917

Chapter 4

Meat, fish and dairy products

Meat, fish and dairy products

Palli D.

Molecular and Nutritional Epidemiology Branch, Epidemiology Unit, Centro per lo Studio e la Prevenzione Oncologica (CSPO), Florence, Italy.

In the last 50 years, since the Second World War, widespread changes in the availability of food have occurred and the populations of most affluent western countries have modified their dietary habits. Overall, animal sources have replaced plant-derived foods, particularly for protein and total energy intake. In addition, as often happens in a rapidly changing situation, it has been difficult to keep a balance with the reduced levels of physical activity, and a high proportion of subjects may be considered overfed. This upward trend of consumption is in fact particularly evident for energy- and fat-dense foods (meat, cheese, and processed foods). Thus, overweight and moderate or severe obesity are now common conditions in developed societies, possibly contributing to an increased risk of chronic diseases, including cancer and premature death. In the last decades, however, epidemiological studies have consistently reported associations between cancer risk at specific sites and dietary patterns rich in meat and dairy products independently from overweight. In particular, an increased risk of colorectal cancer has been consistently linked to excessive red meat consumption.

Epidemiological research in this area has been particularly productive and numerous studies, often with contrasting results, are available. A working group of the World Cancer Research Fund, the American Institute for Cancer Research (WCRF-AICR 1997) has recently summarized the available evidence from epidemiological studies and what still needs to be further explored. Some of the panel conclusions, including those on meat, fish and dairy products, are presented in Fig. 1. The evidence supporting the relation between a "probable increased risk" of colorectal cancer and high consumption of meat and processed meat, was considered particularly convincing; this has been confirmed by a recent meta-analysis (Sandhu *et al.*, 2001). There was also support for a possible link between an increased risk of colorectal cancer and frequent consumption of grilled and barbecued meats and saturated or animal fats; specific mechanisms have been proposed. A link between salt (particularly from salted meat and fish) and gastric cancer was considered probable, while the evidence of a link between gastric cancer and N-nitrosocompounds, mostly derived from meat and fish, was judged still insufficient. Despite the general decline of stomach cancer in western countries, higher risks of this disease are seen in areas where meat consumption is higher, particularly processed, grilled or barbecued meat. Specific mechanisms have been recently suggested (Palli *et al.*, 2001), in analogy with the model of colorectal carcinogenesis. The risk of breast cancer has been linked to increased consumption of red meat and saturated and animal fat, although many studies reported conflicting results. A similar pattern has been more consistently described for prostate cancer, with an additional role for the consumption of dairy products. Interestingly enough, there are no animal products among those listed in the summary table of WCRF-AICR evaluations as clearly linked to a protection from cancer at any site.

In recent years, the fear for the variant Creutzfeldt-Jakob disease (linked to the epidemic of bovine spongiform encephalopathy (BSE) in cattle, also known as mad cow disease) led, at least temporarily, to a widespread reduction in meat consumption. This effect was clearly evident in most European populations, as soon as the media described in detail the increasing number of human vCJ cases, and national governments were forced to take decisions in order to ban or limit cattle imported from suspect areas. The BSE epidemic has been directly linked to the practice of recycling nonedible cattle tissues for animal feed. A Swiss survey compared meat consumption in two periods immediately before and after the first BSE crisis in a representative sample of 1190 men and 1154 women. In 1996,

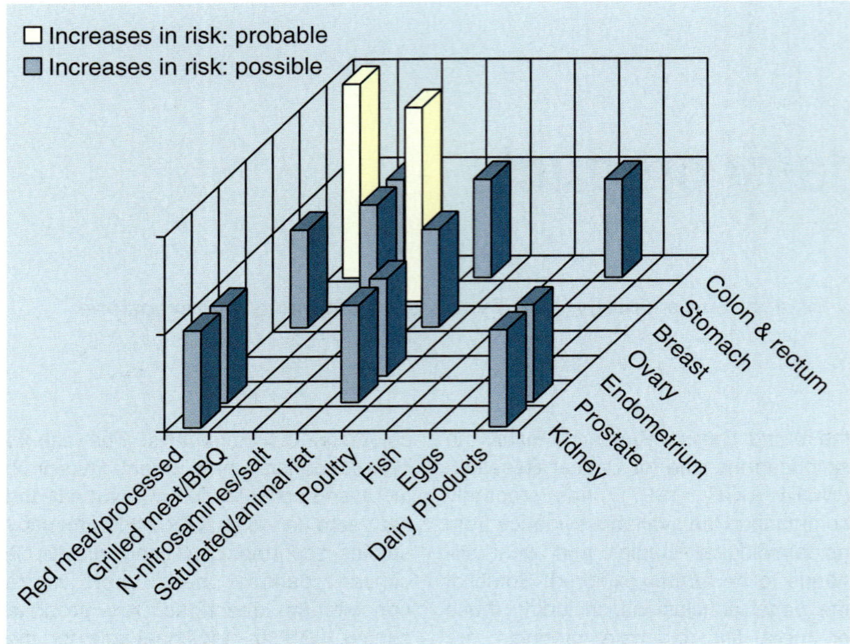

Figure 1
Food items in the meat/fish/dairy products section that have been consistently associated with an increase in the risk of cancer at different sites (modified from WCRF-AACR 1997)

14.6% of interviewed subjects reported not having consumed meat, as compared with 7.7% of subjects in the 1993–1995 survey. Among meat eaters, the amount of beef consumed decreased significantly in women, but not significantly in men (Morabia *et al.*, 1999). It is probably too early to understand whether the even stronger reduction in meat consumption that followed the most recent BSE crisis will last or not. Many scientists, cancer prevention agencies and nutritional recommendations have been trying for a long time to achieve the goal of a permanent reduction in the consumption of meat and other animal products, to be replaced by plant-derived foods. On the other hand, epidemiologists will be interested in understanding whether this large scale modification of dietary habits will significantly affect cancer risk in the near future.

Data gathered in the EPIC study will offer the unique opportunity to observe differences in cancer risk in populations with very different dietary patterns and nutrient intakes and with different risk profiles (smoking history and physical activity, for example); both components differ in the various countries because of different traditions and the genetic heterogeneity of the various populations. Nutritional epidemiological data need to be strengthened by specific analytical and laboratory work in the fields of molecular biology and individual susceptibility; the centralized EPIC biological specimen databank will provide a series of great opportunities in this exciting field.

References

Morabia, A., Bernstein, M.S., Heritier, S. & Beer-Borst, S.A. (1999) Swiss population-based assessment of dietary habits before and after the March 1996 'mad cow disease' crisis. *Eur. J. Clin. Nutr.*, **53**, 158–163

Palli, D., Russo, A., Ottini, R., Masala, G., Saieva, C., Amorosi, A., Cama, A., D'Amico, C., Falchetti, M., Palmirotta, R., Decarli, A., Mariani Costantini, R. & Fraumeni, J.F. Jr. (2001) Red meat, family history and increased risk of gastric cancer with microsatellite instability. *Cancer Res.*, **61**, 5415–5419

Sandhu, M.S., White, I.R. & McPherson, K. (2001) Systematic review of the prospective cohort studies and meat consumption and colorectal cancer risk: a meta-analytical approach. *Cancer Epidemiol. Biomarkers Prev.*, **10**, 439–446

World Cancer Research Fund and American Institute for Cancer Research. (1997) *Food, Nutrition and the Prevention of Cancer: A Global Perspective.* Washington, D.C., WCR-AICR

Meat cooking and cancer risk

Sinha R.[1], Norat T.[2]

[1]Division of Cancer Epidemiology and Genetics, National Cancer Institute, National Institutes of Health, Executive Plaza North, Rm. 443, 6130 Executive Blvd., Rockville, MD 20892. [2]Unit of Nutrition and Cancer, International Agency for Research on Cancer, 150, Cours Albert Thomas, 69372, Lyon Cedex 08, France.

A report by an international panel of experts entitled *Food, Nutrition and the Prevention of Cancer: A Global Perspective* concluded that "diets containing substantial amounts of red meat probably increase the risk of colorectal cancer" and "that such diets possibly increase the risk of pancreatic, breast, prostate, and renal cancers" (World Cancer Research Fund, 1997). The association with red meat intake may be due to a combination of factors such as content of fat, protein, and iron, and/or meat preparation (e.g. cooking or preserving methods).

Laboratory results have shown that meats cooked at high temperatures contain heterocyclic amines (HCAs) and polycyclic aromatic hydrocarbons (PAHs), which are mutagenic and carcinogenic in animals (Ohgaki *et al.*, 1985; Adamson,1990; Felton & Knize, 1990; Skog, 1993; Ito *et al.*, 1991; Ghoshal *et al.*, 1994; Culp *et al.*, 1998). Epidemiological studies (Schiffman *et al.*, 1990; Gerhardsson De Verdier *et al.*, 1991; Steineck *et al.*, 1993; Knekt *et al.*, 1994; Muscat & Wynder, 1994; Ronco *et al.*, 1996) have found a suggestive but inconsistent relationship between the way meat is cooked and colon cancer risk (Table 1). Cooking methods or meat doneness have been examined in epidemiological studies as a surrogate measure of mutagens formed during high-temperature cooking of meat, e.g. HCAs and PAHs. The techniques of meat cooking associated with increased cancer risk were high-temperature cooking methods (frying, broiling, or grilling/barbecuing) and doneness level or surface browning of meat and intake of gravy made from meat drippings. In these studies, the information obtained on meat cooking practices could not differentiate between factors that had an important influence on the production of HCAs and PAHs.

We will describe our approach to estimating meat-cooking mutagens and the main results we have obtained on the association of cancer risk with meat intake, meat cooking methods and certain mutagens formed during cooking.

Assessing exposure to HCAs and PAHs

We set up a multidisciplinary approach to develop tools to estimate dietary intake of HCAs and PAHs. The first step was to develop databases for HCA and PAH content in meat. Approximately 2500 individual pieces of meat were cooked to provide data for 120 categories by cooking method and doneness that were ultimately used to create the HCA database (Knize *et al.*, 1995, 1996; Sinha *et al.*, 1995a; Sinha *et al.*, 1998a,b).

We found that the measured values of the specific HCAs varied with meat type, cut of meat, cooking method, and doneness level and that the different HCAs were formed in varying amounts. The results suggest that questions on meat intake not including details of type or cut of meat, cooking technique, and doneness level are likely to misclassify HCA exposure. For example, for the same level of doneness, steaks, hamburger patties, and roast beef had substantially different levels of HCAs. The three high-temperature cooking methods (pan-frying, oven broiling, and grilling/barbecuing) produced varying levels of HCAs (Fig. 1). We also measured mutagenic activity in the meat samples using the Ames salmonella test (strain 98). Mutagenic activity has the advantage of being a biological measure that integrates all classes of mutagens according to their mutagenic potential.

HCA production resulted from two important elements: temperature and time. By developing the HCA database, we found that cooking technique could serve as a reasonable proxy of temperature and doneness level as a surrogate for time. Using existing Food Frequency Questionnaires (FFQs), we embedded the cooking methods and doneness levels within each meat line item. As doneness can be subjective, we included photographs of different levels of doneness showing both the inside and outside for various meat items (Sinha & Rothman, 1997).

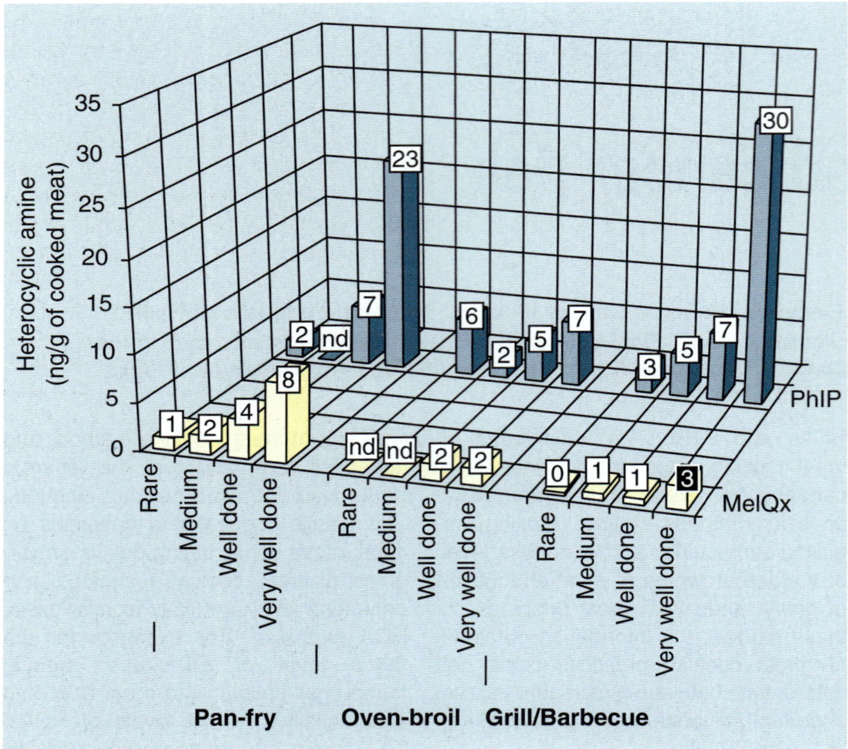

Figure 1
Meat cooking and content in heterocyclic amines

PhIP is 2-amino-1-methyl-6-phenylimidazo[4,5-b]pyridine
MeIQx is 2-amino-3,8-dimethylimidazo[4,5-f]quinoxaline

Development of biomarkers of HCA exposure

In a metabolic study we collected multiple biological samples to test for new biological markers and examine HCA metabolism pathways in individuals who consumed meats containing known amounts of HCAs. We evaluated several markers of HCA intake in the urine by measuring mutagenic activity (free and acid hydrolysed), HCAs (free and acid hydrolysed) and metabolites of HCA (Sinha *et al.*, 1995b ; Stillwell *et al.*, 1997, 1999a, 1999b;). Urinary free HCAs or total (acid-hydrolysed urine samples includes free, N2-glucuronide and sulfamate metabolites) correlated modestly with the amount of HCA consumed in the metabolic study, with the Spearman correlation coefficients between 0.4 and 0.6. HCAs and mutagenic activity in the urine were not detectable 12 h after consuming the high-HCA meal. This indicates that HCAs in urine may not be ideal measures of usual intake in etiological studies. We measured DNA adducts to examine if they could be used as a marker of biologically effective dose of HCAs, but DNA adducts were not sensitive enough, even in subjects who consumed high levels of MeIQx (2-amino-3,8-dimethylimidazo[4,5-f]quinox aline) and PhIP (2-amino-1-methyl-6-phenylimidazo[4,5-b]pyridine). Thus, at present, it is unlikely with current methods that we will be able to measure HCA adducts in a free-living population, whose intake is likely to be much lower than that of subjects in the metabolic study.

The cancer risk posed to humans from HCAs in the diet may depend upon the extent to which the compounds are activated *in vivo*. The initial activation step is thought to be N-oxidation by liver CYP1A2. The N-hydroxylamine metabolite is O-acetylated in the liver itself or transported to the appropriate target organ, where it is acetylated by the polymorphic acetyltransferases, *NAT1* or *NAT2*. The acetylated compound can form adducts and cause DNA damage. CYP1A2 and *NAT2* activities can be measured by evaluating excretion of caffeine metabolites in urine after caffeine consumption. In the metabolic study, CYP1A2 and *NAT2* activities were measured at baseline and at the end of the low- and high-temperature cooked-meat periods. *NAT2* activity remained unchanged throughout the study, while CYP1A2 activity increased in most of the subjects after consuming high-temperature cooked meat, suggesting induction by some compound(s) formed during high-temperature cooking. There was a high within-person correlation for CYP1A2: subjects with low enzymatic activity after eating low-temperature cooked meat tended to have relatively low activity even after consuming high-temperature cooked meat and the subjects who had high enzymatic activity tended to stay relatively high. This suggests a fixed component in the regulation of CYP1A2 and the need to consider both a fixed and an inducible component of this enzyme in epidemiological studies.

Due to the ubiquitous nature of PAHs in foods, estimating dietary consumption is considerably more challenging than estimating intake of HCAs, which are formed in large

Table 1. Epidemiological evidence of the possible association between cooked meat and cancer

Author	Cooking method	RR (CI)	a
Relative risk for very well done meat/high browning vs rare meat/not browning			
Schiffman *et al.*, 1990		3.5 (1.3–9.6)	a
Gerhardsson *et al.*, 1991		2.0 (1.2–3.6)	a
Lang *et al.*, 1994		2.1 (1.1–4.1)	
Muscat *et al.*, 1994		1.2 (0.6–2.4)	
Kampmann *et al.*, 1999		1.2 (0.9–1.5)	
Relative risk for high vs low consumption of meat according to cooking methods			
Lyon *et al.*, 1988	Frying	1.2 (0.8–1.9)	
	Broiling	0.7 (0.8–2.1)	b
Young *et al.*, 1988	Frying	1.3 (1.0–1.8)	b
	Broiling	0.7 (0.5–1.0)	
Peters *et al.*, 1989	Deep frying	2.1 (1.0–4.6)	b
Wohlebb *et al.*, 1990	BBQ	3.3 (1.2–9.2)	a

[a]Statistically significant.
[b]Borderline statistically significant.

Table 2. HCA carcinogenicity in animal and epidemiologic studies

Site	Animal studies	Epidemiological studies
Colon	IQ, MeIQ, PhIP	MeIQx, PhIP[a]
Lung	IQ, MeIQx	MeIQx
Mammary/breast	PhIP	PhIP

PhIP is 2-amino-1-methyl-6-phenylimidazo[4,5-b]pyridine.
MeIQx is 2-amino-3,8-dimethylimidazo[4,5-f]quinoxaline.

[a]Borderline statistically significant.

quantities only in high-temperature cooked meat. Humans can be exposed to PAHs via grilled and smoked foods, foods grown in polluted environments, ambient air contact, and tobacco smoking. Thus, in estimating exposure to PAHs, it is crucial to develop biomarkers that integrate exposures from different sources. We are currently investigating a number of possible biomarkers: urinary PAH metabolites as a measure of dietary exposure and Benzo(a)pyrene-DNA adduct as a marker for long-term PAH exposure from all sources.

Epidemiologic studies

Colorectal adenomas

We investigated the role of meat intake, meat-cooking techniques, and meat-cooking mutagens in a hospital-based case–control study of colorectal adenomas in Bethesda (Sinha *et al.*, 2001). This was the first study to use the detailed FFQ meat-cooking module. We found a nonsignificant increased risk of colorectal adenomas of 4% per 10 g/day (or 2.5 oz/week) of total meat intake. This increased risk for total meat partitioned into a significant 11% per 10 g/day risk increase for consumption of red meat and a nonsignificant decrease in risk of 5% per 10 g/day for white meat intake. The partitioned risk associated with well done/very well done red meat was 29% risk increase per 10 g/day. High-temperature cooking methods were also associated with increased risk; 26% per 10 g/day of grilled red meat and 15% per 10 g/day of pan-fried red meat consumption. The risk was further elevated to 85% per 10 g/day among subjects who ate well done/very well done grilled meat. Risk of colorectal adenomas was doubled in the highest compared to the lowest quintile of intake of DiMeIQx, MeIQx, and PhIP. The excess risk was confined to the fifth quintile for DiMeIQx and MeIQx, and to both the fourth and fifth quintiles for PhIP. When adjusting each HCA for the other two, the risk estimates became attenuated for all three because they were modestly to highly correlated. However, the trend for MeIQx intake remained statistically significant. There was an increase in colorectal adenoma risk in relation to estimated total meat-derived mutagenic activity. The risk associated with mutagenic activity was minimally affected when adjusted for PhIP (which became nonsignificant) and was weakened when adjusted for MeIQx (which was attenuated to an even greater extent; data not shown). Mutagenic activity remained significantly associated with increased risk even when adjusted for intake of red meat or well-done red meat. In contrast, the red meat and well-done red meat associations were no longer statistically significant when adjusted for total mutagenic activity, suggesting that mutagenic activity explained the meat relationships.

Lung cancer

Some epidemiological studies have found that diets high in fat, saturated fat, or cholesterol are associated with an increased risk of lung cancer. Meat consumption is highly correlated with the intake of saturated fat and cholesterol. In the Missouri Women's Study, a population-based lung cancer case–control study, lung cancer was associated with higher intake of total meat, red meat, well-done red meat, and fried red meat (Sinha *et al.*, 1998c). Because MeIQx has been found to induce lung tumours in rodents, we compared risks for the 90th and 10th percentiles of intake (95% confidence interval, CI). We observed significant excess risks for MeIQx (OR, 1.5; CI, 1.1–2.0) but not for DiMeIQx (OR, 1.2; CI, 0.9–1.6) or PhIP (OR, 0.9; CI, 0.8–1.1). Interestingly, MeIQx consumption was associated with an increased risk of lung cancer for the non-smokers and the light/moderate smokers but not for the heavy smokers (Sinha *et al.*, 2000b). The increased risk of lung cancer associated with higher intake of meat, well-done/fried meat, and MeIQx consumption needs to be viewed in the context of other risk factors such as smoking. Smoking is by far the strongest risk factor for lung cancer and its impact cannot be minimized even when other modest risk factors are found. Therefore, we remain concerned about residual confounding from smoking.

Breast cancer

In carcinogenicity experiments with rodents, PhIP consistently induced mammary tumours. In a nested case–control study within the Iowa Women's Health Study, subjects completed the meat-cooking module and preference for level of doneness by using a series of colour photographs. Breast cancer risk was associated with well-done/very well-done red meat (Zheng *et al.*, 1998). We estimated HCA intake and found that risk of breast cancer was elevated across increasing quintiles of PhIP consumption, whereas MeIQx and DiMeIQx were not associated in these analyses (Sinha *et al.*, 2000a). When PhIP and very well-done red meat were adjusted for each other, PhIP remained significantly associated with breast cancer risk but very well-done meat did not, indicating that PhIP may be the relevant component of very well-done red meat.

In a case–control study among women (Susceptibility to Breast Cancer: Dietary and other Factors (Delphina *et al.*, 2000) with suspicious breast masses, no significant associations between red meat intake and breast cancer were found for any doneness preference. White meat intake was significantly protective (for >67 g/day vs <26 g/day (OR, 0.46; CI, 0.23–0.94), as were well-done, pan-fried or barbecued chicken, and other chicken. The subjects with estimated intakes of PhIP in the highest quartile (>240 ng/day) versus the lowest quartile (<31 ng/day) were at a significantly decreased risk of breast cancer (OR, 0.42; CI, 0.02–0.88). The protective effect of PhIP was no longer significant after adjusting for chicken intake. Furthermore, there was no association between *NAT2* genotype and breast cancer.

These two studies appear to contradict each other: PhIP was associated with increased risk of breast cancer in the Iowa Women's Health study, whereas intake of chicken and PhIP were protective in the Californian study. The types of meats consumed and the control subjects used in the two studies, however, were quite different. In Iowa, the risk of breast cancer was associated with very well-done red meat consumption and the HCAs were estimated from three red meats only (steak, hamburger, and bacon). In the California study, the women ate very small amounts of red meat, so PhIP intake was mainly from chicken. Our estimate of PhIP intake in the California study may be a surrogate for chicken consumption rather than an accurate estimate of this compound. Results from the FFQ validation study and database development work indicate that there may be substantial misclassification in estimating PhIP intake from chicken. Estimating chicken intake using the existing FFQs may not be optimal and variability in PhIP content of cooked chicken can be substantial. Better methods to estimate PhIP in chicken are needed.

Stomach cancer

In a population-based case–control study (Ward *et al.*, 1997), high intake of red meat was associated with an increased risk of stomach cancer. Overall, broiling or frying of beef, chicken, or pork was not associated with risk of this tumour. Barbecuing/grilling, reported as the usual cooking method for a small number of study participants, was associated with an elevated risk. After excluding those who reported usually barbecuing/grilling, a source of both PAHs and HCAs, the doneness level was evaluated as a surrogate for HCA exposure. Compared to a preference for rare/medium rare beef, ORs were 2.4 for medium, 2.4 for medium-well and 3.2 for well-done beef preferences, with a significant positive trend. The finding that well-done and grilled meats are associated with an increased risk of stomach cancer suggests that dietary HCAs and PAHs play an etiological role. To assess the role of HCA and PAH intake, future studies of stomach cancer will need more detailed questions on meat-cooking techniques.

Final considerations

We have found that red meat intake is associated with increased risk of colorectal adenomas as well as lung and stomach cancers. Grilled meat intake, a possible surrogate for HCAs and PAHs, increased the risk of colorectal adenomas and stomach cancer, whereas intake of fried meat, which contains mainly HCAs, was associated with lung cancer. With greater degrees of red meat doneness, a proxy for a higher level of meat-cooking carcinogens, an increase in risks for colorectal adenomas, lung, breast, and stomach cancers was observed. The data suggest some degree of organ specificity for HCAs and are consistent with those obtained in animal carcinogenicity studies (Table 2).

To elucidate the relationship between meat-cooking mutagens/carcinogens and cancer risk further, future research should also be conducted in populations with a wide range of consumption of different types of meat and cooking methods, such as in different European countries (European Prospective Investigation on Cancer), groups characterized by rapidly changing diets with increasing meat consumption, such as in Japan and China, and groups with high meat intake using high-temperature cooking methods, such as in some South American countries and Australia/New Zealand.

Using 24-h recalls from the EPIC calibration study, we began to collaborate in the development of meat-cooking modules tailored to country-specific cohorts in the overall study.

References

Adamson, R.H. (1990) Mutagens and carcinogens formed during cooking of food and methods to minimize their formation. In: DeVita, V.T., Hellman, S. & Rosenberg, S.A., eds, *Cancer Prevention*. Philadelphia, J.B. Lippincott Company, pp 1–7

Culp, S.J., Gaylor, D.W., Sheldon, W.G., Goldstein, L.S. & Beland, F.A. (1998) A comparison of the tumor induced by coal tar and benzo[a]pyrene in a 2-year bioassay. *Carcinogenesis*, **19**, 117–124

Delfino, R.J., Sinha, R., Smith, C., West, J., White, E., Lin, H.J., Liao, S.Y., Gim, J.S., Ma, H.L., Butler, J. & Anton-Culver, H. (2000) Breast cancer, heterocyclic aromatic amines from meat and N-acetyltransferase 2 genotype. *Carcinogenesis*, **21**, 607–615

Felton, J.S. & Knize, M.G. (1990) New mutagens from cooked food. *Prog. Clin. Biol. Res.*, **347**, 19–38

Ghoshal, A., Preisegger, K.H., Takayama, S., Thorgeirsson, S.S. & Snyderwine, E.G. (1994) Induction of mammary tumours in female Sprague-Dawley rats by the food-derived carcinogen 2-amino-1-methyl-6-phenylimidazo[4,5-b]pyridine and effect of dietary fat. *Carcinogenesis*, **15**, 2429–2433

Ito, N., Hasegawa, R., Sano, M., Tamano, S., Esumi, H., Takayama, S., Tamano, S., Esumi, H., Takayama, S. & Sugimura, T. (1991) A new colon and mammary carcinogen in cooked food, 2-amino-1-methyl-6-phenylimidazo[4,5-b]pyridine (PhIP). *Carcinogenesis*, **12**, 1503–1506

Gerhardsson De Verdier, M., Hagman, U., Peters, R.K., Steineck, G. & Overvik, E. (1991) Meat, cooking methods and colorectal cancer: a case-referent study in Stockholm. *Int. J. Cancer*, **49**, 520–525

Knekt, P., Steineck, G., Jarvinen, R., Hakulinen, T. & Aromaa, A. (1994) Intake of fried meat and risk of cancer: a follow-up study in Finland. *Int. J. Cancer*, **59**, 756–760

Knize, M.G., Sinha, R., Rothman, N., Brown, E.D., Salmon, C.P., Levander, O.A., Cunningham, P.L. & Felton, J.S. (1995) Fast-food meat products have relatively low heterocyclic amine content. *Food Chem. Toxicol.*, **33**, 545–551

Knize, M.G., Sinha, R., Salmon, C.P., Mehta, S.S., Dewhirst, K.P. & Felton, J.S. (1996) Formation of heterocyclic amine mutagen/carcinogens during cooking of muscle meat. *J. Muscle Food*, **35**, 433–441

Muscat, J.E. & Wynder, E.L. (1994) The consumption of well-done red meat and the risk of colorectal cancer. *Am. J. Public Health*, **84**, 856–858

Ohgaki, H., Hasegawa, H., Kato, T., Suenaga, M., Sato, S., Takayama, S. & Sugimura, T. (1985) Carcinogenicities in mice and rats of IQ, MeIQ, and MeIQx. *Princess Takamatsu Symp.*, **16**, 97–105

Ronco, A., De Stefani, E., Mendilaharsu, M. & Deneo-Pellegrini, H. (1996) Meat, fat and risk of breast cancer: a case–control study from Uruguay. *Int. J. Cancer*, **65**, 328–331

Schiffman, M.H., Van Tassell, R. & Andrews, A.W. (1990) Epidemiologic studies of fecal mutagenicity, cooked meat ingestion, and risk of colorectal cancer. *Prog. Clin. Biol. Res.*, **340**, 205–214

Sinha, R., Rothman, N., Brown, E.D., Salmon, C.P., Knize, M.G., Swanson, C.A., Rossi, S.C., Mark, S.D., Levander, O.A. & Felton J.S. (1995a) High concentrations of the carcinogen 2-amino-1-methyl-6-phenylimidazo[4,5-b]pyridine (PhIP) occur in chicken but are dependent on the cooking method. *Cancer Res.*, **55**, 4516–4519

Sinha, R., Rothman, N., Mark, S.D., Murray, S., Brown, E.D., Levander, O.A., Davies, D.S., Lang, N.P., Kadlubar, F.F. & Hoover, R.N. (1995b) Lower levels of urinary 2-amino-3,8-dimethylimidazo[4,5-f]-quinoxaline (MeIQx) in humans with higher CYP1A2 activity. *Carcinogenesis*, **16**, 2859–2861

Sinha, R. & Rothman, N. (1997) Exposure assessment of heterocyclic amines (HCAs) in epidemiologic studies. *Mutat. Res.*, **376**, 195–202

Sinha, R., Knize, M.G., Salmon, C.P., Brown, E.D., Rhodes, D., Felton, J.S., Levander, O.A. & Rothman, N. (1998a) Heterocyclic amine content of pork products cooked by different methods and to varying degrees of doneness. *Food Chem. Toxicol.*, **36**, 289–297

Sinha, R., Rothman, N., Salmon, C.P., Knize, M.G., Brown, E.D., Swanson, C.A., Rhodes, D., Rossi, S., Felton, J.S. & Levander, O.A. (1998b) Heterocyclic aromatic amine content of beef cooked by different methods and degrees of doneness and beef gravy made from roast. *Food Chem. Toxicol.*, **36**, 279–287

Sinha, R., Kulldorff, M., Curtin, J., Brown, C.C., Alavanja, M.C.R. & Swanson, C.A. (1998c) Fried, well-done red meat and risk of lung cancer in women (United States). *Cancer Causes Control*, **9**, 621–630

Sinha, R., Gustafson, D.R., Kulldorff, M., Wen, W.Q., Cerhan, J.R. & Zheng, W.

(2000a) 2-Amino-1-methyl-6-phenylimidazo [4,5-b]pyridine, a carcinogen in high-temperature cooked meat and breast cancer. *J. Natl. Cancer Inst.*, **92**, 1352–1354

Sinha, R., Kulldorff, M., Swanson, C.A., Curtin, J., Brownson, R.C. & Alavanja, M.C.R. (2000b) Dietary heterocyclic amines and the risk of lung cancer among Missouri women. *Cancer Res.*, **60**, 3753–3756

Sinha, R., Kulldorff, M., Chow, W.H., Denobile, J. & Rothman, N., (2001) Dietary intake of heterocyclic amines, meat derived mutagenic activity, and risk of colorectal adenomas. *Cancer Epidemiol. Biomarkers Prev.* **10**, 559–562

Skog, K. (1993) Cooking procedures and food mutagens: a literature review. *Food Chem. Toxicol.*, **31**, 655–675

Steineck, G., Gerhardsson De Verdier, M. & Overvik, E. (1993) The epidemiological evidence concerning intake of mutagenic activity from the fried surface and the risk of cancer cannot justify preventive measures. *Eur. J. Cancer Prev.*, **2**, 293–300

Stillwell, W.G., Kidd, L.C., Wishnok, J.S., Tannenbaum, S.R. & Sinha, R. (1997) Urinary excretion of unmetabolized and phase II conjugates of 2-amino-1-methyl-6-phenylimidazo[4,5-b]pyridine and 2-amino-3,8-dimethylimidazo[4,5-f]quinoxaline in humans: relationship to cytochrome P4501A2 and N-acetyltransferase activity. *Cancer Res.*, **57**, 3457–3464

Stillwell, W.G., Turesky, R.J., Sinha, R., Skipper, P.L., & Tannenbaum, S.R. (1999a) Biomonitoring of heterocyclic aromatic amine metabolites in human urine. *Cancer Lett.*, **143**, 145–148

Stillwell, W.G., Turesky, R.J., Sinha, R. & Tannenbaum, S.R. (1999b) N-oxidative metabolism of 2-amino-3,8-dimethylimidazo[4,5-f]quinoxaline (MeIQx) in humans: excretion of the N2-glucuronide conjugate of 2-hydroxyamino-MeIQx in urine. *Cancer Res.*, **59**, 5154–5159

Ward, M.H., Sinha, R., Heineman, E.F., Rothman, N., Markin, R., Weisenburger, D.D., Rothman, N., Markin, R., Weisenburger, D.D., Correa, P. & Zahm, S.H. (1997) Risk of adenocarcinoma of the stomach and esophagus with meat cooking method and doneness preference. *Int. J. Cancer*, **71**, 14–19

World Cancer Research Fund/American Institute for Cancer Research. (1997) *Food, Nutrition and the Prevention of Cancer: A Global Perspective.* Washington, D.C., World Cancer Research Fund/American Institute for Cancer Research

Zheng, W., Gustafson, D.R., Sinha, R., Cerhan, J.R., Moore, D., Hong, C.P., Anderson, K.E., Kushi, L.H., Sellers, T.A. & Folsom, AR. (1998) Well-done meat intake and the risk of breast cancer. *J. Natl. Cancer Inst.*, **90**, 1724–1729

Fish and cancer

Lund E.
Institute of Community Medicine, University of Tromsø, Norway.

Introduction

The impact of fish consumption on cancer risk has not been a major issue in studies of nutrition and cancer even though fish is a major source of animal proteins and fat in many countries. Per capita food fish supply has increased slowly over many years, reaching about 15 kg per capita per year worldwide (FAO, 2001). While there has been a levelling off of global fishery capture, agricultural production is increasing. Fish has been considered healthy food, but the scientific documentation is limited. The strongest evidence has been the finding of a reduced risk for death from coronary artery disease (Marckman *et al.*, 1999; Schmidt *et al.*, 2000).

In this article the main focus will be on the methodological problems related to definitions of fish exposure in most epidemiological studies. There will be no attempt to summarize the present knowledge for all sites of cancer.

Fish and cancer: published studies

The report from the World Cancer Foundation/American Society of Cancer Research (World Cancer Research Fund,1997) published in 1997 noted that there was insufficient evidence of decreased risk for breast and ovary cancer with increasing fish consumption. There was possible evidence of no relationship for colon and rectum cancer. In the same report, data on the relationship between cancer and the essential omega-3 fatty acids from fish were considered insufficient. Similarly, a review article published later found no evidence of any effect of the essential fatty acids (De Deckere, 1999).

In nutritional epidemiology, several different approaches have been used. Prospective cohort studies have been advocated in order to reduce the risk of differential information bias, which could exist in case–control studies of dietary habits and cancer (Giovannucci *et al.*, 1993b). There is a substantial number of case–control studies that have included fish. Few prospective studies have been undertaken in order to test hypotheses regarding fish consumption and cancer. As an example, for breast cancer only, four cohort studies have been published (Stampfer *et al.*, 1987; Mills *et al.*, 1989; Vatten *et al.*, 1990; Toniolo *et al.*, 1994), summarized in Table 1. Three of four studies reported no association. The fourth study had one positive subgroup finding.

Information from prospective studies is also limited for other sites of cancer, such as prostate cancer (Terry *et al.*, 2001; Le Marchand *et al.*, 1994; Schuurman *et al.*, 1999; Giovannucci *et al.*, 1993a; Hsing *et al.*, 1990), colon cancer (Gaard *et al.*, 1996; Kato *et al.*, 1997; Giovannucci *et al.*, 1994; Goldbohm *et al.*, 1994; Bostick *et al.*, 1994) and lung cancer (Breslow *et al.*, 2000). In most areas, the studies published after the 1997 report (World Cancer Research Fund, 1997) have not changed the weight of the evidence.

Fish exposure

One major methodological problem has been the treatment of fish as an exposure category. In most studies, fish has been considered a single unit with no attempts to discriminate between different species according to fat

Table 1. A review of fish consumption and breast cancer, prospective studies

Study	*n*	Results	Number of fish questions/total
Stampfer	89 538	No	1/61
Mills	20 341	No	–
Vatten	14 500	No overall, poached negative	5/60
Toniolo	14 291	No	–

content. This lack of discrimination between species could severely bias any estimates for the relationship between essential omega-3 fatty acids and cancer since the fat content in fish varies from near 0% to 25%. Since each country has its local mix of fish species, dependent on local and remote sources, total fish consumption is potentially meaningless in pooled analyses. In the prospective studies of fish consumption and breast cancer, the number of questions were few (Table 1). Even in the Norwegian study, only five questions considered fish consumption. They allowed no discrimination between lean and fatty fish. The lack of detailed exposure information has not been restricted only to cohort studies. As an example, in the pooled analysis of Italian case–control studies, a substantial reduction in risk was found for all cancer of the gastrointestinal tract based on a single question of fish exposure. In the pooled analysis of 13 case–control studies of thyroid cancer (Bosetti *et al.*, 2001), six had only one question about total fish, three had two and three questions, respectively, two had six and ten questions, respectively, and only two studies had more than ten questions covering salt and fresh water fish, fish products, shellfish and different species.

Another example of the lack of exposure classification could be the 1987 U.S. National Health Interview Survey cohort where meat, poultry and fish were analysed together based on 12 separate questions. The only question about fish was fried fish or fish sandwiches.

This is only one of several analyses where fish has been aggregated together with white meat. Further, fish does not have the same composition of amino acids as beef or pork. In addition, fish is a source of several minerals, vitamins and other compounds.

This lack of interest for the relationship between one of the major food groups on a worldwide basis and cancer could have many reasons. There could be a lack of plausible biological hypotheses. Or, since most studies of diet and cancer have been conducted in countries with a low consumption of fish, then fish has not been an important issue in the questionnaires.

Future research

In the future, studies on fish consumption and cancer should take into account not only the content of fatty acids in the fish from different study areas, but also the content of fat-soluble vitamins such as A, D and E in the fish fat. In some regions, people even eat the fish liver, which is extremely rich in vitamins A and D. Additional information has to be collected about the common use of supplements of fish oil, cod liver oil, or purified omega-3 fat as capsules.

A substantial part of the fish is processed before eating, most of it through heating. In many regions fish is smoked, salted or dried. Consumption of salted or smoked fish has been suspected as a risk factor for development of stomach cancer in parts of the world where these processing methods are common. Chinese salted fish has been considered as carcinogenic to humans by IARC (International Agency for Research on Cancer, 1993). The cooking methods differ between different populations such as boiling or steaming, as well as high-temperature methods such as grilling or frying, which could generate carcinogenic pyrolysis products. In addition, fish consumption is seasonal in many areas, and this might need to be considered in exposure measurements.

A new interesting area of research will be the effect of farmed fish versus captured fish. When the agricultural production of fish increases, the food for the farmed fish will be produced not only from marine sources, but also from plant products. Lastly, fat fish could harbour persistent organic pollutants such as dioxin and DDT. In some areas mercury levels are high in fish.

Conclusion

Improvement of the analysis of fish consumption and cancer will depend upon better classification of exposure. In epidemiological research a fish is not a fish.

References

Bosetti, C., Kolonel, L., Negri, E., Ron, E., Franceschi, S., Dal Maso, L., Galanti, M.R., Mark, S.D., Preston-Martin, S., McTiernan, A., Land, C., Jin, F., Wingren, G., Hallquist, A., Glattre, E., Lund, E., Levi, F., Linos, D. & La Vecchia, C. (2001) A pooled analysis of case–control studies of thyroid cancer. VI. Fish and shellfish consumption. *Cancer Causes Control*, **12**, 375–382

Bostick, R.M., Potter, J.D., Kushi, L.H., Sellers, T.A., Steinmetz, K.A., McKenzie, D.R., Gapstur, S.M. & Folsom, A.R. (1994) Sugar, meat, and fat intake, and non-dietary risk factors for colon cancer incidence in Iowa women (United States). *Cancer Causes Control*, **5**, 38–52

Breslow, R.A., Graubard, B.I., Sinha, R. & Subar, A.F. (2000) Diet and lung cancer: a 1987 National Health Interview Survey. *Cancer Causes Control*, **11**, 419–431

De Deckere, E.A.M. (1999) Possible beneficial effect of fish and fish n-3 poly-unsaturated fatty acids in breast and colorectal cancer. *Eur. J. Cancer Prev.*, **8**, 213–221

Food and Agriculture Organisation (FAO). http://www.FAO.org/docrep003/x8002E/ Accessed 15 October 2001

Fernandez, E., Chatenoud, L., La Vecchia, C., Negri, E. & Franceschi, S. (1999) Fish consumption and cancer risk. *Am. J. Clin. Nutr.*, **70**, 85–90

Gaard, M., Tretli, S. & Løken, E.B. (1996) Dietary factors and risk of colon cancer: a prospective study of 50,535 young Norwegian men and women. *Eur. J. Cancer Prev.*, **5**, 445–454

Giovanucci, E., Rimm, E.B., Colditz, G.A., Stampfer, M.J., Ascherico, A., Chute, C.C.

& Willett, W. (1993a) A prospective study of dietary fat and risk of prostate cancer. *J. Natl. Cancer Inst.*, **85**, 1571–1579

Giovannucci, E., Stampfer, M.J., Colditz, G.A., Manson, J.E., Rosner, B.A., Longnecker, M., Speizer, F.E. & Willett, W. (1993b) A comparison of prospective and retrospective assessment of diet in the study of breast cancer. *Am. J. Epidemiol.*, **137**, 502–511

Giovanucci, E., Rimm, E., Stampfer, M.J., Colditz, G.A., Ascherico, A. & Willett, W. (1994) Intake of fat, meat, and fiber in relation to risk of colon cancer in men. *Cancer Res.*, **54**, 2390–2397

Goldbohm, R.A., van den Brandt, P.A., van't Veer, P., Brants, H.A.M., Dorant, E., Sturmans, F. & Hermus, R.J.J. (1994) A prospective study on the relationship between meat consumption and the risk of colon cancer. *Cancer Res.*, **54**, 718–723

Hsing, A.W., McLaughlin, J.K., Schuman, L.M., Bjelke, E., Gridley, G., Wacholder, S., Chien, H.T. & Blot, W.J. (1990) Diet, tobacco use, and fatal prostate cancer: results from the Lutheran Brotherhood Cohort Study. *Cancer Res.*, **50**, 6836–6840

Kato, I., Akmedkhanov, A., Koenig, K., Toniolo, P.G., Shore, R.E. & Riboli, E. (1997) Prospective study of diet and female colorectal cancer: the New York University Women's Health Study. *Nutr. Cancer*, **28**, 276–281

Le Marchand, L., Kolonel, L.N., Wilkens, L.R., Myers, B.C. & Hirohata, T. (1994) Animal fat consumption and prostate cancer: a prospective study in Hawaii. *Epidemiology*, **5**, 276–282

Marckman, P. & Grønbæk, M. (1999) Review. Fish consumption and coronary heart disease mortality. A systematic review of prospective cohort studies. *Eur. J. Clin. Nutr.*, **53**, 585–590

Mills, P.K., Beeson, W., Phillips, R.L. & Fraser, G.E. (1989) Dietary habits and breast cancer incidence among Seventh-Day Adventists. *Cancer*, **64**, 582–590

Schmidt, E.B., Skou, H.A., Christensen, J.H. & Dyerberg, J. (2000) N-3 fatty acids from fish and coronary artery disease: implications for public health. *Publ. Health Nutr.*, **3**, 91–98

Schuurman, A.G., van den Brandt, P.A., Dorant, E. & Goldbohm, R.A. (1999) Animal products, calcium and protein and prostate cancer risk in the Netherlands Cohort Study. *Br. J. Cancer*, **80**, 1107–1113

Stampfer, M.J., Willett, W., Colditz, G.A. & Speizer, F.E. (1987) Intake of cholesterol, fish and specific types of fat in relation to risk of breast cancer. In: Lands, W.E.M. (ed.), *Proceedings of the AOCS short course on polyunsaturated fatty acids and eicosanoids.* AOCS, Champaign, IL, pp. 248–252

Terry, P., Lichtenstein, P., Feychting, M., Ahlbom, A. & Wolk, A. (2001) Fatty fish consumption and risk of prostate cancer. *Lancet*, **357**, 1764–1766

Toniolo, P., Riboli, E., Shore, R.E. & Paternack, B.S. (1994) Consumption of meat, animal products, protein, and fat and risk of breast cancer: a prospective cohort study in New York. *Epidemiology*, **5**, 391–397

Vatten, L.J., Solvoll, K. & Løken, E.B. (1990) Frequency of meat and fish intake and risk of breast cancer in a prospective study of 14,500 Norwegian women. *Int. J. Cancer*, **46**, 12–15

World Cancer Research Fund, American Institute for Cancer Research Expert Panel. (1997) *Food, Nutrition and the Prevention of Cancer: A Global Perspective*. Washington D.C., American Institute for Cancer Research

Dairy foods and colorectal cancer: epidemiological evidence

Kampman E.

Division of Human Nutrition & Epidemiology, Wageningen University, Wageningen, The Netherlands.

Introduction

In 1984, Newmark, Wargowich and Bruce were among the first to suggest that dairy products, which are the main source of calcium in our diet, may protect against colorectal cancer among populations with a high intake of saturated fat. Their "calcium soap hypothesis" proposed that calcium might induce saponification of free fatty acids and bile acids, thereby diminishing the proliferative stimulus of these compounds on the colon mucosa (Newmark *et al.*, 1984). Indeed, those susceptible to colon cancer, e.g. those with a positive family history of colorectal cancer, those with inflammatory bowel diseases and the elderly, do exhibit in their normal-appearing mucosa both an increased colonic epithelial cell proliferation rate and an upward shift of the proliferative zone. Also, it has been observed that a high-fat diet produces proliferative changes in both rodents and humans (Newmark *et al.*, 1984). However, calcium supplementation has been observed to decrease the cytotoxicity of faecal water (Van der Meer *et al.*, 1997), and a decrease in faecal bile acids has not been shown consistently (Alder *et al.*, 1993).

Calcium or low-fat milk can also directly inhibit experimental colorectal carcinogenesis induced by azoxymethane or 1,2-dimethyl-hydrazine. Potential non-luminal mechanisms have been summarized by Pence (Pence, 1993). Vitamin D, which is present in fortified dairy products and effects calcium absorption, might in its hormonally active form (1,25 $(OH)_2D^3$), also inhibit cell proliferation and induce cell differentiation (e.g. Cross *et al.*, 1992).

In epidemiological studies, although inconsistently, high intake of dairy products is associated with a modest decreased risk of colorectal cancer, while it may increase risk of prostate cancer (as recently reviewed by Chan & Giovannucci, 2001). For other cancers, evidence relating dairy products to cancer is limited. This paper provides an overview of epidemiological studies and human intervention studies on the association between the intake of dairy foods, calcium, vitamin D and colorectal cancer risk. Previously published review articles will be used and updated with recent publications.

Observational epidemiological evidence

Dairy products

Epidemiological studies that investigated intake of milk products in relation to colorectal cancer were previously reviewed by Bostick and colleagues (Bostick *et al.*, 1993). This review included 11 case–control and two cohort studies with odds ratios or relative risks ranging from 0.4 to 1.3. Nine studies suggested an inverse association, four of which showed a statistically significant association. Three of the studies showed a nonsignificant positive association.

Of the studies published after the review, the Iowa Women's Health Study reported a RR of 0.7 (95% CI, 0.4–1.4) for total dairy intake and colorectal cancer (Bostick *et al.*, 1993). In the cohort of Finnish men enrolled in the ATBC Study, a relative risk of 0.6 (95% CI, 0.4–0.9) was observed among those in the highest quartile of intake of milk products (median: 1089 g/day) versus those within the lowest quartile of intake (median: 318 g/day). The relatively high consumption of dairy products in this population may explain this inverse association, or, as the authors propose, dairy products may be more important among smokers (Pietinen *et al.*, 1999). In a US case–control study with a relatively wide range in dairy product intake, an inverse association with dairy products was observed among men (OR highest vs lowest category of intake 0.8; 95% CI, 0.6–1.1) and women (OR 0.7; 95% CI, 0.5–0.9) (Kampman *et al.*, 2000).

As far as specific products are concerned, none of the studies published thus far has observed consistent inverse or positive associations with colorectal cancer risk.

Yoon and colleagues recently reviewed the available evidence of total dairy products, milk and colorectal adenoma risk (Yoon *et al.*, 2000). Six case–control and two cohort studies examined the effects of dairy products. In four of the case–control studies, no associations were observed while in two small studies a positive association was reported. Neither of the two cohort studies (Health Professionals Follow-up Study in men, Nurses Health Study in women) observed a significant association between milk (whole, low-fat or skimmed) and the risk for colorectal adenomas after 4 and 8 years of follow-up (see review Yoon *et al.*, 2000). No consistent associations were observed for specific dairy products. Based on the reviewed studies, Yoon and colleagues conclude that dairy product consumption was not markedly associated with small or large adenoma occurrence (Yoon *et al.*, 2000).

Calcium

In 1985, Garland and colleagues were one of the first groups to publish epidemiological results on calcium and colorectal cancer. Their prospective Western Electric Health Study included 1954 men for whom 28-day dietary histories were available. After 19 years of follow-up, calcium intake from diet and supplements was inversely associated with colorectal cancer risk: relative risk was 0.32 (95% CI, 0.13–0.49; 49 cases) (Garland *et al.*, 1985). Many others have investigated this association; a meta-analysis (Bergsma-Kadijk *et al.*, 1997) and a review of these studies (Martinez & Willett, 1998) have been published. The meta-analysis included 16 case–control studies and 8 cohort studies. Overall, a RR of 0.89 was calculated with a 95% CI of 0.79–1.01. For studies focusing on ultimate colorectal cancer, a RR of 0.86 (CI 95%, 0.74–0.98) was found, while adenomas were slightly positive, but not statistically significant, associated with calcium intake (RR 1.13; 95% CI, 0.91–1.39). An inverse association was only observed for the proximal part of the colon (RR 0.79; 95% CI, 0.33–1.47). No important differences were observed for case–control versus cohort studies, men versus women, dietary versus supplemental intake of calcium, high- versus medium- or low-fat diets (Bergsma-Kadijk *et al.*, 1997). The review by Martinez and Willett (1998) discussed the results of 15 case–control and 8 cohort studies, also included in the meta-analysis. Of these studies, 13 showed a nonsignificant inverse association, 5 showed an inverse significant association and in five studies, a nonsignificant positive association was observed. The authors conclude that "calcium intake is not associated with a substantially lower risk of colorectal cancer" (Martinez & Willett, 1998).

Misclassification of intake and an insufficient range of intake may partly explain the weak and inconclusive evidence of epidemiological studies. The range of intake in the previously reviewed studies was between 500 and 1200 mg/day. In the Finnish study connected to the ATBC trial including men with a high intake of dairy products, the relative risk started to decrease already at the second quartile level (RR 0.7; 95% CI, 0.5–1.0) corresponding to over 1000 mg of calcium.

Also, in the US multicentre case–control study with a wide range of dairy product intake (differences in median dietary calcium values between the lowest and highest quintile of intake were 1601 mg for men and 1236 mg for women), a statistically inverse association with colon cancer risk was observed (men: OR 0.7; 95% CI, 0.5–0.9; women: OR 0.6; 95%CI, 0.4–0.9) (Kampman *et al.*, 2000).

In summary, although recent studies in populations with relatively high intakes of calcium do indeed suggest a protective role of calcium in colorectal cancer prevention, the epidemiological evidence for a moderate intake of calcium remains inconsistent.

Vitamin D

As reviewed by Martinez and Willett (1998), epidemiological data on vitamin D and colorectal cancer are sparse and suggest protective rather than harmful effects of vitamin D on colon cancer risk. Of the three case–control studies reviewed, two showed an inverse association, of which one was statistically significant. Of the five cohort studies, four showed an inverse association, only one was statistically significant. In the cohort studies, the inverse associations between dietary vitamin D and colorectal cancer are between 0.59 (Martinez *et al.*, 1996) and 0.98 (Bostick *et al.*, 1993). In most studies, stronger inverse associations were observed with supplemental vitamin D (Martinez & Willett, 1998). In the Finnish prospective study, no important association with vitamin D intake was observed (Piettinen *et al.*, 1999). The US case–control study did not show an association between dietary vitamin D and colon cancer (Kampman *et al.*, 2000). Vitamin D from supplements appeared to be protective, which may point to better measurement of supplement intake or could be indicative of other protective behaviours with supplement use (Kampman *et al.*, 2000). In a case–control study nested in the prospective Nurses' Health Study (Platz *et al.*, 2000), women whose plasma 1,25$(OH)_2$D concentration was below 26.0 pg/mL were at increased risk of distal colon adenoma (OR 1.6; 95% CI, 1.0–2.4). The relationship between its precursor 25(OH)D and distal adenomas of the colon and rectum was U-shaped (ORs second to fourth quartile: 0.64, 0.58 and 1.04, respectively) (Platz *et al.*, 2000). Three previous studies showed no association between 1,25$(OH)_2$D concentration and colorectal cancer, while two studies showed an inverse association with 25(OH)D (reviewed by Martinez and Willett, 1998).

Besides factors related to study design, levels and variation of intake, population characteristics may explain the inconsistencies of epidemiological studies. For instance, inherited variants (*polyA* (short), *BsmI* (*BB*), and *TaqI* (*tt*)) in the vitamin D receptor gene (*VDR*) have been associated with reduced risk of colon cancer (OR 0.5; 95% CI, 0.3–0.9) (Slattery *et al.*, 2001). Vitamin D as well as calcium intake are observed to modify the association between *BsmI* (*BB*) genotype and colorectal adenomas (Kim *et al.*, 2001).

Human experimental studies

Whether supplementation with calcium is indeed beneficial for the colonic mucosa and could influence the recurrence of colorectal adenomas has been studied in several human experimental studies.

Colorectal epithelial cell proliferation

The results of human trials of calcium and colorectal epithelial proliferation have been previously reviewed (Bostick, 1997). Most studies supplemented with calcium carbonate, representing levels of 1200–2000 mg elemental calcium per day. Of the five uncontrolled trials, all suggested substantial and significant (28%–56%) decreases in the rate of proliferation of colon crypt epithelial cells. Of the nine small controlled trials, three found statistically significant decreases and the remainder were inconclusive because of insufficient sample size. The three full-scale trials observed no effect on proliferation rate. One of these studies observed a decrease in the proportion of labelled cells in the upper 40% of the crypt, while another observed an increase. Bostick concludes that "the current literature indicates that in humans, it is unlikely that calcium supplementation can substantially lower proliferation rates, but it may normalize the distribution of proliferating cells within colon crypts" (Bostick, 1997).

Only a few studies have evaluated the effects of dairy product consumption on epithelial proliferation. A randomized, single-blinded study found that high intake of low-fat dairy foods (containing up to 1200 mg/day of calcium) reduced colonic epithelial cell proliferation and restored differentiation after 6 and 12 months among 70 individuals at risk for colonic neoplasia (Holt *et al.*, 1998). Increased consumption of dairy products over a 12-week period was not observed to change rectal mucosal proliferation in a randomized cross-over trial including 40 individuals at risk for colorectal neoplasia (Karagas *et al.*, 1998).

In a recent intervention study (Holt *et al.*, 2002), 39 subjects were supplemented for 6 months with calcium (1500 mg of elemental calcium), calcium (1500 mg) and 400 IU vitamin D_3 or 1,25$(OH)_2D^3$ (0.50 µg). Results support an important role for vitamin D in determining the effects of calcium on colorectal epithelial proliferation. Significant correlations were shown between circulating levels of 25$(OH)D^3$ with indices of colorectal epithelial cell proliferation. According to the authors, some of the variation in colorectal cell proliferation occurring after calcium administration reported in previous studies might have been attributable to lower serum 25(OH)vitamin D levels. They suggest that future studies of the chemopreventive action of calcium and vitamin D should take into account the levels of circulating 25$(OH)D^3$ and probably the activity of the colonic enzyme that converts 25$(OH)D^3$ to 1,25$(OH)_2D^3$.

The *BsmI VDR* variant was not associated with indices of colorectal epithelial cell proliferation in this study (Holt *et al.*, 2002)

Whether altered epithelial cell proliferation indeed predicts future colorectal neoplasia is, however, still under debate. Colorectal adenomas may be more reliable as a surrogate marker for ultimate cancer (Sandler *et al.*, 2000).

Colorectal polyp recurrence

Baron and colleagues (1999) conducted a multicentre, randomized, placebo-controlled intervention study on the effect of supplementation with calcium carbonate (1200 mg elemental calcium) on the risk of recurrence of colorectal adenomas. Among the 832 subjects who completed the study, at least one colorectal adenoma was diagnosed between the first (after about 1 year) and the second (after about 4 years) examination in 127 subjects in the calcium group (31%) and 159 subjects in the placebo group (38%). After adjustment for age, sex, clinical centre, number of previous adenomas and length of follow-up, a moderate but statistically significant reduction in recurrence of adenomatous polyps was observed (OR 0.81; 95% CI, 0.67–0.99). The ratio of the average number of adenomas in the calcium group to that of the placebo group was 0.76 (95% CI, 0.60–0.96). Interestingly, this reduced risk became apparent as early as the first follow-up, which was 9 months after the start of the trial. There was no indication of a greater effect among subjects with a low base-line dietary intake of calcium or a high intake of fat (Baron *et al.*, 1999).

Bonithon-Kopp and colleagues, with data from the European Cancer Prevention Organisation intervention study, support a modest inverse association between calcium supplementation (2000 mg elemental calcium) and adenoma recurrence.

Adjusting for age, sex, adenoma history and number and location of polyps, they observed an overall OR of 0.66 (95% CI, 0.38–1.17) after 3 years of follow-up. However, this protective effect was only apparent among men (OR 0.58; 95% CI, 0.29–1.18), women (OR 1.01) and for those with adenomas at the right colon at inclusion (OR 0.26; 95% CI, 0.08–0.84; left colon: RR 0.97) (Bonithon-Kopp *et al.*, 2000).

Concluding remarks

Epidemiological and human experimental studies published to date show inconsistent findings on the potential inverse association between dairy foods and colorectal cancer. Whether calcium may indeed reduce the risk of colorectal cancer or whether other constituents of dairy products such as vitamin D in fortified milk may be involved needs to be confirmed. Conflicting evidence between epidemiological studies on dairy product consumption and colorectal cancer and human experimental studies with calcium may be explained by methodological issues, levels of intake and genetic differences between populations.

Also, milk intake may modestly raise levels of human insulin-like growth factor-I (IGF-I) (Ma *et al.*, 2001), which is a potent mitogen and inhibits apoptosis in normal and malignant intestinal epithelial cells. Elevated levels of IGF-I have been positively associated with colorectal cancer (e.g. Ma *et al.*, 2001). Thus, any increase in IGF-I levels may counteract the potentially beneficial effects of calcium and/or vitamin D of dairy foods. However, it has also been observed that those with high levels of circulating IFG-I/IGFBP-3 benefit most from a high dairy product intake (Ma *et al.*, 2001).

The hypothesis that the association between calcium intake and colorectal cancer varies according to IGF-I levels should be studied in more detail. Studies among those susceptible for a potential effect of dairy products, e.g. those with high cell proliferation rates, smokers, those with high IGF-1/IGFBP-3 levels or individuals with a polymorphism in the vitamin D receptor gene may help to unravel underlying mechanisms.

The studies reviewed do not support a strong effect of dairy foods in the prevention of colorectal tumours. Efforts to increase calcium intake to prevent other chronic diseases such as osteoporosis should take the potential increased risk of prostate cancer with high intake of dairy products (Chan & Giovannucci, 2001) into consideration, particularly for ageing men.

References

Alder, R.J., McKeown-Eyssen, G. & Bright-See, E. (1993) Randomized trial of the effect of calcium supplementation on fecal risk factors for colorectal cancer. *Am. J. Epidemiol.*, **138**, 804–814

Baron, J.A., Beach, M., Mandel, J.S., van Stolk, R.U., Haile, R.W., Sandler, R.S., Rothstein, R., Summers, R.W., Snover, D.C., Beck, G.J., Bond, J.H. & Greenberg, E.R. (1999) Calcium supplementation for the prevention of colorectal adenomas. Calcium Polyp Prevention Study Group. *N. Engl. J. Med.*, **340**, 101–107

Bergsma-Kadijk, J., van't Veer, P., Kampman, E. & Burema, J. (1996) Calcium does not protect against colorectal neoplasia. *Epidemiology*, **7**, 590–597

Bonithon-Kopp, C., Kronborg, O., Giacosa, A., Rath, U. & Faivre, J. (2000) Calcium and fibre supplementation in prevention of colorectal adenoma recurrence: a randomised intervention trial. European Cancer Prevention Organisation Study Group. *Lancet*, **356**, 1300–1306

Bostick, R.M. (1997) Human studies of calcium supplementation and colorectal epithelial cell proliferation. *Cancer Epidemiol. Biomarkers Prev.*, **6**, 971–980

Bostick, R.M., Potter, J.D., Sellers, T.A., McKenszie, D.R., Kushi, H. & Folsom, A.R. (1993) Relation of calcium, vitamin D, and dairy food intake to incidence of colon cancer in older women. *Am. J. Epidemiol.*,**137**, 1302–1317

Chan, J.M. & Giovannucci, E.L. (2001) Dairy products, calcium, and vitamin D and risk of prostate cancer. *Epidemiol. Rev.*, **23**, 87–92

Cross, H.S., Pavelka, M., Slavik, J. & Peterlik, M. (1992) Growth control of human colon cancer cells by vitamin D and calcium in vitro. *J. Natl. Cancer Inst.*, **84**, 1355–1357

Garland, C., Shekelle, R.B., Barrett-Connor, E., Criqui, M.H., Rossof, A.H. & Paul, O. (1985) Dietary vitamin D and calcium and risk of colorectal cancer: a 19-year prospective study in men. *Lancet* ,**1**, 307–309

Holt, P.R., Atillasoy, E.O., Gilman, J., Guss, J., Moss, S.F., Newmark, H., Fan, K., Yang, K. & Lipkin, M. (1998) Modulation of abnormal epithelial cell proliferation and differentiation by low-fat dairy foods: a randomized controlled trial. *JAMA*, **280**, 1074–1079

Holt, P.R., Arber, N., Halmos, B., Forde, K., Kissileff, H., McGlynn, K.A., Moss, S.F., Fan, K., Yang, K. & Lipkin, M. (2002) Colonic epithelial cell proliferation decreases with increasing levels of serum 25-hydroxy vitamin D. *Cancer Epidemiol. Biomarkers Prev.*, **11**,113–119

Kampman, E., Slattery, M.L., Caan, B. & Potter, J.D. (2000) Calcium, vitamin D, sunshine exposure, dairy products and colon cancer risk (United States). *Cancer Causes Control*, **11**, 459–466

Karagas, M.R., Tosteson, T.D., Greenberg, E.R., Rothstein, R.I., Roebuck, B.D., Herrin, M. & Ahnen, D. (1998) Effects of milk and milk products on rectal mucosal cell proliferation in humans. *Cancer Epidemiol. Biomarkers Prev.*, **7**, 757–766

Kim, H.S., Newcomb, P.A., Ulrich, C.M., Keener, C.L., Bigler, J., Farin, F.M., Bostick, R.M. & Potter, J.D. (2001) Vitamin D receptor polymorphism and the risk of colorectal adenomas: evidence of interaction with dietary vitamin D and calcium. *Cancer Epidemiol. Biomarkers Prev.*, **10**, 869–874

Ma, J., Giovannucci, E., Pollak, M., Chan, J.M., Gaziano, J.M., Willett, W. &

Stampfer, M.J. (2001) Milk intake, circulating levels of insulin-like growth factor-I, and risk of colorectal cancer in men. *J. Natl. Cancer Inst.*, **93**, 1330–1336

Martinez, M. & Willett, W. (1998) Calcium, vitamin D, and colorectal cancer: a review of the epidemiologic evidence. *Cancer Epidemiol. Biomarkers Prev.*, **7**, 163–168

Martinez, M.E., Giovannucci, E.L., Colditz, G.A., Stampfer, M.J., Hunter, D.J., Speizer, F.E., Wing, A. & Willett, WC. (1996) Calcium, vitamin D, and the occurrence of colon cancer among women. *J. Natl. Cancer Inst.*, **88**, 1375–1382.

Newmark, H.I., Warovich, M.J. & Bruce, W.R. (1984) Colon cancer and dietary fat, phosphate, and calcium: a hypothesis. *J. Natl. Cancer Inst.*, **72**,1323–1325

Pence, B.C. (1993) Role of calcium in colon cancer prevention: experimental and clinical studies. *Mut. Res.*, **290**, 87–95

Pietinen, P., Malila, N., Virtanen, M., Hartman, T.J., Tangrea, J.A., Albanes, D. & Virtamo, J. (1999) Diet and risk of colorectal cancer in a cohort of Finnish men. *Cancer Causes Control*, **10**, 387–396

Platz, E.A., Hankinson, S.E., Hollis, B.W., Colditz, G.A., Hunter, D.J., Speizer, F.E. & Giovannucci, E. (2000) Plasma 1,25-dihydroxy- and 25-hydroxyvitamin D and adenomatous polyps of the distal colorectum. *Cancer Epidemiol. Biomarkers Prev.*, **9**,1059–1065

Sandler, R.S., Baron, J.A., Tosteson, T.D., Mandel, J.S. & Haile, R.W. (2000) Rectal mucosal proliferation and risk of colorectal adenomas: results from a randomized controlled trial. *Cancer Epidemiol. Biomarkers Prev.*, **9**, 653–656

Slattery, M.L., Yakumo, K., Hoffman, M. & Neuhausen, S. (2001) Variants of the VDR gene and risk of colon cancer (United States). *Cancer Causes Control*, **12**, 359–364

Van der Meer, R., Lapre, J.A., Govers, M.J.A.P. & Kleibeuker, J.H. (1997) Mechanisms of the intestinal effects of dietary fats and milk products on colon carcinogenesis. *Cancer Lett.*, **114**, 75–83

Yoon, H., Benamouzig, R., Little, J., François-Collange, M. & Tome, D. (2000) Systematic review of epidemiological studies on meat, diary products and egg consumption and risk of colorectal adenomas. *Eur. J. Cancer Prev.*, **9**, 151–164

Prostate cancer: rates in Europe, dietary hypotheses, and plans for EPIC

Key T.J.
(for the EPIC working group on prostate cancer)

Cancer Research UK Epidemiology Unit, University of Oxford, Gibson Building, Radcliffe Infirmary, Oxford, OX2 6HE, UK.

Prostate cancer rates in Europe

Prostate cancer is the second most common cancer among men in the EU, accounting for approximately 135 000 cancer cases and 56 000 deaths each year (data for 1996; EUCAN 2000). The commonest cancer among men in the EU is lung cancer, which is largely caused by smoking, whereas smoking has little if any effect on prostate cancer risk; among non-smokers, therefore, prostate cancer must be the commonest cancer in men in the EU.

Prostate cancer rates vary substantially among countries in the EU. Among the eight EU countries contributing to the EPIC analyses of nutrition and prostate cancer (France is not included because the French cohort is all women), the highest incidence rate is in Sweden (age-standardized rate 63.58 cases per 100 000 per year) and the lowest is in Greece (18.91 cases per 100 000 per year), giving a range of over threefold (EUCAN 2000; Fig. 1). For prostate cancer mortality, the highest rates are again in Sweden and the lowest in Greece, but the difference in rates is less than that for incidence, with just over a twofold range between the extremes (Fig. 2).

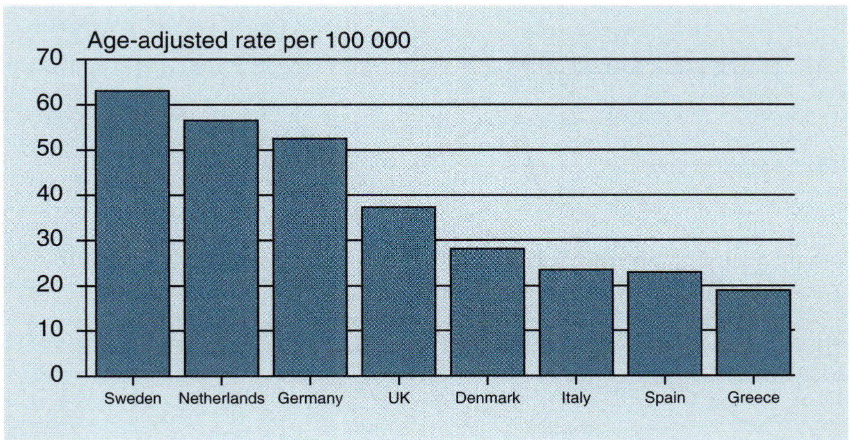

Figure 1
Prostate cancer incidence rates in eight EPIC countries. 1996 rates, EUCAN 2001

The recorded incidence of prostate cancer has increased markedly during the last 20 years in many Western countries; it is clear, however, that much of this rise may be explained by increased detection of small prostate tumours due to increased use of transurethral resection of the prostate in the 1980s (Potosky *et al.*, 1990) and of prostate specific antigen (PSA) testing in the 1990s. To investigate time trends in prostate cancer, therefore, it is currently better to look at mortality rates, although these too must be interpreted with caution. Figure 3 shows trends in prostate cancer mortality in the eight EPIC countries during the last 50 years. Overall, mortality has increased in all the countries, and the ranking of the countries has changed little, with the highest mortality rates in Sweden, Denmark and the other northern European countries, and the lowest rates in Spain, Italy and Greece. An interesting departure from the overall

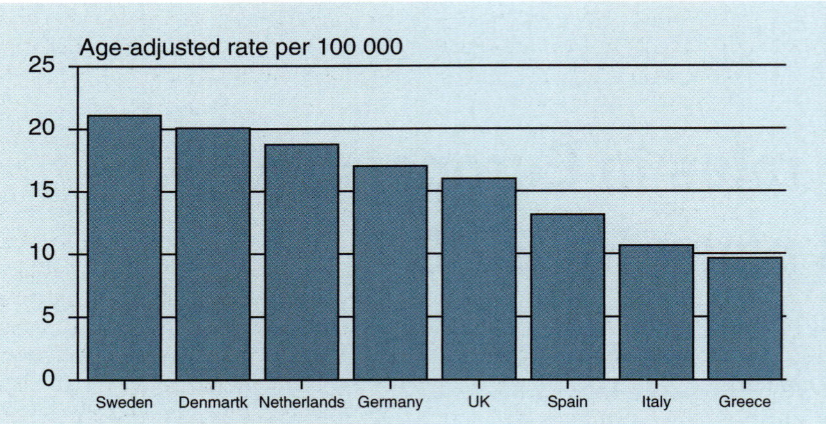

Figure 2
Prostate cancer mortality rates in eight EPIC countries. 1996 rates, EUCAN 2001

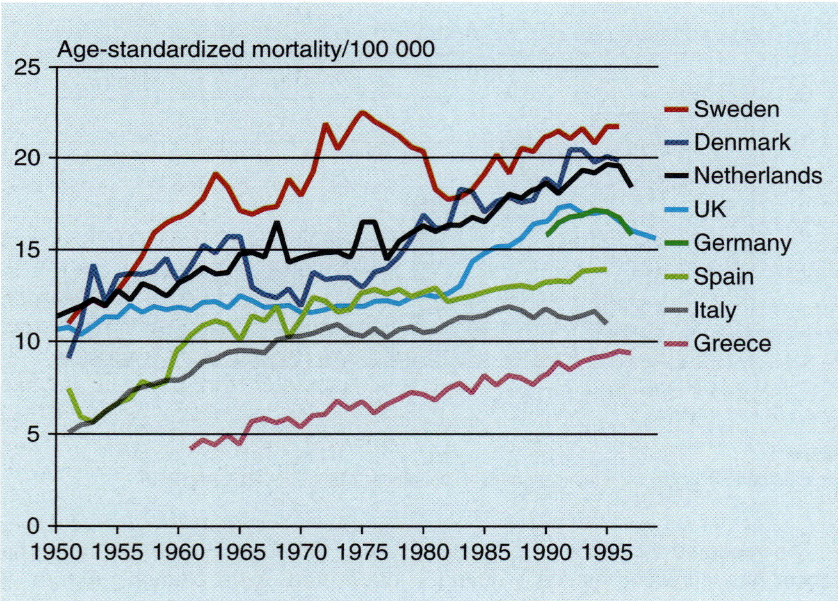

Figure 3
Prostate cancer mortality trends in eight EPIC countries. Adapted from WHO databank, 2001

upward trend is that in some countries, notably the Netherlands, the UK and Germany, there was a small decrease in mortality in the mid-1990s; a similar decrease has also been observed in the US, and may indicate improvements in treatment.

Prostate cancer is a very important cause of morbidity and death throughout the EU. Both incidence and mortality rates are currently lower in Southern Europe than in Northern Europe, but the time trends suggest that over the coming decades the rates in Southern Europe may continue to rise. As discussed below, the causes of prostate cancer are largely unknown; research within EPIC will investigate a range of dietary and hormonal hypotheses, with particular emphasis on factors which might underlie the current variation in disease rates across the EU.

Established risk factors

The only well-established risk factors for prostate cancer are age, population group/ethnicity, and a family history of the disease (Key, 1995). Prostate cancer incidence increases markedly with increasing age, more so than for any other cancer starting later in life. This pattern may reflect the very slow growth of some prostate tumours, and may be expected to change with increased use of PSA testing to detect small tumours at an early stage.

Prostate cancer rates vary greatly between countries worldwide. The variation is very large for incidence rates, but this is partly due to variations in diagnostic practices. For mortality rates, which are less affected by diagnostic practices, there is an approximately tenfold variation between countries, with the lowest rates in Japan and other areas in East Asia, high rates in Western countries, especially northern Europe, and the highest rates among US blacks. Prostate cancer rates increase among migrants from low-risk countries to high-risk countries (for example Japanese migrants to the US), indicating that environmental factors are important determinants of risk; however, whereas for breast and colon cancer there are large international variations in disease rates but the rates among ethnic groups within the US have become rather similar, for prostate cancer there remain substantial differences within the US, with relatively low rates among Asian-Americans and high rates among black Americans. These persistent differences between ethnic groups living in a broadly similar environment suggest that genetic differences between ethnic groups may play a significant role in determining risk, and a promising area of research has already suggested that some of these ethnic differences may be explained by differences in the prevalence of polymorphisms in genes involved in androgen metabolism (Makridakis & Reichardt, 2001).

A family history of prostate cancer is a strong risk factor for this disease. Clinical and epidemiological studies of familial risk of prostate cancer show a trend of increasing risk with an increasing number of affected relatives and with an earlier age of onset in affected relatives. Evidence suggests that one or more high-risk genes may lead to early-onset prostate cancer and recent studies have identified several candidate genes (Stanford & Ostrander, 2001). Although it has been estimated that such high-risk genes account for only a small proportion of prostate cancer in the general population, a study of twins in Northern Europe indicated that heritable factors may contribute to as much as 40% of prostate cancer risk (Lichtenstein *et al.*, 2000). Genetic factors that carry a moderate effect and are not manifested in a family history may therefore play a significant role in prostate cancer development. Of most interest are polymorphisms found in genes that encode for enzymes involved in androgen metabolism and genes that encode for hormone receptors. Several polymorphisms in these genes have been found to differ between prostate cancer cases and controls (Makridakis & Reichardt 2001).

Dietary hypotheses

Ecological analyses show strong positive associations between prostate cancer rates and Western-type diets rich in animal products (Armstrong & Doll, 1975). This observation led to the hypotheses that risk for prostate cancer might be increased by high intakes of meat, dairy products, fat, and refined carbohydrates. Analytical studies published over the last 20 years have provided some support for these and a number of other hypotheses, but at present no dietary factor has been established to be important in the etiology of prostate cancer (World Cancer Research Fund, 1997; Committee on Medical Aspects of Food Policy, 1998; Kolonel, 2001). The main hypotheses which will be investigated in EPIC are discussed briefly below.

Fat

Fat has been the nutrient most frequently studied as a potential risk factor for several cancers, including breast and colon as well as prostate. For prostate cancer, the main basis for this hypothesis is the ecological association of fat intake with prostate cancer, and there is no well-defined mechanism by which high-fat diets might increase prostate cancer risk. It has been suggested that high-fat diets might increase risk by increasing testosterone levels, but direct studies have not shown that dietary fat alters hormone levels in men (Allen & Key, 2000). The results of analytical studies of fat intake and prostate cancer risk have so far been varied (Kolonel, 2001); several case–control studies have suggested that high intakes of total fat, animal fat or saturated fat may increase risk, but the associations reported from prospective studies have been weaker and not statistically significant. These inconsistencies may be partly due to the biases inherent in case–control studies of diet and cancer, as well as to the limited accuracy of measurement of fat intake in epidemiological studies. More data are required, particularly on the possible associations of individual polyunsaturated fatty acids with prostate cancer risk.

Meat, dairy products, animal protein

Similar to the evidence for fat, ecological observations have suggested that risk might be increased by a high intake of meat and dairy products. The results of several large prospective studies have given some support to this hypothesis, especially for red meat and for dairy products (Kolonel, 2001; Chan & Giovannucci, 2001). The possible association with dairy products has led to the hypothesis that a high dietary intake of calcium may increase prostate cancer risk by suppressing the formation of the active form of vitamin D, since some further evidence suggests that vitamin D might reduce prostate cancer risk (Giovannucci, 1998). Alternatively, high intakes of animal protein might increase prostate cancer risk by increasing serum levels of IGF-I (Allen & Key, 2001).

Fruit, vegetables and specific anti-oxidants

Antioxidants have been purported to be protective against prostate cancer, although there is now strong evidence from three large randomized trials that β-carotene, an antioxidant carotenoid, has no beneficial effect (Hennekens *et al.*, 1996; Omenn *et al.*, 1996; Heinonen *et al.*, 1998). Vitamin E supplementation was found to be associated with a significant reduction in prostate cancer rates in a controlled trial in Finland (Heinonen *et al.*, 1998), although observational studies have shown rather mixed results (e.g. Chan *et al.*, 1999). There is some evidence that other antioxidants such as lycopene (Giovannucci *et al.*, 1995; Gann *et al.*, 1999) and selenium (Clark *et al.*, 1996; Yoshizawa *et al.*, 1998) have a protective effect on prostate cancer, although the data are inconsistent (Thomas, 1999; Kristal & Cohen, 2000).

Plans for EPIC

Preliminary results from the EPIC working group on prostate cancer were presented at the European Conference on Nutrition and Cancer, June 2001.

At this time, data were available for 123 000 men from eight countries. The mean follow-up time was 3.3 years, and there was a total of 351 cases of prostate cancer (Britain 103, Sweden 96, Germany 73, Denmark 41, Italy 20, Spain 15, Netherlands 3, Greece 0). These numbers were considered too small for any substantive analyses. Examination of incidence rate ratios by country showed that the highest incidence rates were in Sweden and Germany and the lowest in Spain and Greece. This variation in incidence is similar to that shown by the nationally representative incidence rates published by EUCAN (EUCAN 2000; Fig. 1). Exploratory analyses of fruit and vegetable consumption in relation to prostate cancer risk did not show any clear associations (results not shown).

During the next 4 years, a series of analyses of potential risk factors for prostate cancer will be conducted within the EPIC collaboration. These analyses will include foods and nutrients as discussed above, as well as endogenous sex hormones and growth factors and related genetic polymorphisms.

References

Allen, N.E. & Key, T.J. (2000) The effects of diet on circulating sex hormone levels in men. *Nutr. Res. Rev.*, **12**, 1–27

Allen, N.E., Key, T.J. (2001) Re: plasma insulin-like growth factor-I, insulin-like growth factor-binding proteins, and prostate cancer risk: a prospective study. *J. Natl. Cancer Inst.*, **93**, 649–651

Armstrong, B. & Doll, R. (1975) Environmental factors and cancer incidence and mortality in different countries, with special reference to dietary practices. *Int. J. Cancer*, **15**, 617–631

Chan, J.M. & Giovannucci, E.L. (2001) Dairy products, calcium, and vitamin D and risk of prostate cancer. *Epidemiol. Rev.*, **23**, 87–92

Chan, J.M., Stampfer, M.J., Ma, J., Rimm, E.B., Willett, W.C., & Giovannucci, E.L. (1999) Supplemental vitamin E intake and prostate cancer risk in a large cohort of men in the United States. *Cancer Epidemiol. Biomarkers Prev.*, **8**, 893–899

Clark, L.C., Combs, G.F.J., Turnbull, B.W., Slate, E.H., Chalker, D.K., Chow, J., Davis, L.S., Glover, R.A., Graham, G.F., Gross, E.G., Krongrad, A., Lesher, J.L.J., Park, H.K., Sanders, B.B.J., Smith, C.L., & Taylor, J.R. (1996) Effects of selenium supplementation for cancer prevention in patients with carcinoma of the skin: a randomized controlled trial. *JAMA*, **276**, 1957–1963

Committee on Medical Aspects of Food and Nutrition Policy (1998) Nutritional Aspects of the Development of Cancer. London, The Stationery Office

EUCAN Database 2001. http://www-dep.iarc.fr/encr/dbdown.htm

Gann, P.H., Ma, J., Giovannucci, E., Willett, W., Sacks, F.M., Hennekens, C.H. & Stampfer, M.J. (1999) Lower prostate cancer risk in men with elevated plasma lycopene levels: results of a prospective analysis. *Cancer Res.*, **59**, 1225–1230

Giovannucci, E., Ascherio, A., Rimm, E.B., Stampfer, M.J., Colditz, G.A. & Willett, W.C. (1995) Intake of carotenoids and retinol in relation to risk of prostate cancer. *J. Natl. Cancer Inst.*, **87**, 1767–1776

Giovannucci, E. (1998) Dietary influences of 1,25$(OH)_2$ vitamin D in relation to prostate cancer: a hypothesis. *Cancer Causes Control*, **9**, 567–582

Heinonen, O.P., Albanes, D., Virtamo, J., Taylor, P.R., Huttunen, J.K., Hartman, A.M., Haapakoski, J., Malila, N., Rautalahti, M., Ripatti, S., Maenpaa, H., Teerenhovi, L., Koss, L., Virolainen, M. & Edwards, B.K. (1998) Prostate cancer and supplementation with alpha-tocopherol and beta-carotene: incidence and mortality in a controlled trial. *J. Natl. Cancer Inst.*, **90**, 440–446

Hennekens, C.H., Buring, J.E., Manson, J.E., Stampfer, M., Rosner, B., Cook, N.R., Belanger, C., LaMotte, F., Gaziano, J.M., Ridker, P.M., Willett, W. & Peto, R. (1996) Lack of effect of long-term supplementation with beta carotene on the incidence of malignant neoplasms and cardiovascular disease. *N. Engl. J. Med.*, **334**, 1145–1149

Kristal, A.R. & Cohen, J.H. (2000) Tomatoes, lycopene, and prostate cancer. How strong is the evidence? *Am. J. Epidemiol.*, **151**, 124–127

Key, T.J. (1995) Risk factors for prostate cancer. *Cancer Sur.*, **23**, 63–77

Kolonel, L.N. (2001) Fat, meat, and prostate cancer. *Epidemiol. Rev.*, **23**, 72–81

Lichtenstein, P., Holm, N.V., Verkasalo, P.K., Iliadou, A., Kaprio, J., Koskenvuo, M., Pukkala, E., Skytthe, A. & Hemminki, K. (2000) Environmental and heritable factors in the causation of cancer analyses of cohorts of twins from Sweden, Denmark, and Finland. *N. Engl. J. Med.*, **343**, 78–85

Makridakis, N.M. & Reichardt, J.K. (2001) Molecular epidemiology of hormone-metabolic loci in prostate cancer. *Epidemiol. Rev.*, **23**, 24–29

Omenn, G.S., Goodman, G.E., Thornquist, M.D., Balmes, J., Cullen, M.R., Glass, A., Keogh, J.P., Meyskens, F.L.J., Valanis, B., Williams, J.H.J., Barnhart, S., Cherniack, M.G., Brodkin, C.A. & Hammar, S. (1996) Risk factors for lung cancer and for intervention effects in CARET, the Beta-Carotene and Retinol Efficacy Trial. *J. Natl. Cancer Inst.*, **88**, 1550–1559

Potosky, A., Kessler, L., Gridley, G., Brown, C.C. & Horm, J.W. (1990) Rise in prostatic cancer incidence associated with increased use of transurethral resection. *J. Natl. Cancer Inst.*, **82**, 1624–1628

Stanford, J.L. & Ostrander, E.A. (2001) Familial prostate cancer. *Epidemiol. Rev.*, **23**, 19–23

Thomas, J.A. (1999) Diet, micronutrients, and the prostate gland. *Nutr. Rev.*, **57**, 95–103

WHO Cancer mortality database 2001.

http:\\www.dep.iarc.fr/dataava/globocan/who.htm

World Cancer Research Fund (1997) *Food, Nutrition and the Prevention of Cancer: A Global Perspective.* Washington D.C., American Institute for Cancer Research

Yoshizawa, K., Willett, W.C., Morris, S.J., Stampfer, M.J., Spiegelman, D., Rimm, E.B. & Giovannucci, E. (1998) Study of prediagnostic selenium level in toenails and the risk of advanced prostate cancer. *J. Natl. Cancer Inst.*, **90**, 1219–1224

Very-long-chain ω-3 fatty acids as markers for habitual fish intake in Spain

Amiano P.[1], Dorronsoro M.[1], Larrañaga N.[1], Renobales M.[2], Ruiz de Gordoa J.C.[2]

(the Spanish EPIC cohort of Gipuzkoa, in the Basque Country)

[1]Public Health Division, Health Department of the Basque Country. [2]Faculty of Pharmacy and Sciences, University of Basque Country, Spain.

Background

It is well known that the source of dietary fat determines the fatty acid composition of the blood and adipose tissue and that the biochemical variables are used as complements to dietary assessment methods or to validate these methods (Nikkari *et al.*, 1995). The consumption of fish and other sea products is the primary source of the major ω-3 polyunsaturated fatty acids (PUFA), eicosapentaenoic acid (C20:5) and docosahexaenoic acid (C22:6). The association between habitual fish and marine ω-3 PUFA intake and the fatty acid composition of plasma lipids, cell membranes, and adipose tissue has been demonstrated in intervention studies, principally with dietary supplements, and in studies carried out in populations that traditionally consume large amounts of fish and other sea products such as the Eskimos in Greenland, who show a blood fatty acid profile that is dominated by C20:5 and C22:6 (Dyerberg *et al.*, 1978; Bjerve *et al.*, 1993). As a result of its fishing tradition, cultural habits and geographic location, people of the Basque Country consume a large quantity of fish.

Purpose

The aim of the present study was to assess the relationship between habitual fish intake in the general population with a wide range of fish intake and very long-chain fatty acid levels in serum and in the LDL phospholipids and cholesteryl ester fractions.

Methods

We studied a random sample of 102 healthy volunteers of both sexes aged 35–65 from the cohort recruited in the province of Gipuzkoa (Basque Country, northern Spain) between 1992 and 1995 as part of the European Prospective Investigation into Cancer and Nutrition (EPIC) in the EPIC Spanish project (Grupo EPIC de España 1994). Subjects were divided into four categories of daily fish intake according to results of the dietary survey. The information on habitual intake over the previous year was collected by trained interviewers by means of a computerized questionnaire based on the Diet History method, which had been previously validated (EPIC Group of Spain 1997). Total fish was classified into lean fish, fatty fish, crustacea fish and other fish. The portion size was assessed by means of a photograph series, natural units and house -hold measurements. Anthropometric measurements, height and weight, were taken following a standard protocol. Fasting venous blood samples were drawn and stored in liquid nitrogen at –190°C until analyses and the different fatty acids were determined in serum and in phospholipids and cholesteryl esters of isolated LDL by gas-liquid chromatography.

The data were expressed as an adjusted mean and standard deviation. The means were compared by analysis of variance. Linear regression analyses were conducted to asses the associations between dietary intakes and blood fatty acids.

Results

Mean fish intake for each group was 19.2, 51.1, 83.6 and 146.0 g/day and white fish consumption was higher than fatty fish consumption in all groups (Table 1). Mean concentrations of ω-3 polyunsaturated fatty acids, eicosapentaenoic acid (C20:5), and

Table 1. Main characteristics of the subjects according to habitual fish intake

	≤31 g/d	32–64 g/d	65–115 g/d
Number	26	24	27
Age (years)	50.4 (9.9)	50.6 (8.1)	47.2 (6.8)
Fish intake (g/d)	19.2 (3.7)	51.1 (14.3)	83.6 (16.9)
White fish (g/d)	11.6 (10.4)	27.8 (14.9)	52.3 (23.1)
Fatty fish (g/d)	5.2 (6.5)	16.4 (12.9)	20.7 (23.5)

Table 2. Results of simple linear regression analysis

r	C20:5	C22:6	Ω-3
Serum	0.39[a]	0.38[c]	0.41[a]
Phospholipids	0.31[b]	0.32[c]	0.35[b]
Cholesteryl esters	0.44[b]	0.23[b]	0.39[b]

[a] $P<0.001$.
[b] $P<0.005$.
[c] $P<0.05$.

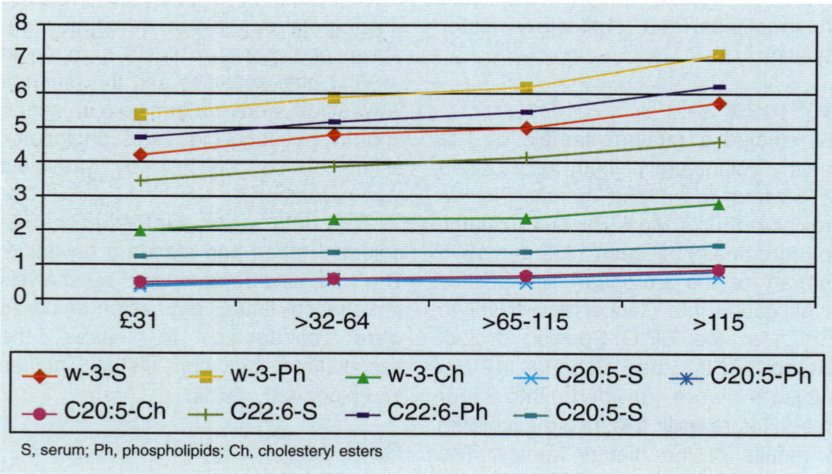

Figure 1
Percentage of total fatty acids in serum, LDL phospholipids and cholesteryl esters according to habitual fish intake (g/d)

docosahexaenoic acid (C22:6) in serum as well as in the LDL fractions of serum phospholipids and cholesteryl esters increased significantly from the lowest (<31 g/d) to the highest (>115 g/d) fish consumption category (Figure 1). In serum, C20:5 increased from 0.39% to 0.73% (P=0.000), a rise of 86% from the lowest to the highest fish consumption group, and C22:6 increased from 3.47% to 4.61% (P=0.000), a rise of 33%.

The simple linear regression analysis showed a statistically significant relationship between the explanatory variable fish intake (g/day) and the response variable concentrations of very long-chain fatty acids in serum and LDL phospholipids and cholesteryl esters (Table 2).

Conclusions

This study shows that in a population with a great tradition of fish consumption, the habitual fish intake is reflected in the content of fatty acids, eicosapentaenoic acid (C20:5) and docosahexaenoic acid (C22:6), in serum and in the LDL phospholipid and cholesteryl ester fractions. The concentrations of very-long-chain ω-3 fatty acids could be useful as biomarkers for habitual dietary fish intake.

References

Bjerve, K.S., Brubakk, A.M., Fougner, K.J., Johnsen, H., Midthjell, K. & Vik, T. (1993) Omega-3 fatty acids: essential fatty acids with important biological effects, and serum phospholipid fatty acids as markers of dietary ω3-fatty acid intake. *Am. J. Clin. Nutr.*, **57**, Suppl, 801S–806S

Dyerberg, J., Bang, H.O., Stoffersen, E., Moncada, S. & Vane, J.R. (1978) Eicosapentaenoic acid and prevention of thrombosis and atherosclerosis? *Lancet*, **2**, 117–119

EPIC Group of Spain (1997) Relative validity and reproducibility of a diet history questionnaire in Spain II. Nutrients. *Int. J. Epidemiol.*, **26**, Suppl 1, S100–S109

Grupo EPIC de España (1994) Estudio prospectivo europeo sobre dieta, cáncer y salud. *Med. Clin. (Barc.)*, **102**, 781–785

Nikkari, T. Luukkainen, P., Pietinen, P. & Puska, P. (1995) Fatty acid composition of serum lipid fractions in relation to gender and quality of dietary fat. *Ann. Med.*, **27**, 491–498

Conjugated linoleic acid and the risk of breast cancer

Chajès V.[1], Lavillonnière F.[1], Ferrari P.[2], Jourdan M.L.[1], Pinault M.[1], Maillard V.[1], Sébédio J.L.[3], Bougnoux P.[1]

[1]Nutrition, Croissance, Cancer, UPRES-E.A. 2103, Université François Rabelais, Tours. [2]International Agency for Research on Cancer, Unit of Nutrition and Cancer, Lyon. [3]Unité de Nutrition Lipidique, INRA, Dijon, France.

Introduction

Conjugated linoleic acid (CLA) refers to a group of octadecadienoic acid isomers that contain two conjugated double bonds. CLA can be found in dairy products or meat of ruminant animals. Attention has recently been directed to CLA based on their ability to act as preventive agents in experimental rat mammary carcinogenesis (Ip *et al.*, 1996). This suggests that dietary CLA might also be used in humans for chemoprevention of breast cancer. The feasibility of increasing the CLA content of foods has already been considered to increase CLA intake in humans (O'Shea *et al.*, 1998). In spite of such a potential, few data are available in humans. One study conducted in Finland found dietary or serum CLA to be significantly lower in cases than in controls, suggesting a protective effect of CLA on breast cancer risk, but only in postmenopausal patients (Aro *et al.*, 2000). Since CLA accumulates in body fat stores, we used the CLA content of breast adipose tissue as a qualitative biomarker of CLA dietary intake and we conducted a case–control study among 297 women treated for breast cancer or benign breast disease at the University Hospital of Tours, in France, to evaluate the hypothesis that CLA protects against breast cancer.

Methods

This study was carried out on a population of patients which was initially selected at the University Hospital of Tours, between 1992 and 1996, for a study on fatty acids and breast cancer risk (Maillard *et al.*, in press). It included 213 patients with invasive breast carcinoma (cases) and 84 patients with benign breast pathologies (controls) (Table 1). Patients had surgery as a first treatment step, during which a specimen of adipose tissue was retained and kept frozen in liquid nitrogen until analysis. Total lipids were extracted from adipose tissue samples, triglycerides were purified by adsorption chromatography and fatty acids and CLA were converted to fatty acid methyl esters (FAME) with sodium methoxyde. CLAs were first concentrated using a

Table 1. Descriptive characteristics of study population

Variables	Controls *n*=84 [Mean (SE)]	Cases *n*=213 [Mean (SE)]	P^a
Age (years)	42.7 (1.49)	55.4 (0.85)	0.0001
BMI (kg/m^2)	22.4 (0.41)	24.5 (0.32)	0.0009
Age at menarche (years)			0.51
≤ 12	33.8%	41.2%	
13–14	49.4%	43.1%	
≥ 15	16.8%	15.7%	
Menopausal status			0.001
Pre-menopausal	77.4%	41.8%	
Post-menopausal	22.6%	58.2%	

^{a}*P* value for chi-square test or Student *t* test.

Table 2. Estimated relative risk (ORs, crude and adjusted[a]) of breast cancer and 95% CIs by adipose tissue CLA levels from the entire population (*n*=97).

Fatty acids	ORs (95% CIs)			*P* for trend
	Tertile 1 (low)	Tertile 2	Tertile 3 (high)	
CLA: crude	1.00	1.29 (0.68–2.45)	1.42 (0.77–2.65)	0.273
CLA: adjusted		1.65 (0.80–3.37)[a]	1.83 (0.90–3.71)[a]	0.101

[a]Adjusted for age at diagnosis, BMI and menopausal status.

high performance liquid chromatography step. Then, the FAME composition of adipose tissue was determined by gas chromatography. Total CLA was calculated as the sum of the isomers and was expressed as a percentage of total fatty acids. Patients were categorized into tertiles according to the percentage composition of CLA. Odds ratios (ORs) and 95% confidence intervals (CIs) were calculated for each tertile using an unconditional logistic regression analysis; estimates were adjusted for age, body mass index (BMI) and menopausal status.

Results

We found that the mean CLA level was 0.44% of total fatty acids in cases (range, 0.19–0.75; SD, 0.10) and 0.43% in controls (range, 0.14–0.70; SD, 0.11). No significant difference in mean CLA levels between control and case patients was found (P=0.35 by Student t test). Within patients, partial Spearman correlation coefficients were calculated between CLA levels and a number of clinical characteristics. We found that CLA levels were not associated with age at diagnosis (n=297; r=0.05; P=0.35) but were inversely associated with BMI (n=297; r=–0.13; P=0.02). No significant association was found between CLA levels in breast adipose tissue and breast cancer risk (Table 2).

Discussion

In contrast to previous data derived from a case–control study based on serum CLA content (Aro *et al.*, 2000), we were not able to document a negative association between adipose tissue CLA and the risk of breast cancer. There are several potential limitations in our study:

1. It was carried out in a geographically limited area in central France, where the ethnic diversity is low and cultural habits are very homogeneous. This might be reflected by the narrow range of CLA distribution among the population. This narrow range may be insufficient to detect a significant association with breast cancer risk.
2. The validity of adipose tissue CLA levels as a biomarker of its past dietary intake is not known since no dietary questionnaires are available.
3. Experimental studies on animals have shown that the feeding of CLA only during pubertal development of the mammary gland, prior to carcinogen administration, led to a reduction in chemically induced mammary carcinogenesis (Thompson *et al.*, 1997). Thus, the timing of CLA exposure may be inappropriate in our study. Before any lack of association can be concluded, other studies based on an identical approach should be carried out in more heterogeneous populations.

Acknowledgements

This work was supported by grants from the CERIN.

References

Aro, A., Männistö, S., Salminen, I., Ovaskainen, M.L., Kataja, V. & Uusitupa, M. (2000) Inverse association between dietary and serum conjugated linoleic acid and risk of breast cancer in postmenopausal women. *Nutr. Cancer*, **38**, 151–157

Ip, C., Briggs, S.P., Haegele, A.D., Thompson, H.J., Storkson, J. & Scimeca, J.A. (1996) The efficacy of conjugated linoleic acid in mammary cancer prevention is independent of the level or type of fat in the diet. *Carcinogenesis*, **17**, 1045–1050

Maillard, V., Bougnoux, P., Ferrari, P., Jourdan, M.L., Pinault, M., Lavillonnière, F., Body, G., Le Floch, O. & Chajès, V. (2002) N-3 and n-6 fatty acids in breast adipose tissue and relative risk of breast cancer in a case–control study in Tours, France. *Int. J. Cancer*, **98**, 78–83

O'Shea, M., Lawless, F., Stanton, C. & Devery, R. (1998) Conjugated linoleic acid in bovine milk fat: a food-based approach to cancer chemoprevention (1998) *Trends Food Sci. Tech.*, **9**, 192–196

Thompson, H., Zhu, Z.J., Banni, S., Darcy, K., Loftus, T. & Ip, C. (1997) Morphological and biochemical status of the mammary gland as influenced by conjugated linoleic acid: implication for a reduction in mammary cancer risk. *Cancer Res.*, **57**, 5067–5072

Red meat and colorectal cancer risk: the effect of dietary iron and haem on endogenous *N*-nitrosation

Cross A.J.[1], Pollock J.R.A.[2], Bingham S.A.[1]

[1]MRC Dunn Human Nutrition Unit, Hills Rd, Cambridge, CB2 2XY, UK. [2]Pollock & Pool Ltd, Ladbroke Close, Woodley, Reading, RG5 4DX, UK.

Background

Epidemiological studies have implicated a high red meat diet as a risk factor for sporadic colorectal cancer, although white meat appears to have no such association (Armstrong & Doll, 1975).

Previous human metabolic studies have shown that an increase in red meat consumption results in an increased production of potentially carcinogenic *N*-nitroso compounds (NOCs). This effect is reproducible (Silvester *et al.*, 1997) and has been shown to occur in a dose-dependent manner (Hughes *et al.*, 2001). Subsequent studies have shown a lack of effect of both a high white meat diet (Cross *et al.*, 2000) and a high vegetable protein diet (unpublished data).

The major contrasting characteristics of red and white meat are the iron and haem content, approximately four times and ten times greater in red meat, respectively.

The aim of this study was to determine the effect of haem and iron independently on the endogenous formation of NOCs in human volunteers.

Methods

Study design

Nine healthy, non-smoking, male volunteers (age range, 24–74 years), who had not been taking antibiotics for 3 months prior to the study, were recruited.

The volunteers were required to live in the metabolic suite of the Dunn Human Nutrition Unit for the duration of the study, where all food and drink was provided and specimens collected.

Body weight was maintained constant throughout the study by adjusting the diets to each individual's energy requirements. Compliance to the study protocol was assessed by faecal and urinary biomarkers.

Volunteers were randomly assigned in a cross-over design to each of the three 15-day dietary periods:

- Low red meat diet (60 g/day)
- Low red meat diet supplemented with 29 mg/day haem iron, in the form of liver and black pudding
- Low red meat diet supplemented with 35 mg/day inorganic iron, in the form of a 300 mg ferrous gluconate tablet

Only six of the volunteers were assigned to all three dietary periods, three volunteers were only able to take part in two dietary periods.

The diets consisted of normal food, weighed to the nearest gram and purchased in advance of the study, from the same batch, to minimize daily variation. The diets were matched for energy, each providing 10 MJ/day, and fat by adjusting intakes of ice cream and a low electrolyte glucose drink (Polycal, Nutricia). To maintain constant nitrate levels, low nitrate vegetables were used and ultra-pure water was used for cooking and drinking. Tea and coffee consumption was maintained at a constant level throughout the study.

Sample collection

Faecal samples were frozen on dry ice to minimize degradation, and analysed on days 10, 13 and 15 of each dietary period. The NOC content was determined by chemical denitrosation with hydrogen bromide and chemiluminescence detection of the released nitric oxide, using a thermal energy analyser to detect the apparent

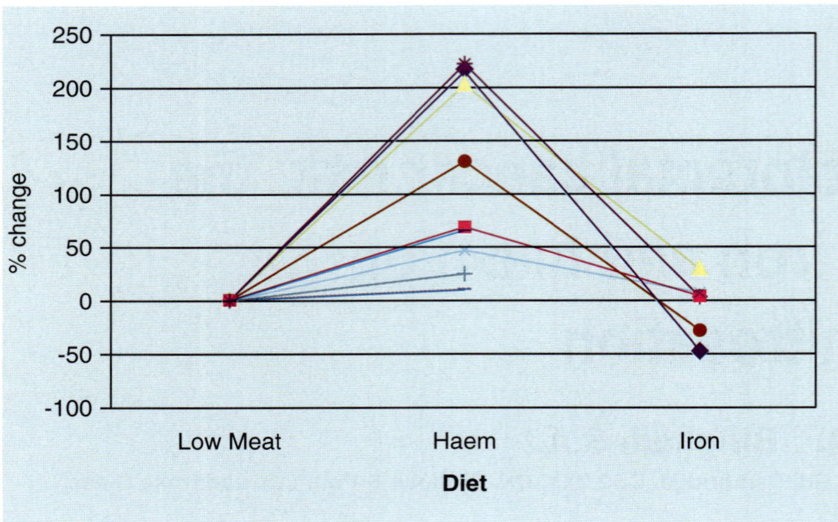

Figure 1
Percentage change in faecal ATNC (µg/kg) from the low meat diet

total *N*-nitroso compounds (ATNC) present (Pignatelli *et al.*, 1987).

Results

All volunteers showed an increase in faecal ATNC on the haem-supplemented diet (Fig. 1), with an average increase from the low meat diet of 109.4%. The mean faecal ATNC level on the low meat diet was 766 mg/kg, increasing significantly (P=0.006) to 1438 mg/kg on the haem-supplemented diet.

Iron supplementation did not significantly enhance faecal ATNC levels (mean level of 852 mg/kg). Therefore there is a significant difference between the effect of haem and inorganic iron in the diet on the formation of ATNC (P=0.004).

The consumption of red meat appears to enhance endogenous *N*-nitrosation by providing a source of haem.

References

Armstrong, B. & Doll, R. (1975) Environmental factors and cancer incidence in different countries. *Int. J. Cancer*, **15**, 617–631

Cross, A.J., Pollock, J.R.A. & Bingham, S.A. (2000) Increased endogenous *N*-nitrosation in the human colon: a response to red and white meat? *Br. J. Cancer*, **83**, (Suppl. 1), 81

Hughes, R., Cross, A.J., Pollock, J.R.A. & Bingham, S. (2001) Dose-dependent effect of dietary meat on endogenous colonic *N*-nitrosation. *Carcinogenesis*, **22**, 199–202

Pignatelli, B., Richard, I., Bourgade, M.C. & Bartsch, H. (1987) Improved group determination of total NOC in human gastric juice by chemical denitrosation and thermal energy analysis. *Analyst*, **112**, 945–949

Silvester, K.R., Bingham, S.A., Pollock, J.R., Cummings, J.H. & O'Neill, I.K. (1997) Effect of meat and resistant starch on faecal excretion of apparent *N*-nitroso compounds and ammonia from the human large bowel. *Nutr. Cancer*, **29**, 13–23

Mercury intake associated with fish consumption in a cohort of Gipuzkoa, Basque Country, Spain

Larrañaga N., Amiano P., Dorronsoro M., Sanzo J.M.
(for the EPIC working group of Spain)

Public Health Division of Gipuzkoa, Health Department of the Basque Country, Spain.

Background

Mercury can be found in three forms: elemental mercury, inorganic mercury salts and organic mercury. Any of them can undergo a methylation process and turn into methylmercury through saprophyte micro-organisms found in soil and water, reaching its highest concentrations in the edible tissues of larger fishes. Among organic mercury compounds, methylmercury is the most toxic form, a neurotoxic agent present in the environment that can easily pass through cellular membranes. The proportion of methylmercury to inorganic mercury in fish has been stated to be 9:1 (Agency for Toxic Substances and Disease Registry, 1992). The 90% of methylmercury in human beings is found in the red blood cells. As a result, the mercury level in erythrocytes can be used as an indicator of methylmercury.

Several studies have shown the variability in mercury content of sea and fresh water fish. Others suggest that human exposure to mercury has been increasing in recent years. Overall, the amount of fish intake is fundamental in estimating exposure to mercury, due to the high rate of retention of methylmercury (Stern *et al.*, 1996).

The Basque country, due to its fishing tradition, sociocultural customs and geographic location, has always had a very high consumption of fish and is thus potentially at risk of high mercury intake.

Purpose

To estimate mercury intake, we used data on fish consumption among participants of Gipuzkoa's cohort of the European Prospective Investigation into Cancer and Nutrition (EPIC). We also validated the estimation by measuring the blood mercury level in a sample of individuals.

Methods

In order to ascertain the most frequently consumed species of fish, the daily amount consumed of each species by the EPIC Gipuzkoa cohort was calculated, along with the daily number of individual consumers. Individual diet was assessed through personal interview using the Diet History method, in a computerized questionnaire specially designed and validated for the study, and a blood sample was taken in the 8417 volunteers constituting the EPIC Gipuzkoa cohort (Grupo EPIC de España, 1994). The mercury content of fish was supplied by the Food Chemical Surveillance Programme (Urieta *et al.*, 1991). For some species, an ad hoc sampling was performed using a similar methodology, in order to complete the number of fish samples analysed. Mercury concentration in red blood cells of a random sample of 120 individuals stratified by fish intake was used for validation. To estimate methylmercury intake, it was assumed that the amount of methylmercury in fish was 90% (Agency for Toxic Substances and Disease Registry, 1992). The statistical tests used for studying the relationship between fish consumption, mercury intake and mercury in erythrocytes were the Kendall correlation coefficient and the Kruskal-Wallis test.

Results

The average consumption of fish was 73.9 g/day in the Gipuzkoa cohort, the highest fish consumption of the different

Table 1. Selected characteristics of the EPIC Spain cohort

	Gipuzkoa		Asturias		Navarra		Granada		Murcia	
	Men (*n*=4158)	**Women** (*n*=4259)	**Men** (*n*=3085)	**Women** (*n*=5459)	**Men** (*n*=3908)	**Women** (*n*=4176)	**Men** (*n*=1797)	**Women** (*n*=6083)	**Men** (*n*=2687)	**Women** (*n*=5837)
Age groups (%)										
<45	23.8	38.6	27.6	42.7	26.5	36.6	25.5	35.7	29.1	40.1
45–54	45.4	38.2	44.1	35.5	44.5	38.3	38.2	35.0	40.0	35.3
55+	30.9	23.2	28.2	21.8	28.9	25.0	36.2	29.3	30.7	24.3
Mean caloric intake (kcal)	2878	2048	2579	1936	2923	2114	2514	1770	2802	2156
Range	(703–10 187)	(605–6178)	(893–7858)	(506–5138)	(1050–7429)	(607–5141)	(771–9211)	(323–6058)	(556–9293)	(395–5989)
Fish intake (g/d)	85.9	60.9	73.8	57.2	78.8	51.6	79.7	52.2	68.3	51.2
Range	(0–478.4)	(0–321.4)	(0–471.0)	(0–358.9)	(0–445.8)	(0–315.6)	(0–436.5)	(0–413.3)	(0–350.9)	(0–326.3)

EPIC regions in Spain (Table 1), with 99% of consumers. Males consumed, on average, 85.9 g/day of fish and women 60.9 g/day.

The average amount of mercury in red blood cells was 17.9 μg/kg, with 19.8 μg/kg in men and 16.3 μg/kg in women. The mercury content in red cells followed an upward slope as fish consumption increased (Table 1) with a statistically significant relationship between fish consumption and the amount of mercury in red blood cells.

The relationship between fish consumption and mercury intake (Kendall correlation coefficient: 0.69, $P<0.001$) as well as mercury in erythrocytes (Kendalls correlation coefficient: 0.39, $P<0.001$) was confirmed.

The average amount of mercury ingestion was estimated for men at 48.3 μg/week, 12% of the WHO's Provisional Tolerable Weekly Intake (PTWI), and the maximum intake was 350.3 μg/week (82% of the PTWI). In women, the average intake was 32.8 μg/week (10% of the PTWI) and the maximum 249.2 (56% of the PTWI). Almost all individuals' intake was below 75% of the PTWI. The average intake of methylmercury for men, assuming that 90% of the mercury was methylmercury, was 43.4 μg/week (16% of the PTWI) and in women 29.5 μg/week (13% of the PTWI). The highest amount consumed was 315.3 μg/week, which corresponds to 112% of the PTWI.

Conclusions

The pattern of very high fish consumption in the Basque Country was confirmed by the fish intake data of the EPIC Gipuzkoa cohort. No individuals from the cohort exceeded WHO's Provisional Tolerable Weekly Intake (U.S. Environmental Protection Agency, 1995). Nevertheless, certain individuals come close to the recommended limits. Mercury in fish should be monitored in order to assess the risk for the population.

References

Agency for Toxic Substances and Disease Registry. (1992) Mercury toxicity. *Am. Fam. Physician*, **46**, 1731–1741

Grupo EPIC de España. (1994) Estudio prospectivo Europeo sobre dieta, cáncer y salud. *Med. Clin. (Barc.)*, **102**, 781–785

Stern, A.H., Korn, L.R. & Ruppel, B.E. (1996) Estimation of fish consumption and methylmercury intake in the New Jersey population. *J. Expo. Anal. Environ. Epidemiol.*, **6**, 503–525

Urieta, I., Jalón, M., García, J. & González de Galdeano, L. (1991) Food surveillance in the Basque Country (Spain). The design of a total diet study. *Food Addit. Contam.*, **3**, 371–380

U.S. Environmental Protection Agency (USEPA). *Oral Reference Dose for Methylmercury*. IRIS (Integrated Risk Information System). On-line5/01/95 http://www.epa.gov/IRIS/subst/0073.htm#oralrfd

Meat consumption in Europe – results from the EPIC study

Linseisen J.[2], Kesse E.[2], Slimani N.[1]
(for the EPIC working group on dietary pattern, subgroup meat)

[1]International Agency for Research on Cancer (IARC), Lyon, France. [2]German Cancer Research Center, Heidelberg, Germany.

Purpose

Consumption of meat – most likely red meat and processed meat – is reported to modulate cancer risk of different sites, e.g. colorectal cancer and breast cancer. In this evaluation, meat consumption patterns will be compared across all European cohorts participating in EPIC (European Prospective Investigation into Cancer and Nutrition). The data given should provide valid information on the exact exposure level for meat and meat subgroups in the different EPIC cohorts. Moreover, the results might be used for calibration of the dietary instruments used to assess usual dietary intake in all EPIC participants.

Methods

In a representative subsample of the EPIC cohorts (27 centres) across 10 Western European countries (France, Italy, Spain, United Kingdom, Germany, The Netherlands, Greece, Sweden, Denmark, Norway), 24-h dietary recalls were assessed by means of the standardized computer program EPIC-SOFT. Single dietary recalls of 22 924 women and 13 031 men (age range, 35–74 years) were evaluated. The given mean intake results for total meat and meat subgroups (e.g. red meat, processed meat) were adjusted for the age of the participants as well as for the recall weekday and season. Factors influencing meat intake were identified by means of analysis of variance. Over the whole study population, about 400 EPIC participants stated they were vegetarian (vegans, ovo-lacto vegetarians, fish eaters with no or low meat intake), most of them originating from the health-conscious cohort in the UK.

Results

Mean total meat intake was lowest in the health-conscious cohort in the United Kingdom (15 g/day and 21 g/day in women and men, respectively), followed by EPIC Greece (47 g/day and 79 g/day, respectively). The highest meat intake was observed in the Northern Spanish EPIC cohorts, especially in San Sebastian, with 124 g/day and 243 g/day in women and men, respectively. Besides Greece, most other Mediterranean EPIC centres in Spain and Italy (except EPIC Naples) also revealed comparably low meat intake data. At the county level, the highest mean meat intake in women was found for the French EPIC participants.

Differences in the intake of meat subgroups across EPIC were even higher than found for total meat intake. The EPIC cohorts in The Netherlands, Germany and the Nordic countries (Denmark, Sweden, Norway) showed, to a certain extent, comparable meat consumption patterns, with a high proportion of processed meat (sausages) and a lower intake of poultry as compared to most Mediterranean EPIC centres and the EPIC UK cohorts. Additionally, in most Mediterranean centres, less pork and more veal/beef was consumed than elsewhere in EPIC. Except EPIC Ragusa, the most pork was consumed in the German, Swedish, Danish, and Dutch centres. In contrast, ruminant meat intake was highest in the EPIC centres of Northern Spain, Italy and France. Overall, mean red meat intake varied between 2 and 57 g/day in female participants and between 8 and 121 g/day in male participants of the different EPIC cohorts. The highest sausage intake was observed for the German EPIC participants, followed by the Nordic cohorts and the Dutch. Also, rarely consumed types of meat were evaluated, with the results indicating that meat from rabbits was more frequently consumed in French, Italian and Spanish EPIC cohorts while game consumption was higher in the Swedish and Norwegian centres.

Saturday and especially Sunday were the weekdays with the highest meat consumption; meat intake on Friday was the lowest. A higher body mass index as well as smoking was associated with a higher meat intake; older age and better education are predictive of a lower overall meat intake (all adjusted for energy intake).

Conclusions

The given high variation in total meat consumption as well as in the consumption of different meat subgroups demonstrate the heterogeneity within EPIC. Therefore, it is likely that results from EPIC will substantially contribute to our knowledge of the role of dietary meat in the etiology of chronic diseases, especially cancers of different sites.

Consumption of added fats and oils in EPIC

Linseisen J.[2], Bergström E., Gafá L.[2], González C., Thiébaut A.[1], Trichopoulou A., Tumino R.
(for the EPIC working group on dietary pattern)

[1]International Agency for Research on Cancer (IARC), Lyon, France. [2]German Cancer Research Center, Heidelberg, Germany.

Purpose

The discussion on the health consequences of dietary fat intake in terms of quantity and quality (fatty acid composition) continues today. Added fats and oils provide an important contribution to the total fat intake. This evaluation aims at describing the differences in the intake of added dietary fats and oils between centres participating in EPIC (European Prospective Investigation into Cancer and Nutrition).

Methods

Single 24-h recalls were assessed in 22 924 women and 13 031 men aged 35–74 years. The participants constitute a representative subsample of each of the EPIC cohorts located in 10 European countries. The amount of added fats and oils consumed was calculated in total as well as for several food subgroups. Furthermore, the intake of lipids originating from the consumption of added fats and oils, including fats and oils used for sauce preparation, was analyzed. All results were adjusted for age of the participants as well as the recall weekday and season. Analysis of variance was applied to identify factors significantly modulating the intake results.

Results

Mean daily intake of total added fats and oils varied between 16.2 g (Varese, Italy) and 41.1 g (Malmo, Sweden) in women and between 24.7 g (Ragusa, Italy) and 66.0 g (Potsdam, Germany) in men. Expressed in terms of lipid (nutrient) intake, it was possible to further include fats and oils used for sauce preparation. Total mean lipid intake by consumption of added fats and oils, including those used for sauces, ranged from 18.3 g/day (Norway) to 37.2 g/day (Greece) in female EPIC participants and from 28.4 g/day (Heidelberg, Germany) to 51.2 g/day (Greece) in males.

In the Mediterranean EPIC centres, a rather high lipid intake was observed, with an overwhelming contribution of olive oil and a low intake of animal fats. This contrasts with the Central and Nordic European EPIC centres where few vegetable oils, more animal fats, and a high proportion of margarine were chosen. The consumption patterns in EPIC France included both a high contribution of animal fats and vegetable oils. The German EPIC centres were at the top in animal fat (butter) consumption and revealed the highest animal fat:vegetable fat ratio.

Among all EPIC centres, the contribution of added fats and oils (including sauces) to total energy intake was lowest in Norwegian women (8.3% of energy) and highest in Greek women (21.8% of energy). In most EPIC centres, female and male participants revealed mean values in the range of 11%±1% and 12%±1% of energy intake, respectively, Spanish centres being an exception with about 15% of energy intake originating from fat and oils.

Besides total energy intake, the consumption of added fats and oils was significantly ($P<0.001$) affected by the following factors: centre, gender, age, smoking and education. Higher age as well as smoking were predictive for a higher consumption of added fats and oils (with energy adjustment), while a higher educational level was associated with a lower intake.

Conclusions

The data demonstrate a high variability in the consumption of added fats and oils across all EPIC centres. Although added fats and oils represent only one of the main lipid sources in the diet, the differences at the nutrient level observed are high as well. This provides a good chance for EPIC to give further insight into the relationship between dietary fat intake and chronic disease risk.

Plasma concentrations of fatty acids in nine European countries: cross-sectional study within the European Prospective Investigation into Cancer and Nutrition (EPIC)

Saadatian-Elahi M.[1], Norat T.[1], Bueno-de-Mesquita H.B., Clavel F., Gonzalez C.A., Hallmans G., Key T.J.T., Krogh V., Miller A.B., Tjonneland A., Trichopoulou A., Riboli E.[1]

(for the EPIC working group on dietary patterns)

[1]International Agency for Research on Cancer, Lyon, France.

Introduction

Dietary fats, which are the major source of energy for human tissues, play several structural and metabolic roles. Fatty acids, and in particular unsaturated fatty acids, form part of cell membranes, providing membrane fluidity and keeping the balance between external and internal exchanges in cells. Lipids also act as cell mediators (prostaglandin, thromboxane, leukotrienes), detergents (bile salts) and hormones (sex hormones).

Dietary fat intake is reflected by the concentration of particular fatty acids in adipose tissue, triglycerides, phospholipids and cholesteryl esters, fractions of serum, plasma or erythrocyte membranes as well as free fatty acids (Melchert *et al.*, 1987; Dougherty *et al.*, 1987).

The present study evaluates the fatty acid composition of plasma phospholipids in 16 geographical areas in nine European countries covered by the European Prospective Investigation into Cancer and Nutrition (EPIC). For this purpose, we used the fatty acid profile of plasma phospholipids as a biomarker of fat intake because it is believed to reflect the quality of medium-term dietary fat intake (Riboli *et al.*, 1987). We compared the fatty acid profile of plasma phospholipids in 3003 subjects, including men and women from 16 geographical areas involved in EPIC.

Materials and method

Three thousand and eighty nine EPIC study subjects were randomly selected from those for whom complete information on food frequency questionnaires (FFQ) and 24-h diet recall was available. Except for France, where only women were recruited, 100 men and 100 women were chosen from each EPIC center. For the Oxford center, 156 vegans (68 men and 88 women) and 46 vegetarians (35 men and 11 women) were included. The final population study included 3003 subjects because blood samples were missing for four subjects, extraction of fatty acids failed for 76 subjects because of technical problems, and six subjects were excluded from the study for other reasons. The sample was stratified by age into four groups (45–49, 50–54, 55–59 and 60–64 years) with an equal number of men and women in each group. Men and women were analysed separately.

Samples were analysed in the Nutrition Laboratory at the International

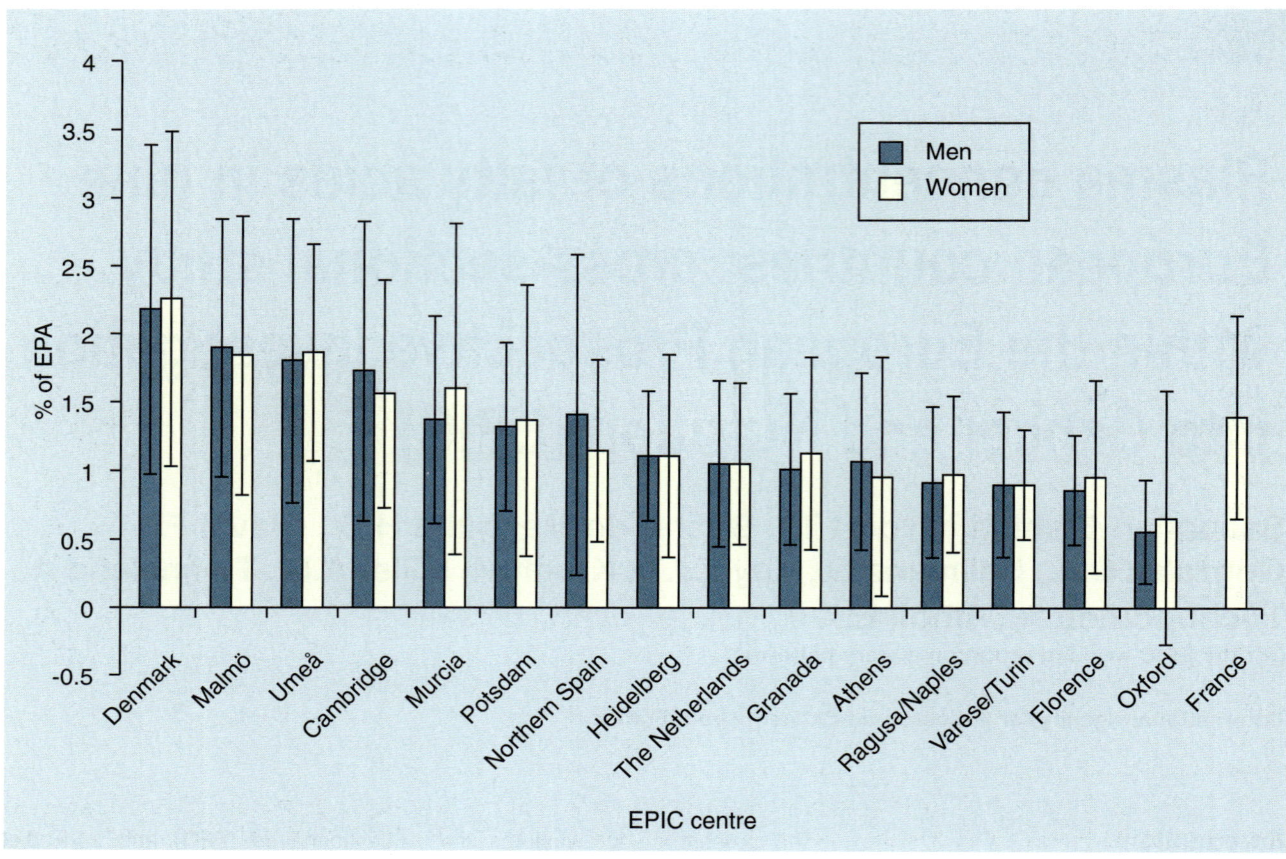

Figure 1
Mean of eicosapentaenoic acid as percent of total fatty acids among EPIC population

Agency for Research on Cancer (IARC), Lyon, France. The fatty acid composition of plasma phospholipids was determined by gas chromatography using the method of Chajès *et al.* (1999). Twenty-two individual fatty acids belonging to different classes (saturated, monounsaturated and polyunsaturated fatty acids) were analysed. Identification of the individual fatty acid methyl ester (FAME) was based on comparison of relative retention times with authentic standard methyl ester fatty acids (Sigma, St. Louis, MO, USA). The relative amount for each fatty acid was expressed as the percentage of total area.

Results

The mean percentages of the three major fatty acid families in both men and women are presented in Tables 1 and 2. UK vegans presented the lowest mean percentage of total saturated fatty acids and the highest levels of total PUFAs. The high level of PUFAs in vegans was mainly due to higher amounts of linoleic acid (C18:2, n-6) in the plasma of these subjects compared to the rest of the study subjects. The highest levels of MUFAs and particularly oleic acid were found in Florence.

Figure 1 shows the mean percentage of some fatty acids across EPIC centres. Alpha linolenic acid (C18:3, n-3) levels were two or three times higher in northern Europe than in southern Europe, with almost the same distributions in men as in women. The highest levels were presented in Sweden. This fatty acid accounted for 0.1%–0.3% of total plasma fatty acids. The analysis of quintile means showed distributions skewed to high extreme values in Nordic countries.

The levels of eicosapentaenoic acid (EPA, C20: 5 n-3) were two to three times higher in Denmark, Sweden and Cambridge than in Italy and Oxford.

Docosahexaenoic acid (DHA, C:22 6 n-3) levels ranged between 2% of total plasma fatty acids in UK vegans and more than 6% in Denmark. Except for Malmö, women generally had a higher percentage of DHA than men.

Table 1. Fatty acid composition of plasma phospholipids in EPIC centres (men)[a]

Region	*n*	Total SFA		Total MUFA		Total n-6		Total n-3	
		Mean	SD (min-max)	Mean	SD (min–max)	Mean	SD (min–max)	Mean	SD (min-max)
Athens	91	39.97	(37.53–41.75)	14.03	(10.22–18.6)	38.27	(33.86–43.34)	7.07	(4.79–11.40)
Florence	94	40.40	(38.26–42.58)	14.98	(11.74–18.56)	38.05	(33.31–42.96)	6.10	(4.05–9.20)
Varese/Turin	96	40.96	(39.18–42.57)	13.95	(10.52–18.16)	38.32	(33.77–43.81)	6.12	(3.76–10.10)
Ragusa/Naples	90	40.66	(38.06–42.46)	14.15	(9.71–19.24)	37.99	(33.10–43.70)	6.34	(4.23–10.54)
Northern Spain	94	40.17	(37.62–42.34)	13.00	(8.89–18.43)	38.15	(30.82–44.69)	7.75	(4.89–14.50)
Granada	93	40.12	(37.55–42.54)	14.16	(10.22–19.19)	37.88	(33.03–43.25)	7.28	(4.77–10.94)
Murcia	96	40.17	(37.72–42.57)	13.51	(9.22–18.33)	37.44	(32.32–43.43)	8.26	(5.60–12.66)
Cambridge	95	40.69	(38.52–42.70)	12.82	(9.77–15.75)	37.52	(29.78–43.90)	8.05	(4.36–16.52)
UK vegetarians	32	40.03	(36.19–42.91)	12.52	(9.79–18.44)	41.84	(36.50–47.39)	4.76	(3.00–7.89)
UK vegans	61	38.82	(34.94–42.15)	12.34	(9.44–15.48)	44.44	(37.14–49.26)	3.49	(1.58–8.00)
The Netherlands	95	41.19	(38.92–43.70)	11.44	(8.70–16.00)	40.3	(34.36–45.49)	6.34	(3.89–10.91)
Heidelberg	95	41.19	(39.11–42.19)	12.68	(9.94–16.60)	39.19	(34.00–44.02)	6.31	(4.54–9.29)
Potsdam	96	41.43	(39.89–43.17)	12.99	(10.28–16.98)	37.90	(32.63–42.92)	7.09	(4.76–10.49)
Malmö	100	40.24	(37.40–42.77)	13.38	(11.34–16.77)	36.48	(30.18–41.60)	9.27	(5.75–14.61)
Umeå	94	40.92	(38.66–42.89)	14.23	(11.54–16.39)	35.58	(29.42–39.99)	8.59	(5.92–13.28)
Denmark	96	41.25	(39.25–43.18)	12.90	(10.10–16.46)	35.63	(29.55–40.32)	9.28	(6.07–16.87)

[a]Means are expressed as a percentage of total area.

In multivariate regression analysis, the geographical region turned out to be the most important parameter of variability for plasma fatty acid profiles. It explained more than 80% of variability seen across EPIC centres for oleic, linoleic and alpha linolenic acid and more than 90% of EPA variability.

Conclusion

This is the first cross-sectional study including a large number of different European populations. The results of this study showed large variations in the fatty acid profile of plasma phospholipids among different regions of Europe. The region was the most important determinant of plasma fatty acid composition, which suggests that the variations observed are largely due to differing dietary patterns. This dietary heterogeneity observed in 22 EPIC centres involved in our cross-sectional study will be a good basis in the future for investigating the relationship between dietary fat intake and the incidence of cancer and cardiovascular diseases.

References

Melchert, H.U., Limsathayourat, N., Mihajlovic, H., Eichberg, J., Thefeld, W. & Rottka, H. (1987) Fatty acid patterns in triglycerides, diglycerides, free fatty acids, cholesteryl esters and phosphatidylcholine in serum from vegetarians and non-vegetarians. *Atherosclerosis*, **65**, 159–166

Dougherty, R.M., Galli, C., Ferro-Luzzi, A., & Lacono, J.M. (1987) Lipid and phospholipid fatty acid composition of plasma, red blood cells, and platelets and how they are affected by dietary lipids: a study of normal subjects from Italy, Finland, and the USA. *Am. J. Clin. Nutr.*, **45**, 443–455

Riboli, E., Rönnholm, M., & Saracci, R. (1987) Biological markers of diet. *Cancer Surv.*, **6**, 685–718

Chajes, V., Hulten, K., Van Kappel, A.L., Winkvist, A., Kaaks, R., Hallmans, G., Lenner, P., & Riboli, E. (1999) Fatty-acid composition in serum phospholipids and risk of breast cancer: an incident case–control study in Sweden. *Int. J. Cancer*, **83**, 585–590

Table 2. Fatty acid composition of plasma phospholipids in EPIC centres (women)[a]

Region	*n*	Total SFA		Total MUFA		Total n-6		Total n-3	
		Mean	SD (min–max)	Mean	SD (min–max)	Mean	SD (min–max)	Mean	SD (min-max)
Athens	100	39.19	(35.91–41.20)	13.31	(9.46–19.89)	39.31	(33.44–44.76)	7.40	(3.78–13.59)
Florence	99	39.50	(36.81–41.73)	14.84	(11.35–20.96)	38.58	(31.75–42.93)	6.46	(4.44–10.23)
Varese/Turin	100	39.77	(37.96–42.08)	13.78	(10.08–16.76)	39.43	(35.72–44.32)	6.54	(4.47–10.29)
Ragusa/Naples	99	39.47	(37.21–41.80)	13.46	(9.62–16.50)	39.20	(32.73–43.92)	7.23	(4.59–12.94)
Northern Spain	100	38.97	(36.61–40.97)	12.11	(8.17–17.46)	40.03	(33.14–46.25)	8.13	(5.16–13.16)
Granada	100	38.81	(36.07–40.95)	13.38	(9.87–18.45)	38.99	(33.15–44.11)	8.18	(5.02–13.36)
Murcia	100	39.15	(36.60–41.15)	12.00	(8.03–17.38)	39.12	(33.21–45.06)	8.90	(5.83–15.89)
Cambridge	100	39.69	(36.74–42.03)	12.95	(10.39–16.33)	38.33	(32.88–43.69)	8.26	(5.17–14.71)
UK vegetarians	12	38.77	(37.57–40.69)	12.76	(9.12–16.15)	41.50	(33.43–47.17)	5.94	(3.92–15.03)
UK vegans	86	37.62	(34.80–40.62)	12.12	(9.40–15.70)	45.34	(37.92–50.15)	4.20	(2.43–8.44)
The Netherlands	100	40.06	(37.40–42.19)	11.90	(8.40–15.81)	40.63	(35.51–45.25)	6.82	(4.53–11.25)
Heidelberg	96	40.58	(37.69–42.52)	12.40	(10.07–15.55)	39.61	(34.50–44.00)	6.82	(4.56–11.23)
Potsdam	99	40.5	(38.30–42.54)	12.45	(9.38–15.38)	38.99	(32.69–43.84)	7.42	(4.83–12.83)
Malmö	95	40.93	(39.06–42.74)	13.52	(11.11–17.06)	36.16	(30.26–39.96)	8.74	(5.74–13.94)
Umeå	99	39.95	(37.40–42.24)	14.20	(11.76–16.88)	35.89	(30.93–39.50)	9.32	(6.24–14.23)
Denmark	100	40.14	(36.91–42.41)	12.70	(9.93–15.88)	36.42	(31.68–41.19)	10.09	(6.41–17.91)
France	96	39.94	(36.57–42.50)	11.64	(8.85–15.89)	39.06	(33.27–44.34)	8.71	(5.35–13.97)

[a]Means are expressed as a percentage of total area.

Use of high-temperature cooking methods in preparation of meat and fish in European countries

Rohrmann S.[1], Linseisen J.[1], Becker N.[1], Sinha R.[2]
(for the EPIC working group on dietary patterns)

[1]Deutsches Krebsforschungszentrum, Heidelberg, Germany. [2]National Cancer Institute, Rockville, MD, USA.

Background

High-temperature cooking methods such as barbecuing (cooked on grill bars over burning charcoal or wood), grilling (cooked rapidly without moisture, on grill bars under or over intense direct heat), and frying (cooked in heated fat, usually over a direct source of heat) are associated with elevated cancer risk in different case–control studies. These cooking methods are thought to be surrogates for carcinogens, e.g. heterocyclic amines or polycyclic hydrocarbons.

A systematic analysis of differences in the use of high-temperature cooking methods for meat and fish preparation used within Europe has not been reported so far. In this short report, we describe the differences in meat and fish cooking techniques in different regions of the European Prospective Investigation into Cancer and Nutrition (EPIC).

Methods

A single 24-h recall was obtained in a representative subgroup of about 10% of all EPIC cohorts. Information about type and quantity of foods consumed as well as details on cooking methods were obtained by means of this method. To ensure that 24-h recalls were conducted in a standardized manner in each EPIC centre, a computer program, EPIC-SOFT, was developed.

Using 24-h recalls of 35 644 persons (22 727 women and 12 917 men, 35–75 years old), we obtained the amount of meat and fish consumed as well as the cooking methods used. The intake of fried, grilled, and barbecued meat and fish and their relative contribution to the overall cooking of meat and fish was calculated per region. The EPIC centres were grouped into regions according to similar patterns in meat and fish cooking. The calculated intake of meat and fish was adjusted for age, weekday and season.

Results

The relative contribution of these three cooking methods to the overall applied cooking methods for meat and fish cooking ranged from a low of 11.5% in North Italian centres to a high of 46.5% in the Dutch cohort. In the northern parts of Europe and North Spain, these high-temperature cooking methods were more often used in contrast to the centres in France, Greece, Italy, and Great Britain. Between 0% and 12% of meat and fish were grilled, 4%–43% were fried and 1%–9% were barbecued. Frying was more often observed in North and Central Europe and less in the South. Although barbecuing was rarely used in most EPIC regions, over 8% of meat and fish was barbecued in Greece.

Mean daily intake of fried, grilled, and barbecued meat and fish varied between 11 g/day (South Spain) and 55 g/day (The Netherlands) for women and between 20 g/day (North Italy) and 91 g/day (North Spain) for men. Most of cooked meat and fish was fried. The lowest amounts were consumed in Greece (1 g/day in women, 2 g/day in men), the highest amounts in the centres of The Netherlands (50 g/day in women, 80 g/day in men) and North Spain (43 g/day in women, 88 g/day in men). The consumption of fried meat and fish was generally lower in the centres of France, Greece, Spain, Italy, and Great Britain than in the northern and middle European centres. The intake of grilled meat and fish ranged from less than 1 g/day (Germany, Naples, Denmark) to 15 g/day among women in Ragusa and 20 g/day among men. A higher intake was observed in the French, Greek, and Italian EPIC cohorts than in the North of Europe. No grilled meat was consumed in the EPIC centres of Spain. Barbecued meat consumed was between 1 g/day and 11 g/day; less than 5 g/day were consumed in most regions.

Conclusion

The consumption of meat and fish prepared by high-temperature cooking methods (frying, grilling, and barbecuing) varies considerably in EPIC. EPIC, therefore, provides the opportunity to further investigate the possible relationship between high-temperature cooking methods, meat and fish cooking carcinogens and cancer risk in a large prospective cohort study. In order to study the variation in meat and fish cooking methods and their impact on cancer risk in the full EPIC cohort, a questionnaire on meat and fish cooking methods was developed. This questionnaire also assesses the degree of browning and doneness of meat and fish consumed.

Variability in fish consumption in 10 European countries

Welch A.A.[1], Lund E.[2], Amiano P.[3], Dorronsoro M.[3]

(for the EPIC working group on dietary patterns)

[1]Department of Public Health and Primary Care, University of Cambridge, Institute of Public Health, Strangeways Research Laboratory, Cambridge, UK. [2]Institute of Community Medicine, University of Tromsø, Norway. [3]Department of Health of the Basque Government, Basque Country, Spain.

Introduction

Consumption of fish (including all marine seafoods) may be important in the etiology of disease by conferring protection against cardiovascular disease and cancer. Fish are important sources of a number of nutrients, particularly protein, retinol, vitamin D, vitamin E and the essential long-chain n-3 fatty acids (N3PUFA) α linolenic acid (18:3n-3), eicosapentaenoic acid (20:5n-3, EPA) and decosahexaenoic acid (22:6n-3, DHA). Fish are the main source of intake of these essential fatty acids (Connor, W.E., 2001). We have investigated the variability of consumption of fish in 10 countries in Europe.

Methods

Fish consumption was estimated using the EPIC-SOFT 24-h recall method and standardized interviewing procedure in 35 955 men and women participating in the EPIC (European Prospective Investigations into Cancer and Nutrition) Calibration Study (Slimani, N. *et al.*, 2000). The countries of France and Norway recruited women only. The 10 countries represent recruitment from a total of 27 centres. Within the UK, participants were recruited both from the general population and a health-conscious group.

Total fish (fish, fish products, crustacea) was classified into white fish, fatty fish, crustacea and roe (roe and roe products) to estimate consumption of the types of fish containing different proportions of fat.

Means were calculated using the STATA statistical package.

Results

Mean consumption of fish is illustrated graphically in Fig. 1 and 2 for 22 924

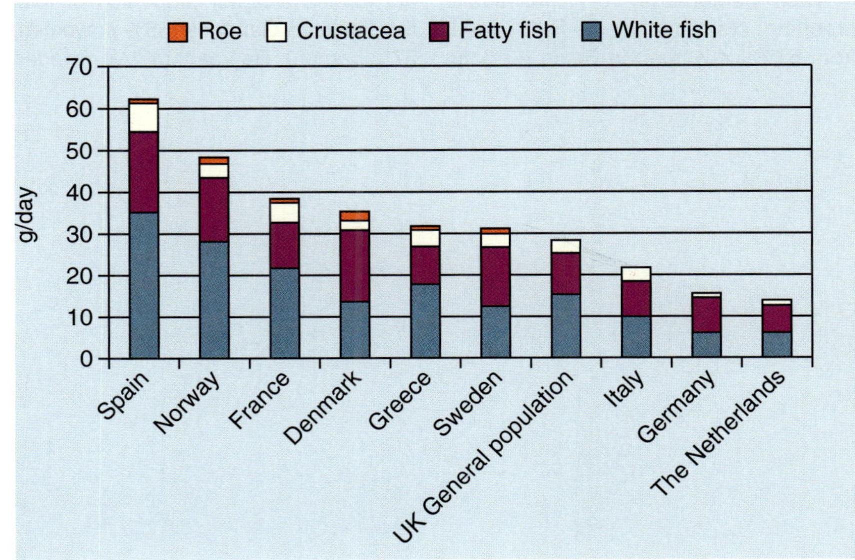

Figure 1
Consumption of different types of fish in women in 10 European countries

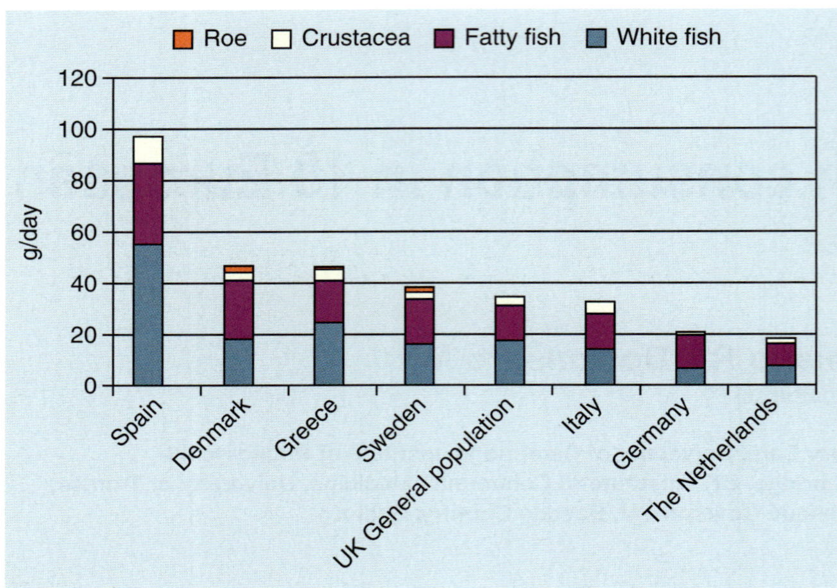

Figure 2
Consumption of different types of fish in men in 8 European countries

women and 13 031 men, respectively. For the UK, only the general population are represented. Total fish intake varied by a factor of five, being the highest in Spain and the lowest in the Netherlands.

The percentage of individuals reporting consumption of fish varied from 57% for women in Spain (67% in men) to 15% in the Netherlands and Germany, reflecting the average consumption of total fish in each country.

The consumption of fatty fish followed the same trends as total fish but formed a larger proportion of total fish intake in Germany (55% in women, 67% in men), Denmark (47%), Sweden (47%) and the Netherlands (47%). Consumption of fatty fish was lowest in women from Norway and France: 28% and 30%, respectively. Spain was the highest and Germany the lowest consumer of crustacea. The highest consumption of roe was in Denmark, although the amount consumed was small: 2.1 g per day in women and 2.6 g per day in men.

Conclusion

Total fish consumption varies substantially across Europe, as does the consumption of different types of fish. Future work will investigate the role these differences play in determining cancer incidence.

References

Connor, W.E. (2001) N-3 fatty acids from fish and fish oil: panacea or nostrum? *Am. J. Clin. Nutr.*, **74**, 415–416

Slimani, N., Ferrari, P., Ocké, M., Welch, A., Boeing, H., Liere, M., Pala, V., Amiano, P., Lagiou, A., Mattisson, I., Stripp, C., Engeset, D., Charrondière, R., Buzzard, M., Staveren, W. & Riboli, E. (2000) Standardization of the 24-hour diet recall calibration method used in the European Prospective Investigation into Cancer and Nutrition (EPIC): general concepts and preliminary results. *Eur. J. Clin. Nutr.*, **54**, 900–917

Meat consumption and colorectal cancer risk: an estimate of attributable and preventable fractions

Norat T., Lukanova A., Ferrari P., Riboli E.

Unit of Nutrition and Cancer, International Agency for Research on Cancer, Lyon, France.

Experimental and epidemiological studies have shown that food and nutrition modify colorectal cancer risk. The scientific evidence has been evaluated and summarized in recommendations by different expert groups that conclude that red meat consumption is likely to be related to increased risk of colorectal cancer (Riboli *et al.*, 1996; AICRF/WCRF,1997; COMA, 1998). Several hypotheses have been developed to explain the association between colorectal cancer risk and red meat. These hypotheses are mainly based on the fat, protein and iron contents of meat, the nitrogen metabolism and the formation of potential carcinogens when meat is cooked or processed (Potter, 1999).

Purpose

To evaluate the possible association between meat consumption and colorectal cancer risk and to estimate the risk fraction that could be attributable to current levels of red meat consumption in different populations. To estimate the potential reduction in colorectal cancer incidence following a reduction in red meat consumption to 10 g/day in populations where the consumption is higher than this value.

Methods

The study comprised a meta-analysis of published results of case–control and cohort studies, with inclusion criteria of case–control or cohort studies evaluating the relationship between total meat, red meat or processed meat consumption and risk of colorectal cancer; providing the information required for the statistical analysis; published in English between 1973 and 2000; and referenced in the Medline database. The statistical methods comprised two overall effect-size statistics, estimating the average of the logarithm of the observed relative risks (estimated as the odds ratio in most of the studies) associated with the highest versus the lowest level of consumption, as reported in the papers. In addition, the pooled coefficient *b* in the dose–response model $\ln RR=bX$ (Greenland and Longnecker's method) was used. When consumption was expressed as frequency, it was multiplied by the mean portion sizes published in previous studies. When consumption was expressed qualitatively, mean and variance derived from published studies were applied to the distribution of the study population. The attributable proportion was estimated as proposed by Miettinen. The pooled slope *b* was used to estimate relative risks associated with quartiles of consumption of red meat in different populations using non-consumption as the reference category. As estimates of the prevalence of red meat intake by geographical area, per caput intakes provided in Food Balance Sheets (F.A.O., 1994) were used, corrected for overestimation with data published from national dietary surveys.

Results

- High intakes of red meat and of processed meat were associated with a moderately increased risk of colorectal cancer. No significant association was found for total meat consumption and colorectal cancer risk. This result is consistent for case–control and cohort studies (Fig. 1).
- Results were more heterogeneous for case–control than for cohort

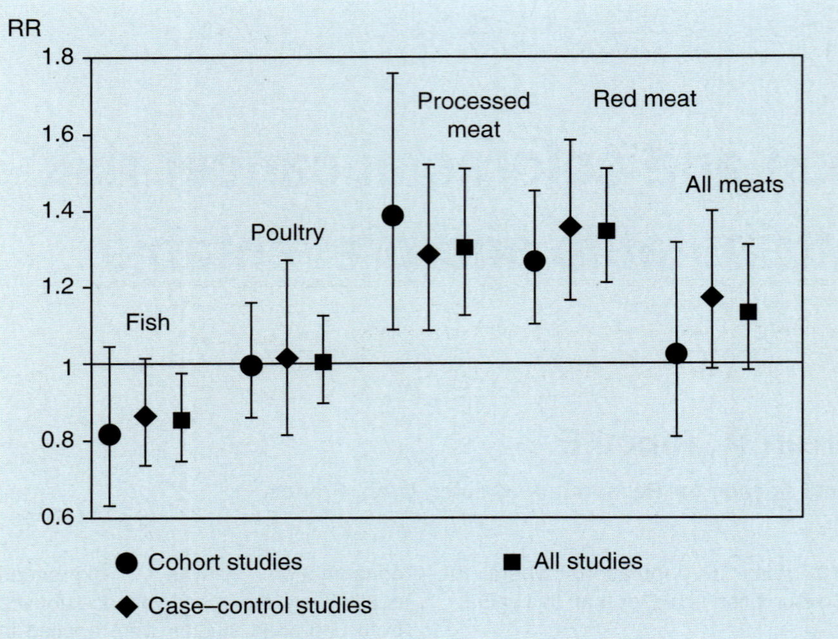

Figure 1
Dose–response relationship between fruit and vegetable consumption and risk of cancers

studies. The risk increase for red meat consumption was lower in cohort than in case–control studies. For processed meat consumption, inversely, the estimated risk increase was higher in cohort than in case–control studies.

- The dose–response association was stronger for processed meat than for red meat. Pooled relative risk estimates were more elevated in studies that included processed meat in the definition of meat groups than in studies defining them as fresh meat or fresh red meat.
- The risk fraction attributable to red meat consumption was between 12% and 25% in world regions where red meat intake is high. Most of the attributable risk fraction could potentially be avoided if red meat intake did not exceed 10 g/day on average in world regions where the consumption is currently high (Fig. 2).

In estimating attributable and preventable fractions, it was assumed that the association between red meat consumption and colorectal cancer is causal and free from bias. However, other dietary and non-dietary factors such as vegetable and fruit intake, smoking habits, reproductive history, physical activity and infectious agents may also contribute to risk differences between areas and be associated with meat consumption habits.

There are no epidemiological data available which would allow an estimation of whether reducing meat consumption after exposure at varying levels for varying duration at different ages would prevent colorectal neoplasia. Nor is it possible to determine after which latency a reduction in incidence might be achieved following a reduction in red meat consumption.

References

COMA Report. (1998) Nutritional aspects of the development of cancer. Report of the Working Group on Diet and Cancer of the Committee on Medical Aspects of Food and Nutrition Policy (COMA). **48**, Norwich, HMSO

Food and Agriculture Organization of the United Nations, Statistical Division. (1994) *Compendium of Food Consumption Statistics from Household Surveys in Developing Countries. Volume 1: Asia. Volume 2: Africa, Latin America and Oceania*. Rome, Food and Agriculture Organization

Potter, J.D. (1999) Colorectal cancer: molecules and populations. *J. Natl. Cancer Inst.*, **91**, 916–932

Riboli, E., Decloitre, F. & Collet-Ribbing, C., eds. (1996) *Alimentation et Cancer. Evaluation des Données Scientifiques*. Paris, Lavoisier

World Cancer Research Fund/American Institute for Cancer Research. (1997) *Food, Nutrition and the Prevention of Cancer: A Global Perspective*. Washington, D.C. WCRF/AICR

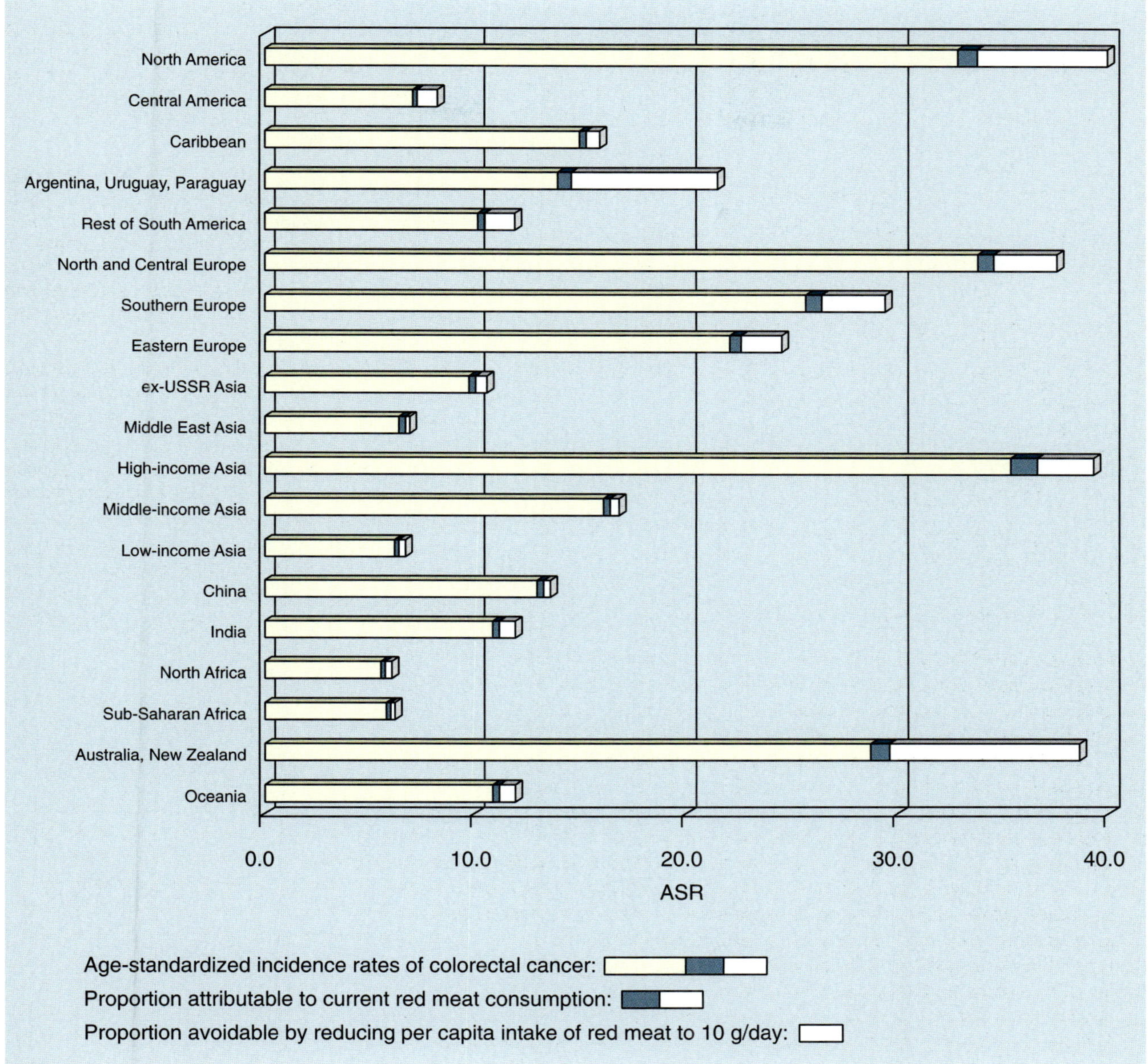

Figure 2
Attributable and avoidable proportion of colorectal cancer risk by red meat consumption in men

Serum fatty acids and risk of breast cancer in a nested case–control study of the New York University Women's Health Study

Saadatian-Elahi M.[1], Toniolo P.[3], Ferrari P.[1], Goudable J.[2], Akhmedkhanov A.[3], Zeleniuch-Jacquotte A.[3], Riboli E.[1]

[1]International Agency for Research on Cancer, Lyon, France. [2]Laboratoire de biochimie, Hôpital Edouard-Herriot, 69437 Lyon Cedex 03. [3]Dept. of Obstetrics and Gynecology and Kaplan Comprehensive Cancer Center, New York University School of Medicine, New York, USA.

Introduction

Experimental animal studies in rodents (Fay *et al.*, 1997) indicate that differences in breast cancer rates are partly related to dietary fat intake and especially to the quantity and the quality of fat ingested. These studies suggest that n-6 polyunsaturated fatty acids (PUFA) stimulate both mammary tumour growth and metastasis whereas n-3 polyunsaturated fatty acids have a tumour-inhibiting effect. On the contrary, results from epidemiological studies are inclusive (Hunter *et al.*, 1996).

We carried out a nested case–control study within the cohort of the New York University Women's Health Study (NYUWHS). We analyzed the fatty acid composition of serum phospholipids of women with clinically identified breast cancer and their matched controls. We focused on 22 individual fatty acids belonging to the four major fatty acid families: saturated fatty acids (SFA), monounsaturated fatty acids (MUFA), and polyunsaturated n-6 and n-3 fatty acids (PUFA).

Material and methods

Subjects

Subjects were participants in a prospective cohort study on hormones, diet and cancer, the New York University Women's Health Study, between 1985 and 1991 (Toniolo *et al.*, 1995). In this study, we included subjects diagnosed with breast cancer 6 or more months after cohort recruitment and prior to 1995. Controls were cohort members free of cancer, randomly selected among those who matched a case by age at recruitment (±3 months), menopausal status at baseline (pre- or postmenopausal), date of baseline blood sampling (±3 months), and number of blood samplings prior to a case's date of diagnosis. If premenopausal, controls were matched also by phase and day of the menstrual cycle at the time of baseline blood collection. One control was identified for each case.

Analysis of fatty acid composition in serum samples

Samples were analysed in the Nutrition Laboratory of the International Agency for Research on Cancer (IARC), Lyon, France.

Lipids were extracted from serum samples according to the method of Chajès *et al.* (Chajès *et al.*, 1999). Phospholipids were purified by adsorption chromatography on silica tubes and then converted to fatty acid methyl esters (FAME) using 25 μL of methyl-prep II.

FAMEs were separated on a gas chromatograph (Hewlett Packard, Palo Alto, CA) equipped with an on-column injector and a capillary column (length, 30 m; diameter, 0.32 mm, Supelco, Bellefonte, PA) and were identified by their equivalent chain length in comparison with standards (Sigma, St.

Table 1. Relative risk[e] (95% confidence intervals) of breast cancer for quartiles of serum phospholipids fatty acid levels

Fatty acids	Menopausal status	RR (95% CI)				
		Quartile			*P* for trend continuous variable	*P* for trend categorical variable
		2nd	3rd	4th		
Saturates						
14:0	Pre	0.48 (0.20–1.14)	1.27 (0.52–3.08)	2.22 (0.78–6.31)	0.07	0.14
	Post	0.59 (0.24–1.44)	0.72 (0.28–1.88)	0.57 (0.23–1.41)	0.62	0.37
	Total	0.59 (0.33–1.07)	0.97 (0.52–1.81)	0.91 (0.49–1.67)	0.27	0.86
18:0	Pre	1.01 (0.39–2.61)	1.27 (0.51–3.28)	2.31 (0.69–7.78)	0.53	0.19
	Post	1.62 (0.64–4.11)	0.88 (0.34–2.29)	1.01 (0.42–2.47)	0.59	0.65
	Total	1.24 (0.66–2.36)	1.04 (0.55–1.97)	1.18 (0.60–2.30)	0.91	0.79
Total SFA[a]	Pre	0.62 (0.24–1.71)	0.85 (0.33–2.14)	1.66 (0.56–4.89)	0.40	0.45
	Post	1.26 (0.49–3.21)	3.91 (1.41–10.87)	1.96 (0.73–5.25)	0.05	0.09
	Total	0.89 (0.46–1.70)	1.75 (0.92–3.34)	1.46 (0.74–2.83)	0.18	0.11
Monounsaturates						
16:1 n-7	Pre	1.31 (0.53–3.24)	1.36 (0.55–3.37)	1.07 (0.41–2.79)	0.91	0.77
	Post	0.96 (0.37–2.36)	1.11 (0.47–2.59)	1.27 (0.54–3.09)	0.92	0.53
	Total	1.09 (0.59–1.99)	1.25 (0.69–2.27)	1.16 (0.62–2.16)	0.90	0.53
18:1 n-9c	Pre	0.41 (0.16–1.06)	0.52 (0.18–1.52)	0.96 (0.37–2.45)	0.24	0.91
	Post	1.18 (0.49–2.82)	2.06 (0.84–5.05)	1.84 (0.72–4.71)	0.38	0.13
	Total	0.75 (0.41–1.39)	1.25 (0.66–2.37)	1.23 (0.65–2.32)	0.41	0.33
Total MUFA[b]	Pre	0.44 (0.18–1.08)	0.57 (0.21–1.58)	1.13 (0.42–3.04)	0.18	0.82
	Post	1.01 (0.42–2.44)	1.55 (0.65–3.72)	1.38 (0.55–3.49)	0.71	0.37
	Total	0.71 (0.39–1.29)	1.02 (0.54–1.94)	1.15 (0.60–2.18)	0.43	0.45
Polyunsaturates						
PUFA n-6, 18:2 n-6	Pre	1.23 (0.45–3.37)	1.25 (0.41–3.84)	1.11 (0.42–2.94)	0.97	0.93
	Post	0.9l (0.40–0.36)	0.83 (0.36–1.88)	1.04 (0.40–2.67)	0.96	0.94
	Total	1.03 (0.55–1.92)	0.99 (0.51–1.90)	1.01 (0.52–1.95)	0.99	0.98
PUFA n-6, 20: 4 n-6	Pre	0.69 (0.25–1.91)	1.68 (0.59–4.73)	0.62 (0.23–1.69)	0.18	0.68
	Post	0.78 (0.34–1.80)	0.61 (0.27–1.38)	0.89 (0.40–1.94)	0.67	0.64
	Total	0.79 (0.43–1.46)	0.99 (0.55–1.81)	0.81 (0.45–1.47)	0.80	0.66
Total, n-6 PUFA[c]	Pre	1.31 (0.46–3.77)	0.73 (0.27–1.98)	0.64 (0.22–1.86)	0.50	0.22
	Post	1.45 (0.65–3.25)	1.09 (0.49–2.41)	0.69 (0.28–1.73)	0.48	0.49
	Total	1.39 (0.75–2.58)	0.97 (0.53–1.78)	0.70 (0.36–1.36)	0.23	0.20
PUFA n-3, 18:3 n-3	Pre	0.86 (0.35–2.10)	1.37 (0.54–3.46)	0.97 (0.41–2.26)	0.76	0.84
	Post	1.46 (0.64–3.36)	0.86 (0.32–2.28)	0.64 (0.26–1.57)	0.35	0.23
	Total	1.14 (0.63–2.06)	1.14 (0.59–2.15)	0.80 (0.44–1.46)	0.65	0.48

Table 1 cont. Relative risk[e] (95% confidence intervals) of breast cancer for quartiles of serum phospholipids fatty acid levels

Fatty acids	Menopausal status	RR (95% CI) Quartile 2nd	3rd	4th	*P* for trend[e] continuous variable	*P* for trend categorical variable
PUFA n-3, 20:5 n-3	Pre	1.09 (0.48–2.46)	0.56 (0.20–1.58)	0.82 (0.32–2.11)	0.67	0.46
	Post	0.86 (0.33–2.22)	1.14 (0.43–3.01)	0.91 (0.32–2.62)	0.90	0.99
	Total	0.95 (0.53–1.69)	0.87 (0.47–1.63)	0.85 (0.44–1.65)	0.96	0.61
PUFA n-3, 22:6 n-3	Pre	0.48 (0.19–1.19)	0.40 (0.14–1.13)	0.83 (0.27–2.58)	0.25	0.51
	Post	1.21 (0.49–2.99)	1.23 (0.52–2.94)	0.67 (0.27–1.70)	0.47	0.41
	Total	0.76 (0.41–1.41)	0.79 (0.41–1.49)	0.70 (0.35–1.40)	0.76	0.49
Total, n-3 PUFA[d]	Pre	0.49 (0.20–1.21)	0.51 (0.19–1.39)	0.79 (0.29–2.18)	0.35	0.52
	Post	1.30 (0.52–3.27)	1.14 (0.44–2.95)	0.68 (0.26–1.74)	0.45	0.30
	Total	0.79 (0.43–1.44)	0.80 (0.41–1.56)	0.69 (0.35–1.34)	0.73	0.30
Total n-3 and n-6	Pre	0.52(0.18–1.47)	0.47 (0.17–1.26)	0.60 (0.24–1.54)	0.48	0.39
	Post	0.86 (0.39–1.87)	0.85 (0.34–2.16)	0.42 (0.17–1.08)	0.31	0.09
	Total	0.77(0.42–1.41)	0.68 (0.36–1.30)	0.59 (0.31–1.09)	0.42	0.09
PUFA/SFA	Pre	0.43 (0.15–1.25)	0.51 (0.19–1.30)	0.45 (0.17–1.23)	0.37	0.21
	Post	0.98 (0.44–2.21)	0.63 (0.28–1.43)	1.17 (0.49–2.76)	0.52	0.27
	Total	1.11 (0.62–2.00)	0.82 (0.45–1.51)	0.65 (0.34–1.22)	0.34	0.12

[a]Included C15:0, C16:0, C17:0 and C20:0.
[b]Included C18:1 n-9t, C18:1 n-7c and C20:1 n-9c.
[c]Included C18:3, C20:2, C20:3, C22:4 and C22:5.
[d]Included C22:5.
[e]RR adjusted for age at first full-term pregnancy, family history of breast cancer, history of benign breast disease and total cholesterol.
Pre, premenopausal women; post, postmenopausal women; Total, entire population (pre- + postmenopausal women); SFA, saturated fatty acids; MUFA, monounsaturated fatty acids; PUFA, polyunsaturated fatty acids.

Louis, MO, USA). The relative amount for each fatty acid was expressed as the percentage of total area.

Statistical Analyses

In statistical analyses, the paired *t* test was used to compare anthropometric values of cases and controls. Conditional logistic regression analysis evaluated the association between fatty acid composition of serum phospholipids and breast cancer risk.

Results

The study included 197 cases and 197 controls (182 pre- and 212 postmenopausal women). There were no significant differences between cases and controls in age at menarche, age at first full-term pregnancy, age at menopause and body mass index.

The odds ratio for the association between breast cancer and serum levels of different fatty acids are given in Table 1.

No significant associations were found between individual or total monounsaturated fatty acids and the risk of breast cancer.

Neither the essential n-6 polyunsaturated fatty acid, linoleic acid, nor other long-chain n-6 fatty acids were associated with cancer risk.

Individual n-3 fatty acids of marine origin, eicosapentaenoic acid (C20:5 n-3), docosahexaenoic acid (C22:6 n-3), and other individual or total n-3 fatty acids were not associated with the risk of breast cancer.

Overall, total polyunsaturated fatty acids (n-6 and n-3) were found to be protective for breast cancer risk.

Total saturated fatty acids were positively and significantly associated with the risk of breast cancer after menopause (*P* for trends = 0.05).

Conclusion

In this prospective study, we examined the fatty acid composition of phospholipids in the serum of 394 subjects in order to determine the role of different types of fatty acids in the incidence of breast cancer. Our results, in conjunction with other epidemiological studies (Howe *et al.*, 1990) suggest that saturated fatty acids are related to the risk of breast cancer after menopause. On the contrary, this study does not lend support to the hypothesis that n-3 fatty acids, either total or long-chain polyunsaturated fatty acids of marine origin, are protectors against mammary carcinogenesis. Further epidemiological studies on biomarkers of fat intake are needed in order to clarify the role of different subtypes of dietary fat in breast cancer development.

References

Chajès, V., Hulten, K., Van Kappel, A.L., Winkvist, A., Kaaks, R., Hallmans, G., Lenner, P. & Riboli, E. (1999) Fatty-acid composition in serum phospholipids and risk of breast cancer: an incident case–control study in Sweden. *Int. J. Cancer*, **83**, 585–590

Fay, M.P. & Freedman, L.S. (1997) Meta-analyses of dietary fats and mammary neoplasms in rodent experiments. *Breast Cancer Res. Treat.*, **46**, 215–223

Howe, G.R., Hirohata, T., Hislop, T.G., Iscovich, J.M., Yuan, J.M., Katsouyanni, K., Lubin, F., Marubini, E., Modan, B. & Rohan, T. (1990) Dietary factors and risk of breast cancer: combined analysis of 12 case–control studies. *J. Natl. Cancer Inst.*, **82**, 561–569

Hunter, D.J., Spiegelman, D., Adami, H.O., Beeson, L., van den Brandt, P.A., Folsom, A.R., Fraser, G.E., Goldbohm, R.A., Graham, S. & Howe, G.R. (1996) Cohort studies of fat intake and the risk of breast cancer – a pooled analysis. *N. Engl. J. Med.*, **334**, 356–361

Toniolo, P.G., Levitz, M., Zeleniuch-Jacquotte, A., Banerjee, S., Koenig, K.L., Shore, R.E., Strax, P. & Pasternack, B.S. (1995) A prospective study of endogenous estrogens and breast cancer in postmenopausal women. *J. Natl. Cancer Inst.*, **87**, 190–197

Dietary factors and multiple myeloma. Case–control study in Belgrade

Pekmezovic T.[1], Vlajinac H.[1], Adanja B.[1], Marinkovic J.[2], Kanazir M.[1], Suvajdzic N.[3], Colovic M.[3]

[1]Institute of Epidemiology, School of Medicine, University of Belgrade, Yugoslavia. [2]Institute of Social Medicine, Statistics and Health Research, School of Medicine, University of Belgrade, Yugoslavia. [3]Institute of Hematology, Clinical Center of Serbia, Belgrade, Yugoslavia.

Introduction

The etiology of multiple myeloma (MM) is little known. Several reports have indicated an increased risk associated with farming and agriculture (Pearce *et al.*, 1986) and food processing. However, evidence relating the increased risk with the exposure to pesticides or with exposure to some virus or antigen associated with meat is inconsistent. Radiation and various chemicals, besides pesticides, and wood dust have been suggested as risk factors for myeloma (Ichimaru *et al.*, 1982). Chronic antigenic stimulation and defective immune response are also postulated to be of importance in development of myeloma.

The aim of this study was to test the existing hypotheses about factors related to occurrence of myeloma, as well as to investigate the possible relationship between dietary factors and this malignancy. In this report only results relating to dietary factors are presented.

Material and methods

The investigation was performed in Belgrade (Yugoslavia) during the period 1994–1998. The case group consisted of 100 newly diagnosed and histologically confirmed MM patients at the Institute of Hematology, University Clinical Center, Belgrade. The same number of controls was recruited among hospital patients. About 50% of controls had ischialgia and the other half were patients with light injuries and skin infections. Cases and controls were interviewed by two physicians using a standard questionnaire including questions on demographic characteristics, habits, personal history, family characteristics, and consumption frequency of main food groups and food items. In the data analysis, univariate and multivariate logistic regression were used.

Table 1. Demographic characteristics of cases and controls

Variable	Cases (*n*=100)	Controls (*n*=100)
Sex		
Male	55	55
Female	45	45
Age (years)		
≤44	10	7
45–54	14	15
55–64	32	37
65–74	39	36
75+	5	5
Residential area		
Rural	24	25
Urban	76	75

Results

Demographic characteristics of cases and controls are presented in Table 1. In both case and control groups, there were 55 men and 45 women. The vast majority of them were 45 years old or older. Patients and controls lived mainly in urban areas.

Out of the main food groups and food items (Table 2), cases more frequently than controls consumed meat (OR, 1.92; 95% CI, 0.95–3.89; P=0.051), yogurt (OR, 2.42; 95% CI, 1.26–4.69; P=0.004) and butter (OR, 1.99; 95% CI, 1.09–3.63; P=0.016). Consumption of fruit and

Table 2. Consumption of food groups and food items of cases and controls

Food groups and food items	Cases (n=100)	Controls (n=100)	OR (95%CI)	P
Meat, 7 times per week	31	19	1.92 (0.95–3.89)	0.051
Milk, 7 times per week	41	30	1.62 (0.87–3.04)	0.104
Yogurt, 4–7 times per week	42	23	2.42 (1.26–4.69)	0.004
Cheese, 7 times per week	24	20	1.26 (0.61–2.61)	0.494
Eggs, 4–7 times per week	35	43	0.71 (0.39–1.31)	0.246
Fruit, 4–7 times per week	62	73	0.60 (0.32–1.15)	0.097
Vegetables, 4–7 times per week	81	92	0.37 (0.14–0.96)	0.023
Juice, >1 time per week	79	70	1.61 (0.81–3.23)	0.144
Butter, >1 time per week	57	40	1.99 (1.09–3.63)	0.016
Sweets, >1 time per week	75	73	1.11 (0.56–2.19)	0.747
Nitrate-treated meat, >1 time per week	63	54	1.45 (0.79–2.66)	0.196
Canned food, >1 time per week	32	29	1.15 (0.60–2.20)	0.645
Lard for food preparation	10	10	1.0(0.36–2.75)	1.00
Alcohol consumption	37	30	1.37 (0.73–2.58)	0.294
Coffee consumption	84	79	1.40 (0.64–3.04)	0.362

vegetables was more frequently reported by controls (OR, 0.60; 95% CI, 0.32–1.15; P=0.098 and OR, 0.37; 95% CI, 0.14–0.96; P=0.026). There were no significant differences between groups for alcohol and coffee consumption.

According to multivariate analysis, consumption of yogurt, 4–7 times per week, (OR, 3.12; 95% CI, 1.64–5.96; P=0.001) and vegetables (with the same frequency of consumption) (OR, 0.37; 95% CI, 0.14–0.96; P=0.022) were associated with MM, after adjustment for other factors significantly related to MM in the present study.

Discussion

According to the literature, etiological investigation of MM in the some countries has placed major emphasis on exposure to various chemicals, particularly pesticides. In recent studies, diet has also been associated with lymphoid neoplasms (Tavani *et al.*, 1997; Brown *et al.*, 2001).

This study comprised 100 MM patients and the equal number of controls. With respect to yogurt as a risk factor for multiple myeloma, cases in the present study consuming not only yogurt, but also milk, butter and meat more frequently than controls could point to animal fat as a dietary factor related to MM. An elevated risk of non-Hodgkin lymphoma was found among men with high milk consumption in Nebraska (Ward *et al.*, 1994) as well as in the study of Tavani *et al.* (1997). In this latter study, butter intake was also an indicator of the risk of myeloma. The association found between animal fat and some other malignant diseases is most probably affected through changes in the hormonal environment. It is also known that some hormones have a strong influence on the immune system (Hunt, 1992). The protective effect of fruit and vegetable consumption has been suggested for many malignant diseases. In a population-based case–control study of MM in three areas of the United States, Brown *et al.* (2001) found that a reduced risk of MM was related to frequent intake of cruciferous vegetables (OR, 0.7; 95% CI, 0.6–0.99) in both races combined, and vitamin C supplements in whites (OR, 0.6; 95% CI 0.5–0.9) and blacks (OR, 0.8; 95% CI, 0.5–1.4). In the investigation of Tavani *et al.* (1997), the highest tertile of intake of beta-carotene was inversely related to lymphoid neoplasms.

Despite the relatively small number of cases and controls in the present study and drawbacks of investigations based on retrospective data and the use of frequency instead of quantitative diet history method, the results obtained are in accordance with other investigators. Additional studies are needed to confirm these findings.

References

Brown, L.M., Gridley, G., Pottern, L.M., Baris, D., Swanso, C.A., Silverman, D.T., Hayes, R.B., Greenberg, R.S., Swanson, G.M., Schoenberg, J.B., Schwartz, A.G. & Fraumeni, J.F Jr. (2001) Diet and nutrition as risk factors for multiple myeloma among blacks and whites in the United States. *Cancer Causes Control*, **12**, 117–125

Hunt, J.S. (1992) Immunology of pregnancy. *Curr. Opin. Immunol.*, **4**, 591–596

Ichimaru, M., Ishimaru, T., Mikami, M. & Matsunaga, M. (1982) Multiple myeloma among atomic bomb survivors in Hiroshima and Nagasaki 1950–76. Relationship to radiation dose absorbed by marrow. *J. Natl. Cancer Inst.*, **69**, 323–327

Pearce, N.E., Smith, A.H., Howard, J.K., Sheppard, R.A., Giles, H.J. & Teague, C.A. (1986) Case–control study of multiple myeloma and farming. *Br. J. Cancer*, **54**, 493–500

Tavani, A., Pregnolato, A., Negri, E., Franceschi, S., Serraino, D., Carbone, A. & La Vecchia, C. (1997) Diet and risk of lymphoid neoplasms and soft tissue sarcomas. *Nutr. Cancer*, **27**, 256–260

Ward, M.H., Zahm, S.H., Weisenburger, D.D., Gridley, G., Cantor, K.P., Saal, R.C. & Blair, A. (1994) Dietary factors and non-Hodgkin's lymphoma in Nebraska (United States). *Cancer Causes Control*, **5**, 422–432

Chapter 5

Body weight, physical activity and cancer

Body weight, physical activity and cancer

Overvad K.

Department of Epidemiology and Social Medicine, Aarhus University, Vennelyst Boulevard 6, DK-8000 Aarhus C, Denmark.

Recently an IARC Handbook of Cancer Prevention was prepared addressing the importance of obesity and physical activity in cancer development, to be published in the year 2002. The most important aspects of body build and physical activity have not yet been identified and the causal pathways linking body build, physical activity and diet are very complex, as was also illustrated during this conference.

Physical activity is reported to be important in the development of cancer in the colon, breast and lung (World Cancer Research Fund, 1997). Physical activity is an important determinant of body weight and therefore presumably also important in the development of other cancers where obesity is a risk factor. In the context of a conference on nutrition and cancer, physical activity is therefore a potential confounder in studies on diet and cancer in the colon, breast, lung and possibly other organs.

Obesity is presumably important in the development of cancer in the endometrium, breast, colon, kidney and oesophagus (World Cancer Research Fund, 1997). When studying the importance of diet in the development of cancer in these organs, obesity is often considered an important confounder to be controlled for in the data analyses. Diet is, however, also important in weight control and in the development of obesity. In studies on diet and cancer, obesity thus appears as both a potential confounder and as a possible intermediate variable between diet and cancer. Therefore, the results of statistical analyses must be interpreted carefully. Results regarding associations between diet and cancer may be biased due to confounding from obesity. Controlling for confounding in multivariate analyses eliminates confounding from obesity from other etiologies but also eliminates the possible causal pathway from diet through obesity to cancer. The results of the bivariate analyses and the multivariate analyses thus no longer reflect the same biological setting. The bivariate analyses reflect all possible mechanisms from diet to cancer whereas the multivariate analyses reflect the associations between diet and cancer through mechanisms other than those involving body weight.

Physical activity and obesity are presumably also independent risk factors for cancer development. Physical activity is a complex exposure and aspects such as duration, frequency and intensity of the activity have been investigated. It has not been well established, however, which of these are the most important aspects in cancer development. Furthermore, assessing levels of physical activity either by questionnaires or by diaries is difficult and only recent calibration studies using heart rate monitors or accelerometers provide insight into the validity of the exposure assessment.

When studying the importance of physical activity in cancer development, both obesity and diet often have to be taken into account. As in its relation to diet, obesity may appear both as a potential confounder and as an intermediate variable between physical activity and cancer. Obesity thus has to be taken into account, considering the statistical analyses and the interpretation of the results in detail. Furthermore, some studies have indicated that obesity may also modify the importance of physical activity in cancer development (Thune *et al.*, 1997).

The importance of diet is often considered, taking into account total energy intake in analyses also including variables of gender and age as well as measures of height and weight. When studying physical activity including these variables, the statistical modelling and interpretation of the results must be considered carefully. In a multivariate model, the variations in physical activity are now variations in disease risk between individuals of the same gender and age, with the same body build and with the same total energy intake. If the variables are simply included in the model together with measures of physical activity the variable physical activity no longer describes the importance of physical activity but more likely, given that the participants have a stable weight, the importance of the metabolic efficiency. In this situation, the bivariate analyses and the multivariate analyses thus assess the importance of completely different exposures.

In studies regarding body build and cancer, a number of anthropometric measures have been used, including height and weight in absolute terms and changes in weight, together with ratio measures such as BMI and the waist-hip ratio. Skin folds and waist circumferences have been measured and recently assessment of lean body mass, total fat mass or fat percentages based on bioelectrical impedance measurements have been introduced. The many different anthropometric measures used illustrates the complexity of describing body build and also the uncertainty about the most relevant mechanisms regarding the importance of body build in cancer development.

Despite the relatively strong conclusions and the suggested population attributable risks assigned to excess body weight and physical activity in the coming IARC Handbook of Cancer Prevention, there is still a need for further studies. Hopefully, the large populations included in the EPIC studies and the substantial variation in body build, levels of physical activity, and dietary habits will provide further insight into this complex and seemingly important area of research

References

Thune, I., Brenn, T., Lund, E. & Gaard, E. (1997) Physical activity and the risk of breast cancer. *N. Engl. J. Med.*, **336**, 1269–1275

World Cancer Research Fund/American Institute for Cancer Research. (1997) *Food, Nutrition and the Prevention of Cancer: A Global Perspective.* Washington, D.C., American Institute for Cancer Research

Anthropometry, physical activity and cancer of the breast and colon

Berglund G.

Department of Medicine, Lund University, University Hospital, Malmö, Sweden.

Introduction

Cancer of the breast is the most common cancer and the most common cause of death from cancer in women, and the third most common cancer overall. Cancer of the colon and rectum is the fourth most common cancer and cause of death from cancer, throughout the world. Greater adult height, obesity and low physical activity are often cited as risk factors for both types of cancer (for review see World Cancer Research Fund, 1997). In this book, data until the mid-1990s are reviewed in a very comprehensive way. The purpose of the present paper is to extend the review of published reports on the association between anthropometry, physical activity and cancer of the breast and colon, up to 2000. Anthropometric variables were height, body mass index (BMI) and waist-hip ratio (WHR). Physical activity was reported separately for activity at work and during leisure time.

Methods

A structured search (e.g. Pub Med) and a review of original reports on anthropometry and/or physical activity in relation to one or both cancers, published until 2000, was carried out. For breast cancer, the analyses were divided into pre- and postmenopausal cancers. Where possible, physical activity was divided into physical activity at work and during leisure time. Colon cancer and rectal cancer were kept separately if so reported. Where appropriate, case–control and cohort studies are presented separately. Due to the limited space allowed, this presentation only gives examples of central publications between 1995 and 2000 in an attempt to analyse new data adding to the picture given in the above-cited review. The structured analyses followed the scheme presented in the 1997 review. It should, thus, be understood that this work deals with a simplified review of the literature, adding a more specific review of more recent date.

Results

Height and risk of breast cancer

In some early cohort studies, height was found to be positively associated with risk of breast cancer (de Ward 1974; Vatten & Kvinnsland, 1990), with a risk ratio of approximately 2 for a 15–20 cm increase in height. The Harvard Pooling Project – the largest anthropometric study of risk of breast cancer so far – confirmed these findings (van den Brandt, 2000). This large nested case (n=4385)–control (10:1) study pooling seven cohorts showed a positive relationship between height and risk of breast cancer both in premenopausal and postmenopausal women, although

Table 1. Data from the Harvard Pooling Project[a]

Anthropometric variable		Premenopausal women		Postmenopausal women	
		RR	*P* for trend	RR	*P* for trend
Height (m)	>1.75 vs <1.60	1.42	0.41	1.22	0.001
Weight (kg)	>80 vs < 60	0.58	0.02	1.25	0.003
BMI (kg/m^2)	>33 vs <21	0.58	0.007	1.27	0.001

[a]This is a nested case (n=4385)–control (10:1) study of seven large cohorts. Adjustments were made for menopausal status, age at menarchy, parity, age at birth of first child, hormonal replacement therapy, oral contraceptive drugs, benign breast disease, maternal history of breast cancer, breast cancer in sister, smoking, education, body mass index or height and intake of fat, fibre, energy and alcohol (From van den Brandt, 2000).

the *P* for trend was significant only in postmenopausal women (Table 1).

BMI and risk of breast cancer

A large number of early case–control studies have examined BMI in relation to risk of breast cancer. The majority of these studies show an association between degree of obesity and risk in postmenopausal women. Several of the studies in premenopausal women indicate a decreased risk of breast cancer in obese women (World Cancer Research Fund, 1997). This inverse relationship between BMI and premenopausal breast cancer could be due to an effect of obesity on anovulatory cycles, in turn associated with decreased risk of breast cancer. For postmenopausal women, obesity may increase risk by affecting estrogen levels through increased conversion in adipose tissue.

The Harvard Pooling Project also analysed BMI in relation to breast cancer risk (van den Brandt, 2000). In premenopausal women, weight and BMI were both inversely associated with risk of breast cancer, while in postmenopausal women the relationship was significantly positive (Table 1). Most relevant confounders were adjusted for with little evidence of interactions.

WHR and risk of breast cancer

This association was examined in the Nurses Health Study (Huang *et al.*, 1999). Over a 6-year period of follow-up, 1037 invasive breast cancers were gathered. WHR was found to be significantly associated with risk in postmenopausal women, especially those who had never taken hormone replacement therapy. There was no significant relationship among HRT users or among premenopausal women.

Weight gain and risk of breast cancer

Several cohort studies (Barnes-Josiah *et al.*, 1995; Huang *et al.*, 1996) have shown a positive association between adult weight gain and risk of breast cancer. Recent analyses from The Malmö Diet and Cancer Study confirm the significant association between weight gain and risk of breast cancer (Lahmann *et al.*, unpublished data).

Table 2. Data from the Health Professionals Study[a]

Anthropometric variable		RR	*P* for trend	RR	*P* for trend
BMI (kg/m^2)	Q5 vs Q1	1.82	0.001	1.48	0.02
Height (m)	Q5 vs Q1	1.96	0.002	1.76	0.02
WHR (cm)	Q5 vs Q1			3.41	0.02
Physical activity (METs)	Q5 vs Q1	0.44	0.002	0.53	0.03

[a]This study of male health professionals performed a baseline examination during 1986 and had a 6-year follow-up yielding 203 cases of colon cancer. Physical activity was expressed in metabolic equivalents (METs) (From Giovannucci *et al.*, 1995).

RR, relative risk adjusted for age; multivariate RR, adjusted for BMI, physical activity, age, history of endoscopic screening or polyp diagnosis, parental history of colorectal cancer, pack-years of smoking, aspirin use, and intake of folate, alcohol, dietary fibre, red meat, and total energy; Q, quintile.

Physical activity and risk of breast cancer

In the NHANES-I (Albanes *et al.*, 1989), a cohort study with a mean follow-up time of 10 years with 122 cases of postmenopausal breast cancer, nonrecreational physical activity (quite inactive vs very active) was significantly associated with the risk of breast cancer. The Nurses' Health Study II (Rockville *et al.*, 1998) studied women aged 25–42 at entry during 6 years of follow-up, yielding 372 premenopausal breast cancer cases. Recreational physical activity was determined in high school, between age 18 and 22 and current physical activity at baseline examination. The authors found no significant relationship between any of these measures of recreational physical activity and risk of breast cancer. The Nurses' Health Study I (Rockhill *et al.*, 1999) found, however, a modest but significant protection from physical activity in mainly postmenopausal women, RR 0.82 (0.70–0.97) with a *P* for trend of 0.004. The very large Swedish Nationwide cohort study (Moradi *et al.*, 1999), where physical demand at work defined by type of occupation was used as a proxy for physical activity, showed that jobs with higher physical demand protected from breast cancer. However, the association disappeared when adjusted for socio-economic factors. The Iowa Women's Health Study (Moore *et al.*, 2000) confirmed a protective effect of physical activity in postmenopausal women.

Height and risk of colon cancer

Two major studies The NHANES I (Albanes *et al.*, 1988) and The Nurses' Health Study (Chute *et al.*, 1991) both found significant positive relationships between adult height and risk of colon cancer (RR Q4 versus Q1, varying between 1.6 and 2.1) in men and women. It is noteworthy that most case–control studies have not shown significant associations (World Cancer Research Fund, 1997).

BMI and risk of colon cancer

It has been suggested that excess body weight increases risk of colon cancer, but the study results are not consistent. Some cohort studies (e.g. Nomura *et al.*, 1985) and also some case–control studies (Peters *et al.*, 1989; Gerhardsson de Verdier, 1990; Le Marchand, 1994) have found that men with high BMI (upper quartile) have a significant (twofold) increase in risk of colon cancer. However, there have been other studies (Thun *et al.*, 1992; Kune *et al.*, 1990) who could not find an association.

Data for women are less consistent. One cohort study (Chute *et al.*, 1991) was unable to find a significant relationship while two other cohort studies (Bostick *et al.*, 1994; Gerhardsson de Verdier, 1990) found significant positive associations, the latter for both right and left colon but not for rectal cancer.

WHR and risk of colon cancer

In the Iowa Women's Health Study (Bostick *et al.*, 1994), the WHR was not found to be significantly associated with colon cancer during a 4-year follow-up rendering 212 cases of colon cancer. A similar study in male health professionals (Giovanucci *et al.*, 1995), the WHR was strongly and positively associated with risk of colon cancer (RR Q5 versus Q1, 3.41 (1.52–7.66, P for trend 0.001) even after adjustment for possible confounders. Data from The Malmö Diet and Cancer Study (Lahmann *et al.*, unpublished data) points in the same direction.

Physical activity and risk of colon cancer

The majority of both case–control and cohort studies have shown a significant protective effect of high physical activity at work and during leisure time (for review, see World Cancer Research Fund, 1997). Occupational studies have examined physical activity during usual lifetime occupation, while leisure-time activity studies have examined activity long before diagnosis. High levels of physical activity throughout life seem to carry the lowest risk of colon cancer. Analyses of specific associations with various subsites hint at a relationship that is stronger for distal than for proximal colon cancer. Evidence for a decreased risk of cancer of the rectum in subjects with high physical activity is not as clear as that for colon cancer (see World Cancer Research Fund, 1997).

A number of recent studies add to the above picture. The Health Professionals Follow-up Study (Giovanucci *et al.*, 1995) analysed the association of physical activity and risk of colon cancer in 203 cases. Physical activity during leisure time (Q5 versus Q1) decreased age-adjusted risk significantly (RR, 0.44; 0.27–0.71; *P* for trend 0.002). Even after adjustment for other possible confounders, the association was significant (RR, 0.53; 0.32–0.88, *P*=0.03). The association found was significant only for distal colon cancers. The Nurses' Health Study (Martinez *et al.*, 1997) reported 87 cases of colon cancer during 6 years of follow-up. They found a significant inverse relationship between physical activity and incidence of colon cancer (RR, 0.54; 0.33–0.90) after multivariate adjustments including BMI. The association was limited to distal colon. The Physicians' Health Study (Lee *et al.*, 1997) gathered 217 cases of colon cancer over 11 years of follow-up. They found no significant relationship between leisure-time activity and risk of colon cancer (RR,1.1); it was nonsignificant after adjustment for age, BMI and alcohol intake. When using a compound variable of physical activity at baseline and after 36 months, the findings were similar. The recent publication from The ATBC Cancer Prevention Study (Colbert *et al.*, 2001) regarding 12 years of follow-up of male Finnish smokers yielding 152 colon cancer cases, found that both light and moderate/heavy occupational physical activity decreased risk of distal but not proximal colon cancer. The authors found no significant relationship with leisure-time physical activity.

Comments and Conclusions

Adult height seems to be positively associated with risk of breast cancer, with a doubling of the risk with a 15–20 cm increase in height. Some studies indicate a stronger relationship in postmenopausal women but this needs to be further studied. The mechanism by which the association works is not clear. Rapid growth at a young age leading to early menarchy has been suggested. However, early menarchy is often associated with shorter adult stature and hence would not fit into the proposed mechanism. The relationships between early menarchy, adult height and risk of breast cancer deserve further research, where also socio-economic status is taken into account.

BMI is negatively associated with premenopausal breast cancer risk and positively associated with postmenopausal risk. An inverse relation between BMI and risk of breast cancer might be due to the effect of obesity on anovulatory cycles. For postmenopausal women, on the contrary, obesity may increase risk by increasing levels of endogenous estrogens. However, the metabolic consequences of obesity with an increase in several growth factors that might influence the progression of breast tumours deserve further studies.

WHR, waist circumference and weight gain are less studied in relation to breast cancer risk but the overall findings favour a positive association in postmenopausal women, especially those taking oral contraceptive therapy. In the majority of studies, high physical activity seems to protect against breast cancer, especially among postmenopausal women. However, the association is reduced when adjusted for socio-economic variables and further analyses are needed before the questions can be answered. The mechanisms through which the protection occurs are not known, but biological pathways involving decreased levels of estrogens has been suggested.

Height is positively and significantly associated with risk of colon cancer in both men and women in a majority of cohort studies, while positive associations have been more difficult to find in case–control studies. The mechanism by which adult height is related to risk of colon cancer is far from established, although the same hypothesis as for breast cancer – rapid growth at a young age – has been suggested.

High adult BMI seems to increase risk of colon cancer both in cohort and in case–control studies. The relationship seems to be stronger for the left than for the right colon, while most studies show no significant association with rectal cancer. The data are more consistent for men than for women and less consistent for childhood BMI. In studies where adjustments for physical activity and dietary factors have been made, these adjustments seem to have little effect on the strength of the associations. The same seems to be true for abdominal obesity – reflected by a high adult WHR – which also is positively associated with colon cancer and where adjustments for physical activity and diet had only minor effects.

Lastly, physical activity, whether reflected by occupational or recreational activity, seems to be inversely related to risk of colon cancer, although the findings vary somewhat between studies. The relation is stronger for the left than for the right colon and there seems to be no significant relationship to rectal cancer.

Thus, there is rather strong epidemiological evidence indicating that tall height, obesity and low physical activity increase the risk of postmenopausal breast cancer and colon cancer. This review of publications since 1995 strengthens this picture.

References

Albanes, D., Jones, D.Y., Schatzkin, A., Micozzi, M.S. & Taylor, P.R. (1988) Adult stature and risk of cancer. *Cancer Res.*, **48**, 1658–1662

Albanes, D., Blair, A. & Taylor, P.R. (1989) Physical activity and risk of cancer in the NHANES I population. *Am. J. Public Health*, **79**, 744–750

Barnes-Josiah, D., Potter, J.D., Sellers, T.A. & Himes, J.H. (1995) Early body size and subsequent weight gain as predictors of breast cancer incidence. *Cancer*, **6**, 112–118

Bostick, R.M., Potter, J.D., Kushi, L.H., Sellers, T.A., Steinmetz, K.A., McKenzie, D.R., Gapstur, S.M. & Rolsom, A.R. (1994) Sugar, meat, and fat intake, and non-dietary risk factors for colon cancer incidence in Iowa women (United States). *Cancer Causes Control*, **5**, 38–52

Chute, C.G., Willett, W.C., Colditz, G.A., Stampfer, M.J., Baron, J.A., Rosner, B. & Speizer, F.E. (1991) A prospective study of body mass, height, and smoking on the risk of colorectal cancer in women. *Cancer Causes Control*, **2**, 117–124

Colbert, L.H., Hartman, T.J., Malila, N., Limburg, P.J., Pietinen, P., Virtamo, J., Taylor, P.R. & Albanes, D. (2001) Physical activity in relation to cancer of the colon and rectum in a cohort of male smokers. *Cancer Epidemiol. Biomarkers Prev.*, **10**, 265–268

De Waard, F. & Baanders-van Halewijn, E.A. (1974) A prospective study in general practice on breast-cancer risk in postmenopausal women. *Int. J. Cancer*, **14**, 153–160

Gerhardsson de Verdier, M., Hagman, U., Steineck, G., Rieger, Å. & Norell, S.E. (1990) Diet, body mass and colorectal cancer: a case-referent study. *Int. J. Cancer*, **46**, 832–838

Giovannucci, E., Ascherio, A., Rimm, E.B., Colditz, G.A., Stampfer, M.J. & Willett, W.C. (1995) Physical activity, obesity, and risk for colon cancer and adenoma in men. *Ann. Intern. Med.*, **122**, 327–334

Huang, Z., Hankinson, S., Colditz, G., Stampfer, M., Hunter, D., Manson, J., Hennekens, C., Speizer, F. & Willett, W. (1996) Body mass index, weight change and risk of breast cancer among women. *Am. J. Epidemiol.*, **143**, S85

Huang, Z., Willett, W.C., Colditz, G.A., Hunter, D.J., Manson, J.E., Rosner, B., Speizer, F.E. & Hankinson, S.E. (1999) Waist circumference, waist:hip ratio, and risk of breast cancer in the Nurses' Health Study. *Am. J. Epidemiol.*, **150**, 1316–1324

Kune, G.A., Kune, S. & Watson, L.F. (1990) Body weight and physical activity as predictors of colorectal cancer risk. *Nutr. Cancer*, **13**, 9–17

Lee, I.M., Manson, J.E., Ajani, U., Paffenbarger, R.S. Jr., Hennekens, C.H. & Buring, J.E. (1997) Physical activity and risk of colon cancer: the Physicians' Health Study. *Cancer Causes Control*, **8**, 568–574

Lee, I.M., Manson, J.E., Ajani, U., Paffenbarger, R.S. Jr., Hennekens, C.H. & Buring, J.E. (2001) Physical activity and breast cancer risk: the Women's Health Study. *Cancer Causes Control*, **12**, 137–145

Le Marchand, L., Wilkens L.R. & Mi, M.-P. (1994) Obesity in youth and middle age and risk of colorectal cancer in men. *Cancer Causes Control*, **3**, 349–354

Martínez, M.E., Giovannucci, E., Spiegelman, D., Hunter, D.J., Willett, W.C. & Colditz, G.A. (1997) Leisure-time physical activity, body size, and colon cancer in women. *J. Natl. Cancer Inst.*, **89**, 948–955

Moore, D.B., Folsom, A.R., Mink, P.J., Hong, C.P., Andersson, K.E. & Kushi, L.H. (2000) Physical activity and incidence of postmenopausal breast cancer. *Epidemiology*, **11**, 292–296

Moradi, T., Adami, H.O., Bergstrom, R., Gridley, G., Wolk, A., Gerhardsson, M., Dosemeci, M. & Nyren, O. (1999) Occupational physical activity and risk for breast cancer in a nation-wide cohort study in Sweden. *Cancer Causes Control*, **10**, 423–430

Nomura, A., Heilbrun, L.K. & Stemmermann, G.N. (1985) Body mass index as a predictor of cancer in men. *J. Natl. Cancer Inst.*, **74**, 319–323

Peters, R.K., Garabrant, D.H., Yu, M.C. & Mack, T.M. (1989) A case–control study of occupational and dietary factors in colorectal cancer in young men by subsite. *Cancer Res.*, **49**, 5459–5468

Rockhill, B., Willett, W.C., Hunter, D.J., Manson, J.E., Hankinson, S.E., Spiegelman, D. & Colditz, G.A. (1998) Physical activity and breast cancer risk in a cohort of young women. *J. Natl. Cancer Inst.*, **90**, 1155–1160

Rockhill, B., Willett, W.C., Hunter, D.J., Manson, J.E., Hankinson, S.E. & Colditz, G.A. (1999) A prospective study of recreational physical activity and breast cancer risk. *Arch. Intern. Med.*, **159**, 2290–2296

Thun, M.J., Calle, E.E., Namboodiri, M.M., Flanders, W.D., Coates, R.J., Byers, T., Boffetta, P., Garfinkel, L. & Heath, C.W. Jr. (1992) Risk factors for fatal colon cancer in a large prospective study. *J. Natl. Cancer Inst.*, **84**, 1491–1500

Van den Brandt, P.A., Spiegelman, D., Yaun, S.S., Adami, H.O., Beeson, L., Folsom, A.R., Fraser, G., Goldbohm, R.A., Graham, S., Kushi, L., Marshall, J.R., Miller, A.B., Rohan, T., Smith-Warner, S.A., Speizer, F.E., Willett, W.C., Wolk, A. & Hunter, D.J. (2000) Pooled analysis of prospective cohort studies on height, weight, and breast cancer risk. *Am. J. Epidemiol.*, **152**, 514–527

Vatten, L.J. & Kvinnsland, S. (1990) Body mass index and risk of breast cancer. A prospective study of 23 826 Norwegian women. *Int. J. Cancer*, **45**, 440–444

World Cancer Research Fund and American Institute for Cancer Research. (1997) *Food, Nutrition and the Prevention of Cancer: A Global Perspective*, Washington, D.C., American Institute for Cancer Research

Leisure-time sport physical activity and dietary intake of foods in Spain

Chirlaque M.D., Tormo M.J., Navarro C.
(for the EPIC working group of Spain)

Regional Health Council, Department of Epidemiology, Murcia, Spain.

Purpose

The objective of the present work is to evaluate the consumption of food groups according to levels of vigorous leisure-time physical activity seen within the EPIC cohort of Spain at recruitment (EPIC Group of Spain, 1994).

Methods

The EPIC cohort of Spain is composed of 25 813 females and 15 634 males, 29–69 years of age, and with an average age of 50.9 (SD±7.2) and 48.4 (SD±8.4) years, respectively. Participants were healthy volunteers, mainly blood donors. In the data analyses we only included those people who declared that they had not had dietary changes during the year up to the interview and those with all anthropometric measures performed, resulting in 37 287 people (90% out of the entire cohort) as suitable for inclusion.

We used a validated questionnaire of physical activity (Pols *et al.*, 1997) to measure the weekly frequency and duration of different kinds of sport activities. Following previous work (Matthews *et al.*, 1997), we categorized the cohort members exclusively by their weekly time spent on physical sport activities. Thus, we considered inactive those people who accumulated ≤30 min/week of physical activity and active those who completed >30 min/week. Furthermore, the latter were split into three progressively active categories of physical activity: a) low: 30 min to 2 h/week, b) moderate: 2–3h/week and, c) intensive: > 3h/week.

For dietary assessment, we used a validated diet history questionnaire (EPIC Group of Spain, 1997) that included all items eaten with a frequency of at least twice a month. It is structured by meals and administered by trained nutritionists.

Anthropometric indexes measured were body mass index (BMI: weight (kg)/height $(m)^2$) and waist:hip ratio (calculated by taking into account both circumferences and expressed without units).

Other non-dietary factors included in the analyses were age, percentage of people with secondary or university studies, percentage of people involved in sedentary work, current smoking, high–excessive drinking (Encuesta Nacional de Salud, 1993) (≥ 526 ml of pure alcohol/week), and whether they had had previous chronic diseases such as acute myocardial infarction, angina pectoris, stroke, cerebrovascular diseases, high blood pressure, hyperlipidemia and diabetes mellitus.

We tested differences in food intake according to physical activity duration by means of an analysis of variance and an analysis of covariance adjusted for confounding factors (age, BMI, current smoking, high–excessive alcohol drinking, secondary and higher education, and sedentary physical activity at work). Linear increases or decreases in food intake across physical activity levels were tested by means of a regression analysis.

Results

Physical inactivity (0–0.5 h/week) was significantly associated with older age, higher waist/hip ratio and lower level of education, current smoking, high–excessive alcohol drinking, sedentary physical activity and having had previous diseases (Table 1). BMI decreased significantly and steadily from lowest to highest physical activity categories, being extremely high on average (mean: 28; SD ± 4.2). These findings hold for both genders except for current smoking, which was less frequent among sedentary women.

Food group intakes showed a different pattern across different physical activity levels. Thus, more vegetables (men, from 233.9 g/day in

Table 1. Distribution of subjects: characteristics according to levels of sport physical activity: mean (SD) and frequency (%) comparisons

Males 0–0.5 (*n*=10 382)	0.5–2 (*n*=1548)	2–3 (*n*=686)	>3 (*n*=1612)	Total (*n*=14 228)	Females Sport physical activity (h/week)	0–0.5 (*n*=18 258)	0.5–2 *n*=2280)	2–3 (*n*=1172)	>3 (*n*=1349)	Total (*n*=14 228)
51.5 (7.2)	48.9 (6.9)[b]	49.4 (7.0)[b]	49.3 (7.2)[b]	50.9 (7.2)[c]	Age (years); mean (SD)	48.9 (8.4)	46.9 (8.2)[b]	46.9 (8.2)[b]	46.5 (8.1)[b]	48.4 (8.4)[c]
28.7 (3.4)	27.8 (3.1)[b]	27.7 (3.0)[b]	27.6 (3.7)[b]	28.4 (3.4)[c]	BMI (m/kg^2); mean (SD)	28.5 (4.8)	26.6 (4.1)[b]	26.3 (3.8)[b]	26.3 (4.3)[b]	28.1 (4.7)[c]
0.95 (0.56)	0.93 (0.50)[b]	0.93 (0.49)[b]	0.92 (0.58)[b]	0.95 (0.57)[c]	Waist:hip ratio; mean (SD)	0.83 (0.78)	0.81 (0.61)[b]	0.81 (0.58)[b]	0.80 (0.61)[b]	0.82 (0.75)[c]
17.7	32.9	35.7	37.1	22.4[c]	≥ Secondary education(%)	12.4	23.5	22.9	30.1	15.1[c]
30.4	42.2	44.6	42.4	33.7[c]	Sedentary PA at work (%)	11.6	17.9	14.2	18.5	12.7[c]
32.0	29.2	28.7	26.1	30.9[c]	Current smoking (%)	17.6	22.6	22.0	24.9	18.8[c]
17.7	16.1	13.0	13.2	16.8[c]	High–excessive alcohol(%)	0.3	0.1	0.1	0.4	0.3[c]
46.5	40.0	37.4	38.4	44.4[c]	Concurrent diseases[a] (%)	35.1	26.5	23.2	25.3	33.0[c]
0.0 (0.01)	1.5 (0.5)[b]	2.9 (0.2)[b]	6.8 (4.1)[b]	1.1 (2.6)[c]	Sport physical activity (h/week); mean (SD)	0.0 (0.1)	1.5 (0.4)[b]	2.9 (0.2)[b]	6.2 (4.0)[b]	0.7 (1.8)[c]

[a]Acute heart attack, angina, stroke, other ischaemic or haemorragic cerebral accidents, high blood pressure, hyperlipidaemia, diabetes.
[b]$P \leq 0.05$ for ANOVA comparing the mean value of each PA category with that of the reference level (0–0.5).
[c]Significant ($P \leq 0.05$) linear trend tests across means and, for percentages, overall chi-square significance tests.
SD, standard deviation; PA, physical activity.

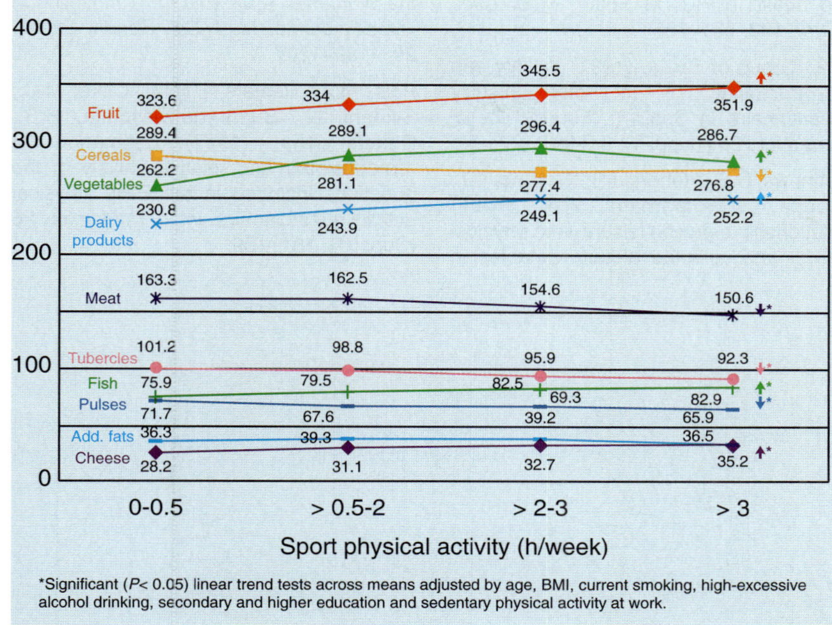

Figure 1
Mean intake of different food groups (g/day) for males according to levels of sport physical activity

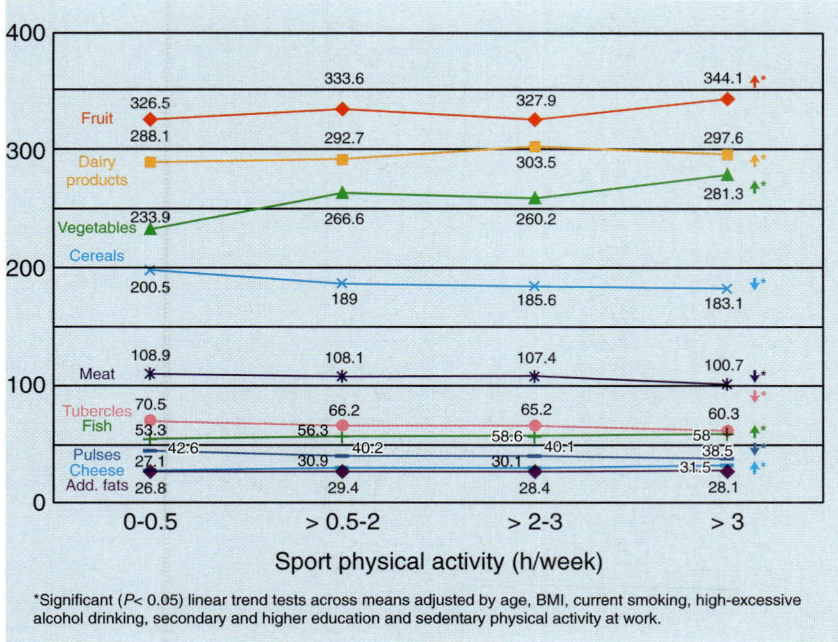

Figure 2
Mean intake of different food groups (g/day) for females according to levels of sport physical activity

0–0.5 h/week of sport physical activity to 281.3 g/day in >3 h/week), fruit, fish, dairy products and cheese were taken with increasing physical activity. Physically active people ate less tubercles, pulses, meat and cereals, and similar quantities of added fats than less active people. The average gender-weighted percentage change in the intake of some food groups increased when moving from the lowest levels of physical activity to the highest; this increase was 15.9% for vegetables, 9% for fish, 6.7% for fruit, and 5.6% for dairy products (Fig. 1 gives information separately by gender).

The comparisons across levels of intake remained significant when the other possible confounding factors were adjusted (age, BMI, current smoking, high–excessive alcohol drinking, secondary and higher education, and sedentary at work), and showed a linear trend ($P \leq 0.05$) of increasing or decreasing intake with increasing physical activity. Further adjustment by total energy intake did not change the results appreciably; thus, the final adjusted model did not include total energy intake as an independent term.

Total energy intakes were similar across different physical activity levels (<2% change in total energy intake between extreme physical activity categories).

Conclusions

Differences between physical activity groups are more qualitatively (food groups) than quantitatively (kilocalories) driven, with caloric intake apparently similar across different demanding levels of physical activity. People engaged in sport physical activity follow healthier lifestyles, with a greater possibility for changing their dietetic habits in a healthier way.

Acknowledgements

Project financed by European Union Europe Against Cancer Programme, by

Spanish Health Research Fund (FIS) and participating Autonomous Regions.

References

Encuesta Nacional de Salud 1993. Ministerio de Sanidad y Consumo. (1994) *Rev. Sanid. Hig. Pública (Madr)*, **68**, 121–178

EPIC Group of Spain. (1994) European prospective investigation on diet, cancer and health (EPIC) in Spain. *Med. Clin., (Barc)*, **102**, 781–785

EPIC Group of Spain. (1997) Validity and reproducibility of a diet history questionnaire in Spain (I. Foods). *Int. J. Epidemiol.*, **26** (Suppl 1), 91–99

Matthews, C.E., Hebert, J.R., Ockene, I.S., Saperia, G., Merriam, P.A. (1997) Relationship between leisure-time physical activity and selected dietary variables in the Worcester Area Trial for Counseling in Hyperlipidemia. *Med. Sci. Sports. Exerc.*, **29**, 1199–1207

Pols, M.A., Peeters, P.H.M., Ocké, M.C., Slimani, N., Bueno-de-Mesquita, H.B., Colette, H.J. (1997) Estimation of reproducibility and relative validity of the questions included in the EPIC physical activity questionnaire. *Int. J. Epidemiol.*, **26** (Suppl 1), 181–189

Energy intake, energy expenditure and BMI influence the risk of endometrial cancer in a prospective study in Norway

Furberg A.S., Thune I.
University of Tromsø, The Norwegian Cancer Society, Norway.

Background

Endometrial cancer is the sixth most common cancer among women worldwide and the incidence is increasing in the Nordic countries. Migrant studies indicate that lifestyle influences the risk of this malignancy. The female sex hormones are thought to be the most important effectors, with the potential to induce malignant transformation of the endometrial glandular cells when present at serum concentrations above the physiologically optimal level in certain sensitive periods of a woman's life. Inactivity, high body weight and weight gain might contribute to an unfavourable hormonal profile (Jasienska & Thune, 2001) and have been associated with increased risk of endometrial cancer in cohort studies (Le Marchand *et al.*, 1991; Moradi *et al.*, 1998; Terry *et al.*, 1999; Thune & Furberg, 2001). However, several aspects of these associations remain to be clarified, including the impact of body size in different periods of life and the independent effect of physical activity.

Aim

The aim of this study was to determine whether energy intake, energy expenditure and body mass index (BMI) independently influence the risk of endometrial cancer in a general population.

Materials and methods

The women included in our study participated in a population-based screening survey conducted between 1977 and 1983 in three counties of Norway. A total of 31 209 women aged 20–54 years participated in this survey. The response rate was 90.8%.

Energy intake was estimated from a self-instructive semi-quantitative food frequency questionnaire including information on 80 food items. The women marked their level of physical activity in leisure time and during work hours on a four-grade scale, where each higher level of activity corresponded to higher energy expenditure. Height and weight were measured, and an estimate of relative weight, BMI, was obtained by dividing the body weight in kilograms by the squared height in meters (kg m^{-2}).

Every incident case of endometrial cancer was identified through record linkage to the Cancer Registry of Norway until the end of follow-up (31 December 1996). Women with malignant disease diagnosed before baseline or within the first year of the study and women with incomplete information on the relevant variables were excluded from the analyses.

Cox's proportional hazard regression analysis was used to investigate the simultaneous effects of energy intake, physical activity, BMI and changes in BMI, and co-variates on endometrial cancer incidence. Analyses were adjusted for potential risk factors (age, parity, age at first birth, geographical area, height, BMI, energy intake, energy expenditure, smoking and alcohol) when appropriate.

Results

We observed 144 incident cases of endometrial cancer among 24 665 women during a mean follow-up time of 15.9 years. The median age at baseline was 45 years and the oldest half of the population was diagnosed with 73% of the cancers. Mean age at diagnosis was 57 years.

The majority had given birth to three or more children and on average the first child was born when the mother was 24.4 years old. Mean daily energy intake was approximately 5700 kJ. Median BMI was 24 kg m^{-2}. Among the study population, 68% and 15% spent

Table 1. Adjusted relative risk (RR)[a] of endometrial cancer according to BMI and level of occupational activity in a prospective cohort study in Norway (*n*=24 665)

Level of occupational activity	BMI < 23.8 kg m^{-2}			BMI > 23.8 kg m^{-2}		
	Cases	RR	95% CI	Cases	RR	95% CI
Sedentary	16	1.0		13	1.0	
Walking	25	0.46	(0.25–0.88)	56	0.85	(0.46–1.56)
Lifting/heavy manual	8	0.39	(0.16–0.93)	26	0.84	(0.43–1.66)
P for trend		0.03			0.76	

[a]Adjusted for age at entry, geographical region, height, parity, leisure-time activity. Also considered age at first birth, smoking habit and alcohol consumption.

4 hours or more of their leisure time in physical activities of moderate intensity and high intensity, respectively. About 60% of the women walked a lot during work hours and 26% were engaged in both walking and lifting or heavy manual work.

High energy intake was suggestive of an increased risk of endometrial cancer. Physical activity in the workplace was inversely associated with risk (relative risk [RR] = 0.63, 95% confidence interval [CI]: 0.42–0.96 for active versus sedentary work) and was especially protective among lean women (BMI <23.8 kg m^{-2}); the categories were: mostly engaged in walking (RR=0.46, 95% CI: 0.25–0.88), or lifting/heavy manual work (RR=0.39, 95% CI: 0.16–0.93) (Table 1). We also observed a risk reduction by recreational physical activity. High BMI was associated with an overall increased risk (RR=2.45, 95% CI: 1.46–4.11 for top versus bottom quartile, *P* for trend =0.0002).

Conclusion

This study indicates that physical activity per se reduces the risk of endometrial cancer, beyond the effect of consequently low BMI.

Acknowledgements

This study was supported by a grant (TP 49 258) from the Norwegian Cancer Society.

References

Jasienska, G. & Thune, I. (2001) Lifestyle, hormones and risk of breast cancer. *BMJ*, **322**, 586–587

Le Marchand, L., Wilkens, L.R. & Ming-Pi, M. (1991) Early-age body size, adult weight gain and endometrial cancer risk. *Int. J. Cancer*, **48**, 807–811

Moradi, T., Nyrén, O., Bergström, R., Gridley, G., Linet, M., Wolk, A., Dosemeci, M. & Adami, H.-O. (1998) Risk of endometrial cancer in relation to occupational physical activity: a nationwide cohort study in Sweden. *Int. J. Cancer*, **76**, 665–670

Terry, P., Baron, J.A., Weiderpass, E., Yuen, J., Lictenstein, P. & Nyrén, O. (1999) Lifestyle and endometrial cancer risk: a cohort study from the Swedish Twin Registry. *Int. J. Cancer*, **82**, 38–42

Thune, I. & Furberg, A.-S. (2001) Physical activity and cancer risk: dose–response and cancer, all sites and site-specific. *Med. Sci. Sports Exerc.*, **33**, 530–550

Prevalence of overweight, general and central obesity in 50- to 64-year-olds involved in the EPIC cohort

Haftenberger M.[1], Lahmann P.H.[2], Panico S.[3], Gonzalez C.[4], Seidell J.[5], Boeing H.[1]

[1]Department of Epidemiology, German Institute of Human Nutrition, Potsdam-Rehbrücke, Germany. [2]Lund University, Department of Medicine, Malmö University Hospital, Sweden. [3]Department of Clinical and Experimental Medicine, Federico II University, Naples, Italy. [4]Department of Epidemiology, Catalan Institute of Oncology, Barcelona, Spain. [5]Department for Chronic Disease Epidemiology, National Institute of Public Health and the Environment, Bilthoven, The Netherlands.

Introduction

Anthropometric measures have been shown to be related to risk for many chronic diseases (WHO, 2000). This includes the growing evidence that excessive body weight increases risk of cancer at several sites such as the breast in postmenopausal women, the colon, endometrium, kidney, prostate, and adenocarcinoma of the oesophagus and thyroid (IARC, 2002).

Further evidence on the role of anthropometric characteristics associated with the risk of cancer and other diseases is needed. EPIC, as a large multicentre prospective study, may contribute to this in the future.

The present paper describes the distribution of overweight, general and central obesity in adults aged 50–64 years from different EPIC centres using baseline data, which were collected between 1992 and 1999.

Methods

Study populations, sample sizes and sources of populations are described in more detail elsewhere (Riboli & Kaaks, 1997). This description was restricted to 83 178 men and 163 851 women aged 50–64 years with anthropometric data available. This age group was represented in all centres.

Anthropometric examinations were mostly undertaken by trained observers using standardized methods and included measurements of weight, height, and waist and hip circumferences. The centres from France and the United Kingdom also included self-reports. In the health-conscious group (United Kingdom), self-reports were converted into estimations of measured values using prediction equations, which were determined by linear regression in subjects from this sample with both measurements and self-reports. The description of the French data will be restricted to the participants with anthropometric examination. In Umeå (Sweden), only weight and height were measured.

Body mass index (BMI) was calculated as weight (kg) divided by height (m) squared. World Health Organization guidelines were used to categorize subjects into BMI groups: underweight (BMI <18.5 kg/m^2), normal weight (18.5≤ BMI <25.0 kg/m^2), overweight (25.0≤ BMI <30.0 kg/m^2) and obesity (BMI ≥ 30.0 kg/m^2) (WHO, 2000). Waist circumference (WC), was used to identify subjects with central obesity, which was defined as WC ≥ 102 cm in males and WC≥ 88 cm in females (NIH, 1998).

Age-adjusted prevalences of normal weight, overweight, general and central obesity are presented for men and women in each centre.

Results

Prevalence of normal weight varied from 7.4% (Navarra, Spain) to 51.1% (health-conscious group, United Kingdom) in men (Table 1) and from 8.5% (Granada, Spain) to 70.5% (south coast of France) in women (Table 2). Prevalence of normal weight exceeded 50.0% in men and women from the health-conscious group (United Kingdom) and in women from France, Turin (Italy), Utrecht (The Netherlands), Malmö (Sweden) and Denmark. Prevalence of overweight varied from 40.9% (health-conscious group, United Kingdom) to 61.4% (San Sebastian, Spain) in men and from 20.9% (south coast of France) to 48.2% (Asturias, Spain) in women. Prevalence of obesity was less than 10% in women from France, the men and women from the health-conscious group and in men from Umeå (Sweden) and exceeded 25% in the Spanish and Greek centres, as well as in Ragusa and Naples (Italy).

Prevalence of central obesity varied between 8.9% (health-conscious group, United Kingdom) and 52.3% (Murcia, Spain) in men (Table 1) and between 9.4% (health-conscious group, United Kingdom) and 76.3% (Murcia, Spain) in women (Table 2). The proportion of centrally obese subjects was lowest in the British health-conscious group and among the French women. The prevalence of central obesity exceeded 30.0% in men and women from Spain and Greece, and in women from Bilthoven (The Netherlands), Germany, Ragusa and Naples (Italy).

Table 1. Age-adjusted prevalence of underweight, normal weight, overweight, general and central obesity in men aged 50–64 years in the different EPIC centres

	Weight status					Central obesity	
EPIC centre	*n*	Under-weight %	Normal weight %	Overweight %	General obesity %	*n*	%
Italy							
Florence	1708	0.2	31.9	53.5	14.2	1449	14.1
Varese	1587	0.4	32.1	53.4	14.1	1558	14.6
Ragusa	1057	0.0	20.2	54.8	25.0	1057	29.2
Turin	2841	0.2	36.8	50.9	12.1	2747	18.9
Spain							
Asturias	1352	0.0	12.1	56.7	31.2	1357	34.1
Granada	879	0.1	10.5	49.3	40.1	891	49.7
Murcia	1264	0.1	11.6	55.9	32.4	1287	52.3
Navarra	1907	0.0	7.4	55.2	37.4	1915	51.6
San Sebastian	2143	0.0	12.8	61.4	25.8	2145	34.8
UK							
General	6473	0.4	39.2	49.1	11.3	6470	16.2
Health-conscious	2415	0.6	51.1	40.9	8.0	2434	8.9
Netherlands							
Bilthoven	3232	0.4	31.6	53.5	14.5	3226	23.9
Greece	3662	0.3	19.3	50.6	29.9	3668	38.8
Germany							
Heidelberg	7100	0.2	26.5	53.6	19.7	7218	29.3
Potsdam	6086	0.3	26.3	54.4	19.0	6123	25.0
Sweden							
Malmö	7299	0.7	41.0	47.1	11.2	7295	18.4
Umeå	5154	0.3	43.3	47.1	9.3	no data	no data
Denmark							
Aarhus	8320	0.2	33.4	51.3	15.1	8323	25.2
Copenhagen	18 511	0.3	35.1	49.3	15.3	18 526	23.5

Discussion

The EPIC study populations were not intended to be representative for general populations. Our observations may therefore deviate from results of other regional studies considering general populations.

Overall, more than 50% of the EPIC participants aged 50–64 years were overweight or obese. Prevalence of both general and central obesity was lowest among the French females and the British subjects with a health conscious lifestyle and was highest among the most southern EPIC centres (Granada, Murcia and Navarra, Spain; Naples and Ragusa, Italy; Greece). However, central obesity was also frequently observed in women from Bilthoven (The Netherlands) and Germany.

Table 2. Age-adjusted prevalence of underweight, normal weight, overweight, general and central obesity in women aged 50–64 years in the different EPIC centres

	Weight status					Central obesity	
EPIC centre	*n*	Under-weight %	Normal weight %	Overweight %	General obesity %	*n*	%
France							
North East	5476	4.0	64.9	23.6	7.6	5479	14.7
North West	1746	2.8	67.7	22.7	6.7	1764	12.9
South	2901	3.6	69.9	21.5	5.0	2900	11.9
South coast	1668	3.4	70.5	20.9	5.2	1669	11.3
Italy							
Florence	6505	0.7	44.6	39.5	15.2	6462	19.2
Varese	4469	1.3	41.9	40.4	16.4	4470	22.9
Ragusa	943	0.3	26.7	44.8	28.2	943	43.9
Turin	2413	1.6	50.4	35.8	12.2	2326	21.7
Naples	2304	0.4	27.2	45.6	26.8	2306	44.7
Spain							
Asturias	1950	0.0	13.7	48.2	38.1	1956	52.7
Granada	2566	0.0	8.5	38.3	53.2	2587	68.3
Murcia	2303	0.0	10.1	41.9	48.0	2329	76.3
Navarra	1730	0.1	15.6	46.9	37.4	1743	60.6
San Sebastian	1637	0.1	24.1	47.2	28.6	1637	44.0
UK							
General	9314	1.4	49.2	34.2	15.2	9326	19.8
Health-conscious	8366	1.4	58.9	30.5	9.2	8233	9.4
Netherlands							
Bilthoven	3559	0.8	40.3	41.0	17.9	3544	36.8
Utrecht	13 461	1.2	51.0	35.6	12.2	13 366	22.5
Greece	5980	0.2	17.7	39.5	42.6	5987	54.5
Germany							
Heidelberg	6387	0.9	42.4	37.4	19.3	6430	33.5
Potsdam	7361	0.5	38.1	39.8	21.6	7411	30.9
Sweden							
Malmö	9318	2.3	54.8	30.8	12.1	9315	15.0
Umeå	5549	1.3	49.9	35.5	13.3	no data	no data
Denmark							
Aarhus	8597	1.3	50.6	34.7	13.5	8597	25.8
Copenhagen	20 864	1.5	50.1	34.3	14.1	20 861	25.7

The notable high prevalences of general and central obesity in the southern Mediterranean centres do not (yet) coincide with risk of obesity-related diseases in the Mediterranean countries. In the future, it will be interesting to study the interaction between obesity, diet, lifestyle factors and disease risk in the different EPIC centres.

References

IARC (2002) *IARC Handbooks of cancer Prevention*, Vol. 6, *Weight Control and Physical Activity*, Lyon, IARC Press

National Institutes of Health (1998) Clinical guidelines on the identification, evaluation, and treatment of overweight and obesity in adults – the evidence report. National Institutes of Health. *Obes. Res.*, **6** (Suppl. 2), 51S–209S

Riboli, E. & Kaaks, R. (1997) The EPIC study: rational and design. *Int. J. Epidemiol.*, **26** (Suppl. 1), S6–S14

World Health Organisation. (2000) *Obesity: Preventing and Managing the Global Epidemic. Report of a WHO Consultation.* WHO Technical Report Series, No. 894

BMI and smoking status in the EPIC cohorts

Kroke A., Haftenberger M., Hoffmann K., Boeing H.
(for the EPIC working group on obesity, physical activity, and SES)

German Institute of Human Nutrition, Dept. of Epidemiology, Potsdam-Rehbruecke, Germany.

Introduction

Body mass index (BMI) and smoking habits are major determinants of chronic disease risk, including cancer. Both lifestyle characteristics are related to dietary habits: smoking and body mass development influence dietary behaviour and vice versa. In addition, BMI and smoking status are similarly related to each other. However, the relation between smoking status and BMI varies between populations (WHO MONICA, 1997). Any analysis of the influence of dietary behaviour on disease risk must therefore take into account these important confounders or effect modifiers. The aim of the present analysis was to describe the relation of BMI to smoking status among middle-aged and older men and women from the EPIC study centres across Europe.

Methods

The present analysis was restricted to men and women between 50 and 64 years of age with complete data for BMI and smoking habits (*n*=220 200). This age group was selected because it was represented in all centres.

Information on lifestyle habits was derived from either questionnaires or personal interviews. Smoking status of cigarette smoking was defined as never-smokers (NSM), ex-smokers (EXSM), and current smokers (CSM). Body height and weight were measured in all study centres except for the UK health-conscious group, where weight and height were self-reported. BMI was calculated as kg/m^2.

NSM, EXSM and CSM from each centre were compared with respect to BMI. Means and 95% confidence limits (upper confidence limit (UCLM) and lower confidence limit (LCLM)) were determined after adjustment for age, educational attainment and physical activity at work and sporting activities (as hours/week). For the adjustment, residuals of linear regression were used. For those centres with missing data for the control variables, crude values are presented. Differences were considered significant when the confidence limits did not include zero. All statistical analyses were performed with SAS®, version 8.0.

Results

Table 1 presents the prevalence of obesity (BMI ≥ 30) and the frequency distribution of smoking status among men and women. In men, the prevalence of cigarette smoking varied from 5% among the health-conscious cohort from the UK to 37.2% in Greece. The prevalence of obesity (BMI ≥ 30) ranged from 7.3% (UK, health conscious) to 40.6% in Granada, Spain. In women, the prevalence of smoking varied between 4% in Granada, Spain, and 33.4% in Naples, Italy. The prevalence of obesity (BMI ≥ 30) ranged from 4.7% in the South of France to 53.5% in Granada, Spain.

In nine centres (out of 19), significant differences in BMI between male NSM and CSM were observed after adjustment for age, educational level, occupational and sport activity (Table 2). BMI of NSM was significantly higher than BMI of CSM except for the Florence centre, where BMI of NSM was lower compared to CSM. Among women, this comparison revealed slightly less heterogeneity. In 15 centres, female NSM had a significantly higher BMI as compared to CSM.

The comparison of EXSM with CSM revealed among men a significantly higher BMI among EXSM in all centres. Among women, in all but three centres, the BMI of EXSM was higher than the BMI of CSM; this difference was significant in 17 out of 25 centres.

The comparison of NSM with EXSM with respect to BMI showed strong differences between men and women by centre. Among men, in all but one centre (San Sebastian), EXSM had a significantly higher BMI as compared to the NSM. In contrast, among women in all centres of France, Germany, the UK, and in Umeå and Florence, EXSM had a significantly higher BMI compared to NSM. In four centres (Asturias, Granada, Navarra, Bilthoven), the opposite was true. Among the remaining

Table 1. Frequency distribution of smoking status and categories of BMI among men and women of the EPIC Study, (n=220 200)

Country	Centre	Men						Women					
		n	Prevalence of obesity[a] %	Smoking status Never %	Ex %	Current %	Other[b] %	n	Prevalence of obesity[a] %	Smoking status Never %	Ex %	Current %	Other[b] %
Denmark	Aarhus	8239	15.1	26.1	38.1	27.5	8.3	8556	13.4	45.5	25.0	29.3	0.1
	Copenhagen	18 242	15.3	25.9	36.6	30.3	7.3	20 701	14.3	43.1	24.6	32.2	0.2
France	North-east	–	–	–	–	–	–	5079	7.4	72.0	20.8	7.2	0.0
	North-west	–	–	–	–	–	–	1659	6.9	76.5	18.1	5.4	0.0
	South	–	–	–	–	–	–	2702	4.7	74.2	19.5	6.3	0.0
	South coast	–	–	–	–	–	–	1561	5.1	76.3	17.2	6.5	0.0
Germany	Heidelberg	6946	20.0	31.6	47.9	18.9	1.6	6352	19.9	58.5	26.6	14.9	0.0
	Potsdam	6001	19.1	29.7	49.8	19.0	1.5	7357	22.4	67.9	20.7	10.8	0.5
Greece	Athens	3459	30.7	27.5	35.2	37.2	0.1	5787	44.3	86.4	4.3	9.4	0.0
Italy	Florence	1650	14.2	25.3	48.4	24.4	2.0	6480	15.0	51.3	21.9	26.8	0.0
	Varese	1564	14.2	27.7	44.8	25.8	1.8	4462	16.6	71.5	13.1	15.4	0.0
	Ragusa	1028	24.9	27.4	45.3	26.0	1.3	930	27.5	71.3	13.2	15.5	0.0
	Turin	2649	11.9	28.6	45.8	23.6	2.0	2284	12.1	63.0	20.4	16.6	0.0
	Naples	–	–	–	–	–	–	2304	26.4	49.5	17.1	33.4	0.0
Netherlands	Bilthoven	3218	14.5	20.9	43.0	31.2	5.0	3550	17.2	40.7	29.0	30.1	0.3
	Utrecht	–	–	–	–	–	–	13 356	12.2	42.1	35.0	22.5	0.4
Spain	Asturias	1350	31.1	32.7	34.4	24.7	8.2	1950	38.4	86.5	4.8	8.7	0.0
	Granada	878	40.6	29.4	41.8	28.6	0.9	2565	53.5	93.1	2.8	4.0	0.0
	Murcia	1263	32.9	25.1	39.7	31.0	4.3	2306	48.1	91.8	3.0	5.1	0.0
	Navarra	1907	37.5	35.3	23.5	26.7	14.4	1726	37.6	88.7	4.2	7.1	0.1
	San Sebastian	2142	26.1	31.7	28.2	22.8	17.3	1635	29.3	88.3	5.6	5.9	0.2
Sweden	Malmö	6896	11.9	30.3	43.6	26.1	0.0	9174	12.8	45.2	27.4	27.4	0.0
	Umeå	4935	9.0	49.7	31.2	16.6	2.5	5405	13.4	63.7	17.2	19.0	0.1
UK	General population	5952	11.3	36.5	46.0	12.4	5.1	8780	15.3	58.5	29.1	12.3	0.1
	Health-conscious	2365	7.3	48.2	43.6	5.0	3.2	8333	9.1	58.9	34.0	7.0	0.1

[a]Obesity defined as BMI ≥ 30.

[b]Other, other than cigarettes (cigars, cigarillos, pipe).

Table 2. Mean differences in BMI between NSM and CSM, CSM and EXSM, NSM and EXSM, stratified by sex. EPIC Study (*n*= 216 142)

	Adjusted[a] mean differences in BMI between																	
	NSM and CSM						EXSM and CSM						NSM and EXSM					
	Men			Women			Men			Women			Men			Women		
	Mean	LCLM[b]	UCLM[c]	Mean	LCLM[b]	UCLM[c]	Mean	LCLM[b]	UCLM[c]	Mean	LCLM[b]	UCLM[c]	Mean	LCLM[b]	UCLM[c]	Mean	LCLM[b]	UCLM[c]
Denmark																		
Aarhus	0.45	0.66	0.87	1.51	1.30	1.73	1.06	0.87	1.25	1.40	1.15	1.64	–0.40	–0.59	–0.21	0.12	–0.11	0.34
Copenhagen	0.66	0.52	0.81	1.29	1.15	1.43	1.04	0.91	1.17	1.14	0.98	1.30	–0.37	–0.51	–0.24	0.15	0.00	0.15
France																		
North-east	–	–	–	0.30	–0.22	0.83	–	–	–	0.75	0.16	1.34	–	–	–	–0.44	–0.77	–0.12
North-west	–	–	–	–0.03	–1.05	1.99	–	–	–	0.59	–0.65	1.83	–	–	–	–0.62	–1.21	–0.03
South	–	–	–	–0.03	–0.68	0.63	–	–	–	0.61	–0.20	1.42	–	–	–	–0.64	–1.05	–0.23
South coast	–	–	–	–0.29	–1.16	0.57	–	–	–	0.50	–0.49	1.50	–	–	–	–0.79	–1.34	–0.25
Germany																		
Heidelberg	0.56	0.32	0.81	1.21	0.89	1.53	1.20	0.97	1.43	1.50	1.16	1.84	–0.64	–0.83	–0.45	–0.28	–0.54	–0.03
Potsdam	0.43	0.16	0.70	0.49	0.16	0.83	1.46	1.22	1.71	1.31	0.91	1.71	–1.03	–1.24	–0.83	–0.81	–1.07	–0.56
Greece																		
Athens	0.92	0.59	1.25	1.00	0.57	1.44	1.13	0.82	0.44	0.98	0.25	1.72	–0.21	–0.53	0.11	0.02	–0.61	0.65
Italy																		
Florence	–0.55	–0.99	–0.20	0.29	0.05	0.52	0.45	0.05	0.45	0.83	0.55	1.12	–1.00	–1.38	–0.61	–0.55	–0.80	–0.29
Varese	0.06	–0.39	0.52	0.78	0.42	1.13	0.49	0.07	0.89	1.01	0.55	1.47	–0.42	–0.81	–0.03	–0.23	–0.62	0.15
Ragusa	–0.01	–0.58	0.57	0.15	–0.65	0.94	0.81	0.27	1.35	0.04	–1.04	1.13	–0.81	–1.30	–0.32	0.10	–0.73	0.94
Turin	0.15	–0.19	0.50	0.74	0.27	1.20	0.46	0.15	0.77	0.95	0.41	1.49	–0.30	–0.60	–0.01	–0.21	–0.64	0.21
Naples	–	–	–	0.73	0.34	1.11	–	–	–	0.69	0.20	1.17	–	–	–	0.04	–0.46	0.53
Netherlands																		
Bilthoven	0.97	0.56	1.38	1.59	1.15	2.02	1.39	1.06	1.73	1.07	0.63	1.50	–0.42	–0.79	–0.05	0.52	0.10	0.94
Utrecht	–	–	–	0.76	0.58	0.93	–	–	–	0.84	0.66	1.03	–	–	–	–0.09	–0.24	0.07
Spain																		
Asturias	–0.25	–0.72	0.23	1.50	0.84	2.16	0.62	0.14	1.10	–0.07	–0.98	0.84	–0.86	–1.30	–0.43	1.57	0.69	2.44
Granada	0.50	–0.17	1.18	0.79	–0.19	1.77	1.23	0.59	1.88	–0.66	–2.08	0.76	–0.73	–1.36	–0.11	1.44	0.32	2.57
Murcia	0.33	–0.21	0.86	0.88	0.06	1.71	1.18	0.66	1.69	1.67	0.10	3.22	–0.85	–1.38	–0.32	–0.78	–1.80	0.24
Navarra	0.12	–0.25	0.48	1.22	0.41	2.03	0.54	0.13	0.95	–0.19	–1.38	0.99	–0.42	–0.79	–0.05	1.42	0.40	2.43
San Sebastian	0.16	–0.22	0.53	0.81	–0.08	1.69	0.49	0.10	0.88	0.70	–0.56	1.96	–0.33	–0.68	0.01	0.10	–0.80	1.01
Sweden																		
Malmö	0.58	0.24	0.91	0.54	0.20	0.88	1.37	1.04	1.69	0.80	0.43	1.17	–0.79	–1.07	–0.51	–0.26	–0.57	0.04
Umeå	0.40	0.15	0.66	0.94	0.64	1.23	1.07	0.79	1.37	1.32	0.94	1.70	–0.68	–0.89	–0.46	–0.38	–0.69	–0.08
United Kingdom																		
General population	0.48	0.13	0.82	0.77	0.38	1.16	1.33	0.97	1.68	1.17	0.72	1.61	–0.85	–1.07	–0.63	–0.39	–0.66	–0.13
Health-conscious	0.18	–0.49	0.89	0.36	–0.13	0.66	1.09	0.39	1.80	0.73	0.29	1.17	–0.91	–1.22	–0.61	–0.47	–0.68	–0.25

[a]Adjusted for age, educational level, occupational and leisure time activity.
[b]LCLM, lower confidence limit.
[c]UCLM,upper confidence limit.
[d]Unadjusted values because adjustment was not possible due to missing data.

centres no significant differences between EXSM and NSM were observed.

Conclusion

Considerable heterogeneity exists across EPIC Study populations and between men and women within each centre or country with respect to the relation between BMI and smoking status. This heterogeneity could not be eliminated by adjustment for important confounding factors. Thus, BMI and changes in BMI reflect, to a varying degree, other determinants of BMI such as energy intake.

It is therefore likely that in the long run also centre-specific heterogeneity will appear in the emerging EPIC results with respect to other risk factors and their relation to disease risk.

References

Molarius, A., Seidell, J.C., Kuulasmaa, K., Dobson, A.J. & Sans, S. (1997) Smoking and relative body weight: an international perspective from the WHO MONICA *Project. J. Epidemiol. Community Health*, **51**, 252–260

Colorectal cancer associated with BMI, physical activity, diabetes, and blood glucose

Lund Nilsen T.I.[1,2], Vatten L.J.[1]

[1]Department of Community Medicine and General Practice, Norwegian University of Science and Technology, University Medical Center, N-7489 Trondheim, Norway. [2]Norwegian Cancer Society, PO Box 5327 Majorstua, N-0304 Oslo, Norway.

Introduction

Obesity, physical inactivity, and consumption of a Western diet high in fat and low in fibre are associated with an increased risk of colorectal cancer. These factors have also been associated with an increased risk of non-insulin-dependent diabetes mellitus. Based on the similarity of risk factors for colorectal cancer and diabetes mellitus, McKeown-Eyssen (1994) and Giovannucci (1995) have proposed that high insulin levels may stimulate the growth of colorectal tumours.

From this background, we prospectively examined the association between obesity, physical activity, diabetes mellitus and blood glucose, and the risk of colorectal cancer in a cohort of 75 219 Norwegian men and women.

Materials and methods

The study cohort was established between 1984 and 1986, when 77 310 subjects in a Norwegian county (90.8% of the total adult population) participated in the HUNT study, which included anthropometric and physiological measures and two questionnaires. For the present study, we included 38 244 women and 36 975 men aged 20 years and over, who had no history of any cancer at study entry. The participants were followed up through the Norwegian Cancer Registry and their data were collected for person-years from the date of study entry until the date of cancer diagnosis (of all sites), death, emigration, or the cut-off date of 1 January 1996, whichever occurred first.

Statistical analyses were conducted separately for males and females. We used Cox regression with each of the study variables and age within 10 categories (<40, 40–44, ..., 75–79, and ≥ 80) to compute age-adjusted incidence rate ratios (RR) with 95% confidence intervals (CIs) and two-sided tests for trend across exposure categories. Multivariable analyses were conducted to assess potential confounding by the other main variables and by marital status and education.

Results

During the 12 years of follow-up (median =10.8), a total of 234 colon and 128 rectal cancers were diagnosed in men, and 277 colon and 91 rectal cancers in women. Mean age at diagnosis of colorectal cancer was 72 years for both men and women.

The results of the combined analysis of colon and rectal cancer are shown in Table 1. Separate analyses for each site (data not shown) showed that the negative association with physical activity among men was slightly stronger for colon cancer (RR=0.47; 95% CI, 0.28–0.80) than for rectal cancer (RR=0.63; 95% CI, 0.36–1.12). Similarly, among women, the positive association with diabetes was slightly stronger for colon (RR=1.60; 95% CI, 1.02–2.51) than for rectal cancer (1.41; 95% CI, 0.61–3.27), while the association with blood glucose was stronger for rectal (RR=2.70; 95% CI, 1.29–5.61) than for colon cancer (RR=1.76; 95% CI, 1.07–2.88). We also found suggestive evidence of a J-shaped association between body mass index (BMI) and colon cancer risk in men, where the point estimates were 0.73, 0.85, and 1.04 for second, third, and highest quartile of BMI, respectively.

Results from multivariable adjusted analyses were not materially different from the age-adjusted results for any of the main variables (data not shown).

Discussion

Several cohort studies have shown that physical activity is negatively associated with risk of colorectal cancer in men. Physical activity may reduce plasma

Table 1. Age-adjusted incidence rate ratios (RRs) for colorectal cancer associated with BMI, physical activity, diabetes and blood glucose

	Men		Women	
Variables	RR	95% CI	RR	95% CI
BMI[a]				
Lowest quartile	1.0	Reference	1.0	Reference
Second quartile	0.90	0.65–1.24	0.89	0.63–1.27
Third quartile	0.96	0.71–1.30	0.80	0.57–1.13
Highest quartile	1.07	0.80–1.42	0.98	0.71–1.34
	P trend[b] = 0.51		*P* trend[b] = 0.96	
Physical activity				
Low	1.0	Reference	1.0	Reference
Medium	0.87	0.65–1.17	0.95	0.68–1.33
High	0.54	0.37–0.79	0.81	0.54–1.23
	P trend[b] = 0.002		*P* trend[b] = 0.34	
History of diabetes				
No	1.0	Reference	1.0	Reference
Yes	0.66	0.35–1.24	1.55	1.04–2.31
Blood glucose (mmol/L)				
< 8.0	1.0	Reference	1.0	Reference
≥ 8.0	0.90	0.58–1.40	1.98	1.31–2.98

[a]Cut-off values for quartiles were 23.0, 24.9, and 27.1 kg/m^2 in men, and 21.8, 24.2, and 27.4 kg/m^2 in women.

[b]Two-sided *P* values for trend from Cox regression when variables were treated as ordinal variables.

insulin, and insulin is a colon tumour promoter in rats and a mitogen for colon carcinoma cells in vitro. Contrary to Thune and Lund (1996), we found no significant association with physical activity in women. Misclassification of physical activity due to energy expenditure in housework rather than in leisure-time activity might contribute to the null finding and little variation in physical activity could mask a difference in risk.

Several possible mechanisms may explain a positive association with diabetes: slower bowel transit, and increased production of bile acids and higher insulin levels (Hu *et al.*, 1999). Nonetheless, these factors cannot explain that a positive association with diabetes is present only among women. In this study, few men with diabetes developed colorectal cancer and the statistical power to examine this question may be too low.

McKeown-Eyssen (1994) has suggested that serum triglycerides and plasma glucose are involved in colorectal carcinogenesis, possibly by increasing insulin secretion. In our study, we found a twofold increased risk among women with the highest blood glucose levels; this is in agreement with a study by Schoen *et al.* (1999). In contrast to our results, they also found a similar association in men.

In summary, these results may, at least in part, support the hypothesis that insulin may act as a promoter in colorectal cancer. However, the gender-specific discrepancy in the results cannot be readily explained and calls for cautious interpretation.

Acknowledgements

Data were made available by the National Health Screening Service, the Cancer Registry of Norway, and the National Institute of Public Health, Community Medicine Research Centre in Verdal, Norway.

References

Giovannucci, E. (1995) Insulin and colon cancer. *Cancer Causes Control*, **6**, 164–179

Hu, F.B., Manson, J.E., Liu, S., Hunter, D., Colditz, G.A., Michels, K.B., Speizer, F.E. & Giovannucci, E. (1999) Prospective study of adult onset diabetes mellitus (type 2) and risk of colorectal cancer in women. *J. Natl. Cancer Inst.*, **91**, 542–547

McKeown-Eyssen, G. (1994) Epidemiology of colorectal cancer revisited: are serum triglycerides and/or plasma glucose associated with risk? *Cancer Epidemiol. Biomarkers Prev.*, **3**, 687–695

Schoen, R.E., Tangen, C.M., Kuller, L.H., Burke, G.L., Cushman, M., Tracy, R.P., Dobs, A. & Savage, P.J. (1999) Increased blood glucose and insulin, body size, and incident colorectal cancer. *J. Natl. Cancer Inst.*, **91**, 1147–1154

Thune, I. & Lund, E. (1996) Physical activity and risk of colorectal cancer in men and women. *Br. J. Cancer*, **73**, 1134–1140

BMI throughout life, intake of vitamin supplements and oral cancer in Spain

Nieto A.[1], Sánchez M.J.[2], Quintana M.J.[3], Castellsagué X.[3], Martínez C.[2], Muñoz J.[3], Bosch F.X.[3], Muñoz N.[4], Herrero R.[4], Franceschi S.[4]

[1]Faculty of Medicine, University of Seville, Spain. [2]Andalusian School of Public Health, Granada, Spain. [3]Catalan Institute of Oncology, Barcelona, Spain. [4]International Agency for Research on Cancer, Lyon, France.

Background

The influences of body mass index (BMI) on colon and lung cancer mortality and morbidity have been explored (Ford, 1999), while several studies have suggested that dietary deficiencies could be associated with an increased risk of oral cancer, the high intake of fruits and vegetables being clearly protective against the appearance of cancer at this site (Bosetti, 2000).

Purpose of the study

The purpose of this study was to asses whether lifetime BMI history was related to the occurrence of oral and oropharyngeal cancer and also to explore the possible protective effect of the intake of vitamin supplements against this cancer.

Materials and methods

The International Agency for Research on Cancer (IARC) coordinated a case–control hospital-based study on cancer of the oral cavity and oropharynx in 14 countries and 18 centres, 3 of them in Spain.

Cases were incident and histologically confirmed cases of oral cancer (codes c01 to c10 of the International Classification of Diseases for Oncology, ICD-O 2nd version), with no age or gender limitations, consecutively diagnosed from 1996 to 1999 in the following Spanish University Hospitals: Santa Creu i Sant Pau and Ciutat Sanitaria de Bellvitge (Barcelona), Virgen de las Nieves (Granada) and Virgen Macarena (Sevilla).

Controls were patients from the same hospitals as the cases, group-matched by age and gender, randomly selected after excluding those patients diagnosed with diseases related to well-known or suspected risk factors for oral cancer.

All the participants were personally interviewed and the study questionnaire included detailed information about socio-demographic characteristics, smoking and drinking habits, frequency of consumption of 25 food items and vitamin supplements, height, weight, oral health and family history of cancer.

BMI was calculated from self-referred height and weight of participants (weight in kilograms divided by squared height in metres). Participants in Barcelona were asked to report their weight at the age of 30 and the participants in Granada and Sevilla were asked to report their weight at the age of 20. Height, weight and BMI distributions were grouped in approximate tertiles and the lowest tertile was used as the reference category for multivariate analysis. Odds ratios (OR) and 95% confidence intervals (95% CI) were calculated by unconditional logistic regression methods, adjusting first for centre, age, gender and education and then introducing variables for smoking, alcohol intake, and frequency of consumption of fruits and vegetables.

Results

Gender and age distributions of the 375 cases and 375 controls in Spain showed that 81% were males and 49% were younger than 60 years. More than 40% of participants had less than 6 years of education. Only 22% were lifetime non-smokers and 15% had always abstained from alcoholic beverages.

Mean height was 165 cm and mean weight was 71 kg at diagnosis, 72 kg 2 years before diagnosis, 66 kg at 30 and 64 kg at 20. Mean BMI was 25.9 (kg/m^2) at diagnosis, 26.3 at 2 years before diagnosis, 24.0 at the age of 30 and 23.4 at 20.

Those patients in the highest tertile of weight or BMI at diagnosis, 2 years before diagnosis and at 30 had a decreased odds ratio of oral cancer after

Table 1. Height, weight and body mass index at diagnosis and 2 years before diagnosis. Odds ratios (OR) and confidence intervals (95% CI) for oral cavity and oropharynx cancer, Spain 1996–1999

	Cases[a]	Controls[a]	OR[b]	95% CI	OR[c]	95% CI
Height (cm)						
≤ 162	123	97	1.0[d]		1.0[d]	
163–169	113	116	0.72	0.49–1.07	0.86	0.56–1.33
≥ 170	101	124	0.56	0.39–0.88	0.72	0.46–1.14
P value for trend			0.007		0.103	
At diagnosis						
Weight (kg)						
≤ 65	179	75	1.0[d]		1.0[d]	
66–75	87	123	0.29	0.20–0.43	0.34	0.22–0.52
≥ 76	75	147	0.21	0.14–0.31	0.28	0.18–0.43
P value for trend			0.000		0.000	
Body mass index						
≤ 22	112	40	1.0[d]		1.0[d]	
23–25	104	88	0.42	0.27–0.67	0.51	0.31–0.84
≥ 26	113	204	0.20	0.13–0.30	0.28	0.17–0.44
P value for trend			0.000		0.000	
2 years before						
Weight (kg)						
≤ 65	159	79	1.0[d]		1.0[d]	
66–75	108	126	0.41	0.28–0.60	0.45	0.29–0.68
≥ 76	80	149	0.26	0.17–0.38	0.34	0.22–0.52
P value for trend			0.000		0.000	
Body mass index						
≤ 22	96	36	1.0[d]		1.0[d]	
23–25	106	88	0.45	0.28–0.72	0.50	0.30–0.85
≥ 26	129	207	0.23	0.15–0.36	0.30	0.19–0.49
P value for trend			0.000		0.000	

[a]Some strata do not add up to the total because of a few missing values.
[b]Estimates from unconditional regression equations including variables for age, gender, centre and education.
[c]Estimates from unconditional regression equations including variables for age, gender, centre, education, smoking and drinking habits, fruit and vegetable intake.
[d]Reference category.

allowing for age, gender, center, education, smoking and alcohol drinking habits, and frequency of consumption of fruits and vegetables (Tables 1, 2). However, neither weight and BMI at 20 years of age nor height had any relationship with the occurrence of oral cancer. Finally, the intake of vitamin supplements, which was reported by 11.7% of cases and 8.3% of controls, did not show any protective effect on the occurrence of oral cavity and oropharynx cancer (Table 2).

Conclusions

A BMI of at least 25 seems to be protective against the development of oral and oropharynx cancer. The results of this study agree, therefore, with other studies that showed an increased odds of smoking-related cancers (Franceschi, 2001; D'Avanzo, 1996) in lean individuals. Leanness antedated cancer diagnosis, being therefore unlikely due to weight loss secondary to cancer symptoms.

In spite of the clearly established protective effect of a high consumption of fruits and vegetables, the intake of vitamin supplements did not decrease the risk of oral cancer. It may, therefore, be important not to replace fruits and vegetables by vitamin supplements.

References

Bosetti, C., Negri, E., Franceschi, S., Conti, E., Levi, F., Tomei, F. & La Vecchia, C. (2000) Risk factors for oral and pharyngeal cancer in women: a study from Italy and Switzerland. *Br. J. Cancer*, **82**, 204–207

D'Avanzo, B., La Vecchia, C., Talamini, R. & Franceschi, S. (1996) Anthropometric measures and risk of cancers of the upper digestive and respiratory tract. *Nutr. Cancer*, **26**, 219–227

Ford, E.S. (1999) Body mass index and colon cancer in a national sample of adult US men and women. *Am. J. Epidemiol.*, **150**, 390–398

Franceschi, S., Dal Maso, L., Levi, F., Conti, E., Talamini, R. & La Vecchia, C. (2001) Leanness as early marker of cancer of the oral cavity and oropharynx. *Ann. Oncol.*, **12**, 331–336

Table 2. Weight and body mass index at the age of 20 and 30 and vitamin intake throughout life. Odds ratios (OR) and confidence intervals (95% CI) for oral cavity and oropharynx cancer, Spain 1996–1999

	Cases[a]	Controls[a]	OR[b]	95% CI	OR[c]	95% CI
At the age of 20[e]						
Weight (kg)						
≤ 60	86	75	1.0[d]		1.0[d]	
61–66	27	36	0.62	0.34–1.13	0.59	0.31–1.13
≥ 67	49	63	0.65	0.39–1.08	0.77	0.43–1.35
P value for trend						
Body mass index						
≤ 22	77	64	1.0[d]		1.0[d]	
23–24	28	42	0.55	0.30–0.99	0.52	0.27–1.01
≥ 25	43	51	0.72	0.42–1.23	0.72	0.40–1.32
P value for trend						
At the age of 30[f]						
Weight (kg)						
≤ 61	71	51	1.0[d]		1.0[d]	
62–69	61	50	0.83	0.49–1.42	1.0	0.53–1.88
≥ 70	49	76	0.43	0.25–0.74	0.50	0.26–0.94
P value for trend						
Body mass index						
≤ 23	93	67	1.0[d]		1.0[d]	
24–25	51	54	0.67	0.41–1.10	0.87	0.48–1.59
≥ 26	33	47	0.50	0.29–0.87	0.50	0.26–0.97
P value for trend						
Vitamin intake						
Never	319	335	1.0[d]		1.0[d]	
Ever	44	31	1.49	0.91–2.45	1.39	0.81–2.39

[a]Some strata do not add up to the total because of a few missing values.

[b]Estimates from unconditional regression equations including variables for age, gender, centre, and education.

[c]Estimates from unconditional regression equations including variables for age, gender, centre, education, smoking and drinking habits, fruit and vegetable intake.

[d]Reference category.

[e]Participants from Granada and Sevilla.

[f]Participants from Barcelona.

Adolescent BMI and cancer risk

Okasha M.[1], Davey Smith G.[1], McCarron P.[2], McEwen J.[3]

[1]Dept. of Social Medicine, Bristol University, UK. [2]National Cancer Institute, National Institute of Health, Bethesda, Maryland, USA. [3]Dept. of Public Health, Glasgow University, UK.

Introduction

The importance of overweight in adult life in relation to cancer risk has recently been highlighted (Bergstrom *et al.*, 2001) This study estimated that in the countries of the European Union, approximately 8% of breast cancers, 10% of colon cancers and 40% of endometrial cancers are attributable to overweight and obesity. The importance of exposures in pre-adult life affecting cancer risk is suggested by observations that height is related to cancers that are not thought to be related to smoking (Gunnell *et al.*, 2001) We therefore explored the association between overweight in early adult life and subsequent cancer risk.

Methods

In 1948, the University of Glasgow initiated annual health checks at the university health service at which height and weight measurements were made by a physician. The students who attended between 1948 and 1968 comprise the Glasgow Alumni Cohort, described in detail elsewhere (McCarron *et al.*, 1999) The cohort members are flagged at the National Health Service Central Register (NHSCR) and we are notified of cancer registrations and deaths. We have recently sent a questionnaire to surviving members of the cohort, requesting information on self-reported cancers.

The current study comprises follow-up to September 2001 for self-reported cancers and mortality and to December 1998 for cancer registrations. Cancers related to smoking are: oropharynx, oesophagus, pancreas, respiratory and urinary tracts. The remainder were classified as cancers not related to smoking (Gunnell *et al.*, 1998). Because of the small numbers of people who were obese in young adulthood, body mass index (BMI) was categorized as lean (<19 kg/m^2), normal (19–22.9 kg/m^2), high normal (23–24.9 kg/m^2) and overweight (≥ 25 kg/m^2). We used logistic regression to compare cancer risk (occurrence or death) among each of these categories.

Results

Of the original 15 322 students, 9199 men and 2528 women with complete data were traced and included in the study (77%). The average age at weight measurement was 20.3 years, and mean BMI was 21.6 kg/m^2 in men and 21.3 kg/m^2 in women. Seven percent of males and females were overweight (*n*=811). In total, 886 cancers were identified. The most frequent site-specific cancers were those of the prostate (*n*=125), breast (*n*=113), lung (*n*=82 men), haematopoietic system (*n*=67 men) and colorectum (*n*=111 men).

There was no association between BMI category and all cancers in men. The age-adjusted odds ratio (OR) and 95% confidence interval (CI) for lean, high normal and overweight individuals compared to normal individuals were 1.01 (CI 95%, 0.77–1.32); 0.92 (CI 95%, 0.73–1.15) and 0.97 (CI 95%, 0.72–1.31). The risk among lean women was reduced compared to normal weight women (0.57, 0.36–0.91). High normal and overweight women were not at increased risk of all cancers compared to normal weight women: OR, 0.83 (CI 95%, 0.56–1.25) and 0.93 (CI 95%, 0.54–1.59), respectively.

The relative risks of the site-specific cancers studied according to categories of BMI are shown in Table 1. A trend of lower risk of lung cancer in heavier men was evident. This was unchanged when controlled for smoking behaviour, but the association was reversed when only non-smokers were considered. Lean men were at risk of haematopoietic cancer compared to normal weight men. There was no association between BMI and prostate, breast or male colorectal cancers.

Comment

The results from this study provide little evidence to support the suggestion that BMI in early life is detrimentally associated with cancer risk.

There are certain limitations with this study that must be acknowledged. Firstly, the analyses are based on 77% of the original cohort, partly because we

Table 1. Association between weight[a] in young adulthood and site-specific cancer risk

	Cases/non-cases	Age-adjusted OR (95% CI)
Colorectal (males)		
Lean	6/975	0.48 (0.21–1.11)
Normal	80/6056	1[b]
High normal	15/1432	0.73 (0.42–1.28)
Overweight	10/625	1.00 (0.51–1.95)
Per 1 kg/m²		1.03 (0.95–1.12); P_{trend} = 0.46
Lung (males)		
Lean	12/969	1.44 (0.77–2.71)
Normal	55/6081	1[b]
High normal	9/1438	0.62 (0.31–1.27)
Overweight	6/629	0.81 (0.35–1.92)
Per 1 kg/m²		0.89 (0.80–0.99); P_{trend} = 0.023
Prostate		
Lean	15/966	1.24 (0.71–2.16)
Normal	80/6056	1[b]
High normal	22/1425	1.05 (0.65–1.70)
Overweight	8/627	0.74 (0.36–1.56)
Per 1 kg/m²		0.96 (0.89 to 1.04); P_{trend} = 0.29
Haematopoietic system (males)		
Lean	12/969	2.28 (1.18–4.41)
Normal	35/6101	1[b]
High normal	13/1434	1.42 (0.75–2.71)
Overweight	7/628	1.50 (0.66–3.43)
Per 1 kg/m²		0.99 (0.89–1.10); P_{trend} = 0.82
Breast (females)		
Lean	12/367	0.61 (0.33–1.14)
Normal	80/1515	1[b]
High normal	13/365	0.67 (0.37–1.22)
Overweight	8/168	0.89 (0.42–1.87)
Per 1 kg/m²		1.00 (0.92–1.08); P_{trend} = 0.99

[a]BMI definitions: lean, <19 kg/m²; normal, 19–22.9 kg/m²; high normal, 23–24.9 kg/m²; overweight, ≥ 25 kg/m².
[b]Reference category.

have only been able to trace 82% of the cohort, and because values for height and weight were missing. However, analyses have indicated that people excluded from the study did not differ importantly in terms of baseline characteristics from those who were included. Secondly, we do not currently have information on health behaviours and patterns of weight fluctuation in adult life. Among a subsample of our cohort who were contacted in mid-adulthood, weight change was more important in determining risk of any cancer than was weight in young adulthood (unpublished results). However, the small numbers of people in that subsample precluded site-specific analyses.

The main strength of the study is that the values of height and weight used to calculate BMI were made prospectively. The majority of studies which have reported on associations between BMI in early life and cancer risk have relied on self-reported measures. These may be poorly reported and subject to bias.

Two interesting results of associations between BMI and cancer risk emerged from this study. The high risk of lung cancer seen among lean men is unlikely to be due to reverse causality (i.e. low weight in men with undetected disease) because of the young age at which the weight measure was made. The observation that non-smoking men, BMI was positively related to lung cancer suggests that the results in Table 1 may be due to error in measurement of smoking behaviour. The association of higher risk of cancers of the haematopoietic system among men who were lean at university was unexpected and needs to be replicated before being accepted as an important finding.

Acknowledgements

We gratefully acknowledge the support of the World Cancer Research Fund International for funding this study. We also thank Helen Davies, Emma Turner and Zoe Wilkins for administrative assistance with the postal questionnaire and data entry.

References

Bergstrom, A., Pisani, P., Tenet, V., Wolk, A. & Adami, H.O. (2001) Overweight as an avoidable cause of cancer in Europe. *Int. J. Cancer*, **91**, 421–430

Gunnell, D., Davey Smith, G., Holly, J., Frankel, S. (1998) Leg length and risk of cancer in the Boyd Orr cohort. *BMJ*, **317**, 1350–1351

Gunnell, D., Okasha, M., Holly, J., Oliver, S., Sandhu, J. & Davey Smith, G. (2001) Height and cancer risk: a systematic review of prospective studies and possible mechanisms. *Epidemiol. Rev.*, in press

McCarron, P., Davey Smith, G., Okasha, M. & McEwen, J. (1999) Life course exposure and later disease: a follow-up study based on medical examinations carried out in Glasgow University (1948–1968) *Public Health*, **113**, 265–271

Physical activity in the EPIC cohort in Italy

Salvini S.[1], Saieva C.[1], Sieri S.[2], Vineis P.[3], Panico S.[4], Tumino R.[5], Palli D.[1]
(the EPIC cohort in Italy)

[1]Molecular and Nutritional Epidemiology Branch, Epidemiology Unit, Centro per lo Studio e la Prevenzione Oncologica, Florence, Italy. [2]National Cancer Institute, Milan, Italy. [3]University of Turin, Turin, Italy. [4]Federico II University, Naples, Italy. [5]Registro Tumori, Azienda Ospedaliera "Civile - M.P. Arezzo", Ragusa, Italy.

Physical activity and body weight are nowadays considered among the most important means to prevent a series of chronic diseases such as diabetes, cardiovascular disease and cancer (Friedenreich, 2001). Body weight is the result of a balance between energy intake and energy expenditure. In the last decades, our average energy expenditure has dropped. Furthermore, food is more easily accessible to the population, easy to prepare, and ready to eat. This results in an increase in total intake of energy, contributing to disrupting the balance.

Dietary and life style habits in Europe show large differences both between and within countries. The present study aims to describe different physical activity patterns within EPIC-ITALY, and to present a method to convert physical activity, as measured by the life style questionnaire in the Italian EPIC centres, into an index of energy expenditure.

Methods

Five centres (Milan, Turin, Florence, Naples and Ragusa) participated in the Italian component of the EPIC study and have enrolled 47 749 volunteers (32 578 women and 15 171 men) from 1993 to 1998. The physical activity section of the EPIC questionnaire is a modification of a validated tool (Pols *et al.*, 1997). Subjects classified themselves in four categories of work activity. In addition, they reported the number of hours spent every week (in summer and in winter, separately) in the following leisure-time activities: walking, biking, gardening and exercising. Do-it-yourself activities were considered independently of the season. Subjects were also asked how many hours per week any of the above activities were performed so intensively as to generate sweat. The number of flights of stairs climbed per day was also requested. Women were asked to report on hours spent each week in household activities. To transform reported activities into energy expenditure we used metabolic equivalents (METs) for types of work (Commission of European Communities, 1993). Different sources (SINU, 1996) were used for translation of leisure-time activities into METs, ranging from 1.8 for do-it-yourself activities to 6.0 for exercise (such as swimming, running, aerobics, etc.). METs were applied to each type of activity and weighted according to the number of hours spent on that activity. All weighted METs were summed to obtain the daily physical activity level (PAL) of each subject and multiplied for the estimated basal metabolic rate of each subject so as to compute a specific daily energy expenditure per subject. We also computed scores of the various types of activity and a cumulative activity score obtained by summing all specific activity scores, and categorized them from zero to three. At the time of the present analyses, information about type of work activity was unavailable for the Naples centre; data in Table 1 are therefore based on four centres. Also, some subjects were excluded due to missing answers.

Results

Figure 1 shows the distribution of hours per week spent in various activities. Very large differences in habits can be observed between centres.

Characteristics of subjects by sex and by activity score are reported in Table 1. Energy intake by cumulative activity score varied from 10.4 (±3.1) MJ for the most sedentary to 13.3 (±3.7) MJ for the most active men, and 8.5 (±2.8) MJ to 9.9 (±3.1) MJ in women. Body mass index was rather stable across different activity score categories, as were other characteristics such as waist-to-hip ratio and blood pressure. Average energy expenditure in the lowest

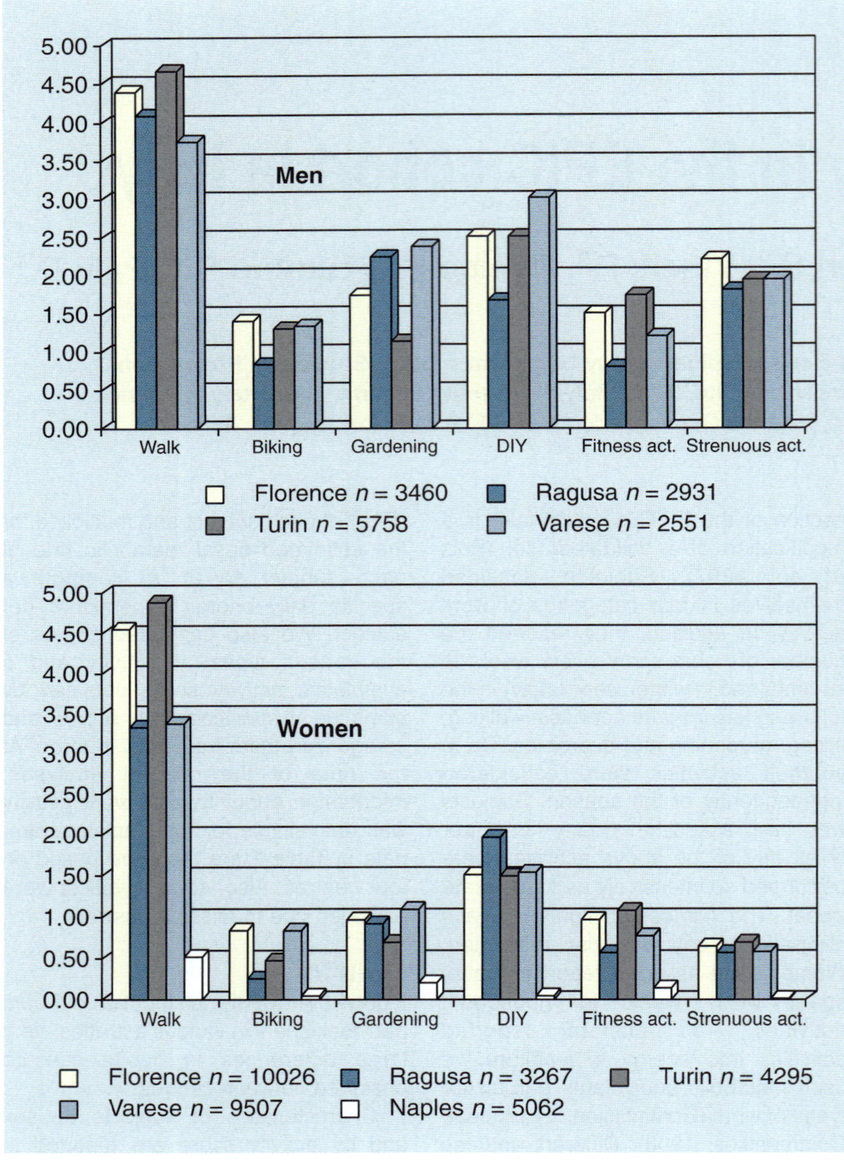

Figure 1
Number of hours per week spent in different leisure-time activities, by centre. EPIC-ITALY 1993-1998.

expenditure category is 10.1 (±1.0) to 16.6 (±2.3) MJ in men and 8.1 (±0.7) MJ to 10.9 (±1.4) MJ in women. The average PAL estimated for this population was 1.60 for men and 1.59 for women. Considering the recommended PAL of 1.75 (WCRF, 1997), only 24% of men and 19% of women met the recommendation (not shown).

Conclusions

The lifestyle questionnaire developed for the EPIC study in Italy allows one to compute indicators of energy expenditure. Energy intake seems to be in some way related to expenditure, although this is more visible in men than in women. In Italian women, house-cleaning activities seem to play an important role in determining energy expenditure; excluding this component, women show very low levels of expenditure. After this very preliminary analysis, more in-depth work is needed to evaluate the best way to use information from the physical activity section of the EPIC questionnaire. A better understanding of activity patterns in the EPIC populations will also be of value in implementing public health initiatives to promote healthy lifestyles in Europe.

References

Commission of European Communities (1993) *Nutrient and Energy Intakes for the European Community, Reports of the Scientific Committee for Food*, (31st Series), Luxembourg, Office for Official Publications of the European Communities

Friedenreich C.M. (2001) Physical activity and cancer prevention: from observational to intervention research. *Cancer Epidemiol. Biomarkers Prev.*, **10**, 287–301

Pols, M.A., Peeters, P.H.M., Ocké, M.C., Slimani, N., Bueno-de-Mesquita, H.B. & Collette, H.J.A. (1997) Estimation of reproducibility and relative validity of the questions included in the EPIC physical activity questionnaire. *Int. J. Epidemiol.*, **26** (Suppl.1), S181–S189

Società Italiana di Nutrizione Umana (SINU) (1998) *Livelli di Assunzione Raccomandata di Energia e Nutrienti per la Popolazione Italiana*, (LARN, revision 1996), Milan, EDRA

World Cancer Prevention Fund and American Institute for Cancer Research (1997) *Food, Nutrition and the Prevention of Cancer: A Global Perspective*, Washington, D.C., WCPF/AICR

Table 1. Characteristics of subjects, expressed as mean (SD), by cumulative activity score. EPIC-ITALY 1993-1998

	Men				Women			
	0	1	2	3	0	1	2	3
Number of subjects[a]	559	4138	9482	521	791	6797	18183	1324
Age (years)	50.7 (7.4)	50.5 (7.5)	49.5(7.6)	48.2 (7.5)	49.5 (8.4)	49.9 (8.3)	50.5 (8.1)	49.4 (7.6)
Body mass index (kg/m^2)	27.5 (3.6)	26.8 (3.5)	26.4 (3.2)	26.8 (3.4)	25.5 (4.6)	25.4 (4.3)	25.5 (4.3)	25.8 (4.4)
Waist-to-hip ratio	0.95 (0.)	0.94 (0.1)	0.93 (0.1)	0.93 (0.1)	0.79 (0.06)	0.79 (0.07)	0.79 (0.07)	0.79 (0.06)
Pulse rate (per min)	70.1 (9.1)	69.5 (9.0)	68.3 (8.7)	67.6 (9.1)	72.0 (9.1)	71.8 (8.9)	71.3 (8.8)	71.2 (8.5)
Blood pressure								
Systolic (mmHg)	134.5 (16.7)	132.9 (16.5)	132.2 (15.8)	132.0 (16.2)	126.6 (17.9)	128.1 (18.8)	128.6 (18.9)	127.8 (18.4)
Diastolic (mmHg)	85.1 (10.0)	84.3 (9.7)	83.9 (9.4)	83.4 (9.2)	80.7 (10.5)	81.0 (10.6)	81.1 (10.4)	80.6 (10.7)
Energy intake								
kcal	2486.7 (734)	2556.7 (741)	2759.4 (774)	3172.9 (895)	2020.5 (684)	2066.7 (617)	2159.0 (645)	2368 (746)
MJ	10.4 (3.1)	10.7 (3.1)	11.5 (3.2)	13.3 (3.7)	8.5 (2.8)	8.7 (2.6)	9.0 (2.7)	9.9 (3.1)
Work (h/day)	4.1 (2.5)	4.1 (2.5)	4.4 (2.3)	5.1 (1.2)	3.6 (2.5)	2.8 (2.7)	2.2 (2.5)	2.8 (2.4)
Leisure-time activity (h/day)	0.3 (0.13)	0.8 (0.5)	1.9 (1.1)	2.7 (1.0)	0.27 (0.1)	0.59 (2.7)	1.37 (0.8)	2.3 (0.9)
House cleaning (h/day)	0	0	0	0	1.29 (0.4)	2.7 (1.7)	4.2 (1.9)	5.5 (1.4)
Flights of stairs (flights/day)	0.92 (0.73)	2.5 (2.8)	6.4 (5.3)	12.1 (5.5)	1.0 (0.7)	2.0 (2.3)	5.2 (5.1)	11.0 (5.5)
Physical activity level	1.34 (0.04)	1.44 (0.12)	1.66 (0.24)	2.06 (0.26)	1.39 (0.04)	1.49 (0.08)	1.62 (0.13)	1.83 (0.18)
Estimated energy expenditure								
kcal	2411.3 (246)	2567.7 (322)	2971.5 (495)	3734.21 (558)	1924.5 (165)	2055.0 (190)	2262.6 (255)	2613.5 (325)
MJ	10.1 (1.1)	10.7 (1.3)	12.4 (2.1)	16.6 (2.3)	8.1 (0.7)	8.6 (0.8)	9.5 (1.1)	10.9 (1.4)

[a]Preliminary data, based on four centres.

Chapter 6

Endogenous hormones and cancer

Hormones and breast cancer

Key T.J., Allen N.E.

Cancer Research UK Epidemiology Unit, University of Oxford, Gibson Building, Radcliffe Infirmary, Oxford OX2 6HE, UK.

Introduction

Breast cancer risk is increased by early menarche and by late menopause (Kelsey, 1979). These relationships indicate that the high serum concentrations of estradiol and/or progesterone in premenopausal women cause a greater increase in breast cancer risk per year than the much lower concentrations of estradiol and progesterone in postmenopausal women. Neither estradiol nor progesterone is genotoxic and it is likely that the high serum concentrations of these hormones in premenopausal women increase breast cancer risk by increasing the mitotic rate of the breast epithelial cells (Pike *et al.*,1993).

Estradiol alone has been shown to stimulate breast cell mitosis in model systems, but the observation that the mitotic rate of human breast epithelial cells is highest during the luteal phase of the menstrual cycle led to the hypothesis that progesterone might augment the mitotic action of estradiol (Key & Pike, 1988; Pike *et al.*, 1993). However, the simplest hypothesis in relation to hormones and breast cancer is that estradiol is the major determinant of the mitotic rate of human breast epithelial cells and that breast cancer risk is increased by relatively high serum concentrations of estradiol in both premenopausal and postmenopausal women. Other sex hormones might also play a role, perhaps through conversion into estradiol within the breast, and recent research has highlighted the potential importance of growth factors such as insulin-like growth factor-I (IGF-I).

Estradiol and breast cancer risk in postmenopausal women

Early studies examined estradiol levels and breast cancer risk by measuring serum concentrations or urinary excretion of estrogens in women diagnosed with breast cancer and in women without breast cancer. Most of these case–control studies showed that postmenopausal women with breast cancer had higher estrogen levels than control women (Key & Pike, 1988), but these findings must be interpreted very cautiously because the estrogen levels in the women with cancer could be affected by the presence of the cancer or by the treatment for cancer. To eliminate this problem it is necessary to conduct prospective studies in which estrogen concentrations are measured in serum samples collected from women before the diagnosis of breast cancer and compared with estrogen concentrations in serum from women of the same age who did not develop breast cancer during the same period.

Results from ten prospective studies have now been published. The earlier studies did not clearly indicate that women who developed breast cancer subsequent to blood collection had higher estradiol concentrations than the control women (Wysowski *et al.*, 1987; Garland *et al.*, 1992; Helzlsouer *et al.*, 1994), but the numbers of cases in these studies were relatively small (39, 15 and 29, respectively). The more recent, generally larger studies have reported that relatively high estradiol concentrations are significantly related to an increased risk for breast cancer (Toniolo *et al.*, 1995; Berrino *et al.*, 1996; Dorgan *et al.*, 1996; Thomas *et al.*, 1997a; Hankinson *et al.*, 1998a; Cauley *et al.*, 1999; Kabuto *et al.*, 2000), with relative risks in the region of 2 to 3 for women with relatively high levels of estradiol compared to women with relatively low levels of estradiol. Overall, therefore, the worldwide data are consistent with the hypothesis that high serum concentrations of estradiol in postmenopausal women increase breast cancer risk.

Bioavailable estradiol and sex hormone-binding globulin

Most of the estradiol in the blood is bound either tightly to sex hormone binding globulin (SHBG) or more loosely to albumin, with only about 2% non-protein-bound or free. A variety of evidence indicates that the fraction of estradiol which is bound to SHBG is not generally available to enter the cells and that the bioavailable fraction of estradiol is either the circa 2% which is free, or perhaps all the estradiol which is not bound to SHBG (i.e. free plus albumin-bound estradiol, sometimes termed non-SHBG-bound estradiol). It would be expected, therefore, that the association of estradiol with breast cancer risk might be stronger for free or non-SHBG-bound estradiol than for total estradiol, and indeed the studies which have examined one or both these indices have generally supported this hypothesis (Helzlsouer *et al.*, 1994; Toniolo *et al.*, 1995; Dorgan *et al.*, 1996; Hankinson *et al.*, 1998a; Cauley *et al.*, 1999; Kabuto *et al.*, 2000). Similarly, most of the prospective studies have also observed SHBG itself to be weakly inversely associated with risk (Berrino *et al.*, 1996; Dorgan *et al.*, 1996; Thomas *et al.*, 1997a; Cauley *et al.*, 1999; Kabuto *et al.*, 2000), although little association was observed in two small studies (Helzlsouer *et al.*, 1994; Garland *et al.*, 1992).

Body mass index, estradiol and breast cancer risk in postmenopausal women

Breast cancer risk is positively associated with body mass index in postmenopausal women; risk is approximately 50% higher in obese than in lean postmenopausal women (Key *et al.*, 2001). The principal source of estradiol in postmenopausal women is via the extraglandular aromatization of androstenedione, and estradiol increases with increasing body mass index in postmenopausal women (Siiteri & MacDonald, 1973). Furthermore, since increasing body mass index is associated with a decrease in SHBG, obesity in postmenopausal women is associated with a marked increase in free estradiol (Key *et al.*, 2001). It is possible that the relationship between body mass index and breast cancer risk can largely be explained by the relationship of body mass index with serum estradiol concentrations, but this has not yet been clearly demonstrated by data from prospective studies.

The possible roles of other sex hormones

The prospective studies which have reported data on estradiol and breast cancer risk have also reported data for several other sex hormones, although the hormones measured have varied between studies. Some data have been published for the estrogens estrone and estrone sulphate and for the androgens dehydroepiandrosterone, dehydroepiandrosterone sulphate, androstenedione and testosterone. The results of individual studies have varied somewhat, but overall have suggested that all these estrogens and androgens are positively associated with breast cancer risk in postmenopausal women (Wysowski *et al.*, 1987; Barrett-Connor *et al.*, 1990; Gordon *et al.*, 1990; Garland *et al.*, 1992; Helzlsouer *et al.*, 1994; Toniolo *et al.*, 1995; Berrino *et al.*, 1996; Dorgan *et al.*, 1996, 1997; Zeleniuch-Jacquotte *et al.*, 1997; Hankinson *et al.*, 1998a; Cauley *et al.*, 1999; Kabuto *et al.*, 2000).

The picture emerging is that, among postmenopausal women, all estrogens and androgens studied may be significantly positively associated with breast cancer risk. These steroid hormones are all closely related to each other metabolically, and typically the serum concentrations of these hormones are positively correlated with each other. It may therefore be difficult to establish from epidemiological studies which of the various sex hormones are most closely associated with risk. Estradiol is probably causally related to risk because it is known to affect breast cell division and because antiestrogenic treatment is effective in early breast cancer; androgens might also be important because they circulate at much higher concentrations than estrogens after menopause and can be converted to estrogens within the breast.

Estradiol and breast cancer risk in premenopausal women

Evaluating the association between breast cancer risk and estradiol concentration among premenopausal women is difficult due to the wide variation in estradiol and progesterone levels throughout the menstrual cycle. To date, five prospective studies have reported on serum estradiol concentrations and breast cancer in premenopausal women. Two earlier, relatively small studies from the Washington County Cohort (Wysowski *et al.*, 1987; Helzlsouer *et al.*, 1994) reported no differences in estradiol concentrations between cases and controls (over the whole menstrual cycle). More recent, slightly larger studies (Rosenberg *et al.*, 1994; Thomas *et al.*, 1997b; Kabuto *et al.*, 2000) have suggested that estradiol concentrations may be higher in cases than controls. In one study it was noted that the difference in estradiol between cases and controls was greatest for women sampled during the mid-part of the menstrual cycle (Thomas *et al.*, 1997b).

Together, these five prospective studies included only 225 women who developed breast cancer after blood collection, and few conclusions can be drawn from such limited data. Although premenopausal women who develop breast cancer do not appear to have grossly elevated estradiol concentrations compared with healthy individuals, it remains unclear whether moderately higher levels of estradiol are associated with an increased breast cancer risk.

Insulin-like growth factor-I

Insulin-like growth factor-I (IGF-I) is a polypeptide hormone which, like estradiol, acts to stimulate cell growth and inhibit cell death in many tissue types, including normal and diseased breast tissue. Two prospective studies have investigated the association between circulating IGF-I concentration and breast cancer risk. These studies have both found a relatively high IGF-I concentration, either as absolute concentrations or relative to levels of its main binding protein, IGF binding protein-3, to be associated with an approximately twofold increased risk of breast cancer in premenopausal women but not in postmenopausal women (Hankinson *et al.*, 1998b; Toniolo *et al.*, 2000). Further data are needed on this possible association of IGF-I with breast cancer risk and on whether the effect of obesity on breast cancer risk may be partly due to the effects of insulin on the bioavailability of IGF-I (Kaaks & Lukanova, 2001).

Prolactin

Prolactin is a polypeptide hormone which is essential for mammary gland development and lactation. Four prospective studies have examined the association between serum prolactin concentration and breast cancer risk, and three have observed an increase in risk with increasing prolactin levels, although this was only statistically significant in the largest study by Hankinson *et al.* (Wang *et al.*, 1992; Hankinson *et al.*, 1999; Kabuto *et al.*, 2000); the small study of Helzlsouer *et al.* observed no association (Helzlsouer *et al.*, 1994). Further data are needed on the possible association of prolactin with breast cancer risk.

Conclusions

Among postmenopausal women, breast cancer risk is strongly related to the serum concentration of estradiol. High risk is also associated with relatively high concentrations of other sex hormones. Mechanistic arguments suggest that estradiol is likely to be the most important hormone in determining risk, but the epidemiological data are currently insufficient to establish this. There are relatively few data for premenopausal women; the data available are inconclusive but are compatible with the hypothesis that breast cancer risk is increased by relatively high estradiol concentrations in premenopausal women. Other sex hormones and IGF-I may also play important roles. To clarify these relationships, the Endogenous Hormones and Breast Cancer Collaborative Group has been established to conduct pooled analyses of prospective studies of endogenous hormones and breast cancer risk.

References

Barrett-Connor, E., Friedlander, N.J. & Khaw, K.-T. (1990) Dehydroepiandrosterone sulfate and breast cancer risk. *Cancer Res.*, **50**, 6571–6574

Berrino, F., Muti, P., Micheli, A., Bolelli, G., Krogh, V., Sciajno, R., Pisani, P., Panico, S. & Secreto, G. (1996) Serum sex hormone levels after menopause and subsequent breast cancer. *J. Natl. Cancer Inst.*, **88**, 291–296

Cauley, J.A., Lucas, F.L., Kuller, L.H., Stone, K., Browner, W. & Cummings, S.R. (for the Study of Osteoporotic Fractures Research Group) (1999) Elevated serum estradiol and testosterone concentrations are associated with a high risk for breast cancer. *Ann. Int. Med.*, **130**, 270–277

Dorgan, J.F., Longcope, C., Stephenson, H.E. Jr., Falk, R.T., Miller, R., Franz, C., Kahle, L., Campbell, W.S., Tangrea, J.A. & Schatzkin, A. (1996) Relation of prediagnostic serum estrogen and androgen levels to breast cancer risk. *Cancer Epidemiol. Biomarkers Prev.*, **5**, 533–539

Dorgan, J.F., Stanczyk, F.Z., Longcope, C., Stephenson, H.E., Jr., Chang, L., Miller, R., Franz, C., Falk, R.T. & Kahle, L. (1997) Relationship of serum dehydroepiandrosterone (DHEA), DHEA sulfate, and 5-androstene-3β,17β-diol to risk of breast cancer in postmenopausal women. *Cancer Epidemiol. Biomarkers Prev.*, **6**, 177–181

Garland, C.F., Friedlander, N.J., Barrett-Connor, E. & Khaw, K-T. (1992) Sex hormones and postmenopausal breast cancer: a prospective study in an adult community. *Am. J. Epidemiol.*, **135**, 1220–1230

Gordon, G.B., Bush, T.L., Helzlsouer, K.J., Miller, S.R. & Comstock, G.W. (1990) Relationship of serum levels of dehydroepiandrosterone and dehydro epiandrosterone sulfate to the risk of developing postmenopausal breast cancer. *Cancer Res.*, **50**, 3859–3862

Hankinson, S.E., Willett, W.C., Manson, J.E., Colditz, G.A., Hunter, D.J., Spiegelman, D., Barbieri, R.L. & Speizer, F.E. (1998a) Plasma sex steroid hormone levels and risk of breast cancer in postmenopausal women. *J. Natl. Cancer Inst.*, **90**, 1292–1299

Hankinson, S.E., Willett, W.C., Colditz, G.A., Hunter, D.J., Michaud, D.S., Deroo, B., Rosner, B., Speizer, F.E. & Pollak, M. (1998b) Circulating concentrations of insulin-like growth factor-I and risk of breast cancer. *Lancet*, **351**, 1393–1396

Hankinson, S.E., Willett, W.C., Michaud, D.S., Manson, J.E., Colditz, G.A., Longcope, C., Rosner, B. & Speizer, F.E. (1999) Plasma prolactin levels and subsequent risk of breast cancer in postmenopausal women. *J. Natl. Cancer Inst.*, **91**, 629–634

Helzlsouer, K.J., Gordon, G.B., Alberg, A.J., Bush, T.L. & Comstock, G.W. (1992) Relationship of prediagnostic serum levels of dehydroepiandrosterone and dehydroepiandrosterone sulfate to the risk of developing premenopausal breast cancer. *Cancer Res.*, **52**, 1–4

Helzlsouer, K.J., Alberg, A.J., Bush, T.L., Longcope, C., Gordon, G.B. & Comstock, G.W. (1994) A prospective study of endogenous hormones and breast cancer. *Cancer Detection Prev.*, **18**, 79–85

Kaaks, R. & Lukanova, A. (2001) Energy balance and cancer: the role of insulin and insulin-like growth factor-I. *Proc. Nutr. Soc.*, **60**, 1–16

Kabuto, M., Akiba, S., Stevens, R.G., Neriishi, K., & Land, C.E. (2000) A prospective study of estradiol and breast cancer in Japanese women. Cancer *Epidemiol. Biomarkers Prev.*, **9**, 575–579

Kelsey, J.L. (1979) A review of the epidemiology of human breast cancer. *Epidemiol. Rev.*, **1**, 74–109

Key, T.J. & Pike, M.C. (1988) The role of oestrogens and progestagens in the epidemiology and prevention of breast cancer. *Eur. J. Cancer. Clin. Oncol.*, **24**, 29–43

Key, T.J., Allen, N.E., Verkasalo, P.K. & Banks, E. (2001) Energy balance and cancer: the role of sex hormones. *Proc. Nutr. Soc.*, **60**, 81–89

Pike, M.C., Spicer, D.V., Dahmoush, L. & Press, M.F. (1993) Estrogens, progestogens, normal breast cell proliferation, and breast cancer risk. *Epidemiol. Rev.*, **15**, 17–35

Rosenberg, C.R., Pasternack, B.S., Shore, R.E., Koenig, K.L. & Toniolo, P.G. (1994) Premenopausal estradiol levels and the risk of breast cancer: a new method of controlling for day of the menstrual cycle. *Am. J. Epidemiol.*, **140**, 518–525

Siiteri, P.K. & MacDonald, P.C. (1973) Role of extraglandular estrogen in human endocrinology. In: Geiger, S.R., Astwood, E.B. & Greep R.O., eds. *Handbook of Physiology*, Vol 2, Washington D.C., American Physiological Society, pp. 615–629

Thomas, H.V., Key, T.J., Allen, D.S., Moore, J.W., Dowsett, M., Fentiman, I.S. & Wang, D.Y. (1997a) A prospective study of endogenous serum hormone concentrations and breast cancer risk in postmenopausal women on the island of Guernsey. *Br. J. Cancer*, **76**, 401–405

Thomas, H.V., Key, T.J., Allen, D.S., Moore, J.W., Dowsett, M. Fentiman, I.S. & Wang, D.Y. (1997b) A prospective study of endogenous serum hormone concentrations and breast cancer risk in premenopausal women on the island of Guernsey. *Br. J. Cancer*, **75**, 1075–1079

Toniolo, P.G., Levitz, M., Zeleniuch-Jacquotte, A., Banerjee, S., Koenig, K.L., Shore, R.E., Strax, P. & Pasternack, B.S. (1995) A prospective study of endogenous estrogens and breast cancer in postmenopausal women. *J. Natl. Cancer Inst.*, **87**, 190–197

Toniolo, P., Bruning, P.F., Akhmedkhanov, A., Bonfrer, J.M., Koenig, K.L., Lukanova, A., Shore, R.E. , Zeleniuch-Jacquotte, A. (2000) Serum insulin-like growth factor-I and breast cancer. *Int. J. Cancer*, **88**, 828–832

Wang, D.Y., De Stavola, B.L., Bulbrook, R.D., Allen, D.S., Kwa, H.G., Fentiman, I.S., Hayward, J.L. & Millis, R.R. (1992) Relationship of blood prolactin levels and the risk of subsequent breast cancer. *Int. J. Epidemiol.*, **21**, 214–221

Wysowski, D.K., Comstock, G.W., Helsing, K.J. & Lau, H.L. (1987) Sex hormone levels in serum in relation to the development of breast cancer. *Am. J. Epidemiol.*, **125**, 791–799

Zeleniuch-Jacquotte, A., Bruning, P.F., Bonfrer, J.M.G., Koenig, K.I., Shore, R.E., Kim, M.Y., Pasternack, B.S. & Toniolo, P. (1997) Relation of serum levels of testosterone and dehydroepiandrosterone sulfate to risk of breast cancer in postmenopausal women. *Am. J. Epidemiol.*, **145**, 1030–1038

Possible mechanisms relating diet to colorectal cancer risk

Bruce W.R., Giacca A., Medline A.

Departments of Nutritional Sciences, Physiology and Pathology, University of Toronto, Canada.

Introduction

The most important environmental risk factor for colorectal cancer is thought to be diet, with diets high in saturated fat and low in fruits, vegetables and fibre believed to increase risk. However, several clinical intervention trials with reduced fat and increased fibre, fruits and vegetables have failed to affect the development of colonic polyps (Schatzkin *et al.*, 2000). This suggests that our understanding of the mechanisms relating diet and colon cancer development is incomplete and that new, clearly defined hypotheses are needed, together with methods for testing them.

Recent developments in epidemiology, experimental carcinogenesis, metabolic and membrane physiology, and tumour genetics suggest that diet composition can affect colon cancer risk through two quite different physiological mechanisms (Bruce *et al.*, 2000a). In the first, dietary excess, through the process of insulin resistance, increases circulating insulin and energy sources and provides a proliferative stimulus that increases cancer risk. In the second, dietary deficiencies and excesses, through processes affecting epithelial permeability, expose focal areas of the colon to intraluminal growth factors and to inflammatory agents which increase proliferation and mutation, and thereby cancer risk. Both mechanisms explain a wide range of epidemiological and experimental data. However, at this time both must be considered hypotheses, with new approaches to cancer prevention studies required.

The insulin resistance mechanism

A highly palatable, energy-dense diet, which is high in fat and low in dietary fibre, may provide insufficient satiety and therefore excess energy for individuals with a sedentary lifestyle (Drewnowsky, 1998). The consequences of consumption of excess calories are that circulating levels of glucose, triglycerides and non-esterified fatty acids (NEFAs) tend to increase, with β-cell production of insulin increasing to reduce circulating glucose. Energy substrates increase in muscle, liver and fat cells. With their accumulating energy, these organs begin to display a resistance to the effect of insulin. As a result, circulating levels of insulin, triglycerides and NEFAs become even more elevated. Thus a full-blown picture of hyperinsulinemia/insulin resistance develops and all the cells in the body are exposed to higher levels of insulin and energy substrates (DeFronzo *et al.*, 1991). In this setting, colonic cells may be more likely to proliferate and suffer oxidative damage. These effects increase the possibility for initiation and promotion of colon cancer (Bruce *et al.*, 2000b).

Many epidemiological studies have shown association of colon cancer risk with levels of insulin and triglyceride (Bruce *et al.*, 2000a). This may merely reflect a concomitant association, since the risk factors for colon cancer and insulin resistance or type 2 diabetes are similar. Both are positively associated with diets that provide excess calories and with lifestyles that are sedentary. Both are also associated with increased levels of saturated fatty acids and perhaps deficiencies of essential fatty acids.

Experimental animal studies, however, suggest that elevated insulin and/or energy substrates are on the pathway between diet and cancer. The first of these studies was made using rats given a colon carcinogen, azoxymethane. Treatment of these animals with exogenous insulin resulted in larger aberrant crypt foci (ACF), putative precursors of colon cancer (Corpet *et al.*, 1997), and increased number and frequency of tumours (Tran *et al.*, 1996), a result consistent with the proposed mechanism but not conclusive, since exogenous insulin has many dietary, hormonal and metabolic effects.

Dietary studies with carcinogen-treated animals provide further support for the importance of insulin resistance in colon carcinogenesis. They show that diets, which increase energy consumption, also increase the degree of both measures of insulin resistance and colonic tumour promotion (Koohestani *et al.*, 1998). Compared with the control diet, a calorie-restricted diet decreased, while a high-fat or cafeteria diet increased glucose intolerance, as measured by area under the glucose tolerance curve. Similarly, calorie-restricted diets decreased and calorie-excess diets increased the growth of ACF. These results are thus consistent with the proposed mechanism.

Experimental studies with infused insulin and energy substrates allow a more specific test of possible mechanisms. Such studies permit separate measure of the effect of insulin, glucose and fatty acids on the colonic epithelium. Early results with this approach indicate that insulin by itself can increase proliferation of colonic epithelial cells. Fatty acids with insulin may increase this effect. Insulin could also have promotional effects through a reduction of apoptosis, and the effects of insulin may be mediated in part through increased levels of free IGFs or increased intracellular energy.

The effects of insulin and energy substrates on colonic cells have not been systematically studied *in vitro*; however, insulin has been shown to stimulate DNA and RNA synthesis (Cezard *et al.*, 1981) and insulin and glucose have been shown to increase reactive oxygen species (ROS) in HT29 colon adenocarcinoma cells (Giulivi & Cadenas, 1998). Studies with other epithelial cell lines have demonstrated possible links of both insulin and energy pathways with epithelial cell proliferation (Bjjork, 1993; Hardy 2000). *In vitro* studies with colonic cells may be particularly valuable for elucidating pathways involving pharmacological agents, which affect insulin resistance.

The genetic properties of human tumours may provide evidence relating to their origin. Many tumours have increased IGF and insulin receptors (Singh & Rubin, 1993). Most show evidence of defects in cell cycle control (Weinstein *et al.*, 1997). These observations are consistent with the proposed insulin resistance mechanism outlined above.

The focal inflammation mechanism

A high-risk diet may increase colonic permeability focally, affecting tight junctions (TJs) between epithelial colonocytes. Some dietary factors increase TJ permeability, while others produce a decrease. The focal increase in colonic permeability exposes the basal and lateral surfaces of adjacent epithelial cells and the cells of the lamina propria to agents in the luminal environment. This includes locally produced growth factors, which can be at high concentration in the lumen (Mullin, 1997). It also includes toxic agents that induce inflammation. Both growth factors and products of inflammation can increase proliferation, affect rates of apoptosis and mutations, thereby increasing the possibility for epithelial cell carcinogenesis. The cycle of increased permeability and inflammation can be perpetuated. Inflammation can further increase colonic permeability and mutations can reduce the effectiveness of TJ closure.

Epidemiological studies support an association between colonic inflammation and colon cancer risk. Colon cancer risk is markedly increased in inflammatory bowel disease (IBD), especially ulcerative colitis and the geographic pattern of risk for IBD and colorectal cancer are similar (Sandler & Eisen, 2000). Recent Norwegian studies with the granulocyte marker protein, calprotectin, also support such an association. Granulocytes are the definitive marker of acute inflammation. Since calprotectin resists breakdown by colonic bacteria, its presence in faeces indicates the presence of an acute inflammatory process in the gastrointestinal tract. The levels of calprotectin in faeces have been measured with an enzyme-linked immunosorbent assay (ELISA) reliably and reproducibly, in 100-mg samples of faeces (Tøn *et al.*, 2000). Such assays have been used in assessing the status and prognosis of IBD. They have also been used to screen for colorectal cancers and polyps (Tibble *et al.*, 2001). Granulocyte marker protein is elevated in faeces of carcinogen-treated rats before the appearance of colonic polyps (Kristinsson *et al.*, 1999). It is also likely the case in human colon carcinogenesis as calprotectin levels are frequently found to be elevated even after the removal of polyps and cancers. These observations are consistent with an association of colon carcinogenesis and colonic inflammation.

At least one component in the diet can affect colonic inflammation. Oral sodium phosphate, as used in the colonic preparation prior to colonoscopy, has been shown repeatedly to induce aphthous ulcers and focal inflammation in the colon approximately 1 day after administration in some patients (Driman & Preiksaitis, 1998). The levels of phosphate used were larger than daily intake of phosphate in the diet and, in the diet, phosphate is usually accompanied by calcium with which it interacts, reducing the concentration of free phosphate (Newmark *et al.*, 1984). Indeed, there is no reported clinical or epidemiological evidence that high concentrations of phosphate represent an increased colon cancer risk in humans. However, diets high in phosphate and low in calcium act as promoters in carcinogen-treated animals (Wargovich *et al.*, 1990) and similar diets, with other potential risk factors associated with the Western diet, produce evidence of hyperproliferation and a small number of tumours in animals not treated with carcinogen (Yang *et al.*, 2001). Furthermore, a recent intervention study found that supplementary calcium reduced the recurrence of colonic polyps (Baron *et al.*, 1999). Supplemental calcium may counter the effect of the large excess of phosphate in meats, leavened breads and potatoes of some diets.

Calcium has been known for more than 30 years to have a striking effect on *in vitro* models of colonic epithelium. In these models epithelial cells are grown to confluence on permeable fibres in specially constructed chambers that allow for the separate control of the basal and apical (or luminal) surfaces of the cells. The TJs of epithelial cells normally form a seal to separate the luminal from basolateral spaces and also act as a "fence", separating the apical from the basal and lateral surfaces of each epithelial cell. The closure of TJs is markedly affected by the calcium concentration on the basal surface (Ma *et al.*, 2000). With decreased calcium, TJs open. With normal calcium, TJs quickly close in a process referred to as the fast calcium switch. Phorbol esters and many other factors can have effects similar to reduced calcium and the study of the molecular biology underlying these phenomena has become an important area of physiological investigation. These investigations have shown that the closure of TJs critically depends on the function of adhesion molecules, including cadherin (Troxell *et al.*, 1999). Open TJs can allow the passage of large molecules such as epidermal growth factor (EGF) and presumably other growth factors from the luminal surface, through the epithelial layer (Mullin *et al.*, 1998). The *in vitro* model of epithelial cell growth may appear rather artificial. However, tight junctions can be identified in colonic epithelium. Macromolecules labelled with heavy metals are excluded by normal epithelium but penetrate through the TJs between epithelial cells in at least some polyps and apparently all cancers (Soler *et al.*, 1999).

A large number of experimental animal studies have examined the effect of dietary supplements and additives on carcinogenesis. Rats and mice have been given a colon carcinogen and the effect of dietary supplements on the yield of subsequent tumours has been observed (Bruce *et al.*, 2000a). Protective effects have been noted with a wide range of additives, in addition to the aforementioned effect of calcium in a high-phosphate diet. Clear protection has been observed with folic acid given to animals receiving a folic-acid-deficient diet, with non-steroidal anti-inflammatory drugs, with n-3 fatty acids, with pre- and probiotics, with the demulcent, polyethylene glycol MW8000, and with a large group of phytochemicals that are thought to reduce inflammation. We have noted that these additives could each inhibit the pathway to inflammation in the colon by reducing colonic epithelial permeability and the degree and toxic effects of focal inflammation (Bruce *et al.*, 2000a).

Most human adenomatous polyps and colon tumours have mutations of the APC gene, known to affect cadherin activity and the closure of TJs (Troxell *et al.*, 1999). This observation is consistent with the proposition that these mutations are selected for during the process of repeated opening and closing of TJs by dietary factors.

Possible tests of the mechanisms

A clear prediction of the dietary excess/insulin resistance hypothesis is that dietary or pharmacological interventions that reduce insulin resistance and the level of insulin will impede the process of colon carcinogenesis. The expected reduction of colon carcinogenesis must follow a demonstration of the control of insulin levels by dietary or pharmacological methods. That is, it is first necessary to identify a particular intervention that reduces hyperinsulinemia/insulin resistance before it is possible to determine if this intervention reduces carcinogenesis. On the basis of the model we have presented here, hyperinsulinemia/insulin resistance might be reduced in several ways:

- By increasing the satiety of food to reduce dietary energy intake.
- By increasing energy expenditure to reduce the excess available.
- By diverting fat to adipocytes through the action of peroxisome proliferator agonist receptor (PPAR) γ activators, thereby reducing triglycerides in muscle and liver.

If such strategies succeed in reducing insulin, the intervention(s) could be tested for colon carcinogenesis. Presumably, this could be done by observing the effect of the intervention on ACF size observed *in vivo*, or through effects on colonic polyp recurrences.

A clear prediction of the increased permeability/focal inflammation hypothesis is that a dietary or pharmacological intervention that decreases colonic permeability or inhibits focal colonic inflammation will reduce colon carcinogenesis. As with the insulin resistance hypothesis, this expectation is conditional. That is, it is first necessary to identify a particular intervention that reduces colonic inflammation before it is possible to assess the effectiveness of the intervention in reducing carcinogenesis. Again, on the basis of the model we have presented here, colonic inflammation might be reduced in several ways:

- By increasing dietary calcium, or reducing dietary phosphate, to reduce the possibility of TJ opening with resultant colonic permeability.
- By providing factors in the diet that increase the osmotic pressure of the faecal stream and the tension on epithelial cell membranes and junctions (Parnaud *et al.*, 2001).
- By inhibiting the process of inflammation directly to reduce the effect of inflammatory products on

epithelial permeability and the possibility of a continuing inflammatory process.

If such strategies are successful in reducing colonic inflammation, the intervention(s) could be tested for effect on colon carcinogenesis, again by observing ACF number and size *in vivo* or through effects on colonic polyp recurrences.

The two-step approach to testing mechanisms has several advantages over more prolonged studies applied directly on colon carcinogenesis: clinical trials to reduce hyperinsulinemia/insulin resistance and to reduce colonic inflammation. Studies focused on processes that increase colon cancer risk could be completed in less time and with less expense than studies directed at the longer-term goal with carcinogenesis endpoints. Finally, combined interventions that reduce insulin resistance and focal colonic inflammation could be tested for their effects on colon carcinogenesis to add to the understanding of the overall process of colon carcinogenesis and its prevention.

Acknowledgements

The mechanisms we have proposed are, of course, based the work of many earlier investigators. We thank especially Gail Eyssen, Thien Tran, Jim Mullin, Denis Corpet and Sol Rabinovich for their continued support and perspective in our attempt to integrate this array of work. We thank the Cancer Research Society for continued support.

References

Baron, J.A., Beach, M., Mandel, J.S., van Stolk, R., Haile, R., Sandler, R., Rothstein, R., Summers, R., Snover, D., Beck, G., Bond, J. & Greenberg, E. (1999) Calcium supplements for the prevention of colorectal adenomas. Calcium Polyp Prevention Study Group. *N. Engl. J. Med.*, **340**, 101–107

Bjjork, J., Nilsson, J., Hultcranz, R. & Johansson, C. (1993) Growth-regulatory effects of sensory neuropeptides, epidermal growth factor, insulin and somatostatin on non-transformed intestinal epithelial cell line IEC-6 and colon cancer cell line HT 29. *Scand. J. Gastroenterol.*, **28**, 879–884

Bruce, W.R., Giacca, A. & Medline, A. (2000a) Possible mechanisms relating diet and risk of colon cancer. *Cancer Epidemiol. Biomarkers and Prev.*, **9**, 1271–1279

Bruce, W.R., Wolever, T.M.S. & Giacca, A. (2000b) Mechanisms linking diet and colorectal cancer: the possible role of insulin resistance. *Nutr. Cancer*, **37**, 19–26

Cezard, J.P., Forgue-Lafitte, M.E., Chamblier, M.C. & Rosselin, G.E. (1981) Growth-promoting effect, biochemical activity, and binding of insulin in human intestinal cancer cells in culture. *Cancer Res.*, **41**, 1148–1153

Corpet, D.E., Jacquinet, C., Peiffer, G. & Tache, S. (1997) Insulin injections promote the growth of aberrant crypt foci in the colon of rats. *Nutr. Cancer*, **27**, 316–320

DeFronzo, R.A. & Ferrannini, E. (1991) Insulin resistance: a multifaceted syndrome responsible for NIDDM, obesity, hypertension, dyslipidemia, and atherosclerotic cardiovascular disease. *Diabetes Care*, **14**, 173–194

Drewnowski, A. (1998) Energy density, palatability, and satiety: implications for weight control. *Nutr. Rev.*, **56**, 347–353

Driman, D.K. & Preiksaitis, H.G. (1998) Colorectal inflammation and increased cell proliferation associated with oral sodium phosphate bowel preparation solution. *Hum. Pathol.*, **29**, 972–978

Giulivi, C. & Cadenas, E. (1998) Extracellular activation of fluorinated aziridinylbenzoquinone in HT29 cells EPR studies. *Chem. Biol. Interact.* **5**, 191–204

Hardy, S., Langelier, Y. & Prentki, M. (2000) Oleate activates phospatidylinositol 3-kinase and promotes proliferation and reduces apoptosis of MDA-MB-231 breast cancer cells, whereas palmatate has the opposite effects. *Cancer Res.*, **60**, 6353–6358

Koohestani, N., Chia, M.C., Pham, N.-A., Tran, T.T., Minkin, S., Wolever, T.M.S. & Bruce, W.R. (1998) Aberrant crypt focus promotion and glucose intolerance: correlation in the rat across diets differing in fat, *n*-3 fatty acids and energy. *Carcinogenesis*, **19**, 1679–1684

Kristinsson, J., Røseth, A.G., Sundseth, K., Nygaard, K., Løberg, M., Paulsen, J.E., Aadland, E. & Fagerhol, M.K. (1999) Granulocyte marker protein is increased in stool from rats with azoxymethane-induced colon cancer. *Scand. J. Gastroenterol.*, **34**, 1216–1223

Ma, T.Y., Tran, D., Hoa, N., Nguyen, D., Merryfield, M. & Tarnawski, A. (2000) Mechanism of extracellular calcium regulation of intestinal epithelial tight junction permeability: role of cytoskeletal involvement. *Microsc. Res. Tech.*, **51**, 156–168

Mullin, J.M. (1997) Potential interplay between luminal growth factors and increased tight junction permeability in epithelial carcinogenesis. *J. Exp. Zool.*, **279**, 484–489

Mullin, J.M., Ginanni, N. & Laughlin, K.V. (1998) Protein kinase C activation increases transepithelial transport of biologically active insulin. *Cancer Res.*, **58**, 1641–1645

Newmark, H.L, Wargovich, M.J. & Bruce, W.R. (1984) Colon cancer and dietary fat, phosphate and calcium: a hypothesis. *J. Natl. Cancer Inst.*, **72**, 1323–1325

Parnaud, G., Corpet, D.E. & Gamet-Payrastre, L. (2001) Cytostatic effect of polyethylene glycol on human colonic adenocarcinoma cells. *Int. J. Cancer*, **92**, 63–60

Sandler, R.S. & Eisen, G.M. (2000) Epidemiology of inflammatory bowel disease. In: Kirsner, B., ed, *Inflammatory Bowel Disease*, 5th ed, Philadelphia, W.B. Saunders Company, pp 89–112

Schatzkin, A., Lanza, E., Corle, D., Lance, P., Iber, F., Caan, B., Shike, M., Weissfeld, J., Burt, R., Cooper, R., Kikendall, W. & Cahill, J. (2000) Lack of effect of a low-fat, high-fiber diet on the recurrence of colorectal cancer. *N. Eng. J. Med.*, **342**, 1149–1155

Singh, P. & Rubin, N. (1993) Insulin-like growth factors and binding proteins in colon cancer. *Gastroenterology*, **105**, 1218–1237

Soler, A.P., Miller, R.D., Laughlin, K.V., Carp, N.Z., Klurfeld, D.M. & Mullin, J.M. (1999) Increased tight junctional permeability is associated with the development of colon cancer. *Carcinogenesis*, **20**, 1425–1431

Tibble, J., Sigthorsson, G., Foster, R., Sherwood, R., Fagerhol, M. & Bjarnason, I. (2001) Faecal calprotectin and faecal occult blood tests in the diagnosis of colorectal carcinoma and adenoma. *Gut*, **49**, 402–408

Tøn, H., Brandnes, Ø., Dale, S., Holtlund, J., Skuibina, E., Schønsby, H. & Johne, B. (2000) Improved method for calprotectin. *Clin. Chim. Acta*, **292**, 41–54

Tran, T.T., Medline, A. & Bruce W.R. (1996) Insulin promotion of colon tumors in rats. *Cancer Epidemiol. Biomarkers Prev.*, **5**, 1013–1015

Troxell, M.L., Chen, Y.-T., Cobb, N., Nelson, W.J. & Marrs, J.A. (1999) Cadherin function in junctional complex rearrangement of post-translational control of cadherin expression. *Am. J. Physiol.*, **276** *Cell Physiol.*, **45**, C404–C418

Wargovich, M.J., Allnutt, D., Palmer, C., Anaya, P. & Stephens, L.C. (1990) Inhibition of the promotional phase of azoxymethane-induced colon carcinogenesis in the F344 rat by calcium lactate: effect of simulating two human nutrient density levels. *Cancer Lett.*, **53**, 17–25

Weinstein, B.I., Begeman, M., Zhou, P., Han, K.-H., Sgambato, A., Doki, Y., Arber, N., Ciaparrone, M. & Yamamoto, H. (1997) Disorders in cell circuitry associated with multistage carcinogenesis: exploitable targets for cancer prevention and therapy. *Clin. Cancer Res.*, **3**, 2696–2702

Yang, K.A., Liu, Y., Shinozaki, H., Fan, K., Yan, H., Newmark, H., Steele, L., Kopelovich, L., Kelloff, G.L. & Lipkin M. (2000) Western-style diet induces intestinal adenomas and carcinomas in normal C57BL/6 mice without carcinogen exposure. *Proc. Am. Assoc. Cancer Res.*, **41**, 476 (Abstract)

Androgenic hormones and prostate cancer risk: status and prospects

Gann P.H.

Northwestern University Medical School, Chicago, IL, USA

Prostate cancer is the most common potentially life-threatening cancer diagnosed among men in Western countries today. The relationship of androgen hormone levels to risk of developing prostate cancer has been an important focus of investigation since the Nobel Prize-winning work of Charles Huggins several decades ago, which demonstrated the effectiveness of castration in the treatment of advanced disease (Lytton, 2001). The issue is relevant to nutrition research, because it is clear from migrant studies that some feature or features of the environment affect prostate cancer risk on the population level and because it is plausible that some degree of the variation in hormone levels between individuals is attributable to dietary differences. Hence the effects of hormones and diet on prostate cancer risk are likely to be inter-related. Despite significant advances in both laboratory technique and knowledge of the underlying biology, the major questions remain unresolved, and thus opportunities for primary prevention are not yet available. The aim of this paper is to briefly review the evidence linking androgens to prostate cancer risk, critically discuss the obstacles faced by past and current research, and present several promising new areas of study.

Nonepidemiological evidence relating androgen levels to prostate cancer risk

Prostate cancer requires a sufficient level of androgens in order to develop. Research thus far in culture systems, animal models and clinical observation has been unable to determine whether this relationship is merely facultative or more subtle variations between men are determinants of risk. The prostate gland needs a constant supply of androgens to develop and maintain itself. Apart from the findings concerning the effect of androgen deprivation on existing cancers, males with a rare inherited defect in 5α-reductase synthesis have small, underdeveloped prostate glands (Thigpen *et al.*, 1992). This enzyme is responsible for the conversion of testosterone to dihydrotestosterone (DHT), which is believed to be the most important intraprostatic androgen. Many literature sources also state that eunuchs (males castrated before or soon after puberty) do not develop prostate cancer. It is more accurate to state, based on limited observation, that eunuchs have underdeveloped glands. Castration was practiced in Imperial China to produce palace guards and in Italy to produce opera singers with unique vocal qualities. But these practices were ended long before cohorts of eunuchs could be observed by modern methods of scientific observation. In 1960, 26 surviving elderly eunuchs in Beijing were examined and all were found to have either non-palpable or very small prostates (Ping & Fang-Liu, 2001).

Studies of cultured prostate cancer cells demonstrate a dose-dependent relationship of androgen to three major processes involved in prostate carcinogenesis: proliferation, differentiation and apoptosis. The dog is the only animal besides man in which prostate cancer is known to occur spontaneously, except in rare instances. Nonetheless, some rodent models for prostate cancer have been informative regarding the role of androgens. Adenocarcinoma of the prostate can be induced in several strains of rat by exogenous testosterone alone, and more strongly by testosterone combined with estrogen (Bosland *et al.*, 1995). Interestingly, concurrent stimulation of cell proliferation by hormonal treatment appears to increase the ability of chemical carcinogens to induce prostate cancer in the rat. It is important to note that the tumour-promoting effects of androgens in these models are quite potent; they can be observed with only a twofold to threefold sustained increase in plasma testosterone (Bosland *et al.*, 1995). This is well within the amount of variation seen in human populations.

For example, in a population of 1418 men aged 28–40 years, we recently observed an approximately threefold difference in serum testosterone between the upper and lower quartile means (unpublished data).

Epidemiologic evidence

The following is a brief summary; several more extensive reviews have been published recently (Eaton *et al.*, 1999; Bosland, 2000; Hsing, 2001; Kaaks *et al.*, 2001). Numerous case–control studies on the relationship of circulating hormone levels to prostate cancer were published from the 1960s through the 1980s, in what might be considered Phase 1 of epidemiological research in this area. These studies had several serious limitations: sample sizes were often small and controls were often selected based on convenience rather than representativeness of the source population for cases. Most importantly, blood samples were collected after diagnosis, which could introduce bias due to the effect of disease on hormone levels, rather than vice-versa. Apart from the suggestion that hormone metabolism could be affected by the stress and lifestyle changes that accompany a diagnosis of cancer, there is evidence to suggest that androgen levels at diagnosis are affected by disease. Men with prostate cancer have increased clearance of androgens and lower levels of androgens at diagnosis are associated with increased stage and an unfavorable prognosis (Harper *et al.*, 1987; Meikle *et al.*, 1987).

The second phase of epidemiological research involves prospective studies, usually with a case–control design, nested within a defined cohort. Approximately 8–10 such studies were conducted during the 1990s. All of these studies evaluated total testosterone and several also measured DHT, 3α-androstanediol glucuronide (a major intraprostatic DHT metabolite) and sex hormone-binding globulin (SHBG). Only one study, which we conducted within the Physicians' Health Study cohort, observed a clear relationship between androgen levels and prostate cancer risk (Gann *et al.*, 1996). In this analysis, which was the largest to date with 222 cases and 390 controls, total testosterone and SHBG were very weakly associated with prostate cancer risk (testosterone positively and SHBG inversely) when evaluated separately. However, as other investigators have observed, there was a substantial correlation between testosterone and SHBG levels (r=0.6), due to the servomechanism operating within the hypothalamic–pituitary axis. Because of this correlation and because androgen bound to SHBG is presumed to be biologically inactive, the results for testosterone and SHBG are mutually confounding. When these analytes were simultaneously adjusted, strong linear associations were apparent (again, positive for testosterone and inverse for SHBG). Two recent prospective studies have attempted to replicate these findings with respect to simultaneous adjustment for testosterone and SHBG. One, conducted with the cohort of male smokers participating in the Finnish antioxidant trial, found no associations with or without adjustment (Dorgan *et al.*, 1998). The other, which used serum collected in another Finnish cohort from 1966 to 1972, found no associations when all 24 years of follow-up were included (Heikkila *et al.*, 1999). However, when the first 8 years of follow-up were excluded, there was evidence for a positive association for testosterone (SHBG-adjusted), with an odds ratio of 2.0 in the highest versus lowest quintile, and a trend across quintiles with a P value of 0.06.

Clearly, further prospective studies such as these are warranted. Several methodological issues will have to be addressed in order to avoid biased results, as listed in Table 1.

Since DHT is most likely a more important androgen than testosterone in the prostate, it would appear important to measure DHT in the circulation. However, blood levels of DHT are strongly influenced by production of DHT in the skin and elsewhere, from the action of type I 5α-reductase. Moreover, DHT is rapidly metabolized to androstanediol, which contributes to a predictably poor correlation between DHT levels in the blood and prostate. Investigators have measured 3α-androstanediol glucuronide as a surrogate for DHT, and although it has a longer half-life in blood than DHT and has been used to identify the presence of clinical disorders affecting DHT metabolism, it can also be produced in tissues other than the prostate (Kaaks *et al.*, 2001).

Protein binding of androgens in the blood presents another challenge. Ideally, one could measure testosterone

Table 1. Methodological limits of second phase, prospective studies on circulating androgens and prostate cancer risk

1. Uncertainty regarding the "active" forms of androgen and lack of consensus regarding how to handle protein binding.
2. The relationship of blood-to-tissue levels of androgens is largely unknown.
3. Potential problems with sample integrity with frozen storage over long periods.
4. Difficulty maintaining assay reproducibility, especially when assaying many batches of samples.
5. Consistency of hormone level over time not well understood; single measures could be a poor reflection of levels at distant time points.
6. Androgen exposure might be more important during certain age periods in life.

in at least two of its three circulating forms: free, albumin-bound, and SHBG-bound. However, assays for free and SHBG-bound testosterone require relatively large amounts of serum or plasma that are often not available in precious archived samples. Calculation of the amount of testosterone in each compartment, using information on the binding constant of testosterone for each protein as well as hormone and protein concentrations has been suggested. In some cases, albumin levels are assumed to be constant, since these do not vary greatly and have little effect on bioavailability due to the weak binding of androgens to albumin. There are surprisingly few data on the correspondence between these calculated values and directly measured ones and hence the suitability of these estimates is open to question (Vermeulen *et al.*, 1999). For the moment, the most accurate and efficient method for considering the effects of SHBG binding on testosterone effects might be simultaneous adjustment using mathematical models.

It is clear that androgen levels within the prostate are more germane than those in the circulation. Given the presence of androgen-metabolizing enzymes with the prostate, serum–tissue discrepancies would not be surprising. There are data indicating that although testosterone and DHT levels decline with aging, they do not necessarily decline in the prostate, particularly in the stromal as opposed to the epithelial compartment (Kreig *et al.*, 1993). Unfortunately, we do not have good methods at present for measuring the amounts of intraprostatic androgen or the specific effects of androgen action. Liquefying tissue samples and relating hormone concentrations to measures of total protein or DNA are not very accurate. Improvement of such methods would provide a great boost.

Most steroid hormones are fairly robust in frozen storage. However, the integrity of samples frozen for very long periods, particularly at temperatures warmer than –70°C, is a concern. In one of the prospective studies mentioned earlier, samples were stored for more than 25 years at –20°C. Storage integrity of proteins such as SHBG is of even greater concern. Our laboratory and others have observed that frequent or rapid thawing of samples can reduce the amount of SHBG measurable by immunoassays. Maintaining immunoassay reproducibility for hormones is not a simple task, especially when large numbers of samples are assayed for epidemiological research. Reproducibility errors can result from factors such as the sticking of steroids to glass or plastic ware, low activity for radioactive or fluorescent tracers, use of a new antibody lot, and inaccurate standard curves. Studies should always strive to minimize the effects of interbatch variance by assaying cases and matched control samples in the same batch. In addition, reproducibility results from identical masked quality control samples, which are indistinguishable from subject samples, are an important method for assessing inter- and intrabatch variability. In our laboratory, we observed a sudden 35% drop in values for SHBG from identical QC samples and were eventually able to trace this to a change in the source of SHBG standards used for development of the standard curves.

Table 2. Consistencv of testosterone and SHBG levels over time: two serum samples, 3 years apart, CARDIA Male Hormone Study

	N, pairs	Var_W	Var_B	R	95% CI, *r*
Total testosterone					
Black	622	1.42	2.19	0.60	0.52–0.67
White	796	0.93	2.25	0.71	0.64–0.76
All	1418	1.14	2.24	0.66	0.59–0.72
SHBG					
Black	622	41.15	129.57	0.76	0.71–0.80
White	796	36.09	137.57	0.80	0.75–0.83
All	1418	38.22	134.17	0.78	0.73–0.82

CARDIA, Coronary Artery Risk Development in Young Adults; Var_W and Var_B, variance within and between persons; *r*, Pearson correlation coefficient; CI, confidence interval.

Only one of the prospective studies conducted to date was able to measure hormone levels at more than one time point, and that study had only 16 cases (Carter *et al.*, 1995; Pearson *et al.*, 1996). Indeed, we have had surprisingly little information on the consistency of androgen levels within the same man over time, yet this can contribute substantially towards attenuation of risk estimates in studies utilizing only a single measure. We recently obtained the following data (Table 2) from the CARDIA Male Hormone Study, which illustrate the correlation among Black and white men aged 28–40 for measurements of total testosterone and SHBG, with samples taken 3 years apart.

Both measurements were obtained in the same assay run. The within-person correlations are somewhat reassuring, yet they indicate the potential for serious attenuation in estimating relatively modest risks. The timing of androgen measurement during the life cycle must also be considered. While it is well known that prostate cancer occurs primarily within ageing men whose androgen levels are declining, androgen levels much earlier in life might affect risk, even during the period *in utero* when imprinting of developing tissues can occur (Ekbom *et al.*, 1996).

Emerging opportunities for future research: genetics, structural biology and androgen action

Several areas of research show promise for developing new insights into the role of hormones in the etiology of prostate cancer, including identification of genetic polymorphisms that could affect androgen action, studies on the determinants of androgen levels and new findings in structural biology and the molecular mechanisms of androgen action. Development of methods for high-throughput genotyping has created an explosion in the amount of information available on human genetic variation. Many prostate cancer investigators have recognized the potential importance of studying polymorphisms among genes involved in the synthesis, action and metabolism of androgens (Ross *et al.*, 1999). While we are still in the early phase of this research, it is well advised to identify several challenges that lie on the road ahead.

First, we do not know which genes are important. Any examination of androgen synthesis and metabolic pathways can reveal a discrete number of obvious candidate genes, but the actual number of potentially relevant genes could be far greater. If, for example, unsuspected genes influence expression of an enzyme involved in the pathway, we have the possibility of an almost unlimited number of relevant genetic variants as the causal web moves outward. Second, within each candidate gene, we are not sure how many polymorphisms exist nor which of them might be functionally significant. The studies required to determine functional significance can be very costly, and perhaps represent a major bottleneck in the research effort. Third, adequate planning and interpretation of epidemiological studies on polymorphisms related to hormone action require specification of plausible gene–hormone interaction models. For example, in the case of CYP17, an enzyme involved in the early steps of steroid biosynthesis, hormone levels would represent an *intervening* variable between the polymorphism and its effect on prostate cancer risk and thus no real interaction could be predicted. In other cases, the genetic and hormonal factors both could bear on a common pathway, which would lead to an additive prediction for joint effects. An example of this could be the effects of a hormone and a gene on a single factor: activation of the androgen receptor. Truly multiplicative interactions have the potential to affect risk most strongly, but these should be specified in advance to the extent possible.

We already know, based on the degree of clustering of prostate cancer within families, that single gene effects and simple Mendelian inheritance will not explain a large percentage of prostate cancer incidence. This means that gene–gene and gene–environment interactions are essential, and not merely *en vogue*. These interactions could easily be beyond second order, i.e. involve more than two factors, leading to an exponential growth in exposure categories. Given this, plus the near certainty that the main effects of any polymorphism on risk are likely to be very small (particularly in genetically heterogeneous populations), we have a situation that demands very large study sizes and an enormous problem with multiple comparisons. These problems apply for the candidate gene approach to research, much less the genomic or anonymous gene approach, for which the problems would be even more constraining. There is even the possibility – taking pessimism to the extreme – that no identifiable set of genetic and hormonal interactions will explain a meaningful proportion of cases. These challenges notwithstanding, research in this area is likely to progress to the extent that it exploits emerging information regarding the biology of prostate cancer.

As stated earlier, interindividual and interpopulation differences in androgen levels are real and substantial. An indirect but potentially useful research strategy is to identify the determinants (both genetic and environmental) of androgen levels and then look for associations between these determinants and prostate cancer risk. Studies aimed at determining the relationship of body size, diet and physical activity to androgen action are of interest, particularly if they include longitudinal measurements at various ages. Finally, new information from molecular and structural biology is likely to have a profound effect on the way we think about androgen action. Changes in mRNA and protein expression that result from androgen exposure to normal prostate tissue are beginning to be elucidated. This could create important opportunities for epidemiologists to develop biomarkers that reflect the proximal effects of androgen in the prostate. For example, gene expression scans have led to the identification of calreticulin as a molecule that is strongly up-regulated by androgens in few tissues except the prostatic epithelium (Zhu *et al.*, 1998). The early model of androgen action that involves primarily a ligand and a receptor is rapidly giving way to a far more complex model, one that allows numerous entry points for influences on androgen action whether receptor-mediated or not. Elaboration of proteins involved in key signal transduction pathways provides just one example.

Structural biologists have solved the three-dimensional structures of two crucial molecules – androgen receptor and SHBG – just within the past two years (Grishkovskaya *et al.*, 2000; Sack *et al.*, 2001). These discoveries will inevitably lead to new hypotheses regarding the regulation of androgen action, and thus new testable hypotheses concerning the role of androgens in prostate cancer etiology.

In conclusion, the hypothesis that interindividual differences in androgen levels affect prostate cancer risk remains viable but not yet established. Research to date has taught us what some of the most important current methodological challenges are. Ongoing basic research is providing us with an ever-expanding array of tools and hypotheses. The finasteride trial for primary prevention of prostate cancer, which will report its results in several years, could by itself provide a major proof-of-principle for the hypothesis (Thompson *et al.*, 1997). Resolution of the hormone-prostate cancer question will have a profound influence on how we approach primary prevention of prostate cancer. It will also affect policies regarding the use of androgen supplements, which are now used by millions of men in the U.S. – with or without medical supervision – since the topical gel form was approved for use in 2000 (Anonymous, 2000).

References

[Anonymous] (2000) Androgel. *Med. Lett. Drugs Ther.*, **42**, 49–51

Bosland, M.C. (2000) The role of steroid hormones in prostate carcinogenesis. *Journal of the National Cancer Institute Monographs*, **27**, 39–66

Bosland, M.C., Ford, H. & Horton, L. (1995) Induction at high incidence of ductal prostate adenocarcinomas in NBL/Cr and Sprague-Dawley Hsd:SD rats treated with a combination of testosterone and estradiol-17 beta or diethylstilbestrol. *Carcinogenesis*, **16**, 1311–1317

Carter, H.B., Pearson, J.D., Metter, E.J., Chan, D.W., Andres, R., Fozard, J.L., Rosner, W. & Walsh, P.C. (1995) Longitudinal evaluation of serum androgen levels in men with and without prostate cancer. *Prostate*, **27**, 25–31

Dorgan, J.F., Albanes, D., Virtamo, J., Heinonen, O.P., Chandler, D.W., Galmarini, M., McShane, L.M., Barrett, M.J., Tangrea, J. & Taylor, P.R. (1998) Relationships of serum androgens and estrogens to prostate cancer risk: results from a prospective study in Finland. *Cancer Epidemiol. Biomarkers Prev.*, **7**, 1069–1074

Eaton, N.E., Reeves, G.K., Appleby, P.N. & Key, T.J. (1999) Endogenous sex hormones and prostate cancer: a quantitative review of prospective studies. *Br. J. Cancer*, **80**, 930–934

Ekbom, A., Hsieh, C.C., Lipworth, L., Wolk, A., Ponten, J., Adami, H.O. & Trichopoulos, D. (1996) Perinatal characteristics in relation to incidence of and mortality from prostate cancer. *BMJ*, **313**, 337–341

Gann, P.H., Hennekens, C., Ma J., Longcope, C. & Stampfer, M.J. (1996) A prospective study of sex hormone levels and risk of prostate cancer. *J. Natl. Cancer Inst.*, **88**, 1118–1126

Grishkovskaya, I., Avvakumov, G.V., Sklenar, G., Dales, D., Hammond, G.L. & Muller, Y.A. (2000) Crystal structure of human sex hormone-binding globulin: steroid transport by a laminin G-like domain. *EMBO J*, **19**, 504–512

Harper, M.E., Wilson, D.W., Jensen, H.M., Pierrepoint, C.G. & Griffiths, K. (1987) Steroid hormone concentrations in relation to patient prognosis and prostate tumour grade. *J. Steroid Biochem.*, **27**, 521–524

Heikkila, R., Aho, K., Heliovaara, M., Hakama, M., Marniemi, J., Reunanen, A. & Knekt, P. (1999) Serum testosterone and sex hormone-binding globulin concentrations and the risk of prostate carcinoma: a longitudinal study. *Cancer*, **86**, 312–315

Hsing, A.W. (2001) Hormones and prostate cancer: what's next? *Epidemiol. Rev.*, **23**, 42–58

Kaaks, R., Lukanova, A. & Sommersberg, B. (2001) Plasma androgens, IGF-1, body size, and prostate cancer risk: a synthetic review. *Prostate Cancer Prostatic Dis.*, **3**, 157–172

Krieg, M., Nass, R. & Tunn, S. (1993) Effect of aging on endogenous level of 5 alpha-dihydrotestosterone, testosterone, estradiol, and estrone in epithelium and stroma of normal and hyperplastic human prostate. *J. Clin. Endocrinol. Metab.*, **77**, 375–381

Lytton, B. (2001) Prostate cancer: a brief history and the discovery of hormonal ablation treatment. *J. Urol.*, **165**, 1859–1862

Meikle, A.W., Smith, J.A. & Stringham, J.D. (1987) Production, clearance, and metabolism of testosterone in men with prostatic cancer. *Prostate*, **10**, 25–31

Pearson, J.D., Luderer, A.A., Metter, E.J., Partin, A.W., Chan, D.W., Fozard, J.L. & Carter, H.B. (1996) Longitudinal analysis of serial measurements of free and total PSA among men with and without prostatic cancer. *Urology*, **48**, 4–9

Ping, W.C. & Fang-Liu, G. (2001) The prostate in eunuchs, In: *Urological Oncology, Reconstructive Surgery, Organ Conservation, and Restoration of Function.* Chichester, UK, Wiley., pp. 249–255

Ross, R.K., Coetzee, G.A., Pearce, C.L., Reichardt, J.K., Bretsky, P., Kolonel, L.N., Henderson, B.E., Lander, E., Altshuler, D. & Daley, G. (1999) Androgen metabolism and prostate cancer: establishing a model of genetic susceptibility. *Eur. Urol.*, **35**, 355–361

Sack, J.S., Kish, K.F., Wang, C., Attar, R.M., Kiefer, S.E., An, Y., Wu, G.Y., Scheffler, J.E., Salvati, M.E., Krystek, S.R. Jr., Weinmann, R. & Einspahr, H.M. (2001) Crystallographic structures of the ligand-binding domains of the androgen receptor and its T877A mutant complexed with the natural agonist dihydrotestosterone. *Proc. Natl. Acad. Sci. U S A*, **98**, 4904–-4909

Sodergard, R., Backstrom, T., Shanbhag, V. & Carstensen, H. (1982) Calculation of free and bound fractions of testosterone and estradiol-17 beta to human plasma proteins at body temperature. *J. Steroid Biochem.*, **16**, 801–810

Thigpen, A.E., Davis, D.L., Gautier, T., McGinley, J.I. & Russell, D.W. (1992) The molecular basis of steroid 5α-reductase deficiency in a large Domincan kindred. *N. Engl. J. Med.*, **327**, 1216–1219

Thompson, I.M., Coltman, C.A.J. & Crowley, J. (1997) Chemoprevention of prostate cancer: the Prostate Cancer Prevention Trial. *Prostate*, **33**, 217–221

Vermeulen, A., Verdonck, L. & Kaufman, J.M. (1999) A critical evaluation of simple methods for the estimation of free testosterone in serum. *J. Clin. Endocrinol. Metab.*, **84**, 3666–3672

Zhu, N., Pewitt, E.B., Cai, X., Lang, S., Chen, R. & Wang, Z. (1998) Calreticulin: an intracellular Ca^{++}-binding protein abundantly expressed and regulated by androgen in prostatic epithelial cells. *Endocrinology*, **139**, 4337–4344

Nutrition, energy balance and colon cancer risk: the role of insulin and insulin-like growth factor-I

Kaaks R.

International Agency for Research on Cancer, Lyon, France.

Introduction

Age-adjusted incidence and mortality rates of colon cancer are many times higher in Western, industrialized societies than in rural Africa or Asia. Strong international correlations between age-standardized incidence or mortality rates and estimated per capita availabilities of foods and nutrients suggest that a Western type of diet – characterized by high intakes of total and saturated fats, meat, and refined carbohydrates – predisposes to colon cancer development. In addition, colon cancer risk is directly related to measures of obesity such as body mass index (BMI) or the ratio of waist-to-hip circumferences (WHR), and relates inversely to physical activity levels. Finally, colon cancer risk has also been found to be associated with adult body height, a marker of growth rates, and indirectly of nutrition, during childhood.

This paper reviews the background and epidemiological evidence for recent theories which stipulate that a Western nutritional lifestyle may increase colon cancer through increases in plasma and tissue levels of insulin and/or as insulin-like growth factor (IGF)-I.

Effects of insulin and IGF-I on cell proliferation, apoptosis, and tumour development

The development of tumours is thought to result from an imbalance between cellular differentiation, proliferation and programmed death (apoptosis), allowing the clonal selection and multiplication of cells that have accumulated somatic mutations in pro-oncogenes and tumour-suppressor genes, making them independent of normal growth control. Hormones and growth factors play a key role in regulating cellular growth control. Among various peptide growth factors involved, insulin, IGF-I and IGF-binding proteins (IGFBPs) are of special interest, as their concentrations in plasma and tissues are intricately related to nutritional status.

Insulin and IGF-I both stimulate the proliferation, and inhibit apoptotis, of normal and neoplastic cells (Jones & Clemmons, 1995; Werner & LeRoith, 1996), including those of the colonic mucosa (Singh & Rubin, 1993). Colon cancer tissue has receptors for both insulin and IGF-I (Guo *et al.*, 1992; MacDonald *et al.*, 1993). Signal transduction pathways mediating the effects of insulin on gene expression and mitosis include the activation of the *ras* oncogen (Burgering *et al.*, 1989; Burgering *et al.*, 1991), which plays a central role in colon carcinogenesis.

IGF-I bioactivity within tissues is modulated by IGFBPs, which may either enhance or inhibit binding of IGF-I to its receptors (Jones & Clemmons, 1995). In addition, some of the IGF-binding proteins may exert growth regulating effects through their own specific binding sites on the cell membrane. For example, IGFBP-3 has been shown to inhibit cellular proliferation and to enhance apoptosis through binding with specific IGFBP-3 binding sites (Jones & Clemmons, 1995; Rajah *et al.*, 1997).

Nutritional determinants of plasma insulin and IGF-I bioactivity

Nutritional determinants of insulin levels

Chronically elevated plasma insulin levels, also in the fasting state, occur when tissues (especially skeletal muscle and liver) have a diminished sensitivity to the physiological actions of insulin.

Insulin resistance is a frequent phenomenon in Western populations. It is partially a consequence of increased hepatic and muscular uptake and oxidation of fatty acids (Randle, 1995) which, in turn, is related to a rise in plasma concentrations of free fatty acids. Another metabolic factor in the circulation that causes insulin resistance and that is also partially derived from adipose tissue is tumour-necrosis factor alpha (TNF-alpha). The development of insulin resistance is thus strongly related to obesity (Reaven, 1988). Nevertheless, insulin resistance is also observed in relatively high proportions of adult men and women with normal weight for height, but with some increase in intra-abdominal fat stores.

Physical activity improves insulin sensitivity and decreases plasma insulin (Mayer *et al.*, 1998). In sedentary subjects, physical activity can improve insulin sensitivity within days and thus independently of any substantial changes in body weight. Over the longer term, physical activity can also improve insulin sensitivity by preventing or reducing obesity.

In addition to insulin resistance, the consumption of foods rich in refined carbohydrates that are rapidly digested and absorbed, elicits elevated glycemic and insulinemic responses. It is possible that especially at such postprandial concentrations, insulin provides a direct stimulus to the development of colon tumours. Furthermore, there is some evidence from cross-sectional and prospective cohort studies that over the long term, the consumption of foods rich in rapidly digestible carbohydrates may also contribute to the development of insulin resistance (Feskens & Kromhout, 1990).

The IGF-I/IGFBP system

The bioactivity of IGF-I within tissues is determined partially by total plasma concentrations of IGF-I and of its major plasmatic binding proteins (IGFBPs), and partially also by the local production of IGF-I and IGFBPs within tissues (Thissen *et al.*, 1994; Jones & Clemmons, 1995). At least six different IGFBPs have been identified so far (Jones & Clemmons, 1995). Most of IGF-I and IGFBPs circulating in plasma is produced in the liver. Over 80% of IGF-I in plasma is complexed with IGFBP-3 plus another glycoprotein, called acid-labile subunit (ALS), and most of the remaining fraction is bound to the other IGFBPs in blood. IGFBP-3 has a very high affinity for IGF-I and the large IGF-I/IGFBP-3/ALS complex cannot pass through the capillary barrier to target tissues. IGFBP-5 has an even higher affinity than IGFBP-3 for IGF-I, and also forms a complex with ALS. The IGFBPs -1, -2, -4 and -6 have lower binding affinities for IGF-I, do not bind ALS, and are small enough to cross the endothelial barrier (Jones & Clemmons, 1995). Among the six or more IGFBPs, the IGFBPs -1, -2 and -3 appear to be most strongly dependent on nutritional status.

Nutritional determinants of IGF-I bio-activity

Growth hormone (GH) provides the primary stimulus for the production of IGF-I and of its major plasmatic binding protein (IGFBP-3), in liver and many other tissue types (Thissen *et al.*, 1994; Jones & Clemmons, 1995). Besides GH, insulin plays a central role in regulating levels of IGF-I and IGFBPs. Insulin improves GH sensitivity of tissues by increasing hepatic GH-receptor levels (Baxter & Turtle, 1978; Mercado & Baumann, 1995) and by enhancing cellular uptake of amino acids for protein (Thissen *et al.*, 1994). Furthermore, insulin reduces concentrations of IGFBP-1 by acute inhibition of its synthesis in liver and other tissues and is also inversely related to levels of IGFBP-2 (Nam *et al.*, 1997). Thus, situations in which endogenous insulin synthesis is low, such as prolonged fasting, chronic malnutrition, but also insulin-dependent diabetes mellitus (IDDM), all cause a decrease in GH receptor levels, resistance to the GH stimulation of IGF-I synthesis, reductions in plasma IGF-I and IGFBP-3, and rises in plasma levels of GH, IGFBP-1 and IGFBP-2. In addition, these situations are related to decreased levels of plasma free IGF-I, a small fraction of IGF-I in blood plasma that is not bound to any IGF-binding protein (Nam *et al.*, 1997). By contrast, situations of chronic hyperinsulinemia, such as obesity, but also non-insulin-dependent diabetes mellitus (NIDDM), are related to reduced levels of IGFBP-1 and IGFBP-2, an increase in free plasma IGF-I, and a reduction in plasma GH. Plasma total IGF-I levels, however, either remain stable (in mildly obese subjects) or decrease only slightly (in more severely obese subjects). The reduction in GH levels in obese and insulin-resistant subjects may be explained by an increased negative feedback on pituitary GH secretion by free IGF-I (Chapman *et al.*, 1998) and by an increased sensitivity to GH, and thus a reduction in GH requirements for synthesis of a given amount of IGF-I (Thissen *et al.*, 1994).

The decreases in absolute plasma IGF-I concentrations, both in conditions of chronic malnutrition (a severe decrease in IGF-I) and obesity (a more modest decrease), suggest a nonlinear relationship between body energy reserves and IGF-I levels. In well-nourished men and women, cross-sectional studies have indeed shown such a nonlinear relationship between BMI and IGF-I levels, with peak levels of IGF-I around a BMI of 25–26 (Kaaks *et al.*, 2001). In addition to energy balance, the intake of animal protein may stimulate IGF-I synthesis, as reflected lower IGF-I levels in vegans compared to lacto/ovo vegetarians and meat eaters (Allen & Key, 2001; Kaaks *et al.*, 2001).

Plasma insulin and colon cancer risk

The insulin-colon cancer hypothesis derives from several lines of evidence. First, as discussed above, experimental studies have shown that insulin can enhance tumour development, either directly by acting itself as a growth factor or indirectly by increasing the biological activity of IGFs. Second, the insulin-colon cancer hypothesis integrates most observations of potential nutritional risk factors for colon cancer, many of the risk factors for colon cancer, including sedentariness, obesity, and high intakes of refined carbohydrates, have also been related to increases in fasting and non-fasting plasma insulin. Based on these various observations, both McKeown-Eyssen (McKeown, 1994) and Giovannucci (Giovannucci, 1995) postulated independently that colon cancer development may be promoted by elevated fasting or postprandial plasma insulin levels (insulin hypothesis).

Indirect epidemiological evidence supporting the insulin hypothesis comes from studies showing an increase in colorectal cancer incidence and mortality in subjects with elevated fasting or post-challenge plasma glucose concentrations (McKeown, 1994; Giovannucci, 1995; Schoen *et al.*, 1999), which is a correlate of insulin resistance and fasting and non-fasting plasma insulin levels. In addition, several studies, but not all, have shown an increased risk of colon cancer in diabetics who, although being glucose-intolerant, generally have high endogenous production and plasma levels of insulin (McKeown, 1994; Giovannucci, 1995; Hu *et al.*, 1999).

More direct evidence for the insulin hypothesis comes from at least two prospective cohort studies. The first of these showed an approximately twofold increase in colorectal cancer risk in men and women who had elevated plasma insulin concentrations 2 hours after having taken a standard oral dose of glucose (Schoen *et al.*, 1999). The second study, in New York women, showed an approximate fourfold increase in colon cancer risk comparing subjects in the top and bottom quartiles of serum C-peptide (Kaaks *et al.*, 2000), a marker of pancreatic insulin secretion. In the latter study, colon cancer risk was also inversely related to serum levels of IGFBP-1 and IGFBP-2, two IGF-binding proteins that generally have lower levels in subjects with comparatively elevated plasma insulin.

Plasma IGF-I and colon cancer risk

Epidemiological studies have shown a direct association of colon cancer risk with body height, which may reflect levels of IGF-I during puberty and adolescence. Furthermore, patients with acromegaly – a pathology due to a GH excess and associated with elevated IGF-I levels – have an increased risk of developing colonic polyps and colon cancer (Giovannucci, 1995). In two case–control studies (Giovannucci *et al.*, 2000; Renehan *et al.*, 2001), the presence of large and high-risk colorectal adenomas, but not of small adenomas, was found to be associated with more elevated IGF-I levels, compared to adenoma-free controls. These observations, plus the known effects of nutritional energy balance on IGF-I levels, lead to the speculation that elevated total plasma IGF-I might be a risk factor for colon cancer (IGF-I hypothesis).

At least three cohort studies (Ma *et al.*, 1999; Kaaks *et al.*, 2000; Giovannucci *et al.*, 2000) have shown mild, statistically nonsignificant increases in risk with increasing plasma or serum levels of total IGF-I. In two of the three studies (Ma *et al.*, 1999; Giovannucci *et al.*, 2000), but not in the third, the risk showed a much stronger and statistically significant increase in relation to IGF-I after adjustment for circulating levels of IGFBP-3. In a fourth study (Palmqvist *et al.*, 2001), absolute plasma IGF-I unadjusted for IGFBP-3 was directly and significantly associated with colon cancer risk but, unexpectedly, showed an inverse (but statistically nonsignificant) association with risk of rectal cancer. Finally, in one case–control study (Manousos *et al.*, 1999), colorectal cancer risk was associated positively with IGF-I and inversely with IGFBP-3, although neither of these relationships reached statistical significance.

Conclusions

Traditional theories about mechanisms relating nutrition to colon cancer risk have focused mostly on effects of diet on the exposure of the colonic mucosa to mutagenic or tumour-promoting compounds within the lumen. Such compounds may be of endogenous origin, for example, bile acids, converted by the colonic microflora into secondary and tertiary bile acids with tumour-promoting activity (Weisburger, 1991) or of exogenous origin such as heterocyclic aromatic amines or polycyclic hydrocarbons formed in meat during grilling or frying (Sugimura & Sato, 1983). A limitation of these theories is that they do not provide an explanation for the associations of colon cancer risk with excess body weight and lack of physical activity.

The present review presents preliminary evidence in favour of complementary theories suggesting that colon cancer risk may be related to chronically elevated insulin levels, as well as to increased levels of IGF-I, either as absolute concentrations or relative to levels of IGFBP-3, IGF's major plasmatic binding protein. The evidence presented, however, is not entirely consistent across studies (e.g., associations with absolute IGF-I concentrations, or only with levels of IGF-I adjusted for IGFBP-3) and requires confirmation from further prospective cohort studies.

Further studies are also needed to better understand the relationships between levels of IGF-I and its various binding proteins in blood plasma and within tissues. It is believed that a decrease in plasma IGFBP-3, with a transfer of IGF-I to IGFBP-1 or IGFBP-2, will result in greater availability of circulating IGF-I to tissues. Decreases in plasma IGFBP-1 or -2 (leading to an increase in plasma free IGF-I) are also believed to increase the bioavailability of IGF-I. In addition, IGFBP-3 itself is believed to exert proapoptotic and antimitogenic effects via its own receptor, thus antagonizing the effects of IGF-I (Thissen *et al.*, 1994; Jones & Clemmons, 1995). Further studies are needed to confirm these various hypotheses and to show possible relationships between levels of circulating IGF-I and IGFBPs and indices of cell proliferation and/or apoptosis within the colonin mucosa and other tissues.

References

Allen, N.E. & Key, T.J. (2001) Re: plasma insulin-like growth factor-1, insulin-like growth factor-binding proteins, and prostate cancer risk: a prospective study. *J. Natl. Cancer Inst.*, **93**, 649–651

Baxter, R.C. & Turtle, J.R. (1978) Regulation of hepatic growth hormone receptors by insulin. *Biochem. Biophys. Res. Commun.*, **84**, 350–357

Burgering, B.M., Medema, R.H., Maassen, J.A., van-de, W.M., van-der, E.A., McCormick, F. & Bos, J.L. (1991) Insulin stimulation of gene expression mediated by p21ras activation. *EMBO J.*, **10**, 1103–1109

Burgering, B.M., Snijders, A.J., Maassen, J.A., van-der, E.A. & Bos, J.L. (1989) Possible involvement of normal p21 H-ras in the insulin/insulinlike growth factor 1 signal transduction pathway. *Mol. Cell. Biol.*, **9**, 4312–4322

Chapman, I.M., Hartman, M.L., Pieper, K.S., Skiles, E.H., Pezzoli, S.S., Hinyz, R.L. & Thorner, M.O. (1998) Recovery of growth-hormone release from suppression by exogenous insulin-like growth factor I (IGF-I): evidence for a suppressive action of free rather than bound IGF-I. *J. Clin. Endocrinol. Metab.*, **83**, 2836–2842

Feskens, E.J. & Kromhout, D. (1990) Habitual dietary intake and glucose tolerance in euglycaemic men: the Zutphen Study. *Int. J. Epidemiol.*, **19**, 953–959

Giovannucci, E. (1995) Insulin and colon cancer. *Cancer Causes Control*, **6**, 164–179

Giovannucci, E., Pollak, M.N., Platz, E.A., Willett, W.C., Stampfer, M.J., Majeed, N., Colditz, G.A., Speizer, F.E. & Hankinson, S.E. (2000) A prospective study of plasma insulin-like growth factor-I and binding protein-3 and risk of colorectal neoplasia in women. *Cancer Epidemiol. Biomarkers Prev.*, **9**, 345–349

Guo, Y.S., Narayan, S., Yallampalli, C. & Singh, P. (1992) Characterization of insulinlike growth factor I receptors in human colon cancer. *Gastroenterology*, **102**, 1101–1108

Hu, F.B., Manson, J.E., Liu, S., Hunter, D., Colditz, G.A., Michels, K.B., Speizer, F.E. & Giovannucci, E. (1999) Prospective study of adult onset diabetes mellitus (type 2) and risk of colorectal cancer in women. *J. Natl. Cancer Inst.*, **91**, 542–547

Jones, J.I. & Clemmons, D.R. (1995) Insulin-like growth factors and their binding proteins: biological actions. *Endocr. Rev.*, **16**, 3–34

Kaaks, R., Soderberg, S., Olsson, T., Hallmans, G. & Stattin, P. (2001) Response: re plasma insulin-like growth factor-1, insulin-like growth factor-binding proteins, and prostate cancer risk: a prospective study. *J. Natl. Cancer Inst.*, **93**, 650–651

Kaaks, R., Toniolo, P., Akhmedkhanov, A., Lukanova, A., Biessy, C., Dechaud, H., Rinaldi, S., Zeleniuch-Jacquotte, A., Shore, R.E. & Riboli, E. (2000) Serum C-peptide, insulin-like growth factor (IGF)-1, IGF-binding proteins, and colorectal cancer risk in women. *J. Natl. Cancer Inst.*, **92**, 1592–1600

Ma, J., Pollak, M.N., Giovannucci, E., Chan, J.M., Tao, Y., Hennekens, C.H. & Stampfer, M.J. (1999) Prospective study of colorectal cancer risk in men and plasma levels of insulin-like growth factor (IGF)-1 and IGF-binding protein-3. *J. Natl. Cancer Inst.*, **91**, 620–625

MacDonald, R.S., Thornton, W.H. Jr. & Bean, T.L. (1993) Insulin and IGE-1 receptors in a human intestinal adenocarcinoma cell line (CACO-2): regulation of Na+ glucose transport across the brush border. *J. Recept. Res.*, **13**, 1093–1113

Manousos, O., Souglakos, J., Bosetti, C., Tzonou, A., Chatzidakis, V., Trichopoulos, D., Adami, H.O. & Mantzoros, C. (1999) IGF-I and IGF-II in relation to colorectal cancer. *Int. J. Cancer*, **83**, 15–17

Mayer, D.E., D'Agostino, R., Karter, A.J., Haffner, S.M., Rewers, M.J., Saad, M. & Bergman, R.N. (1998) Intensity and amount of physical activity in relation to insulin sensitivity: the Insulin Resistance Atherosclerosis Study. *JAMA*, **279**, 669–674

McKeown, E.G. (1994) Epidemiology of colorectal cancer revisited: are serum triglycerides and/or plasma glucose associated with risk? *Cancer Epidemiol. Biomarkers Prev.*, **3**, 687–695

Mercado, M. & Baumann, G. (1995) Characteristics of the somatotropic axis in insulin-dependent diabetes mellitus. *Arch. Med. Res.*, **26**, 101–109

Nam, S.Y., Lee, E.J., Kim, K.R., Cha, B.S., Song, Y.D., Lim, S.K., Lee, H.C. & Huh, K.B. (1997) Effect of obesity on total and free insulin-like growth factor (IGF)-1, and their relationship to IGF-binding protein (BP)-1, IGFBP-2, IGFBP-3, insulin, and growth hormone. *Int. J. Obes. Relat. Metab. Disord.*, **21**, 355–359

Palmqvist, R., Hallmans, G., Rinaldi, S., Biessy, C., Stenling, R., Riboli, E. & Kaaks, R. (2002) Plasma IGF-I, IGF-binding protein-3 and risk of colorectal cancer: a prospective study in northern Sweden. *Gut*, **50**, 642–646

Rajah, R., Valentinis, B. & Cohen, P. (1997) Insulin-like growth factor (IGF)-binding protein-3 induces apoptosis and mediates the effects of transforming growth factor-beta1 on programmed cell death through a p53- and IGF-independent mechanism. *J. Biol. Chem.*, **272**, 12181–12188

Randle, P.J. (1995) Metabolic fuel selection: general integration at the whole-body level. *Proc. Nutr. Soc.*, **54**, 317–327

Reaven, G.M. (1988) Banting lecture 1988. Role of insulin resistance in human disease. *Diabetes*, **37**, 1595-1607

Renehan, A.G., Painter, J.E., Atkin, W.S., Potten, C.S., Shalet, S.M. & O'Dwyer, S.T. (2001) High-risk colorectal adenomas and serum insulin-like growth factors. *Br. J. Surg.*, **88**, 107–113

Schoen, R.E., Tangen, C.M., Kuller, L.H., Burke, G.L., Cushman, M., Tracy, R.P., Dobs, A. & Savage, P.J. (1999) Increased blood glucose and insulin, body size, and incident colorectal cancer. *J. Natl. Cancer Inst.*, **91**, 1147–1154

Singh, P. & Rubin, N. (1993) Insulinlike growth factors and binding proteins in colon cancer. *Gastroenterology*, **105**, 1218–1237

Sugimura, T. & Sato, S. (1983) Mutagens-carcinogens in foods. *Cancer Res.*, **43**, 2415S–2421S

Thissen, J.P., Ketelslegers, J.M. & Underwood, L.E. (1994) Nutritional regulation of the insulin-like growth factors. *Endocr. Rev.*, **15**, 80–101

Weisburger, J.H. (1991) Causes, relevant mechanisms, and prevention of large bowel cancer. *Semin. Oncol.*, **18**, 316–336

Werner, H. & LeRoith, D. (1996) The role of the insulin-like growth factor system in human cancer. *Adv. Cancer Res.*, **68**, 183–223

The effect of diet on serum insulin-like growth-factor-I and its main binding proteins

Allen N.E.[1], Appleby P.N.[1], Davey G.K.[1], Key T.J.[1], Rinaldi S.[2], Kaaks R.[2]

[1]Imperial Cancer Research Fund, Cancer Epidemiology Unit, Oxford, UK. [2]International Agency for Research on Cancer, Lyon, France.

Introduction

Insulin-like growth factor-I (IGF-I) is a polypeptide involved in the control of mitogenesis, cell-cycle regulation and cell survival. Prospective epidemiological studies suggest that elevated circulating levels of IGF-I, either as absolute concentrations or relative to levels of insulin-like growth factor binding protein-3 (IGFBP-3), are a risk factor for the development of several common types of cancer, including cancers of the prostate, breast, colorectum and lung (Yu and Rohan, 2000). Circulating levels of IGF-I and its main binding proteins are known to be sensitive to nutrition and energy balance, but the effect of diet on IGF-I levels in the general population have not been studied in detail. The aim of this study was to examine the nutritional determinants of serum IGF-I and its main binding proteins among a large group of meat-eaters, vegetarians and vegans.

Material and methods

Cross-sectional data were available for 696 men and 294 women participating in the Oxford arm of the European Prospective Investigation into Cancer and Nutrition (EPIC). Subjects were excluded if they had a self-reported history of cancer or were taking medication known to influence hormone levels. Equal numbers of meat-eaters, vegetarians and vegans were included in order to obtain a wide range of nutrient intakes. All participants completed a questionnaire containing questions on age, anthropometric, smoking and other lifestyle factors as well as a detailed semi-quantitative food frequency questionnaire. A 30-mL non-fasting blood sample was taken and serum concentrations of IGF-I were measured in men and serum concentrations of IGF-I and its main binding proteins (IGFBP-1, -2 and -3) were measured in women using immunoenzymatic assays.

Statistical methods

Hormone concentrations were logarithmically or square-root transformed to approximate normal distributions. Mean values of IGF-I and its main binding proteins by dietary group were compared using analysis of variance, adjusted for age, smoking (men only) and for variables associated with blood collection and analysis (batch, time of day at venipuncture, time since last eaten at venipuncture, and days between venipuncture and blood processing).

Results

The mean age was 47 years for men and 44 years for women (67% of women were premenopausal and 33% were postmenopausal). Vegetarians and vegans had a lower weight and BMI than meat-eaters. Examination of nutrient intakes showed that vegetarians and vegans had lower intakes of energy, protein, total fat, saturated and monounsaturated fatty acids, and alcohol (each as percent energy) and dietary cholesterol than meat-eaters. Conversely, vegans had higher intakes of polyunsaturated fatty acids (percent energy), polyunsaturated:saturated fatty acid ratio and non-starch polysaccharides than meat-eaters.

The mean serum IGF-I concentration was significantly lower among vegan men than meat-eaters and vegetarians after adjustment for potential confounders (Allen *et al.*, 2000). Vegan women also had a lower mean IGF-I concentration and a lower ratio of IGF-I:IGFBP-3, used as a marker of biologically active IGF-I, than meat-eaters and vegetarians. Serum IGFBP-1 and IGFBP-2 concentrations were significantly higher among vegan women than meat-eaters and vegetarians. The serum concentration of IGFBP-3 in women was similar across the three dietary groups (Allen *et al.*, submitted for publication).

Discussion

A vegan diet is associated with a lower concentration of IGF-I and ratio of IGF-I:IGFBP-3 and a higher IGFBP-1 and IGFBP-2 concentration compared with an omnivorous or vegetarian diet, suggesting that nutritional factors specific to a vegan diet are important determinants of IGF-I, IGFBP-1 and -2.

The relationship between IGF-I and its binding proteins is complex and not completely understood; however, it is thought that an increase in IGFBP-1 and -2 may lead to an increased binding of IGF-I, thus reducing the proportion of IGF-I that is biologically active (Jones and Clemmons, 1995). These results suggest that both the circulating total IGF-I and the proportion of IGF-I that is biologically available is lower among individuals who adopt a vegan diet.

The mechanisms through which a vegan diet may reduce IGF-I and increase IGFBP-1 and -2 are not known, but may be related to the reduced intake of certain essential amino acids, which may directly suppress growth hormone secretion. This may reduce hepatic production of IGF-I while boosting that of IGFBP-1 and -2 (Harp *et al.*, 1991). It is not known whether differences in insulin sensitivity between dietary groups have an effect on the production of IGF-I and IGFBP-1 (Brismar *et al.*, 1994).

These results suggest that total IGF-I and the proportion of IGF-I that is biologically active is lower among individuals who adopt a vegan diet. Future work is needed to determine the nutritional components of a vegan diet that are associated with lower IGF-I levels and whether this is associated with a subsequent reduction in cancer incidence.

References

Allen, N.E., Appleby, P.N., Davey, G.K. & Key, T.J. (2000) Hormones and diet: low insulin-like growth factor-I but normal bioavailable androgens in vegan men. *Br. J. Cancer*, **83**, 95–97

Brismar, K., Fernqvist-Forbes, E., Wahren, J. & Hall, K. (1994) Effect of insulin on the hepatic production of insulin-like growth factor-binding protein-1 (IGFBP-1), IGFBP-3, and IGF-I in insulin-dependent diabetes. *J. Clin. Endocrinol. Metabol.*, **79**, 872–878

Harp, J.B., Goldstein, S. & Phillips, L.S. (1991) Nutrition and somatomedin. XXIII. Molecular regulation of IGF-I by amino acid availability in cultured hepatocytes. *Diabetes*, **40**, 95–101

Jones, J.I. & Clemmons, D.R. (1995) Insulin-like growth factors and their binding proteins: biological actions. *Endocr. Rev.*, **16**, 3–34

Yu, H. & Rohan, T. (2000) Role of insulin-like growth factor family in cancer development and progression. *J. Nat. Cancer Inst.*, **92**, 1472–1489

Diet and postmenopausal breast cancer in Portugal

Amaral T.[1], de Almeida M.D.V.[1], Barros H.[2]

[1]Faculty of Nutrition and Food Sciences, Porto University, Rua Dr. Roberto Frias, 4200-465 Porto, Portugal.
[2]Faculty of Medicine, Porto University, Portugal.

Purpose

Breast cancer is the most common cancer in Portuguese women. Although Portugal shares some southern European food patterns, it has particular food habits. Identification of foods and nutrients associated with the risk of breast cancer could give etiological clues to the disease and allow the development of preventive strategies.

The aim of this study was to evaluate the effect of diet in the risk of breast cancer independently of the contribution of reproductive factors, tobacco, alcohol intake and other lifestyle factors.

Methods

We conducted a hospital-based case–control study in Porto between 1993 and 1996. Breast cancer cases involved 127 Portuguese Caucasian postmenopausal women with incident histologically confirmed breast cancer (median age, 64 years) consecutively admitted for treatment in the major oncology hospital in Porto. The control group consisted of 158 woman (median age, 62 years) from the same residential area, admitted consecutively for non-tumoral diseases in the major central hospital in Porto during the same period (minor general or osteoarticular surgery).

A questionnaire was used to collect data on socio-demographic characteristics, family history of breast cancer, physical activity, smoking, reproductive and medical history, anthropometry, alcohol intake and other dietary patterns.

A food frequency questionnaire (180 foods and recipes) was developed to measure food intake during the previous year and to classify the participants according to quartiles of daily intake of foods, food groups and nutrients. Trained nutritionists collected data by direct interview. We considered information about food portion sizes, obtained with visual aids, as well as about culinary methods and seasonality. Foods were converted to nutrients using the software package Microdiet® completed with Portuguese data.

Relative validity was assessed in a sample of university students and in a sample of the control group. Results showed that this food frequency questionnaire could be regarded as a reliable source of information for most nutrients (Amaral, 1998).

Cases and controls were distributed in quartiles according to the distribution of each variable of the entire study group. Food groups, foods and nutrients were adjusted for total energy intake by the residual method.

The association between the disease and possible risk factors was calculated by means of odds ratios (OR) and 95% confidence intervals (CI) in univariate analysis and adjusted using non-conditional logistic regression (OR for the highest category versus the lowest).

Results

Total energy intake was independently associated with postmenopausal breast cancer risk (Table 1). Low intake of vitamin C and vegetables and high intakes of white fish and olive oil were also significantly associated with increased breast cancer risk (Table 2). Although non-significant, high intakes of protein, monounsaturated fatty acids and cholesterol and low intake of carotenes and fibre increased breast cancer risk. Other aspects of food habits, including ethanol and alcoholic beverage intake, showed no association with increased risk.

Discussion

As various previous studies, this case–control study showed a protective effect for vitamin C and for vegetables. Our results suggest that total energy intake is more associated with the risk of breast cancer than any source of energy (total fat or types of fat, protein or total carbohydrate). The adverse effect of energy was also reflected in height, a

Table 1. Postmenopausal breast cancer risk – multivariate analysis

	OR	95% CI	*P*
Age (years)	1.06	1.02–1.09	0.002
Education (years)			
0	1.00		
1–4	1.20	0.67–2.15	0.547
≥ 5	2.76	0.86–8.88	0.088
Positive family history of breast cancer			
yes versus no	2.92	0.83–10.30	0.096
Age at first birth (years)			
Nulliparous	1.00		
≤ 21	0.64	0.26–1.57	0.326
22–25	1.06	0.44–2.51	0.903
≥ 26	1.14	0.48–2.73	0.767
Menopause–menarche (years)			
<33	1.00		
33–36	1.48	0.74–2.94	0.267
≥ 37	1.27	0.65–2.46	0.482
Height (metres)			
<1.50	1.00		
1.50–1.54	3.08	1.26–7.52	0.014
1.55–1.60	2.13	0.89–5.09	0.091
≥ 1.61	3.15	1.25–7.96	0.015
Energy intake (kcal/day)			
≤ 1223	1.00		
1224–1553	0.67	0.33–1.37	0.276
1554–1889	1.37	0.65–2.91	0.407
1890–3729	3.16	1.38–7.24	0.006
Non-removal of visible fat in meat			
Never versus ever	1.86	0.93–3.74	0.081

measure suggestive of high intakes of energy in early childhood and adolescence, and independent of memory, as found by others (Männistö *et al.*, 1996).

Cases and controls had a similar pattern in the choice of different types of cooking and seasoning fat (data not shown). Regarding the amount, we found a significant increase of the risk of breast cancer with a high intake of olive oil used in seasoning. Other studies conducted in Mediterranean countries found protection for higher intakes of olive oil (La Vecchia *et al.*, 1995; Moreno *et al.*, 1994). These discrepant results could be explained by differences in content of either protective or adverse components or in some other protective aspect of the lifestyle of these women (Simonsen *et al.*, 1998).

Conclusions

This study confirms, in a southern European population, the protective effect of vitamin C, vegetables and low levels of energy intake on the risk of breast cancer.

We found no relation of ethanol and alcoholic beverages or other dietary patterns with the risk of breast cancer.

Acknowledgements

The first author was funded by the Junta Nacional de Investigação Científica e Tecnológica – Program Ciência (BD/2223/92) and Program Praxis XXI (BD/5481/95).

References

Amaral, T. (1998) Nutritional risk in the epidemiology of breast and colo-rectal cancer. PhD Thesis. Faculty of Nutrition and Food Sciences, Porto University, Portugal

La Vecchia, C., Negri, E., Franceschi, S., Decarli, A., Giacosa, A. & Lipworth, L. (1995) Olive oil, other dietary fats, and the risk of breast cancer (Italy). *Cancer Causes Control*, **6**, 545–550

Mannisto, S., Pietinen, P., Pyy, M., Palmgren, J., Eskelinen, M. & Uusitupa, M. (1996) Body size indicators and risk of breast cancer according to menopause and estrogen receptor status. *Int. J. Cancer*, **68**, 8–13

Martin Moreno, J.M., Willet, W.C., Giorgojo, L., Banegas, J.S., Rodriguez-Artalejo, F., Fernandez-Rodriguez, J.C., Maisonnneuve, P. & Boyle, P. (1994) Dietary fat, olive oil intake and breast cancer risk. *Int. J. Cancer*, **58**, 774–780

Simonsen, N.R., Fernandez-Crehuet Navajas, J., Martin-Moreno, J.M., Strain, J.J., Huttunen, J.K., Martin, B.C., Thamm, M., Kardinaal, A.F., van't Veer, P., Kok, F.J. & Kohlmeier, L. (1998) Tissue stores of individual monounsaturated fatty acids and breast cancer: the EURAMIC study. *Am. J. Clin. Nutr.*, **68**, 134–141

Table 2. Nutrients and foods and postmenopausal breast cancer risk – multivariate analysis.

	Cases/controls (*n*)	OR[a]	95% CI
Protein (g/day)			
26.5–63.7	28/54	1.00	–
63.8–73.1	34/35	1.60	0.74–3.46
73.2–94.0	35/33	2.34	1.07–5.11
94.1–151.4	30/36	1.57	0.71–3.46
Cholesterol (mg/day)			
27.2–158.4	28/55	1.00	–
158.5–203.8	39/35	2.20	1.08–4.47
203.9–258.4	32/34	1.73	0.80–3.71
258.5–484.0	28/34	1.87	0.83–4.19
MUFA (g/day)			
4.4–11.7	29/46	1.00	–
11.8–14.4	39/39	1.98	0.95–4.13
14.5–17.5	26/38	0.91	0.41–2.03
17.6–46.7	33/35	1.50	0.70–3.32
Vitamin C (mg/day)			
27.1–78.4	39/33	1.00	–
78.5–113.5	31/40	0.76	0.35–1.64
113.6–162.5	28/33	0.56	0.25–1.27
162.6–600.5	29/52	0.46	0.22–0.96
Fibre (g/day)			
9.1–15.6	31/32	1.00	–
15.7–18.7	37/35	0.90	0.41–1.97
18.8–22.9	23/41	0.53	0.23–1.22
23.0–37.4	36/50	0.56	0.26–1.22
Carotene (μg/day)			
298.9–1975.7	36/32	1.00	–
1975.8–2897.1	37/36	0.96	0.45–2.06
2897.2–4461.9	29/38	0.78	0.36–1.71
4462.0–20 603.1	25/52	0.48	0.23–1.02
Olive oil (g/day)			
0.0–1.7	19/41	1.00	–
1.8–3.9	34/30	3.81	1.58–9.20
4.0–6.5	34/45	2.02	0.85–4.80
6.6–57.9	40/42	2.45	1.07–5.64
White fish (g/day)			
0.0–3.4	29/47	1.00	–
3.5–11.5	35/24	2.14	0.90–5.07
11.6–20.5	26/43	1.18	0.53–2.64
20.6–123.0	37/44	2.16	0.97–4.81
Vegetables (g/day)			
7.0–125.9	40/31	1.00	–
126.0–182.8	30/39	0.65	0.30–1.43
182.9–288.7	32/40	0.80	0.37–1.74
288.8–693.6	25/48	0.34	0.15–0.76

[a]Adjusted for age, education, height, age at first birth, length of exposure to endogenous estrogens, family history of breast cancer, non-removal of visible fat in meat and total energy.

Use of hormonal therapy for menopause in nine European countries

Banks E.[1], Barnes I.[1], Baker K.[1], Key T.J.[1]

(for the EPIC working group on reproductive and hormonal factors)

[1]**Imperial Cancer Research Fund, Cancer Epidemiology Unit, Gibson Building, Radcliffe Infirmary, Oxford OX2 6HE, UK.**

Introduction

Use of hormonal therapy for menopause has increased in many countries in recent years; however, large-scale comparable data on its use in European countries are lacking. This paper describes and compares patterns of use of hormonal therapy for menopause in countries participating in the European Prospective Investigation into Cancer and Nutrition (EPIC).

Study population

Cross-sectional data from 105 618 women joining EPIC at 11 centres in Britain, Denmark, Germany, Greece, Italy, The Netherlands and Spain from 1993 to 1997 were analysed.

Use of hormonal therapy in Europe

Large variations in the prevalence of current use of hormone replacement therapy (HRT) for menopause were observed between countries. Overall, the prevalence of current HRT use was around 40% in Germany, 30% in Denmark and the United Kingdom, 10%–15% in The Netherlands, Northern Italy and Northern Spain, and 2%–5% in Southern Spain, Southern Italy and Greece (Table 1). This pattern of variation in use was seen at most ages examined (Fig. 1). The prevalence of past use varied from around 5% to 16%. In almost all of the centres examined, the highest prevalences of use were seen in women aged 50–54. Relatively rapid increases in the age-adjusted prevalence of current use of HRT were seen in the United Kingdom, Northern Spain and Northern Italy from 1993 to 1997, while use in Greece decreased over this period.

The prevalence of hysterectomy without oophorectomy varied from 3% to 26% by recruitment region and the

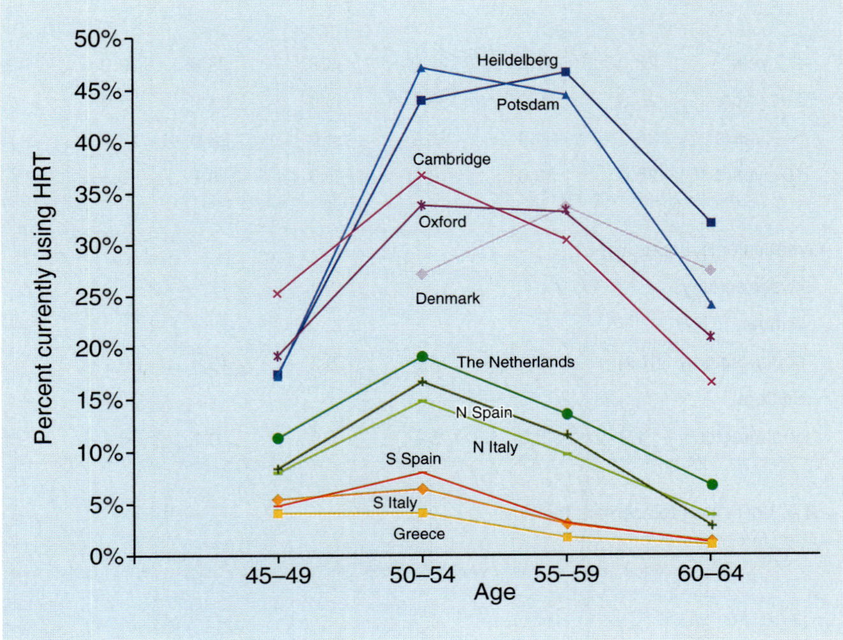

Figure 1
Use of hormonal therapy for the menopause in the EPIC cohort among women aged 50–64, 1993–1997.

Table 1. Use of hormonal therapy for menopause in the EPIC cohort among women aged 50–64, 1993–1997

	Denmark	Heidelberg	Potsdam	Cambridge	Oxford	Netherlands	N. Spain	S. Spain	N. Italy	S. Italy	Greece
	n=29484	*n*=5050	*n*=5980	*n*=7703	*n*=9514	*n*=16940	*n*=5205	*n*=4852	*n*=13262	*n*=3273	*n*=4355
	%	%	%	%	%	%	%	%	%	%	%
HRT use											
Ever user	44.8	54.6	52.7	43.2	46.1	26.3	19.3	12.8	24.1	13.9	7.3
Current user	29.0	40.7	38.6	28.1	30.3	14.3	11.5	4.5	10.3	4.4	2.1
Past user	15.8	14.0	14.2	15.1	15.8	12.0	7.8	8.3	13.9	9.5	5.2
Age at starting HRT use among ever users											
< 45	16.7	9.9	5.6	6.1	8.2	13.0	12.0	19.1	14.0	16.4	33.8
45–49	35.2	30.5	21.5	29.7	34.2	34.7	28.2	28.2	29.3	31.3	33.1
50–54	40.0	46.5	53.0	43.3	43.2	43.1	45.2	42.0	46.4	43.8	25.2
55+	8.1	13.1	19.9	20.9	14.4	9.2	14.6	10.8	10.3	8.6	7.9
Duration of HRT use among ever users											
≤ 1 year	28.0	17.6	22.2	35.8	33.8	39.0	56.1	70.1	56.2	62.2	65.0
2–4 years	25.3	29.0	38.4	33.0	31.0	33.0	33.4	23.3	29.6	26.5	20.1
5–9 years	20.3	31.4	28.9	24.0	26.0	18.7	6.7	3.7	10.7	9.2	10.2
10+ years	26.4	22.0	10.5	7.3	9.2	9.3	3.7	3.0	3.6	2.0	4.8
Gynaecological operations											
Hysterectomy without oophorectomy	10.6	26.4	13.6	16.5	16.8	20.1	3.9	3.7	7.5	4.0	3.3
Bilateral oophorectomy	4.9	5.0	8.1	5.9	6.1	4.2	10.2	9.5	5.9	9.2	8.5

HRT, hormone replacement therapy.

prevalence of oophorectomy ranged from 4% to 10% (Table 1). At all of the centres examined, current use of HRT was substantially more common among women who reported hysterectomy and/or oophorectomy than among women who had not had either of these operations (data not shown).

Comment

The data presented here suggest that large numbers of women in Europe are using hormonal therapy for menopause. Substantial variation in the prevalence of current use exists between countries in Europe, with use being more common in northern versus southern European centres. However, it should be noted that the methods and sampling frame for recruitment into the EPIC study vary according to the centre involved and the prevalences shown here may not directly reflect those in the general population of each country or region. Bearing this in mind, the almost 20-fold range of variation in the prevalence of current use of hormonal therapy observed between countries suggests that real differences in the patterns of use are likely. The reason for the wide variation in use is unclear. The finding of increased use among women who reported having had a hysterectomy and/or oophorectomy was common to all countries and regions examined and is consistent with results from previous studies (Lancaster *et al.*, 1995; Johannes *et al.*, 1994).

References

Johannes, C.B., Crawford, S.L., Posner, J.G. & McKinlay, S.M. (1994) Longitudinal patterns and correlates of hormone replacement therapy use in middle-aged women. *Am. J. Epidemiol.* **140**, 439–452

Lancaster, T., Surman, G., Lawrence, M., Mant, D., Vessey, M., Thorogood, M., Yudkin, P. & Daly, E. (1995) Hormone replacement therapy: characteristics of users and non-users in a British general practice cohort identified through computerised prescribing records. *J. Epidemiol. Community Health* **49**, 389–394

Plasma bile acids and risk of breast cancer

Costarelli V.[1], Sanders T.A.B.[2]

[1]School of Applied Science, South Bank University, 103 Borough Road, London SE1 0AA, UK. [2]Nutrition Food & Health Research Centre, King's College London, Franklin Wilkins Building, London SE1 9NN, UK.

Introduction

Secondary bile acids produced by the action of the colonic microflora may increase the risk of breast cancer (Hill *et al.*, 1971). DCA is found in human breast cyst fluid at concentrations about 50 times greater than those in plasma (Javitt *et al.* 1994). DCA is mutagenic, has a co-carcinogenic activity and promotes the growth, oestrogen receptor and oestrogen-regulated proteins of MCF-7 human breast cancer cells (Baker *et al.*, 1992).

The aim of the present study was to ascertain whether plasma concentrations of DCA were greater in newly diagnosed patients with breast cancer than healthy controls matched for age and body mass index.

Subjects, Materials and Methods

Subjects

Twenty Caucasian postmenopausal women with newly diagnosed breast cancer were recruited from the Oncology Clinics of Guy's and Charing Cross Hospitals in London. Twenty healthy postmenopausal women were recruited from the staff and relatives of staff and students of King's College London and from the general public, using an advertisement in the newspaper *The Guardian*. Exclusion criteria included any treatment for breast cancer or diabetes mellitus, use of hormone replacement therapy in the last 12 months, a history of liver or gall bladder disease or abnormal liver function. A fasting blood sample was obtained for determination of liver function tests and bile acid concentration. Cases were matched by age (mean, 60; range, 50–75 years) and body mass index (mean, 26.1; SD, 3.6 kg/m^2) with postmenopausal women.

Laboratory methods

Blood was collected from an anticubital vein using the vacutainer technique into tubes containing EDTA as anticoagulant for analysis of bile acids. Plasma samples from cases and their respective controls were analyzed in the same batch. Plasma bile acids were analyzed by gas chromatography/mass spectroscopy (Clayton & Muller, 1980).

Statistical analysis

A sample size of 20 subjects had statistical 85% power to detect a 1 SD difference in plasma DCA concentration between groups at $P<0.05$. Comparisons between cases and controls were made using a paired sample *t* test.

Results

Table 1 shows the plasma bile acid concentrations in the cases and the controls. Plasma deoxycholic acid concentrations were 52% higher ($P=0.012$) in patients with breast cancer than in controls. The ratio of plasma

Table 1. Plasma bile acids concentrations (μmol/L) in 20 postmenopausal women with breast cancer compared with age and BMI matched controls

	Breast cancer patients		Controls	
	Mean	SE	Mean	SE
Cholic acid (CA)	0.93	0.10	1.00	0.11
Chenodeoxycholic acid	1.31	0.18	1.04	0.11
Deoxycholic acid (DCA)	1.31[a]	0.17	0.86	0.07
Ursodeoxycholic acid[b]	0.45	0.08	0.36	0.08
Total bile acids	3.95	0.42	3.17	0.27
Ratio DCA:CA	1.61	0.25	1.16	0.21

[a]Significantly different compared with the controls $P<0.05$ (paired sample *t* test).
[b]Detected in 14 cases and 15 controls.

DCA:CA tended to be higher in the cases compared to the controls but the difference was not statistically significant (P=0.105). No other significant differences were noted.

Discussion

There are several possible explanations for the higher plasma concentrations of deoxycholic acid. Plasma bile acids are rapidly cleared from circulation by the liver and one cause of elevated plasma bile acid concentrations is liver disease. However, this is an unlikely explanation in the present study as liver function was normal. Fasting plasma bile acid concentrations were measured in the present study as there is a large increase following meals containing at least 15 g of fat (Costarelli & Sanders, 2001). In contrast, fasting plasma bile acid concentrations did not differ significantly on a day-to-day basis over a 6-week period (the mean within subject deviation for DCA was 0.43 μmmol/L).

These findings support the concept of a relationship between intestinally derived bile acids and risk of breast cancer, but require confirmation from prospective case–control studies. Future studies should also consider determining both fasting and postprandial plasma concentrations of bile acids in cases and controls as well as determining the concentrations of deoxycholic in breast cyst aspirates of cases and controls.

Acknowledgements

We thank Professor Ian Fentiman and Mr Dudley Sinnett from Guy's and Charing Cross Hospitals, respectively, for their valuable assistance in the recruitment of the breast cancer patients.

References

Baker, P.R., Wilton, J.C., Jones, C.E., Stenzel, D.J. Watson, N. & Smith, G.J. (1992) Bile acids influence the growth, oestrogen receptor and oestrogen-regulated proteins of MCF-7 human breast cancer cells. *Br. J. Cancer*, **65**, 566–572

Clayton, P.T. & Muller, D.P. (1980) A simplified gas-liquid chromatographic method for the estimation of non-sulphated plasma bile acids. *Clin. Chim. Acta*, **105**, 401–405

Costarelli, V. & Sanders, T.A.B. (2001) Acute effects of dietary fat composition on postprandial plasma bile acid and cholecystokinin concentrations in healthy premenopausal women. *Br. J. Nutr.*, **86**, 471–477

Hill, M.J., Goddard, P., & Williams, R.E. (1971) Gut bacteria and aetiology of cancer of the breast. *Lancet* **2**, 472–473

Javitt, N.B., Budai, K., Miller, D.G., Cahan, A.C., Raju, U., & Levitz, M. (1994) Breast–gut connection: origin of chenodeoxycholic acid in breast cyst fluid. *Lancet* **343**, 633–635

Age at menarche in relation to adult height in the EPIC cohort

Moret N.C., van Gils C.H., Peeters P.H.M.
(for the EPIC Working Group on Reproductive and Hormonal factors)

Julius Center for General Practice and Patient Oriented Research, UMC Utrecht, The Netherlands.

Introduction

Studies have consistently shown that women having their menarche at an earlier age are at increased risk for breast cancer compared to women who had their menarche at a later age (Key *et al.*, 2001). The role of height as a breast cancer risk factor has been under debate for many years, but the majority of studies show that taller women have a higher breast cancer risk than shorter women (Key *et al.*, 2001).

Since the early nineteenth century, secular changes have been described for age at menarche as well as for adult height. In several European countries, height has increased by about 0.3–3.0 cm per decade in the last half of the twentieth century (Hauspie *et al.*, 1997). Also, the age at menarche has decreased in this same period, although the results from the last 50 years are less consistent (Hauspie *et al.*, 1997).

Although on a population level women seem to grow taller and have their menarche earlier, several studies showed that women who have their menarche earlier stay shorter than women having their menarche at a later age (Biro *et al.*, 2001). The relationship between menarcheal age and adult height on the one hand, and their individual effects on breast cancer risk on the other, shows an intriguing discrepancy. Women with earlier menarche have an increased breast cancer risk, but at the same time these women reach a shorter adult height, which decreases their risk of breast cancer.

The aim of the present paper is to describe secular trends in the last century in height and age at menarche in nine European countries and to investigate whether, on an individual level, adult height is still related to menarcheal age.

Methods

The EPIC study is a multicentre prospective study carried out in 23 study centres from 10 countries. The results of Norway were not yet included in the central database at the time of the analysis. Over 500 000 middle-aged men and women participated between 1992 and 1999. The study design of the EPIC study was described in detail earlier (Riboli & Kaaks, 1997). In the present study, only the data from the female EPIC participants were used (n=307 081). The analyses were restricted to women who had their menarche between age 10 and 18 (n=303 238).

For the description of secular trends, mean age at menarche and height were plotted by 5-year birth cohorts (Fig. 1). Trends were tested using a linear regression model with 5-year birth cohort as the independent variable and either age at menarche or height as the dependent variable. Linear regression models were also used to assess the relationship between age at menarche and adult height on an individual level. Results were adjusted for age at the time of inclusion in the EPIC study. Because there were significant differences in the relationship between age at menarche and adult height between different countries and between women born before 1940 and from 1940 onwards, the analyses were done separately for each country and for these two groups of year of birth.

Results

In all European countries, a significant downward trend in the mean age at menarche of 1–2 months per 5 years was observed (β trend ranges from –0.06 to –0.17 years, P<0.0001, in all countries). In several countries, the decline in the mean age at menarche seems to have stabilized (Italy and Germany) or even reversed (Spain and United Kingdom) in the last decade, although in other countries, a decrease is still visible (Denmark, Sweden, The Netherlands, Greece and France). In France, Germany, The Netherlands and to a lesser extent in Italy, a sudden increase in mean age at menarche was seen in women born between 1920 and 1940. This is probably due to malnutrition during the period in

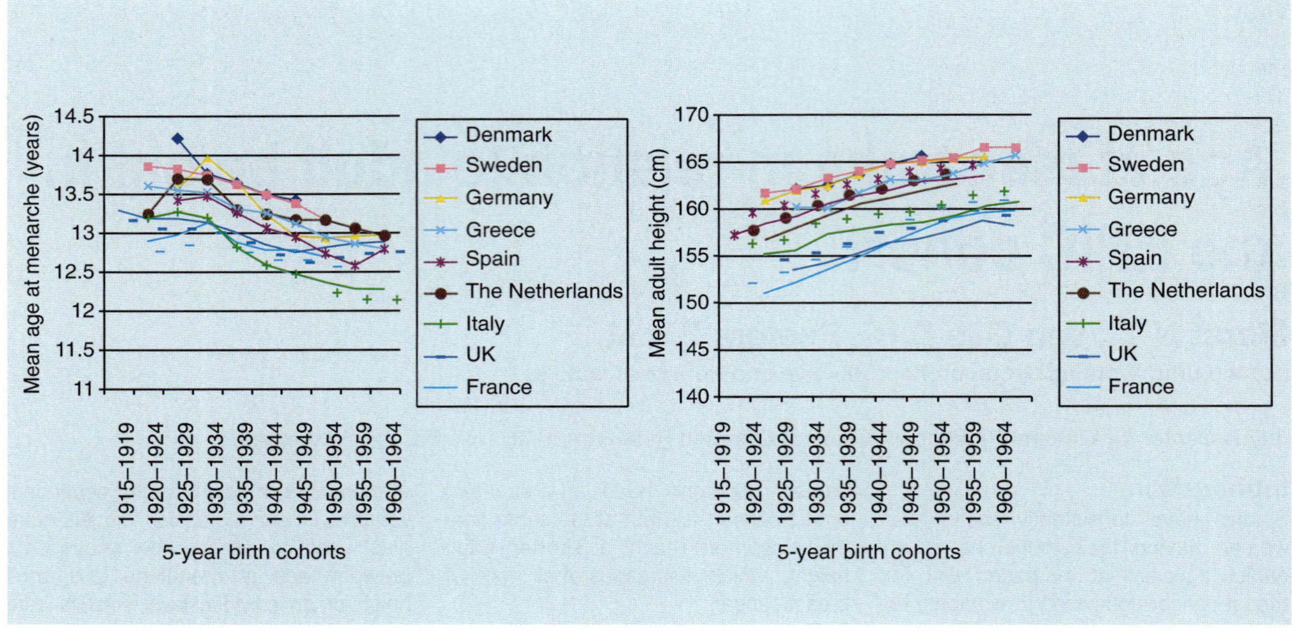

Figure 1
Mean age at menarche and mean adult height for the nine countries in 5-year birth cohorts

which they should reach menarche because of the Second World War.

The mean height for women has increased in all European countries with 0.6–1.3 mm per 5 years (β trend ranges from 0.6 to 1.3, $P<0.0001$, in all countries). In several countries (The Netherlands, Sweden, UK, France, Italy, Greece, Spain), it looks like the increase in mean height is leveling off, indicating that a maximum has been reached.

Table 1. Regression coefficients for the individual relationship between age at menarche and measured height per country and for two birth cohorts, adjusted for age at the inclusion into the EPIC study

	1920–1939		1940–1964	
	β	95% CI	β	95% CI
France	0.44	0.35–0.53	0.55	0.48–0.62
Italy	0.26	0.17–0.34	0.42	0.36–0.48
Spain	0.17	0.09–0.26	0.36	0.31–0.42
United Kingdom	0.33	0.25–0.41	0.37	0.28–0.45
The Netherlands	0.16	0.08–0.23	0.30	0.23–0.37
Greece	0.22	0.13–0.31	−0.03	−0.12 to 0.06
Germany	0.26	0.17–0.35	0.40	0.34–0.46
Sweden	0.22	0.14–0.30	0.26	0.15–0.36
Denmark	0.19	0.13–0.26	0.35	0.29–0.42

Women who had their menarche at a later age reached a taller adult height (Table 1), e.g. for France a delay of menarche of 1 year increased the adult height by 0.44 cm. In the majority of the countries, the association was stronger for women born in 1940 or later.

Discussion

In this study we found that in Europe, mean adult height has increased and mean age at menarche has decreased over the years. The trends observed are probably due to changes in nutritional, hygienic and health status of all populations (Hauspie *et al.*, 1997). Our data support the general belief that women who have their menarche at a later age will eventually grow taller than those with an early menarche. This association is still present for women from the later birth cohorts (1960–1964), who reach menarche earlier but grow taller than older women. Although the associations observed are quite strong, only a small part of the variation in height is explained by the variation in menarcheal age (about 2% in this study). This could be an explanation for the apparent discrepancy between the effect of menarcheal age on adult height and the individual effects of both factors on breast cancer risk.

References

Biro, F.M., McMahon, R.P., Striegel-Moore, R., Crawford, P.B., Obarzanek, E., Morrison, J.A., Barton, B.A. & Falkner, F. (2001) Impact of timing of pubertal maturation on growth in black and white female adolescents: The National Heart, Lung, and Blood Institute Growth and Health Study. *J. Pediatr.*, **138**, 636–643

Hauspie, R.C., Vercauteren, M. & Susanne, C. (1997) Secular changes in growth and maturation: an update. *Acta Paediatr. Suppl.*, **423**, 20–27

Key, T.J., Verkasalo, P.K. & Banks, E. (2001) Epidemiology of breast cancer. *The Lancet Oncology*, **2**, 133–140

Riboli, E. & Kaaks, R. (1997) The EPIC Project: rationale and study design. European Prospective Investigation into Cancer and Nutrition. *Int. J. Epidemiol.*, **26** (Suppl 1), S6–S14

The 1944–1945 Dutch famine and age at natural menopause – the value and validity of individual exposure assessment.

Elias S.G.[1], Van Noord P.A.H.[1], Peeters P.H.M.[1], Den Tonkelaar I.[2], Grobbee D.E.[1]

(the DOM cohort in Utrecht)

[1]Julius Center for General Practice and Patient Oriented Research, University Medical Center Utrecht, The Netherlands. [2]International Health Foundation, Utrecht, The Netherlands.

Introduction

In 1909 Moreschi reported that caloric restriction may reduce cancer risk in rodents, a result that was consistently reproduced in the following years (Moreschi, 1909). This triggered interest in a preventive potential of caloric restriction on cancer risk in humans.

In the Netherlands, at the end of the Second World War, history provided an experiment where one can investigate the effects of extreme caloric restriction in humans: the October 1944–May 1945 Dutch famine.

In September 1944, a railroad strike was ordered by the Dutch government in exile to thwart German transport of troops and ammunition in order to support an Allied attempt to capture the Rhine bridge at Arnhem, the Netherlands. The German occupier reacted with a food embargo, resulting in a fierce famine in the densely populated western parts of The Netherlands. The official daily rations per capita for adults dropped from about 1500 calories in September 1944 to below 700 calories in January 1945. The ratio of proteins, fats and carbohydrates remained practically unchanged during the 6-month famine, which ended with liberation on 5 May 1945 (Burger *et al.*, 1948).

Methods

Between June 1983 and March 1986, all 19 732 women born between 1911 and 1941 and participating at that time in the DOM breast cancer screening project in Utrecht, The Netherlands (De Waard *et al.*, 1984), received a questionnaire regarding their famine experience. They were asked about their wartime place of residence and their experiences of hunger, cold and weight loss during the famine period. These last questions were categorized into three levels: hardly, a little or very much. We combined these answers into an individual 3-point subjective hunger score. Women reporting severe exposure to at least two of the above-mentioned famine characteristics were considered severely exposed. Women reporting no exposure to at least two of the above-mentioned famine characteristics were considered unexposed and all others were considered moderately exposed (after Van Noord & Kaaks, 1991).

Information regarding their place of residence included degree of urbanization: rural area, village, small city, large city, Amsterdam/Rotterdam/The Hague or concentration camp. This distinction was made because people in concentration camps and the densely populated cities of Amsterdam, Rotterdam and The Hague were much more affected by famine than those living in rural areas where in many cases there was still plenty of food (De Jong, 1981). We used this information to validate the subjective hunger score.

Of the 19 732 women, 16 821 (85%) could be classified as to their exposure status and place of residence. As displayed in Figure 1, the proportion of women reporting severe exposure to the famine increased with the degree of urbanization, as expected.

Table 1. Results from linear regression analysis: difference in mean age at natural menopause in years due to famine exposure (age at exposure subgroups)

Famine exposure status	Age at exposure Early childhood 2–6 years (*n*=851)	Middle childhood 7–9 years (*n*=856)	Later childhood 10–12 years (*n*=1037)	Adolescence 13–18 years (*n*=1992)	Adult >18 years (*n*=4735)
Not exposed	Reference				
Moderately exposed					
β[a]	−0.16	0.22	−0.03	0.04	−0.01
95% CI	(−0.69 to 0.36)	(−0.70 to 0.26)	(−0.47 to 0.41)	(−0.37 to 0.29)	(−0.25 to 0.23)
Severely exposed					
β[a]					
95% CI	−1.83	1.30	−0.47	−0.32	0.14
	(−3.03 to −0.63)	(−2.18 to −0.42)	(−1.24 to 0.31)	(−0.84 to 0.21)	(−0.48 to 0.19)

[a]Adjusted for smoking, socio-economic status, body mass index, parity, age at menarche and year of birth.

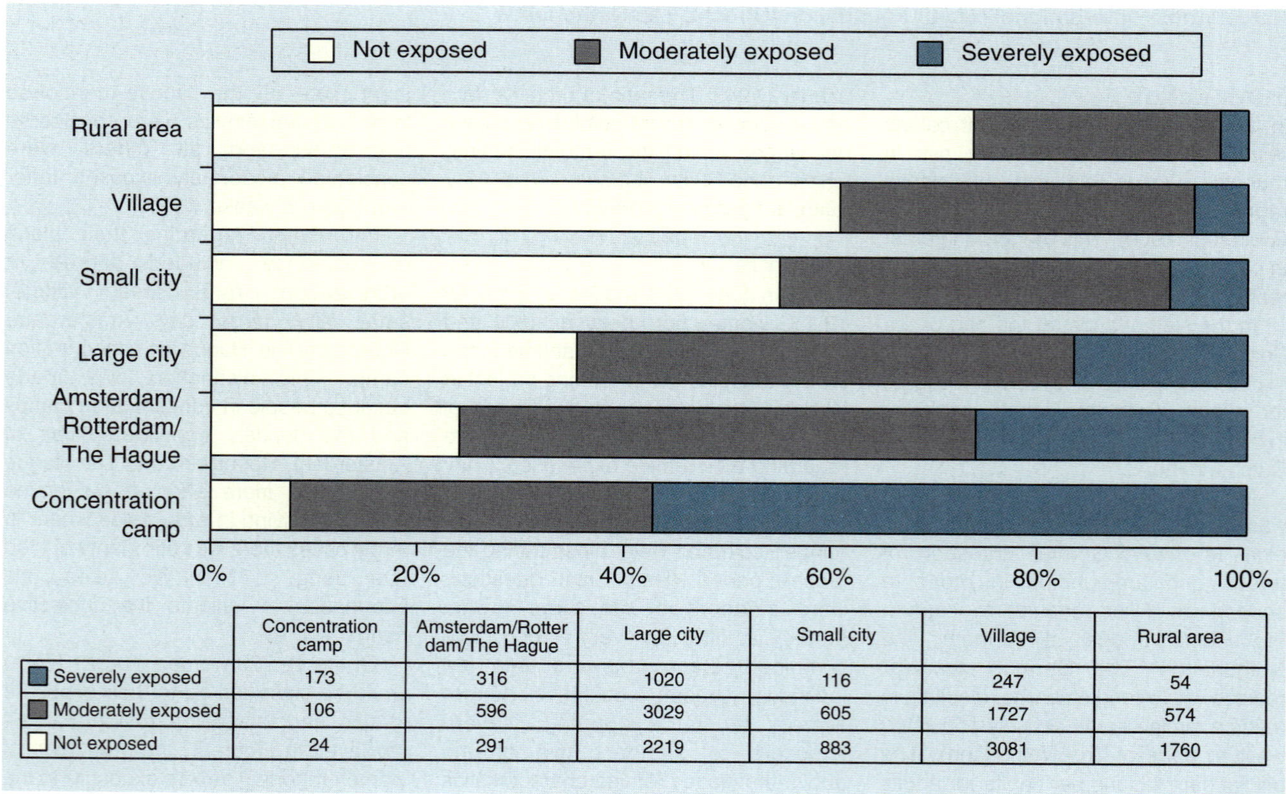

	Concentration camp	Amsterdam/Rotterdam/The Hague	Large city	Small city	Village	Rural area
Severely exposed	173	316	1020	116	247	54
Moderately exposed	106	596	3029	605	1727	574
Not exposed	24	291	2219	883	3081	1760

Figure 1
Distribution of recollected famine exposure status according to place of residence during famine. Numbers in table are number of women within categories

The ability to discriminate between three levels of famine exposure makes it possible to investigate the effects of caloric restriction in a dose–response-like manner and to get quantitatively better estimates of the effects compared to ecological studies.

This individual famine exposure score was used to investigate the effect of caloric restriction on age at natural menopause. Only women with a natural menopause who did not use hormonal replacement therapy were included in this analysis (*n*=9471).

A multivariate linear regression model was fitted on the data to adjust the effect of famine exposure on age at natural menopause for smoking, parity, socioeconomic status, body mass index, age at menarche and year of birth.

The study population was then divided into age groups at exposure, specifically relevant in the female development, to examine time windows in which caloric restriction may have the largest impact.

Results

Overall, severely exposed women experienced age at natural menopause on average 0.36 years earlier (95% confidence interval, –0.60 to –0.11) and moderately exposed women experienced age at natural menopause 0.06 years earlier (95% CI, –0.22 to 0.09) compared to unexposed women. This effect was particularly pronounced in the severely exposed at 2–6 years of age: –1.83 years (95% CI, –3.03 to –0.63) (Table 1).

We were able to show that caloric restriction decreases age at natural menopause, which might reduce subsequent breast cancer risk. Prepuberty seems to be a particularly sensitive period for this effect.

Discussion

We can conclude that the famine exposure score based on individual recollection seems to give a valid discrimination between exposure to famine categories and is capable of measuring an effect of caloric restriction on age at natural menopause.

This score provides us with a tool to investigate the effect of caloric restriction on cancer risk in humans.

This study was supported by grant UU 2000-2313 from the Dutch Cancer Society to Dr. P.A.H. van Noord.

References

Burger, G.C.E., Drummond, J.C. & Sandstead, H.R., eds. (1948) *Malnutrition and Starvation in the Western Netherlands, September 1944 to July 1945, Part I and II*, The Hague, General State Printing Office

De Jong, L. (1981) *Het koninkrijk der Nederlanden in de Tweede Wereldoorlog*, The Hague, General State Printing Office

De Waard, F., Collette, H.J., Rombach, J.J., Baanders-van Halewijn, E.A. & Honing, C. (1984) The DOM project for the early detection of breast cancer, Utrecht, The Netherlands. *J. Chronic Dis.*, **37**, 1–44

Moreschi, C. (1909) Beziehungen zwischen ernahrung und tumorwachstum. *Zeitschrift fur immunitatsforschung Originale BD II*, **2**, 644–675

Van Noord, P.A.H. & Kaaks, R. (1991) The effect of wartime conditions and the 1944–45 'Dutch famine' on recalled menarcheal age in participants of the DOM breast cancer screening project. *Ann. Hum. Biol.*, **18**, 57–70

Effects of maternal age at birth on breast cancer risk factors in daughters. A hypothesis on the role of oocyte, mitochondrial-related chromosomal instability

van Noord P.A.H.
(the DOM cohort in Utrecht)

Julius Center UMC, Utrecht University, The Netherlands.

Introduction

Most cancers show signs of chromosomal instability; however, all genetic defects in nuclear DNA, e.g. BRCA-1 or 2 mutations combined, explain only a small percentage of cancers such as breast cancer. Epigenetic factors influencing chromosomal stability could provide a missing link (Chen & Loeb, 1997). Chromosomal instability is not limited to cancer, but operates already around conception, affecting reproductive fitness. Fecundity declines and oocyte aneuploidy increases with maternal age, reflected in increasing spontaneous abortion, trisomy and twinning rates. Parents of trisomy have a tendency to aneuploidy, which may reflect a more general cellular propensity that is only accentuated by maternal and oocyte age.

Maternal age at birth has consistently been shown to have negative effects on cancer risks. Based on maternal age effects on the menopause of daughters, we put forward a hypothesis that links such preconception maternal/oocyte-related phenomena to cancer as well as its risk factors (van Noord & Dubas, 2001). As for the vulnerable time window, our hypothesis proposes that this period precedes the two early life and uterine growth phase hypotheses put forward by de Waard (De Waard & Trichopoulos, 1988) and by Trichopoulos (Trichopoulos, 1990; Titus-Ernstoff *et al.*, 2002).

Our hypothesis predicts that several breast cancer risk factors may worsen with the "biological" age of the oocyte at conception, reflected by higher maternal ages at birth.

Methods

This study explored correlations and *t*-test differences in maternal/oocyte age and several known breast cancer risk

Table 1. Pearson's correlation coefficient of mother's age at birth (a cohort of 2979, 15–42 years) and breast cancer risk factors

	Range	Pearson's *r*	*P*
Menarche	10–18 years	–0.03	0.36
Interval marriage to first birth	0–18 years	0.02	0.63
Number of live births	0–9	–0.03	0.17
Age first childbirth	16–42 years	0.12	0.00
Body mass index	15–49	–0.09	0.00
Adult height	100–184 cm	0.07	0.00
Age at natural menopause	30–58 years	–0.05	0.00

Table 2. Difference in mother's age at birth for daughters with and without a DY pattern at mammography (suggesting dysplasia)

	Range	*t* test
With DY pattern	26.0	–2.1
Without DY pattern	25.7 (–0.36 y)	

indicators in a cohort of healthy Dutch women. The study was done in a DOM (Diagnostisch Onderzoek Mamma-carcinoom) cohort, from a population-based breast cancer screening project (Collette, 1984) consisting of women born between 1911 and 1926 who participated after 1983 in the fifth screening round when all women had been asked for information about parental characteristics.

Results

Results are shown in Tables 1 and 2. Daughters with no children (n=561) differed from daughter's with children. Non-parous women had mothers that were on average 1 year older at the birth of their daughters (P<0.00). The daughters themselves had a slightly earlier natural menopause (P=0.001), were 1 cm taller (P<0.002) and weighed 3 kg less (P<0.000). They had a lower BMI (P<0.100) and had similar ages at menarche (P<0.52) as daughters with children.

Discussion

The results seem to fit our hypothesis on preconceptional epi-genetic aspects of oocyte-mediated qualities, reflected by maternal age at birth, and affecting breast cancer risk factors in their daughters. Women born of biologically older oocytes show more unfavourable levels of breast cancer risk factors, such as age at first childbirth, parity, height, age at menopause and percentage of daughters with dysplasia.

The later age at the birth of the first child, a lower number of children and an earlier menopause could all be evidence of oocytes that are less fit and therefore of a similar condition of all body cells in daughters of older mothers. A comparable tendency was seen among women who had not conceived or had not been able to conceive. Having no children might, in terms of maternal factors, reflect the contribution of oocyte aneuploidy to infertility, leading to childlessness in some women and a longer interval to first conception in other women who had borne children.

We think that the relevance of our findings is not in the size of the effects, as each separate effect is rather small, but in the consistency of the emerging pattern. Cellular tests (if available) could result in fewer misclassifications of these oocyte-mediated traits than the crude epidemiological risk factors used here, especially since we think that the underlying mechanism operates at the level of mitochondrial DNA. The mtDNA is purely maternally inherited through ooplasm. Mitochondrial DNA, in contrast to nuclear DNA, is especially vulnerable to free-radical-mediated mutations in post-mitotic/meiotic non-dividing resting cells (Ozawa, 1999). Oocytes can remain in such a resting state for decades, covering generations as well as all exposures during that time-span.

Our hypothesis is not germline DNA-mutation-based, but relates to mtDNA as directly responsible for proper functioning of all cellular ATP energy centers, the mitochondria (Ozawa, 1999). Ooplasm donation with young donor-mother mtDNA was shown to revitalize less fit oocytes before conception (Cohen *et al.*, 1998). Particularly during the first post-conception cell divisions, the blastula is entirely dependent on the proper functioning of this energy source, that upon fertilization drives the nuclear spindle, the imprinting process, etc. (Volarcik *et al.*, 1998). All these events happen well before nidation but from there on in all cells divided throughout the rest of life.

Preconception effects might also explain some phenomena covered by the two previous hypotheses on early-life effects. Since our hypothesis could reflect proposed, more general phenomena, we assume that similar relations on cancer risk may exist with the age at which the mother is to experience her own (natural) menopause.

To the extent that ovarian ageing indicates general ageing, we also expect relations with the age at which the mother (but not necessarily the father) dies, thereby fitting the more general disposable soma hypothesis of ageing. Studies in other populations (including animals) are required to test the predictions following from the proposed hypothesis.

References

Cheng, K.C. & Loeb, L.A. (1997) Genomic stability and instability: a working paradigm. *Curr. Top. Microbiol. Immunol.*, **221**, 5–19

Collette, H.J., Day, N.E., Rombach, J.J. & de Waard, F. (1984) Evaluation of screening for breast cancer in a non-randomised study (the DOM project) by means of a case–control study. *Lancet*, **1**, 1224-6

Cohen, J., Scott, R., Alikani, M. & Schimmel, T. (1998) Ooplasmic transfer in mature human oocytes. *Mol. Hum. Reprod.*, **4**, 269–280

Ozawa, T. (1999) Mitochondrial genome mutation in cell death and aging. *J. Bioenerg. Biomembr.*, **31**, 377–390

Titus-Ernstoff, L., Egan, K.M., Newcomb, P.A., Ding, J., Trentham-Dietz, A., Greenberg, E.R., Baron, J.A., Trichopoulos, D. & Willett, W.C. (2002) Early life factors in relation to breast cancer risk in postmenopausal women. *Cancer Epidemiol. Biomarkers Prev.*, **11**, 207–210

Trichopoulos, D. (1990). Is breast cancer initiated in utero? *Epidemiology,* **1**, 95–96

Van Noord, P.A.H., Dubas, J.S. (2001) Maternal/oocyte age effects on age at natural menopause of daughters; observations in the DOM cohort. *Am. J. Epidemiol.*, **153**, S140 (abstract 492)

Volarcik, K., Sheehan, L., Goldfarb, J., Woods, L., Abdul-Karim, F.W. & Hunt, P. (1998) The meiotic competence of in-vitro matured human oocytes is influenced by donor age: evidence that folliculogenesis is compromised in the reproductively aged ovary. *Hum. Reprod.*, **13**, 154–160

de Waard, F. & Trichopoulos, D.A. (1988) Unifying concept of the aetiology of breast cancer. *Int. J. Cancer,* **41**, 666–669

Bone mineral density and subsequent risk of prostate cancer in the NHANES-1 follow-up

Nelson R.L., Turyk M., Kim J., Persky V.

Department of Surgery and Department of Epidemiology and Biostatistics, University of Illinois at Chicago, USA.

Introduction

Increased calcium intake has been associated with increased risk of prostate cancer (Chan *et al.*, 1998; Giovannucci *et al.*, 1998). In this report we use the NHANES-1 follow-up to pursue the hypotheses that (bone mineral density) BMD will correlate directly with subsequent prostate cancer incidence.

Methods

The first National Health and Nutrition Examination Survey (NHANES-1) collected data from a national probability sample of the United States civilian non-institutionalized population between the ages of 1 and 74 years (National Center for Health Statistics, 1973). In addition to the emphasis on nutrition in NHANES-1, a subset sample of persons age 25–74 received a more detailed health examination through October 1975. This additional exam included a hand/wrist X-ray, completed in 6413 subjects. Each X-ray was a posterior/anterior view of the left hand and wrist taken by direct exposure using 10x12 Eastman Industrial Type AA Ready Pak film. The prescribed radiography technique called for a focus-to-film distance of 36 in. with the focal spot centred on the midpoint of the third metacarpal. These hand/wrist X-rays were reread for bone density using a technique called osteogram radiographic absorptiometry (RA) by Compu-Med Incorporated. BMD could not be calculated using this method for 153 of the 6413 subjects with hand X-rays due to improper exposure, poor picture quality or damaged or missing film.

Follow-up data on disease incidence are available through 1993. Outcome date was obtained on these individuals from the NHANES-1 Epidemiologic Follow-up Studies (NHEFS). Those with at least one follow-up record were included in the analysis, resulting in a final sample size of 6046. Disease outcomes were obtained using ICD-9 codes (International Classification of Diseases, 9th Revision) from death certificates and diagnostic codes in NHEFS mortality and health care facility stay data bases. They were, respectively, prostate cancer (185), hip fractures (820.0–820.9) and osteoporosis (733.00–733.03, 733.09).

Person-years of follow-up were computed for each cohort as the amount of time since the NHANES-1 examination to the date of ICD-9 disease code of interest from the health care facility stay file or date of death from the NHEFS mortality file, or the last day of contact from 1992 NHEFS vital status file. For persons with more than one hospital admission listing a disease outcome of interest, the date of the earliest admission was used. Person-years of follow-up were calculated separately for each disease outcome. Cohorts who reported a history of hip fracture at baseline were excluded from the hip fracture analysis (30 women and 27 men) and those who reported a prior malignant tumour or growth were excluded from all the cancer analyses (120 women and 49 men).

Cohorts were divided into four groups according to their RA BMD: <96, 95–105, 105–115, >115 (mass/volume units established by Compu-Med). Incidence rates for each diagnosis of interest were calculated for each BMD group by dividing the number of cases of disease by the number of person-years of follow-up. Analyses of hip fractures and osteoporosis outcomes were adjusted for gender. Cox proportional-hazards models were fitted for disease outcomes with BMD groups, controlling for age at NHANES-1 examination, body mass index at NHANES-1 examination, and race. Similar models, replacing the three indicator variables for RA BMD with a single variable for RA BMD group, were tested to determine the significance of the trend in risk of disease. Body mass index and race were omitted from the final models, as they did not confound the relationships of disease outcomes with BMD.

Results

The BMD sample of NHANES-1 included 6046 individuals who had bone density read by RA with follow-up data in NHEFS. This group included 5252 Caucasians, 742 African-Americans and 52 individuals of Hispanic origin. There were 2818 men and 3228 women. The median age at the time of bone density reading was slightly less than 50 years.

By 1993, a total of 94 cases of prostate cancer had been reported within this subset of the NHANES-1 cohort. In addition, there had been 103 cases of osteoporosis and 84 cases of reported hip fracture. Significant inverse associations were seen with both osteoporosis and hip fracture (Table 1) after adjustment for age and gender.

Prostate cancer risk was not significantly associated with increasing levels of BMD, although there were diminished risks in upper quartiles of BMD, which was in the opposite direction of our hypothesis (Table 2).

Table 1. Bone mineral density and subsequent incidence of osteoporosis and hip fracture in men and women

	Number in cohort	Number of cases	Incidence rate (cases/1000 person-years)	Age & gender: adjusted rate ratio (95% CL)	*P* value for rate ratio
Hip fractures					
All	5989	84	0.87		
RA BMD					
<95	1577	58	2.63	1	
95–105	1352	14	0.64	0.44 (0.24–0.80)	0.008
105–115	1483	7	0.28	0.32 (0.14–0.72)	0.006
>115	1577	5	0.18	0.27 (0.10–0.71)	0.009
Test for linear trend					0.0003
Osteoporosis	All	6046	103	1.06	
RA BMD					
<95	1607	70	3.13	1	
95–105	1363	17	0.77	0.51 (0.30–0.89)	0.02
105–115	1491	8	0.32	0.35 (0.16–0.75)	0.008
>115	1585	8	0.29	0.39 (0.17–0.88)	0.02
Test for linear trend					0.001

Table 2. Bone mineral density and subsequent incidence of prostate cancer

	Number in cohort	Number of cases	Incidence rate (cases/1000 person-years)	Age & gender: adjusted rate ratio (95% CL)	*P* value for rate ratio
Men					
All	2769	94	2.20		
RA BMD					
<95	649	39	4.68	1	
95–105	686	22	2.09	0.65 (0.38–1.09)	0.10
105–115	734	20	1.67	0.88 (0.51–1.53)	0.65
>115	700	13	1.10	0.74 (0.39–1.41)	0.36
Test for linear trend					0.42

Discussion

Hip fracture and osteoporosis

Associations of BMD with hip fracture and the development of osteoporosis were investigated in order to establish the validity of this BMD measurement. As anticipated, in the NHEFS, diminished BMD is significantly associated with the development of osteoporosis and hip fracture (Table 1).

Prostate cancer

As stated above, calcium ingestion has also been associated with an increased risk of prostate cancer (Chan *et al.*, 1998; Giovannucci *et al.*, 1998). The only study to look at BMD and prostate cancer risk was a case–control design. It showed no association, though cases already had prostate cancer when BMD was measured and controls were patients with other urological diseases or presenting for prostate cancer screening (Demark-Wahnefried *et al.*, 1997). Reported herein is the first study to obtain BMD measurement prior to the diagnosis of prostate cancer; no association was found (Table 2).

Acknowledgements and disclaimers

NHANES-1 and NHEFS data were provided from the National Center for Health Statistics (NCHS). All analyses, interpretations and conclusions based upon those data are made by the authors only and not the NCHS.

References

Chan, J.M., Giovannucci, E., Andersson, S.O., Yuen, J., Adami, H.O. & Wolk, A. (1998) Dairy products, calcium, phosphorous, vitamin D and risk of prostate cancer. *Cancer Causes Control*, **9**, 559–566

Demark-Wahnefried, W., Conaway, M.R., Robertson, C.N., Mathias, B.J., Anderson, E. & Paulson, D.F. (1997) Anthropometric risk factors for prostate cancer. *Nutr. Cancer*, **28**, 302–307

Giovannucci, E., Rimm, E.B., Wolk, A., Ascherio, A., Stampfer, M.J., Colditz, G. & Willett, W.C. (1998) Calcium and fructose intake in relation to risk of prostate cancer. *Cancer Res.*, **58**, 442–444

National Center for Health Statistics. (1973) Plan and initial program of the health examination survey. *Vital Health Stat.* **1**, 1–3

Reliability and validity of direct radioimmunoassays for measurement of postmenopausal serum androgens and estrogens

Rinaldi S.[1], Déchaud H.[2], Toniolo P.[3], Kaaks R.[1]

[1]International Agency for Research on Cancer, Unit of Nutrition and Cancer, Lyon, France. [2]Central Laboratory for Biochemistry, Hôpital de l'Antiquaille, Lyon, France. [3]New York University School of Medicine, Department of Obstetrics and Gynecology, New York, NY, USA.

Introduction

Blood levels of sex steroids in postmenopausal women have been associated with risk of different cancers. The main prerequisite for the estimation of relative risks in this population is the accurate ranking of subjects by their hormone levels. Since sex-steroid concentrations in this population are very low, accurate measurements of these hormones in serum samples are a difficult task to achieve. Methods used for these measurements must be very sensitive and in order to be applicable to large-scale epidemiological studies, they must be fast, relatively inexpensive and require a small amount of sample. Direct immunoassays could meet these needs, but since they are mainly designed for clinical use, their validity and precision in this domain must be assessed. We report the results of a study for the validation of commercially available direct assays for testosterone (T), Δ4-androstenedione (A), estrone (E_1) and 17β-estradiol (E_2), in view of their possible use in prospective cohort studies on cancer risk.

Materials and methods

Concentrations of T, A, E_1, and E_2 were measured by direct radioimmunoassays in serum samples from 20 postmenopausal women, who participated in an ongoing prospective study: the New York University Women's Health Study (NYUWHS). These values were compared with those obtained by radioimmunoassays after organic extraction and chromatographic prepurification on celite columns (Celite method). Direct assays for the four steroids were chosen among those commercially available in France and were performed according to the protocols from the manufacturers. Indirect assays of T, A, E_1 and E_2 were based on sample extraction by organic solvent, purification on celite columns and radioimmunoassay. All measurements were done in duplicate in each batch and all assays were performed twice over time (Time 1, Time 2). Direct assays were measured at the International Agency for Research on Cancer (Lyon, France), while the indirect assays were measured at the Central Laboratory for Biochemistry, Hôpital de l'Antiquaille (Lyon, France).

All statistical analyses were performed on log-transformed variables. They included the calculation of means and population standard deviations of the measurements, and calculation of Pearson correlation coefficients.

Results

For each steroid, mean values varied widely between the different kits used and the values obtained by indirect method were systematically lower than those obtained by direct assays (Table 1). In the same batch, the reproducibility of subject ranking by the direct assays was generally high (Pearson correlations all above 0.81). Between batches, Pearson correlations were also high (r >0.80).

The validity of ranking, as judged from the Pearson correlations between direct and indirect assays, was good for all six assays for T (r >0.70), for all four assays for A (r >0.82), and for the

Table 1. Means, confidence intervals and Pearson correlation coefficients within and between batch for testosterone, Δ4-androstenedione, estradiol and estrone measurements by indirect method and direct assays in 20 serum samples of postmenopausal women

Hormone / Method[a]	Time 1		Time 2		Pearson r	
	Mean	CI	Mean	CI	Within batch	Between batch
Testosterone (nmol/L)						
Celite	0.39	(0.28–0.52)	0.41	(0.31–0.55)	–	0.99
Immunotech	0.65	(0.51–0.84)	0.39	(0.28–0.55)	0.95	0.91
Orion	0.72	(0.55–0.95)	1.03	(0.77–1.36)	0.91	0.87
Cisbio	1.22	(1.00–1.50)	0.87	(0.64–1.18)	0.99	0.84
DSL	1.22	(1.00–1.47)	0.85	(0.66–1.09)	0.97	0.80
Sorin	0.73	(0.57–0.94)	0.63	(0.47–0.84)	0.94	0.93
Byk	0.82	(0.62–1.09)	0.96	(0.69–1.34)	0.98	0.80
Androstenedione (nmol/L)						
Celite	1.41	(1.04–1.89)	1.31	(0.99–1.75)	–	0.99
Immunotech	2.28	(1.60–3.25)	4.41	(3.32–5.86)	0.94	0.97
DSL	3.73	(2.98–4.67)	3.93	(3.04–5.08)	0.93	0.90
Sorin	3.28	(2.61–4.12)	3.74	(3.04–4.60)	0.96	0.92
DPC	2.57	(1.89–3.50)	3.12	(2.27–4.28)	0.98	0.98
Estradiol (pmol/L)						
Celite	0.07	(0.05–0.09)	0.10	(0.08–0.14)	–	0.92
Immunotech	0.56	(0.46–0.68)	0.66	(0.55–0.81)	0.94	0.97
Cisbio	0.27	(0.21–0.35)	0.31	(0.26–0.38)	0.89	0.98
DSL	0.28	(0.22–0.36)	0.36	(0.30–0.43)	0.81	0.95
Sorin	1.61	(1.48–1.68)	1.17	(1.03–1.33)	0.97	0.90
Biosource	0.78	(0.63–0.97)	0.88	(0.77–1.00)	0.90	0.94
Estrone (pmol/L)						
Celite	0.32	(0.24–0.42)	0.22	(0.15–0.31)	–	0.97
DSL	0.68	(0.57–0.81)	0.90	(0.79–0.10)	0.81	0.91

[a]Immunotech, Immunotech, Marseille, France; Orion, Orion Diagnostica, Espoo, Finland; Cis-Bio, Cis-Bio International, Gif-sur-Yvette, France; DSL, Diagnostic System Laboratories, Webster, Texas, USA; Sorin, DiaSorin, Saluggia, Italy; Byk, Byk-Sangtec Diagnostica, Dietzenbach, Germany; Bio-Source, Bio-Source Europe, Nivelles, Belgium; DPC, Diagnostica Products Corporation, Los Angeles, USA.

Table 2. Pearson correlation coefficients between direct assays and the indirect method

	DSL	Sorin	Immunotech	CisBio	Byk	Orion	DPC	BioSource
Testosterone	0.76	0.76	0.86	0.70	0.78	0.79	–	–
Δ4-Androstenedione	0.82	0.86	0.89	–	–	–	0.85	–
Estradiol	0.84	0.86	0.29	0.65	–	–	–	0.42
Estrone	0.81	–	–	–	–	–	–	–

assay of E_1 (r=0.81) (Table 2). For E_2, however, only two direct kits gave good correlations with the indirect assay.

Discussion

In this study, the reproducibility and the validity of measurements of sex steroids by direct radioimmunoassays using commercially available kits were evaluated. This evaluation was done by comparing direct radioimmunoassays with indirect assays, requiring sample extraction and chromatographic prepurification before quantification by radioimmunoassay.

Previous studies have addressed the reproducibility of hormonal assays within and between laboratories (Falk *et al.*, 1997; Gail *et al.*, 1996), or correlations over time between hormone assays in blood samples collected at different points in time (Cauley *et al.*, 1991; Hankinson *et al.*, 1995; Muti *et al.*, 1996). To our knowledge, this study is the first to compare direct with indirect assays in samples from a representative sample of women from a well-defined epidemiological study population.

The reproducibility of direct assays tested in this study appeared to be high, both between and within batches. Most of the direct assays for T, A and E_1 showed good correlations with the indirect assays, suggesting little subject misclassification and random error in the direct assays. For E_2, however, correlations with the indirect assays were elevated (>0.84) for only two out of five kits tested.

Absolute mean levels varied substantially for a given hormone, depending on the kit used, and values obtained from the indirect method were always lower than those obtained by direct assays. Even though the absolute levels of measurements is of secondary importance in epidemiological studies compared to the correct ranking of subjects, proper scaling of measurements enhances comparability of results between studies and may also be important for the calculation of levels of bio-available T or E_2.

In conclusion, direct immunoassays have the advantage over indirect assays of requiring smaller volumes of serum or plasma and of being amenable to automation. Our results show that, with careful selection, and depending on the specific study population to be analysed, commercial kits can provide accurate results in terms of relative ranking by hormone level.

References

Cauley, J.A., Gutai, J.P., Kuller, L.H. & Powell, J.G. (1991) Reliability and interrelations among serum sex hormones in postmenopausal women. *Am. J. Epidemiol.*, **133**, 50–57

Falk, R.T., Dorgan, J.F., Kahle, L., Potischman, N. & Longcope, C. (1997) Assay reproducibility of hormone measurements in postmenopausal women. *Cancer Epidemiol. Biomarkers Prev.*, **6**, 429–432

Gail, M.H., Fears, T.R., Hoover, R.N., Chandler, D.W., Donaldson, J.L., Hyer, M.B., Pee, D., Ricker, W.V., Siiteri, P.K., Stanczyk, F.Z., Vaught, J.B. & Ziegler, R.G. (1996) Reproducibility studies and interlaboratory concordance for assays of serum hormone levels: estrone, estradiol, estrone sulfate, and progesterone. *Cancer Epidemiol. Biomarkers Prev.*, **5**, 835–844

Hankinson, S.E., Manson, J.E., Spiegelman, D., Willett, W.C., Longcope, C. & Speizer, F.E. (1995) Reproducibility of plasma hormone levels in postmenopausal women over a 2- to 3-year period. *Cancer Epidemiol. Biomarkers Prev.*, **4**, 649–654

Muti, P., Trevisan, M., Micheli, A., Krogh, V., Bolelli, G., Sciajno, R. & Berrino, F. (1996) Reliability of serum hormones in premenopausal and postmenopausal women over a one-year period. *Cancer Epidemiol. Biomarkers Prev.*, **5**, 917–922

Chapter 7

Mechanisms of nutritional carcinogenesis and anticarcinogenesis

Food and carcinogenesis

Lambert R.

International Agency for Research on Cancer, 150, Cours Albert Thomas, 69372 Lyon Cédex 08, France.

Numerous epidemiological studies have confirmed a link between diet and the risk of cancer. The mucosal lining of the digestive tract is indeed directly exposed to nutrients which may cross the mucosal barrier either through cellular absorption or through an abnormal permeability of the tight junctions between cells. Nutrients undergo metabolic changes during this phase and the resulting metabolites may interact with molecular carcinogenesis at any of the successive steps: initiation linked to the first mutation, then promotion of a benign tumour, and finally progression to malignancy. Metabolized nutrients may be transformed into pro-carcinogens, interacting either at the initiation or at the promotion phase of carcinogenesis. On the other hand, the metabolized nutrients may act as inhibitors. The impact of diet on carcinogenesis and anticarcinogenesis occurs spontaneously in connection with socio-economic factors governing lifestyle. Recommendations for a healthy diet may be suggested by health authorities. A considerable number of studies aim to isolate specific molecules affording protection on animal models. The application of such molecules in chemoprevention protocols for humans requires a sound basis of their point of impact in cell biology and confirmation of their efficacy in randomized trials.

The global energy intake has an impact on the risk for cancer and an excess intake of either carbohydrate or fat has per se a promoting effect on cancer. Concerning fat intake, the luminal content of the colon may achieve genotoxicity in relation to its content in fat. Fatty acids in intimate contact with the epithelium can alter the transcription of *COX-2*, which stimulates cell proliferation in the mucosa. The promoting effect of meat may relate to the presence of high amounts of genotoxic substances in pyrolysis products (heterocyclic amines and polycyclic aromatic hydrocarbons) formed during cooking at high temperatures. It is also modulated by the nature of the fat included in meat. A major role is attributed to intestinal permeability in the passage of promoting agents for cancer, elements protecting the mucosal barrier could reduce the passage of promoting agents, as demonstrated in the experimental model with the protective effect of polyethylene glycol.

Specific protective effects of macronutrients in carbohydrates and fats have been shown. With carbohydrates, protective effects correspond to dietary fibre and their bacterial metabolism in the colon and to lignans, whose chelating properties may block the absorption of some pro-carcinogens. With fat, protection is linked to polyunsaturated fatty acids, mainly of the omega-3 family. The unsaturated fatty acids are present in fish; however, their presence may be influenced by the nutrition of the fish and one may suspect that the protection afforded by the consumption of wild fish should be less with farm fish.

Micronutrients from plants are a major source of studies on anticarcinogenesis factors present in the diet. However, their quantitative and qualitative distribution in a plant depends on its geographical origin, the composition of the soil, the age of the plant, either on the site or after collection. Such factors have proved to play a role with the allyl compounds in garlic. Anticarcinogens can also be destroyed by heating or cooking the plant. Finally, micronutrients undergo alterations in the digestive lumen or after their absorption. A common feature of these studies on vegetal compounds is that the literature advocating protection is rarely supported by a precise analysis of their point of impact on the cell cycle, nor by rigorous trials in human beings. However, a large field of experimental research is now emerging with thousands of plants analysed for isolation of candidate molecules. In addition, numerous studies are conducted on experimental carcinogenesis and its inhibition in rodents, aiming to explore the efficacy of the candidate molecules.

Among mineral micronutrients, selenium has often been considered as protective against cancer. The presence of selenium in various enzymes is the suggested molecular mechanism of action. A number of trials in humans have been conducted, some countries have added selenium to the water supply, some agronomic industries have raised plants in selenium-enriched soils. However, there is persisting doubt about selenium's protective capacity and about the molecular form of action. Indeed, selenium is believed to be less active as a mineral than in organic sulfur compounds (methyl-seller-cysteine). Other organic molecules assumed to be protective are present in the cruciferous vegetables, particularly the isothiocyanates, which occur as conjugates in a variety of cruciferous vegetables. The protecting capacity of garlic is assumed to correlate with the presence of allyl compounds whose concentration is increased in the aged plant and decreased by cooking. Some organosulfur compounds (diallyl-disulfide, diallyl-sulfide) have been demonstrated to inhibit chemical initiation of carcinogenesis while their effect on promotion is still questioned. Currently, most studies on vegetables concern the group of phytoestrogens with three classes of molecules, isoflavones, coumestans and lignans, present in the soybean but also in bean sprouts, and some are studying linseed, whole grains and berries. The best-known compounds are the isoflavones, which have a structural similarity to mammalian estrogens. The soybean is a major source of isoflavones (genistein and daidzein) Protection against breast cancer has been assumed because of the lowest incidence in Asian countries with a diet that is rich in soybean (tofu is an example). There is still conflicting evidence on protection because the flavonoids ingested are believed to undergo metabolic changes to compounds with hormonal activity. They may either act as a natural alternative to tamoxifen blocking the estrogen beta-receptors, or mimic hormonal pro-carcinogen effects. Other molecules are assumed to be protective in relation to antioxidant properties (beta-carotene, lycopene extracted from tomatoes).

Finally, the supposed anticancer activity of some minerals or some nutrients extracted from plants is extensively advertised in the area of nonconventional medicine. Multiple variants of soybean extracts, antioxidants, lycopene, and selenium preparations are available either on the Internet or in healthfood shops. In contrast to pharmaceutical products, these compounds are subject to no control of their content in terms of quality and efficacy in most countries.

This section of the volume groups three kinds of reports:

- minireviews presenting the list of plant-derived anticarcinogens, the relation of phytoestrogens and unsaturated fatty acids with breast cancer and the relation of polysaccharides and meat with colorectal cancer;

- human studies based on the analyses of collected samples. This includes a demonstration that the consumption of red meat increases the faecal content in carcinogenic nitroso compounds and that a diet enriched in vegetables increases the exfoliation of colonic cells. The extracts of human faecal water have been shown to stimulate proliferation on cell lines, with induction of cyclooxygenase-2 activity. The hormonal influence of isoflavones from soy foods has not been confirmed by the analyses of blood and urine samples collected in premenopausal women receiving or not receiving isoflavones.

- results of studies on the experimental animal model (the rat) for mammary and colonic carcinogenesis. For colonic carcinogenesis where the aberrant crypt foci are often the end point of the studies, the modulating effect of the diet on the genotoxicity of an imidazole-quinoline derivative is confirmed. The promoting effect of sucrose and dextrin is confirmed while indigestible carbohydrates are protective. A ranking list of chemopreventive agents introduced in the diet is established in the rat model. For mammary carcinogenesis, there is a complex interaction between antioxidants and polyunsaturated fatty acids in the diet. Depending on the concentration of the fatty acid in the diet, the antioxidant may or may not have a promoting effect on the number of tumours per rat.

Phytoestrogens and breast cancer risk: review of the epidemiological evidence

Peeters P.H.M., Keinan-Boker L., van der Schouw Y.T., Grobbee D.E.
Julius Center for General Practice and Patient-Oriented Research, University Medical Center Utrecht, the Netherlands.

Introduction

Phytoestrogens are natural plant substances (Setchell *et al.*, 1984). The three main classes are isoflavones, coumestans, and lignans. These compounds show structural similarity to mammalian estrogens. Isoflavones, the most frequently studied, are present in large amounts in soybeans and soy products such as miso and tofu. The most important isoflavones are genistein and daidzein. Biochanin A and formononetin are precursors, present in some legumes, which are metabolized to genistein and daidzein, respectively. Coumestans occur in bean sprouts and fodder crops, and they have received little scientific attention so far. Lignans occur as pre-lignans and are more widespread in plants, where they form the building blocks in cell walls. Linseed (flaxseed) especially is a rich source, but lignans also occur in relatively high amounts in whole grains and berries.

The potential preventive actions of phytoestrogens on the occurrence of cancer have been suggested and studied in the 1980s and 1990s (Adlercreutz *et al.*, 1982; Messina *et al.*, 1994). This study will summarize the postulated mechanisms of isoflavones on breast cancer risk and will review the epidemiological evidence for this hypothesis.

Anticarcinogenic mechanism

Isoflavones have received scientific attention largely due to their actions as phytoestrogens: after consumption many metabolic conversions occur in the gut, resulting in hormone-like compounds. The postulated anticarcinogenic mechanism involves a weak estrogen-like activity. Isoflavones bind to estrogen receptors, preferentially to the estrogen beta receptor. They initiate only a modest response and at the same time they block the binding of more potent estrogens. They have a structural similarity to the potent synthetic anti-estrogen, tamoxifen, a drug that is effective in breast cancer treatment and prevention.

There are hundreds of *in vitro* studies showing that genistein, and to a lesser extent daidzein, inhibit the growth of a wide range of both hormone-dependent and hormone-independent cancer cells. It has been shown to inhibit growth in many cell lines, including those without estrogen receptors. Phytoestrogens may act as antioxidants and/or inhibit angiogenesis, the formation of new blood vessels, essential for a tumour to expand (Messina *et al.*, 1994; Bingham *et al.*, 1998; Messina, 1999; Bouker *et al.*, 2000).

In animal studies, soybean products have generally reduced tumours induced by chemical carcinogens, while diets supplemented with soybean revealed lower numbers of tumours in rats (Messina *et al.*, 1994; Bingham *et al.*, 1998; Messina, 1999; Bouker *et al.*, 2000).

Several recent intervention studies in humans show the effects of soy or flaxseed consumption on hormone levels. Although Martini *et al.* (1999) could not find changes in the urinary excretion of hormones after soy supplementation in 36 premenopausal women, there are five studies that do show effects of soy in premenopausal women (Nagata *et al.*, 1998; Xu *et al.*, 1998; Duncan *et al.*, 1999; Lu *et al.*, 2000a; Lu *et al.*, 2000b). These include a decrease in serum 17beta estradiol (Nagata *et al.*, 1998; Lu *et al.*, 2000a), a decrease in plasma FSH and LH (Duncan *et al.*, 1999) or an increase in the urinary 2-hydroxyestrone/16alpha hydroxyestrone ratio (Xu *et al.*, 1998; Lu *et al.*, 2000b). These data suggest that isoflavones may exert cancer-preventive effects in premenopausal women by altering estrogen metabolism away from genotoxic metabolites toward inactive metabolites. Isoflavone consumption, compared with a control diet, decreased urinary excretion of the hypothesized genotoxic estrogen metabolites, 16 alpha-hydroxyestrone, 4-hydroxyestrone, and 4-hydroxyestradiol. An increase in the 2-hydroxyestrone/16 alpha-hydroxyestrone ratio is believed to be beneficial. The same effect was also reported recently for postmenopausal women, although less pronounced (Xu *et al.*, 2000).

Overall, the impression is that phytoestrogens may exert anticarcinogenic potential by altering blood levels of relevant hormones and/or exhibit antioxidant or anti-angiogenic effects. However, phytoestrogens also have significant estrogenic properties in *in vitro* and *in vivo* models (Bingham *et al.*, 1998; Messina, 1999; Bouker *et al.*, 2000). Epidemiological and clinical data support the view that exposure to estrogens has a significant influence on increased breast cancer risk (Key, 1999). Based on findings of studies addressing the estrogenecity or antiestrogenecity of phytoestrogens, it cannot be concluded whether the net result of their consumption will be an inhibition or a stimulation of carcinogenesis. For an evaluation of their net result, we will need additional population data. This review presents the epidemiological studies published so far on isoflavones and breast cancer risk. The review is divided into two sections: 1) studies that assessed the relation through the dietary intake of soy (as a proxy for the intake of isoflavones) in relation to breast cancer, and 2) studies that measured urinary excretion of isoflavones in relation to breast cancer.

Review of epidemiological studies

Dietary measurements of soy intake and breast cancer

Studies on geographical differences in breast cancer occurrence suggest preventive effects for soy products (Bingham *et al.*, 1998; Messina, 1999; Bouker *et al.*, 2000). Women who usually consume large amounts of phytoestrogens due to the natural presence of these compounds in their traditional diets, as is the case in Asian countries, show lower breast cancer rates compared to Western countries. Women from Asian populations overall also have longer menstrual cycle lengths, and have up to roughly 40% lower estrogen levels (Table 1, adapted from Wu *et al.*, 1998).

Until now, five published epidemiological studies have directly assessed relations between dietary intake of soy (as a proxy for isoflavone consumption) and the risk of subsequent breast cancer.

The first study appeared in 1991 (Lee *et al.*, 1991; Lee *et al.*, 1992), showing a significant protective effect only on premenopausal breast cancer risk for women who consumed over 55 g of soy products per day (RR, 0.4; 95% CI, 0.2–0.9). The second case–control study conducted by Hirose *et al.*, (1995) was exceptionally large, including over 1000 breast cancer cases and over 22 000 controls from outpatient clinics. This study again showed the protective effects of consuming bean curd (tofu) three or more times per week (RR, 0.8; 95% CI, 0.6–1.0). Still, the result was borderline statistically significant only in premenopausal women and no effect was seen in postmenopausal women. A third case–control study in China was negative, i.e. it could not disclose any preventive effects of soy intake on breast cancer risk (per 18 g soy protein: RR, 1.0; 95% CI, 0.7–1.4) (Yuan *et al.*, 1995). A study by Wu *et al.* (1996) showed protective effects, but these were only significant in non-US-born Asian Americans (RR per weekly soy product consumption, 0.79; 95% CI, 0.66–0.94). The authors hypothesized that soy intake is protective only when consumed at higher doses and at younger ages. The mean intake of soy products of US-born Asian women is much lower, when compared to non-US-born Asian women who migrated to the US. The mean intake of soy was 10–15 times higher in Chinese women who were born and live in Asia (36–45 g soy products/day), than in Asian-Americans currently residing in California and Hawaii (1.9–4.0 g soy products/day) (Wu *et al.*, 1998). The upper quartile of intake in Asian-Americans is still two to three times lower compared to the lowest quartile of women in Asia. Relations with breast cancer may be different for different parts of the dose–response relation between soy and breast cancer risk (Wu *et al.* 1998).

All these studies used dietary questionnaires to quantify soy intake. It is difficult to accurately measure habitual soy intake. All studies were case–control studies, suffering from an additional problem, i.e. recall bias (cases may remember their diet more or less accurately than healthy controls).

Until now, only one prospective study has been published on Japanese women (Key *et al.*, 1999) and no protective effects of tofu (or miso soup) intake of more than four times per week on pre- or postmenopausal breast cancer risk were found (RR, 1.1; 95% CI, 0.8–1.5). Studies have so far been restricted to Asian populations, because they consume high amounts of soy products that can be determined by questionnaires. Of concern is that soy intake may be homogeneously high in Asia, making it difficult to identify differences in breast cancer risk between moderate and high consumption. No studies were done in Western populations where consumption of soy or soy products is usually low. However, isoflavones are also present in soybean flour, soymilk and soy sauce, and in much smaller amounts in dried beans. Few analyses of isoflavones in food have been done and food composition tables do not usually include values of isoflavones for different food groups.

Urinary isoflavones and breast cancer

When consumed, the plant isoflavones undergo metabolism by bowel microflora and are absorbed to a variable extent.

Table 1. Overview of epidemiological studies on dietary soy and breast cancer risk

Author, journal year, country	Design dietary questionnaire: soy			
Lee (*Lancet*, 1991) Singapore	200 cases, 420 controls, hospital-based case–control	Soy product	Premenopausal	Postmenopausal
		<20 g/day	1.0	1.0
		20.3–54.9 g/day	0.6 (0.3–1.2)	0.9 (0.4–1.9)
		≥ 55 g/d	0.4 (0.2–0.9)	1.1 (0.5–2.3)
Hirose (*Jpn. J. Cancer Res.*, 1995) Japan	1186 cases, 21 295 controls, outpatients, case–control	Bean curd	Premenopausal	Postmenopausal
		≤ 3 times/month	1.0	1.0
		1–2 times/week	0.9 (0.7–1.2)	0.9 (0.6–1.2)
		≥ 3 times/week	0.8 (0.6–1.0)	1.0 (0.7–1.3)
		Miso soup		
		Occasionally	1.0	1.0
		Daily	1.2 (1.0–1.4)	1.0 (0.8–1.2)
Yaun (*Br. J. Cancer*, 1995) China, Shanghai, Tianjin.	Shanghai 534 cases, 534 controls; Tianjin 300 cases, 300 controls; population-based case–control	Soy protein	Pre- and postmenopausal	
		Per 18 g/day (continuous)	1.0 (0.7–1.4)	
Wu (*Cancer Epidemiol. Biomarkers Prev.*, 1996) USA, Chinese, Japanese, Filippino	597 cases, 966 controls, Population-based case–control	Soy product	US-born Asians	No US-born Asians
		Per 1 time/week	0.93 (0.73–1.18)	0.79 (0.66–0.94)
Key (*Br. J. Cancer.*, 1999), Japan	34 759 women, 427 cases, prospective population-based study	Tofu	Pre- and postmenopausal	
		≤ 1/week	1.0	
		2–4 times/week	1.0 (0.8–1.2)	
		≥ 5 times/week	1.1 (0.8–1.5)	
		Miso soup	1.0	
		≤ 1/ week	1.0 (0.8–1.3)	
		2–4 times/week	0.9 (0.7–1.1)	
		≥ 5 times/week		

Intake of foods rich in phytoestrogens is followed by a peak urinary excretion in the subsequent 24 h; excretion turns to its previous rate in 48–72 h (Table 2). Urinary excretion is dose-dependent at low to moderate levels of soy protein intake. Adlercreutz was the first to detect lower urinary excretion of equol (a metabolite of daidzein) in seven postmenopausal breast cancer cases compared to ten healthy American women (Adlercreutz *et al.*, 1982).

The first case–control study was published in 1997 (Ingram *et al.*, 1997). It included a mix of pre- and postmenopausal Australian women and showed protective effects for several types of isoflavones. A statistically significant result was only seen for equol (a metabolite of daidzein) (fourth versus first quartile: RR, 0.3; 95% CI, 0.1–0.7). This study was criticized because isoflavones are short-term biomarkers of dietary intake. Since breast cancer cases in Ingram's study were recently confronted with the diagnosis of a serious illness, they may have changed their dietary intake. Moreover, the participation rate of controls was below 50% and healthy subjects may preferentially have been selected (Lancet, 1998).

A second case–control study, published by Zheng *et al.* (1999), again showed the protective effects of higher excretion levels of the isoflavones daidzein and genistein, although results did not reach statistical significance. Again, the population comprised both pre- and postmenopausal women living in Shanghai, China.

Lower urinary mean levels of daidzein and genistein were observed in 18 Australian postmenopausal breast cancer cases compared to 20 controls in a third very small study (Murkies *et al.*, 2000).

It is difficult to interpret the temporality of the observed associations in these case–control studies. One may question the relevance of phytoestrogen levels in urine samples collected between diagnosis and surgery to induction or progression of the disease many years earlier.

The only prospective study that was done included postmenopausal women in the Netherlands with urine collected 1–9 years prior to disease diagnosis (Tonkelaar den *et al.*, 2001). No association was observed for higher levels of genistein and breast cancer risk (third tertile versus first: RR, 0.8; 95% CI, 0.5–1.5).

Conclusion

The anticarcinogenic potential of phytoestrogens on breast cancer risk was investigated in five studies that measured usual dietary soy (product) intake in relation to breast cancer (Lee *et al.*, 1991; Hirose *et al.*, 1995; Yuan *et al.*, 1995; Wu *et al.*, 1996; Key *et al.*, 1999). Only one of these five studies was prospective and this study did not find a protective effect (Key *et al.*, 1999). All of these studies were done on Asian populations where soy consumption is homogeneously high. Relations with breast cancer may be difficult to find if consumption for the total population is above a threshold value. If there is a protective effect in these populations it seems to be present for premenopausal breast cancer only or for women who consume high amounts of soy at young ages (Lee *et al.*, 1991; Hirose *et al.*, 1995; Wu *et al.*, 1996).

In Western populations, habitual consumption of isoflavones is much lower. Assessment through the diet is difficult due to lack of food composition data. No studies have so far been done that that have assessed dietary intake of isoflavones in Western populations in relation to breast cancer risk. However, there were four studies that measured urinary excretion of isoflavones in relation to breast cancer risk (Ingram *et al.*, 1997; Zheng *et al.*, 1999; Murkies *et al.*, 2000; Tonkelaar den *et al.*, 2001). Again, only one study was prospective and reported a nonsignificant reduction in breast cancer risk (Tonkelaar den *et al.*, 2001).

Levels of phytoestrogens in urine (or blood) do not only reflect dietary intake. The condition of the intestinal flora is crucial for phytoestrogen levels, i.e. the use of antibiotics may affect levels; furthermore genetic influence may also play a role.

We decided not to do a meta-analysis on the published results because we believe that the methodological differences between the studies are too large to allow pooling the results. Studies differed in:

- Study design (case–control, prospective).
- The amounts of isoflavones consumed (Asian, Western populations).
- The measurement method of isoflavones (questionnaire: soy products, urine or blood: tertiles or quartiles of several subclasses).
- The cut-off points used in the analyses of soy consumption (grams of soy product, weekly consumption of miso, etc).
- Menopausal status (pre- or postmenopausal women or mix).

All of these points are relevant for the interpretation of the observed relations.

From the published data we may conclude that overall information about phytoestrogen consumption and breast cancer risk is still scarce: there are only two prospective studies (Key *et al.*, 1999; Tonkelaar den *et al.*, 2001). These studies do not show significant protection. However, we may also conclude that none of the studies so far showed evidence for an increased risk of breast cancer with increased phytoestrogen intake. An absence of risk is important, since the putative physiological effects of phytoestrogens have created a market that has been utilized by the nutrition industry. Soy supplements are on the market now and soy flour is increasingly used in the

Table 2. Overview of epidemiological studies on urinary isoflavone excretion and breast cancer

Author, journal year, country	Design	Isoflavones: urinary excretion	Results: relative risk, 95% confidence interval	
Ingram (*Lancet*, 1997), Australia	144 cases, 144 controls; case–control study	Equol quartile 1 2 3 4	 1.0 0.5 (0.2–1.0) 0.5 (0.2–1.2) 0.3 (0.1–0.7)	Mix of pre- and postmenopausal women; results the same for daidzein, but nonsignificant
Zheng (*Cancer Epidemiol. Biomarkers Prev.*, 1999) Shanghai, China	60 cases, 60 controls; population-based case–control study	Genistein tertile 1 2 3	 1.0 0.5 (0.2–1.1) 0.7 (0.3–1.8)	Mix of pre- and postmenopausal women; results the same for daidzein
Murkies (*Menopause*, 2000) Australia	18 cases, 20 controls Case–control study		nmol/day	Only postmenopausal
		Mean genistein Cases vs. controls	25 (5–132) vs. 155 (43–550)	
		Mean daidzein Cases vs. controls	31 (4–234) vs. 427 (96–1906)	
Tonkelaar den (*Cancer Epidemiol. Biomarkers Prev.*, 2001), the Netherlands	88 cases, 268 controls; prospective (nested case–control) study, urine collection 1–9 years prior to diagnosis	Genistein tertile 1 2 3	 1.0 0.9 (0.5–1.6) 0.8 (0.5–1.5)	Only postmenopausal

nutritional industry due to its FDA (Food and Drug Administration)-approved claim of reducing lipid levels and preventing cardiovascular diseases (October 1999). Women will increasingly consume phytoestrogens, even without knowing it. One should keep in mind that the studies included overall healthy subjects. It is not clear what the effect of increased consumption will be in women at high risk of breast cancer (i.e. previous cancer, genetic predisposition).

Overall, prospective epidemiological studies on phytoestrogens and breast cancer are scarce, limiting our knowledge about the exposure–disease relation.

Acknowledgements

We thank the World Cancer Research Fund (WCRF 2000/30) and Zorg Onderzoek Nederland (ZON, 21000027) for financial support.

References

Adlercreutz, H., Fotsis, T., Heikkinen, R., Dwyer, J.T., Woods, M., Goldin, B.R. & Gorbach, S.L. (1982) Excretion of the lignans enterolactone and enterodiol and of equol in omnivorous and vegetarian postmenopausal women and in women with breast cancer. *Lancet*, **ii**, 1295–1259

Bingham, S.A., Atkinson, C., Liggins, J., Bluck, L. & Coward, A. (1998) Review article. Phyto-oestrogens: where are we now? *Br. J. Nutr.*, **79**, 393–406

Bouker, K.B. & Hilakivi-Clarke, L. (2000) Genistein: does it prevent or promote breast cancer. *Environ. Health Perspect.*, **108**, 701–708

Duncan, A.M., Merz, B.E., Xu, X., Nagel, T.C., Phipps, W.R. & Kurzer, M.S. (1999) Soy isoflavones exert modest hormonal effects in premenopausal women. *J. Clin. Endocrinol. Metab.*, **84**, 192–197

Hirose, K., Tajima, K., Hamajima, N., Inoue, M., Takezaki, T., Kuroishi, T., Yoshida, M. & Tokudome, S. (1995) A large-scale, hospital-based case–control study of risk factors for breast cancer according to menopausal status. *Jpn. J. Cancer Res.*, **86**, 146–154

Ingram, D., Sanders, K., Kolybaba, M. & Lopez, D. (1997) Case–control study of phyto-oestrogens and breast cancer. *Lancet*, **350**, 990–994

Key, T.J. (1999) Serum oestradiol and breast cancer risk (review). *Endocr. Relat. Cancer*, **6**, 175–180

Key, T.J., Sharp, G.B., Appleby, P.N., Beral, V., Goodman, M.T., Soda, M. & Mabuchi, K. (1999) Soya foods and breast cancer risk: a prospective study in Hiroshima and Nagasaki, Japan. *Br. J. Cancer*, **81**, 1248–1256

Lancet. Discussion, comments. Phyto-oestrogens and breast cancer. (1998) *Lancet*, **351**, 137–139

Lee, H.P., Gourley, L., Duffy, S.W., Esteve, J., Lee, J. & Day, N.E. (1991) Dietary effects on breast cancer risk in Singapore. *Lancet*, **331**, 1197–1200

Lee, H.P., Gourley, L., Duffy, S.W., Esteve, J., Lee, J. & Day, N.E. (1992) Risk factors for breast cancer by age and menopausal status: a case–control study in Singapore. *Cancer Causes Control*, **3**, 313–322

Lu, L.-J.W., Anderson, K.E., Grady, J.J., Kohen, F. & Nagamani, M. (2000a) Decreased ovarian hormones during a soya diet: implications for breast cancer prevention. *Cancer Res.*, **60**, 4112–4121

Lu, L.-J.W., Cree, M., Josyula, S., Nagamani, M., Grady, J.J. & Anderson, K.E. (2000b) Increased urinary excretion of 2-hydroxyestrone but not 16 alfa-hydroxyestrone in premenopausal women during soya diet containing isoflavones. *Cancer Res.*, **60**, 1299–1305

Martini, M.C., Dancisak, B.B., Haggans, C.J., Thomas, W. & Slavin, J.L. (1999) Effects of soy intake on sex hormone metabolism in premenopausal women. *Nutr. Cancer*, **34**, 133–139

Messina, M.J. (1999) Legumes and soybeans: overview of their nutritional profiles and health effects. *Am. J. Clin. Nutr.*, **70**, 439S–450S

Messina, M.J., Persky, V., Setchell, K.D.R. & Barnesn, S. (1994) Soy intake and cancer risk: a review of in vitro and in vivo data. *Nutr. Cancer*, **21**, 113–131

Murkies, A., Dalais, F.S., Briganti, E.M., Burger, H.G., Healy, D.L., Wahlqvist, M.L. & Davis, S.R. (2000) Phyto-oestrogens and breast cancer in postmenopausal women: a case–control study. *Menopause*, **7**, 289–296

Nagata, C., Takatsuka, N., Inaba S., Kawakami, N. & Shimizu, H. (1998) Effect of soymilk consumption on serum estrogen concentrations in premenopausal Japanese women. *J. Natl. Cancer Inst.*, **90**, 1830–1835

Setchell, K.D.R., Borriello, S.P., Hulme, P. & Axelson, M. (1984) Nonsteroidal estrogens of dietary origin: possible roles in hormone-dependent disease. *Am. J. Clin. Nutr.*, **40**, 569–578

Tonkelaar den, I., Keinan-Boker, L., Veer van't, P., Arts, C.J.M., Adlercreutz, H., Thijssen, J.H.H. & Peeters, P.H.M. (2001) Urinary phyto-oestrogens and postmenopausal breast cancer risk. *Cancer Epidemiol. Biomarkers Prev.*, **10**, 223–228

Wu, A.H., Ziegler, R.G., Horn-Ross, P.L., Nomura, A.M., West, D.W., Kolonel, L.N., Rosenthal, J.F., Hoover, R.N. & Pike, M.C. (1996) Tofu and risk of breast cancer in Asian-Americans. *Cancer Epidemiol. Biomarkers Prev.*, **5**, 901–906

Wu, A.H., Ziegler, R.G., Nomura, A.M.W., West, D.W., Kolonel, L.N., Horn-Ross, P.L., Hoover, R.N. & Pike, M.C. (1998) Soy intake and risk of breast cancer in Asians and Asian Americans. *Am. J. Clin. Nutr.*, **68**, 1437S–1443S

Xu, X., Duncan, A.M., Merz, B.E. & Kurzer, M.S. (1998) Effects of soy isoflavones on estrogen and phytoestrogen metabolism in premenopausal women. *Cancer Epidemiol. Biomarkers Prev.*, **7**, 1101–1108

Xu, X., Duncan, A.M., Wangen, K.E. & Kurzer, M.S. (2000) Soy consumption alters endogenous estrogen metabolism in postmenopausal women. *Cancer Epidemiol. Biomarkers Prev.*, **9**, 781–786

Yuan, J.M., Wang, Q.S., Ross, R.K., Henderson, B.E. & Yu, M.C. (1995) Diet and breast cancer in Shanghai and Tianjin, China. *Br. J. Cancer*, **71**, 1353–1358

Zheng, W., Dai, Q., Custer, L.J., Shu, X.-O., Wen, W.-Q., Jin, F. & Frank, A.A. (1999) Urinary excretion of isoflavonoids and the risk of breast cancer. *Cancer Epidemiol. Biomarkers Prev.*, **8**, 35–40

n-3 fatty acids and breast cancer

Bougnoux P. *[1], Maillard V.[1], Ferrari P.[2], Jourdan M.L.[1], Chajès V.[1]

[1]Nutrition, Croissance et Cancer, INSERM EMI 02-11, Université François-Rabelais, Tours. [2]International Agency for Research on Cancer, Unit of Nutrition and Cancer, Lyon, France.

Breast cancer is the most frequent cancer among women, with an incidence rate of 88 per 100,000 women in France. International variation in breast cancer incidence rates and changes in incidence among migrant populations have indicated that breast cancer risk is influenced by environmental factors, in particular diet, and therefore may be preventable. Among dietary constituents, data from several case–control studies (Franceschi *et al.*, 1995; Braga *et al.*, 1997) suggested a protective effect of a diet high in fish, but results were generally not confirmed by cohort studies (Vatten *et al.*, 1990; Toniolo *et al.*, 1994). A number of studies would indicate that a diet high in vegetables and/or fruits might protect against breast cancer (Freudenheim *et al.*, 1996; Zhang *et al.*, 1999). While a few studies have failed to document a relation, the finding of a protective effect of vegetables and/or fruits is relatively consistent.

The role of specific food-related nutrients in the risk of breast cancer has yet to be determined. Most data suggest that the association between dietary fat and breast cancer may be more dependent on the type of fat consumed than on total fat intake. Most of the epidemiological studies have concentrated on saturated fat and total unsaturated fatty acids. Limited data is available on the relation of estimated dietary intake of n-3 long-chain polyunsaturated fatty acids (PUFA) originating from fish, or alpha-linolenic acid from vegetables, to the risk of breast cancer. With regard to long-chain n-3 PUFA, no association has been found between estimated dietary intake (Willett, 1997) or energy from long-chain n-3 PUFA (Holmes *et al.*, 1999) and breast cancer risk. Inconsistent data were also found for alpha-linolenic acid, with negative (Franceschi *et al.*, 1996) or positive association (De Stefani *et al.*, 1998) between dietary intake of alpha-linolenic acid and breast cancer risk. However, data derived from animal experiments generally showed that diets high in n-3 long-chain PUFA (Fay *et al.*, 1997) or in alpha-linolenic acid (Thompson *et al.*, 1996) inhibit mammary tumour growth and metastasis. Given the relative consistence of experimental data on the inhibitory effect of n-3 fatty acids, the role of these nutrients in the risk of breast cancer requires further attention.

Conclusive evidence of a role for individual n-3 fatty acids in breast cancer risk may be precluded by the many methodological limitations in measurements of dietary intake of individual fatty acids. In this regard, the use of reliable markers of relatively stable metabolic characteristics related to diet is of major interest. Among all biological markers of qualitative composition of dietary fatty acids, adipose tissue fatty acid composition is particularly advantageous because it reflects qualitative dietary intake of fatty acids on a long-term basis (Kaaks *et al.*, 1996), thereby avoiding the potential bias derived from an effect of the disease on the measured biochemical parameters.

We have previously examined adipose tissue fatty acid levels and the risk of metastasis occurrence in a cohort of 121 patients with an initially localized presentation of breast cancer. Adipose tissue was obtained at the time of initial surgery and its fatty acid content analyzed by capillary gas chromatography. A low level of alpha-linolenic acid (18:3 n-3) in adipose tissue was found to be associated with positive axillary lymph node status and with the presence of vascular invasion. After an average 31 months of follow-up, 21 patients developed metastases. A Cox proportional hazard regression model was used to identify prognostic factors. Low alpha-linolenic acid level and large tumour size were the two factors predictive of metastases (Bougnoux *et al.*, 1994). The probability of remaining metastasis-free subsequent to breast cancer treatment was higher when alpha-linolenic acid level in adipose tissue was elevated at the time of breast cancer diagnosis (Fig. 1). Since metastasis occurrence is one clinical expression of breast cancer regrowth, these data are in line with the possibility that alpha-linolenic acid could

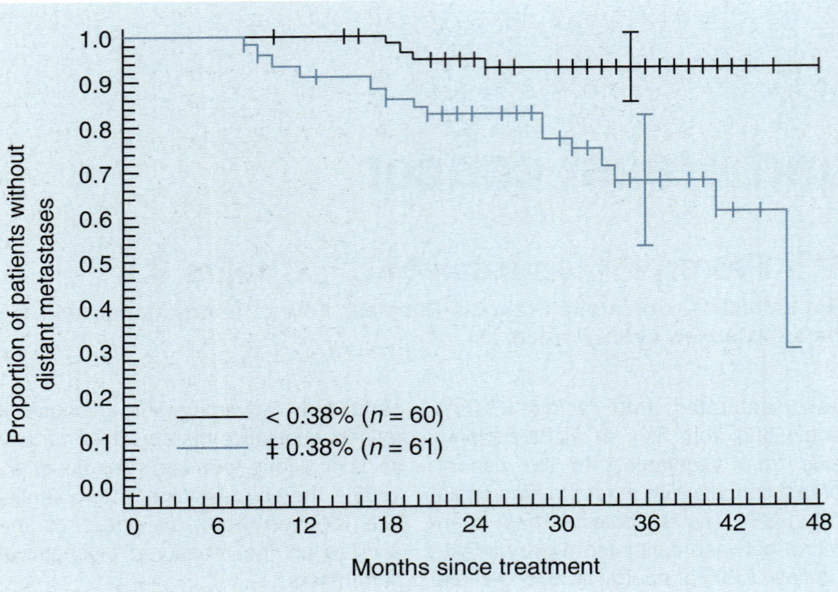

Figure 1
Metastasis-free survival in breast cancer patients according to alpha-linolenic acid level in adipose tissue (Bougnoux *et al.*, 1994). Triglycerides were purified from a sample of adipose tissue obtained at diagnosis during lumpectomy and fatty acids analyzed by capillary gas chromatography. Patients were separated into 2 groups by alpha-linolenic acid level (above or below the median value) and probability of metastasis-free survival calculated in each group according to time following treatment (P<0.01; log-rank)

inhibit or delay tumour growth in breast cancer patients. Therefore alpha-linolenic acid, which is an essential fatty acid exclusively originating from food, may be a link between diet and breast cancer.

We performed a case–control study to explore the hypothesis that alpha-linolenic acid had a protective effect on breast cancer risk. We compared adipose tissue fatty acid levels of 123 breast cancer patients previously used for a prognostic study to those measured in adipose tissue specimen of a population of 59 patients with benign breast tumours as controls. An unconditional logistic regression model was used to obtain odds ratio estimates while adjusting for age, menopausal status and body mass index. We found an inverse association between alpha-linolenic acid in adipose fat and breast cancer risk. Women in the highest quartile of breast adipose tissue alpha-linolenic acid had an odds ratio of 0.36 (95% confidence interval, 0.12–1.02) compared with those in the lowest quartile (P trend, 0.026), suggesting a protective effect of alpha-linolenic on breast cancer risk (Klein *et al.*, 2000).

This finding remained to be confirmed and additional data on the relation of long-chain n-3 PUFA (originating from fish) to the risk of breast cancer are needed. To further examine the role of n-3 fatty acids (alpha-linolenic acid and long-chain n-3 PUFA) in the risk of breast cancer, we conducted a new case–control study among 329 women treated for breast cancer or benign breast disease at the University Hospital of Tours, in France (Maillard *et al.*, 2002). This study involved new patients and was independent of the initial study (Klein *et al.*, 2000). We examined the fatty acid composition in adipose tissue from 241 patients with invasive, nonmetastatic breast carcinoma and from 88 patients with benign breast disease as controls. Unconditional logistic regression modelling was used to obtain odds ratio estimates while adjusting for age, height, menopausal status and body mass index. We found inverse associations between breast cancer risk and n-3 fatty acid levels in breast adipose tissue (Table 1). Women in the highest tertile of alpha-linolenic acid (18:3 n-3) had an odds ratio of 0.39 compared to women in the lowest tertile. In a similar way, women in the highest tertile for docosahexaenoic acid (22:6 n-3) had an odds ratio of 0.31 compared to women in the lowest tertile. Women in the highest tertile of 18:3 n-3/18:2 n-6 ratio had an odds ratio of 0.41 compared to women in the lowest tertile. These data based on fatty acid levels in breast adipose tissue suggest a protective effect of n-3 fatty acids on breast cancer risk.

In contrast to our findings, two case–control studies conducted in North America found no consistent association between adipose tissue n-3 PUFA levels in adipose tissue and breast cancer risk (London *et al.*, 1993; Petrek *et al.*, 1994). In agreement with our finding, a case–control study in postmenopausal women, conducted in five European countries, reported an inverse association between the ratio of long-chain n-3 fatty acids to total n-6 PUFA in adipose tissue and breast cancer in four of five centres (Simonsen *et al.*, 1998). These data support the hypothesis that the balance between n-3 and n-6 fatty acids plays a role in breast cancer and emphasizes the need to take into account all components of lipids.

The possibility that a low level of n-3 PUFA in adipose breast tissue in breast cancer patients reflected a reduced dietary intake of n-3 PUFA rather than metabolic interactions between breast

Table 1. Estimated relative risk (odds ratio, adjusted[a]) of breast cancer and 95% CI by adipose tissue n-3 and n-6 fatty acid levels from the whole population (n=329)

Fatty acids	Odds ratio (95% CI) 1st tertile (low)	2nd tertile	3rd tertile (high)	*P* for trend
18:2 n-6	1.00	1.60 (0.76–3.36)	2.31 (1.15–4.67)	0.06
18:3 n-3	1.00	0.97 (0.50–1.90)	0.39 (0.19–0.78)	0.01
22:6 n-3	1.00	0.84 (0.40–1.75)	0.31 (0.13–0.75)	0.016
Total n-3	1.00	0.91 (0.45–1.87)	0.40 (0.17–0.94)	0.001
Ratios				
18:3n-3/18:2n-6	1.00	0.89 (0.46–1.75)	0.41 (0.20–0.81)	0.0004
Long chain n-3/total n-6	1.00	0.48 (0.23–0.97)	0.33 (0.17–0.66)	0.0002

[a]Adjusted for age at diagnosis, height, BMI (as continuous variables), menopause (pre- and post-) and menopausal status–BMI interaction. Tests for trend were performed by using the means within each category in the logistic regression model.

adipose tissue and breast epithelium deserves consideration. This hypothesis was explored in a rat N-methylnitrosourea (NMU)-induced mammary carcinogenesis model. We reported a lack of an association of n-3 PUFA levels in mammary adipose tissue and tumour growth (Lhuillery *et al.*, 1995), suggesting that a low level of n-3 PUFA as a consequence of interactions between carcinoma and breast adipose tissue is very unlikely.

We explored the role of n-3 PUFA on mammary tumour growth using the experimental system of NMU-induced mammary tumours in rats. Because PUFA are substrates for lipid peroxidation processes, we studied the effects of n-3 PUFA on tumour growth in interaction with anti- or pro-oxidant compounds. We found that dietary 18:3n-3 (rapeseed oil) or n-3 PUFA (fish oil) inhibited tumour development and growth only in the absence of the antioxidant vitamin E (Fig. 2a). This inhibition was even greater in the presence of pro-oxidants (Cognault *et al.*, 2000). Such effects were not found when the lipid diet was low in PUFA. These data suggested that oxidized n-3 PUFA have an inhibiting role on tumour growth and emphasize the importance of the interaction of anti- and pro-oxidant compounds with n-3 PUFA. Other experimental studies on several models of mammary carcinogenesis, *in vivo* (Welsch, 1997) or *in vitro* (Chajès *et al.*, 1995) reported that the inhibitory effects of n-3 on tumour growth were suppressed by vitamin E, and were a function of increased lipid peroxidation.

A critical question was how n-3 PUFA decrease mammary tumour growth and how antioxidant vitamin E suppresses this effect. Tumour growth is the consequence of an imbalance between cell proliferation, which leads to increased tumour mass, and tumour cell loss, which decreases it. When analysing tumour cell proliferation by measuring the proportion of tumour cells in S phase by flow cytometry, we found no difference in tumour cell proliferation between the two different dietary groups (Fig. 2b). In contrast, when we investigated tumour cell loss, based on the comparison between the potential doubling time (Tpot) and the actual doubling time of the tumour, we found more tumour loss in the dietary group with PUFA and without vitamin E than in the group with vitamin E (Fig. 2c). In line with this finding, when we directly quantified the number of apoptotic bodies in tumour sections, we found that n-3 PUFA, in comparison to n-3 PUFA in combination with antioxidant vitamin E, led to an increase in tumour cell loss. These data show that n-3 PUFA decrease mammary tumour growth by increasing tumour cell loss, an effect which is abolished by vitamin E, suggesting the involvement of lipid peroxide formation. These findings fit well with data obtained in several breast cancer cell lines *in vitro*, where PUFA, in the absence of lipid antioxidants, inhibited the growth *in vitro* and induced apoptosis (Hawkins *et al.*, 1998). The extent of PUFA-induced lipid peroxidation also correlated with the proportion of apoptosis (Hawkins *et al.*, 1998).

In conclusion, in patients, elevated n-3 PUFA in body stores are associated with a decreased risk of breast cancer and with better survival. In rats, the interaction of n-3 PUFA with lipid antioxidants in diets seems to be determinant in experimental mammary tumour growth. These studies highlight the importance of the interaction of these lipids with other food components. The presence or absence of effects on tumour growth appears to depend on the background level of antioxidants and may account for previously inconsistent results in experimental carcinogenesis. Recognition of the role of lipoperoxidation in the antitumour effects of these highly peroxidizable fatty acids is a major advance in the field (Bougnoux, 1999). The potential of these promising molecules as nutritional targets for cancer prevention implies that the effects of their interaction be precisely understood.

Acknowledgements

Experimental data presented involved the research group. We acknowledge the participation of C. Couet, who provided his expertise in nutritional

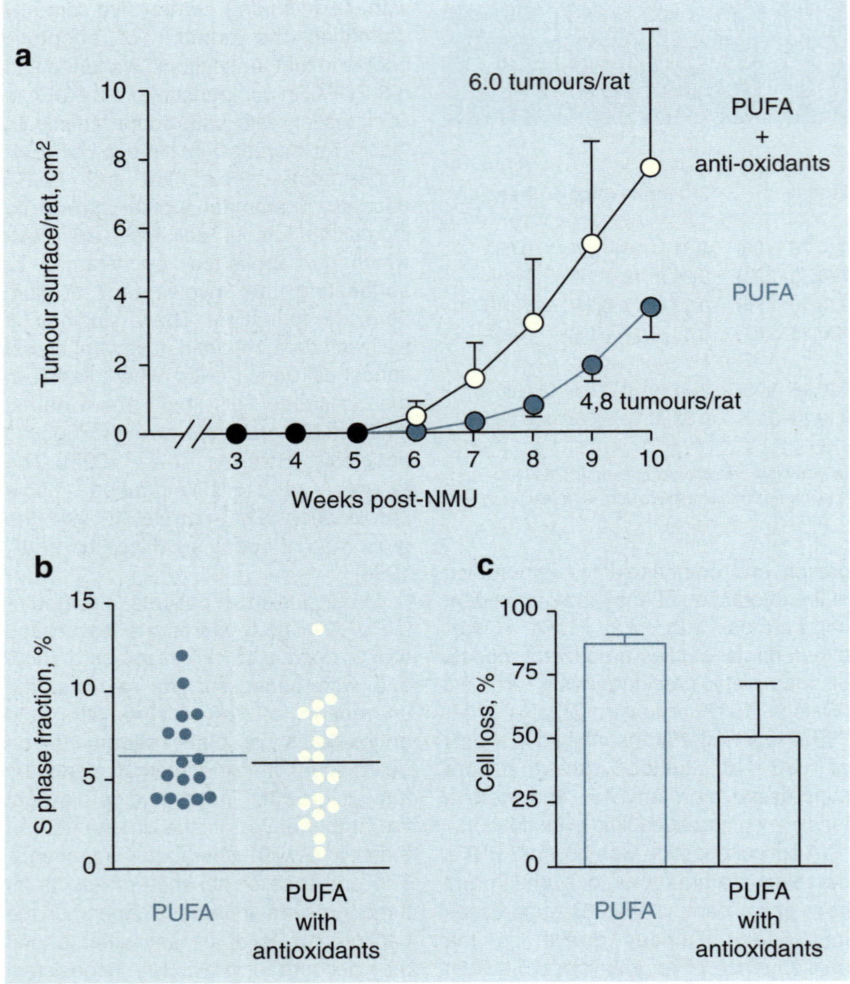

Figure 2
Interaction between n-3 PUFA and antioxidant lipids. Two groups of female rats received a single NMU injection when 50 days old to initiate mammary tumors and were fed diets enriched in alpha-linolenic acid (linseed oil) in the absence (PUFA) or in presence of vitamin E (PUFA + antioxidants). a, Tumour growth according to diet; b, Proportion of tumour cells in S phase; c, Level of cell loss

interventions, and C. Lhuillery (INRA, Jouy-en-Josas, France) who headed the research group where animal experiments were developed. Financial support was from the French Ministry of Research (Nutrialis), INSERM and the Ligue Contre le Cancer. V. Chajès is on a grant from the prevention program of the Agence Régionale d'Hospitalisation, Center Region, France.

References

Bougnoux, P. (1999) n-3 polyunsaturated fatty acids and cancer. *Curr. Opin. Clin. Nutr. Metab. Care*, **2**, 121–126

Bougnoux, P., Koscielny, S., Chajes, V., Descamps, P., Couet, C. & Calais, G. (1994) Alpha-linolenic acid content of adipose breast tissue: a host determinant of the risk of early metastasis in breast cancer. *Br. J. Cancer*, **70**, 330–334

Braga, C., La Vecchia, C., Negri, E., Franceschi, S. & Parpinel, M. (1997) Intake of selected foods and nutrients and breast cancer risk: an age- and menopause-specific analysis. *Nutr. Cancer*, **28**, 258–263

Chajès, V., Sattler, W., Stranzl, A. & Kostner, G.M. (1995) Influence of n-3 fatty acids on the growth of human breast cancer cells *in vitro*: relationship to peroxides and vitamin E. *Breast Cancer Res. Treat.*, **34**, 199–212

Cognault, S., Jourdan, M.L., Germain, E., Pitavy, R., Morel, E., Durand, G., Bougnoux, P. & Lhuillery, C. (2000) Effect of an alpha-linolenic acid-rich diet on rat mammary tumor growth depends on the dietary oxidative status. *Nutr. Cancer*, **36**, 33–41

De Stefani, E., Deneo-Pellegrini, H., Mendilaharsu, M. & Ronco, A. (1998) Essential fatty acids and breast cancer: a case–control study in Uruguay. *Int. J. Cancer*, **76**, 491–494

Fay, M.P., Freedman, L.S., Clifford, C.K. & Midthune, D.N. (1997) Effect of different types and amounts of fat on the development of mammary tumors in rodents: a review. *Cancer Res.*, **57**, 3979–3988

Franceschi, S., Favero, A., La Vecchia, C., Negri, E., Dal Maso, L., Salvini, S., Decarli, A. & Giacosa, A. (1995) Influence of food groups and food diversity on breast cancer risk in Italy. *Int. J. Cancer*, **63**, 785–789

Franceschi, S., Favero, A., Decarli, A., Negri, E., La Vecchia, C., Ferraroni, M., Russo, A., Salvini, S., Amadori, D. & Conti, E. (1996) Intake of macronutrients and risk of breast cancer. *Lancet*, **347**, 1351–1356

Freudenheim, J.L., Marshall, J.R., Vena, J.E., Laughlin, R., Brasure, J.R., Swanson, M.K., Nemoto, T. & Graham, S. (1996) Premenopausal breast cancer risk and intake of vegetables, fruits, and related nutrients. *J. Natl. Cancer Inst.*, **88**, 340–348

Hawkins, R.A., Sangster, K. & Arends, M.J. (1998) Apoptotic death of pancreatic cancer cells induced by polyunsaturated fatty acids varies with double bond number and involves an oxidative mechanism. *J. Pathol.*, **185**, 61–70

Holmes, M.D., Hunter, D.J., Colditz, G.A., Stampfer, M.J., Hankinson, S.E., Speizer, F.E., Rosner, B. & Willett, W.C. (1999) Association of dietary intake of fat and fatty acids with risk of breast cancer. *J.A.M.A.*, **281**, 914–920

Kaaks, R., Riboli, E. & Sinha, R. (1996) Biochemical markers of dietary intake. In: *Applications of Biomarkers in Cancer Epidemiology* (IARC Scientific Publications No. 142), Lyon, IARC, pp. 103–126

Klein, V., Chajès, V., Germain, E., Schulgen, G., Pinault, M., Malvy, D., Pinault, M., Fetissof, F., Fignon, A., Le Floch, O., Lhuillery, C. & Bougnoux, P. (2000) Low alpha-linolenic acid content of adipose breast tissue is associated with an increased risk of breast cancer. *Eur. J. Cancer*, **36**, 335–340

Lhuillery, C., Bougnoux, P., Groscolas, R. & Durand, G. (1995) Time-course study of adipose tissue fatty acid composition during mammary tumor growth in rats with controlled fat intake. *Nutr. Cancer*, **24**, 299–309

London, S.J., Sacks, F.M., Stampfer, M.J., Henderson, I.C., Maclure, M., Tomita, A., Wood, W.C., Remine, S., Robert, N.J. & Dmochowski, J.R. (1993) Fatty acid composition of the subcutaneous adipose tissue and risk of proliferative benign breast disease and breast cancer. *J. Natl. Cancer Inst.*, **85**, 785–793

Maillard, V., Bougnoux, P., Ferrari, P., Jourdan, M.L., Pinault, M., Lavillonnière, F., Body, G., Le Floch, O. & Chajès, V. (2002) N-3 and n-6 fatty acids in breast adipose tissue and relative risk of breast cancer in a case–control study in Tours, France. *Int. J. Cancer*, **98**, 78–83

Petrek, J.A., Hudgins, L.C., Levine, B., Ho, M. & Hirsch, J. (1994) Breast cancer risk and fatty acids in the breast and abdominal adipose tissues. *J. Natl. Cancer Inst.*, **86**, 53–56

Simonsen, N., Van't Veer, P., Strain, J.J., Martin-Moreno, J.M., Huttunen, J.K., Navajas, J.F., Martin, B.C., Thamm, M., Kardinaal, A.F., Kok, F.J. & Kohlmeier, L. (1998) Adipose tissue omega-3 and omega-6 fatty acid content and breast cancer in the EURAMIC study. European Community Multicenter Study on Antioxidants, Myocardial Infarction, and Breast Cancer. *Am. J. Epidemiol.*, **147**, 342–352

Thompson, L.U., Rickard, S.E., Orcheson, L.J. & Seidl, M.M. (1996) Flaxseed and its lignan and oil components reduce mammary tumor growth at a late stage of carcinogenesis. *Carcinogenesis*, **17**, 1373–1376

Toniolo, P., Riboli, E., Shore, R.E. & Pasternack, B.S. (1994) Consumption of meat, animal products, protein, and fat and risk of breast cancer: a prospective cohort study in New York. *Epidemiology*, **5**, 391–397

Vatten, L.J., Solvoll, K. & Loken, E.B. (1990) Frequency of meat and fish intake and risk of breast cancer in a prospective study of 14,500 Norwegian women. *Int. J. Cancer*, **46**, 12–15

Welsch, C. (1997) The role of lipid peroxidation in growth suppression of human breast carcinoma by dietary fish oil. *Adv. Exp. Med. Biol.*, **400B**, 849–860

Willett, W.C. (1997) Specific fatty acids and risks of breast and prostate cancer: dietary intake. *Am. J. Clin. Nutr.*, **66**, 1557S–1563S

Zhang, S., Hunter, D.J., Forman, M.R., Rosner, B.A., Speizer, F.E., Colditz, G.A., Manson, J.E., Hankinson, S.E. & Willett, W.C. (1999) Dietary carotenoids and vitamins A, C, and E and risk of breast cancer. *J. Natl. Cancer Inst.*, **91**, 547–556

Novel plant-derived anticarcinogens

Kosmeder J.W. II, Pezzuto J.M.
(Program for Collaborative Research in the Pharmaceutical Sciences)

Department of Medicinal Chemistry and Pharmacognosy, College of Pharmacy, Department of Surgical Oncology, College of Medicine, and Cancer Center, University of Illinois at Chicago, Chicago, Illinois 60612, USA.

Introduction

Although systemic drug therapy has been the mainstay of pharmaceutical care, the logic of disease prevention is overwhelming. This concept is clearly exemplified by the success of large-scale vaccination programs (e.g. smallpox, polio) as well as drug-based strategies implemented for the reduction of serum cholesterol and subsequent problems associated with heart disease. In a similar manner, the pandemic nature of cancer demands aggressive implementation of therapeutic and preventive measures that are designed for the reduction of this disease.

Cancer chemoprevention is a process that employs dietary or pharmaceutical agents to inhibit or block carcinogenesis in normal or preneoplastic tissues. Some active agents may be endogenous components of the diet, based on epidemiological studies that suggest a diet high in fruit and vegetable consumption correlates with a decreased risk of cancer. A number of compounds have been shown to mediate cancer chemopreventive activity in animal models and various clinical trials are underway, primarily with humans at high risk for developing cancer (Boone *et al.*, 1990). Our efforts in this area are predominantly directed toward drug discovery of novel cancer chemopreventive agents from plant sources using a multidisciplinary approach (Pezzuto, 1995). By means of a programme project mechanism, we are capable of bringing discoveries from the field to the level of establishing *in vivo* efficacy with structurally and mechanistically characterized chemical entities. Plant material is obtained from a variety of locations worldwide, with an emphasis on medicinal and/or edible properties. The plant extracts are evaluated with a panel of *in vitro* bioassays that are designed to monitor three modulation stages of carcinogenesis: 1) initiation, for example, induction of quinone reductase (QR), 2) promotion, such as inhibition of cyclooxygenase-2 (*COX-2*) and ornithine decarboxylase (ODC) or 3) progression, e.g., inhibition of aromatase, induction of HL-60 differentiation, anti-estrogenic activity in Ishikawa cells. Extracts that are deemed active are further evaluated in an *ex vivo* assay system that employs carcinogen-treated mouse mammary glands in culture. An extract that is active in one or more of the *in vitro* assays and the *ex vivo* assay is fractionated into individual compounds, utilizing an *in vitro* bioassay as a monitor. The active individual compounds are re-evaluated in the *ex vivo* assay for efficacy. The lead compounds resulting from this process are then prepared on a large scale for evaluation in an appropriate *in vivo* model, such as a two-stage (initiation/promotion) mouse skin or rat mammary carcinogenesis study.

Utilizing this discovery process, more than 3000 plants have been evaluated, yielding over 15 000 bioassay results. As a result of bioassay-guided fractionation, approximately 200 compounds have been identified as potential cancer chemoprevention leads, and many have shown activity in preventing the formation of 7,12-dimethylbenz(a)anthracene (DMBA)-induced preneoplastic lesions in the *ex vivo* mouse mammary organ culture (MMOC). Of these leads, several compounds have been shown to mediate considerable cancer chemopreventive activity in full-term tumorigenesis models. Several of these promising candidates that are now undergoing further development as chemopreventive agents have been derived from edible plants and may prove to have superior toxicological profiles.

Resveratrol

The discovery of cancer chemopreventive activity mediated by E-resveratrol [**1**; isolated from the Peruvian plant *Cassia quinquangulata* Rich. (Leguminosae)] (Fig. 1) garnished

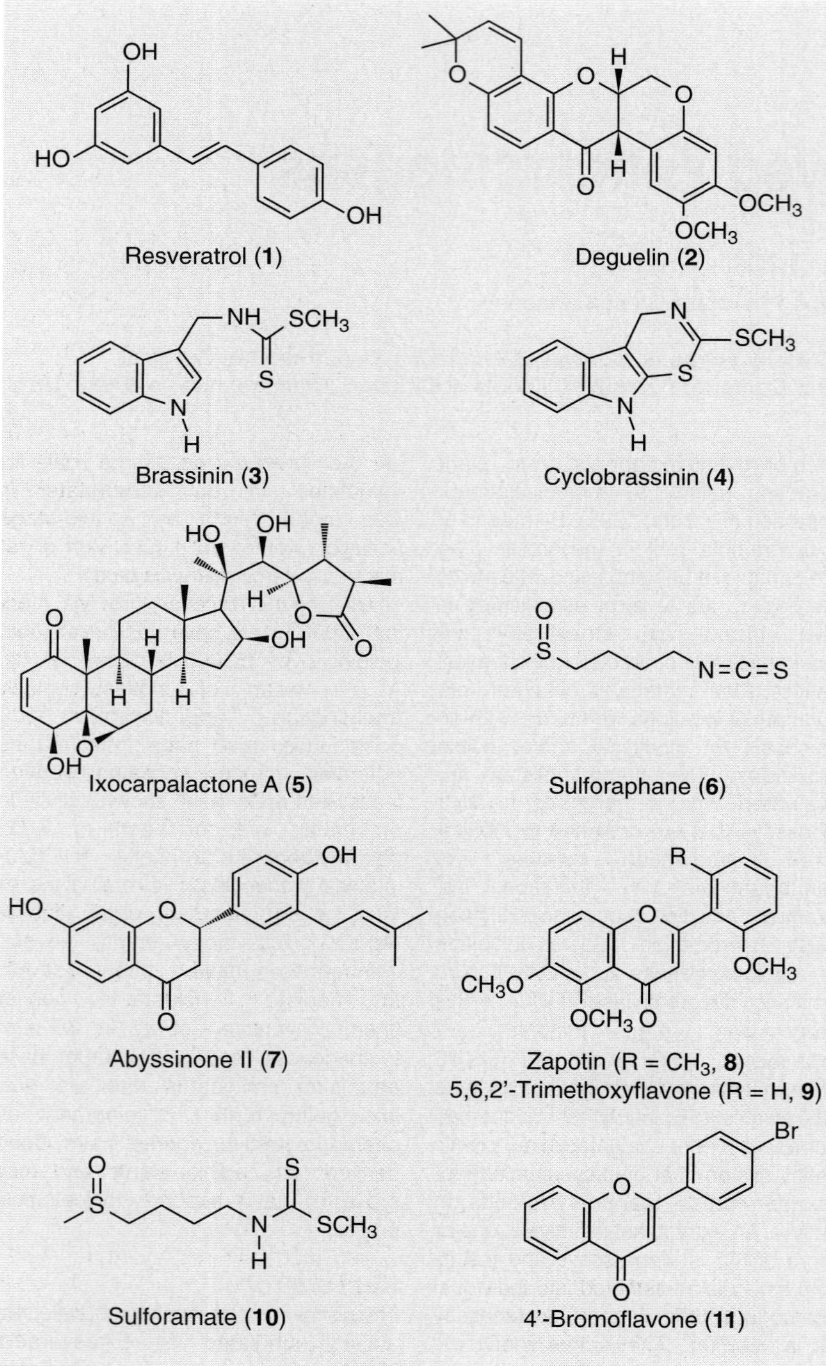

Figure 1
Structures of cancer chemopreventive lead compounds

considerable attention, as this compound is a significant human dietary constituent found in mulberries, peanuts and grapes. Relatively high levels are found in the latter, with 50–100 mg of resveratrol per gram of fresh grape skin or 1.5–3 μg/l in red wine (Goldberg *et al.*, 1995). Resveratrol can also be synthesized on a multi-hundred gram scale, which permits evaluation in animal and human studies. In our earlier work (Jang *et al.*, 1997), resveratrol was found to inhibit cellular events associated with tumour initiation, promotion and progression. The anti-initiating effects were demonstrated by dose-dependent inhibition of free-radical formation of 12-O-tetradecanoylphorbol-13-acetate (TPA)-treated human promyelocytic leukemia cells HL-60 (ED_{50} 27 μM) and an antimutagenic response in DMBA-treated *Salmonella typhimurium* strain TM677 (ED_{50} 4 μM). Additionally, resveratrol induced QR activity in mouse hepatoma cells Hepa 1c1c7 in a monofunctional manner with a concentration to double activity of 21 μM. Resveratrol's anti-promoter effects were exhibited by inhibition of both isoforms of cyclooxygenase (IC_{50} values of 1.1 and 1.3 μM for *COX-1* and *COX-2*, respectively). Resveratrol showed anti-progressional effects by inducing expression of differentiation markers in HL-60 cells for granulocyte formation (ED_{50} 11 μM), macrophage formation (ED_{50} 19 μM), and inhibition of [3H]-thymidine incorporation (ED_{50} 18 μM), which is indicative of terminal differentiation to a non-proliferating phenotype. Resveratrol inhibited DMBA-induced preneoplastic lesions in MMOC (ED_{50} 3.1 μM) without signs of toxicity.

In full-term animal studies, resveratrol has been shown to inhibit tumorigenesis in the two-stage mouse skin model (Jang *et al.*, 1997) as well as mouse colon (Steele *et al.*, 1998) and rat mammary gland (Bhat *et al.*, 2001a) models. Numerous studies have been performed to define the mechanism of action (Bhat *et al.*, 2001b). In our laboratory, the estrogenic/antiestrogenic potential has recently been evaluated with endometrial (Bhat & Pezzuto, 2001) and mammary (Bhat *et al.*, 2001a) models. Overall, resveratrol demonstrates great promise and preclinical toxicological investigations are currently underway that should set the stage for clinical evaluations.

Deguelin

Deguelin (**2**) (Fig. 1) is a rotenoid isolated from the Kenyan medicinal plant *Mundulea sericea* Willd. (Leguminosae), but is commonly found in many other legumes (e.g., *Derris*, *Lonchocarpus*, *Tephrosia* species) from around the world. Deguelin was found to be a potent inhibitor of TPA-induced ODC activity in cultured mouse epidermal 308 cells (IC_{50} 20 nM), which inhibits mammalian polyamine synthesis, thereby acting as an anti-promotor (Gerhäuser *et al.*, 1995). Deguelin was shown to reduce TPA-induced ODC mRNA expression to approximately 25% of the maximal response at 4 h compared to a TPA control. In the MMOC assay, deguelin showed 100% inhibition of DMBA-induced preneoplastic mammary lesions. To enable animal studies, several grams of enantiomerically pure deguelin were synthesized since isolation from natural sources would be too expensive and time-consuming. With this material, evaluations have been performed with the two-stage DMBA/TPA mouse skin model and NMU-induced mammary carcinogenesis model with Sprague Dawley rats (Udeani *et al.*, 1997). The deguelin-treated skin of CD-1 mice showed a decreased tumour incidence of 85% and 100% over control animals at doses of 33 and 330 mg, respectively. In the full-term NMU mammary study, rats had a decrease in tumour multiplicity from 6.8 tumours per rat in the control group to 5.1 and 3.2 tumours per rat in groups treated with 2 and 4 mg/kg body weight (i.g.) of deguelin, respectively. While tumour incidence was unchanged, the group fed 4 mg/kg deguelin showed a significant increase in the tumour latency period. Mechanistic investigations of deguelin and a small library of structurally related rotenoids revealed a link between inhibition of NADH-dehydrogenase and TPA-induced ODC activity (Gerhäuser *et al.*, 1997). Inhibition of NADH-dehydrogenase leads to a rapid depletion in ATP levels and subsequent interference with signal transduction events for TPA- or c-Myc-induced ODC activity.

Brassinin

Brassinin (**3**) (Fig. 1) is a dithiocarbamate-substituted indole phytoalexin found in cruciferous vegetables (e.g., cabbage, broccoli, Brussels sprouts), especially in many *Brassica* species, and is a common component of the human diet. Brassinin was found to be an anti-initiator by potent induction of phase II metabolizing enzymes through QR activity with a concentration required to double activity (CD) of 4.0 μM. A natural analogue, cyclobrassinin (**4**) (Fig. 1) shows stronger inducing capability with a CD of 1.2 μM. A small library of brassinin analogues were examined and all were found to be bifunctional inducers, i.e. they induced both phase I (e.g. cytochrome P450 isozymes) and phase II enzymes. When tested in MMOC, brassinin and cyclobrassinin showed inhibition of 73% and 91%, respectively, at 10 μg/mL (Mehta *et al.*, 1994). Synthetically, cyclobrassinin is difficult to produce on the multi-gram scale. Brassinin, however, is readily synthesized and was subsequently assessed in two-stage mouse skin and rat mammary carcinogenesis *in vivo* studies (Mehta *et al.*, 1995). Mice treated with a 0.5% or 1.0% solution of brassinin showed decreases in tumour incidence of approximately 30% and 50%, respectively, along with decreases in tumour multiplicity of 55% and 70%, respectively, when compared to control groups.

Withanolides

The tomatillo, a green tomato-like fruit produced by *Physallis philadelphica* Lam. (Solanaceae), is commonly used in Mexican and Latin American cuisine. Utilizing induction of QR activity as a guide, we have isolated a steroidal class of compounds called withanolides (e.g. ixocarpalactone A; **5**) (Fig. 1) from *P. philadelphica* extracts. These compounds function as monofunctional inducers with potency similar to sulforaphane (**6**; Kennelly *et al.*, 1997) (Fig. 1). Short-term animal studies have demonstrated potential for enzyme induction in laboratory animals (Song, 2000) but, unfortunately, an economically viable synthesis is not apparent. As a result, we have cultivated a sufficient quantity of the plant to permit isolation of quantities of withanolides that will permit animal testing. These isolation procedures are currently underway.

Flavonoids

A group of flavonoid aromatase inhibitors (e.g. abyssinone II; **7**) (Fig. 1) were isolated from the edible plant *Broussonetia papyrifera* L. (Moraceae), a deciduous tree found in Asia and North America (Lee *et al.* 2001). The aromatase enzyme is the final, rate-limiting step in estrogen biosynthesis and its inhibition may help treat or prevent breast and prostate cancers. Four of these flavonoids were not estrogenic but inhibited aromatase with IC_{50} values in the range of 0.1–0.5 μM. Under the auspices of the RAPID program of the U.S. National Cancer Institute (http://www.cancer.gov/prevention/rapid/), these lead compounds are currently being synthesized in sufficient quantities to permit more advanced testing.

Two unusually substituted flavones [zapotin (**8**), and 5,6,2'-trimethoxyflavone (9)] (Fig. 1) were isolated from the seeds of the edible fruit "zapote blanco" from *Casimiroa edulis* Llave et Lex. (Rutaceae). The tree is distributed widely in Mexico and Central America and the fruits are consumed as a tropical dessert. Both compounds showed moderate anti-initiating activity by inhibiting EROD (phase I enzyme) activity in rat liver microsomes; however, both also had anti-promoting activity by inducing differentiation of cultured HL-60 cells (Ito *et al.*, 1998). When tested in MMOC, compounds **8** and **9** showed inhibitions of 50% and 80%, respectively. Currently, these compounds and their derivatives are being synthesized to prepare quantities necessary for future *in vitro* and *in vivo* evaluation.

Sulforamate

In many cases, modification of a natural product lead may improve efficacy by means of increasing activity or decreasing toxicity. Two promising synthetic compounds, sulforamate (**10**) and 4'-bromoflavone (**11**) (Fig. 1), were conceptualized from natural products (sulforaphane and flavone, respectively). Sulforamate was designed based on the structure of the anti-initiating compound sulforaphane, but the isothiocyanate moiety was modified to the less electrophilic methyl dithiocarbamate group found on brassinin (Gerhäuser *et al.*, 1997). In comparison with sulforaphane, the resulting compound was tested in mouse Hepa 1c1c7 wild-type and mutant cells and found to be equipotent as a monofunctional phase II enzyme inducer (e.g., cytochrome P450s were not induced). Importantly, relative to sulforaphane, toxicity was reduced by approximately threefold. Therefore, it appears the therapeutic range of sulforamate would be much broader than that of sulforaphane and this compound is readily available through chemical synthesis.

4'-Bromoflavone

4'-Bromoflavone (**11**; 4'-BF) was synthesized as part of a library of flavonoid derivatives and subsequently found to be an extremely potent inducer of phase II enzymes (for QR in Hepa 1c1c7 cells, CD 10 nM) (Song *et al.*, 1999). It was found that 4'-BF was non-toxic in Hepa 1c1c7 cells (IC_{50} >166 μM, the solubility limit in cell culture medium). Compared to sulforaphane, 4'-BF was approximately 40 times more active and 15 times less toxic. On the other hand, 4'-BF was a bifunctional inducer (induction of cytochrome P4501A1), but simultaneously, the catalytic activity of P4501A1 was inhibited (IC_{50} 86 nM). Other phase II enzymes were induced as well, such as the α and μ isoforms of glutathione-S-transferases (GST) in H4IIE cells. Rats given a diet containing 300–5000 mg/kg of 4'-BF showed maximal induction of QR at concentrations ranging from 2500 to 5000 mg/kg diet, and maximum induction of glutathione (GSH) at concentrations ranging from 1250 to 2500 mg/kg diet, in the liver, mammary gland, colon, stomach and lung. Based on these results, 4'-BF was assessed in the DMBA-induced rat mammary tumorigenesis model. At concentrations of 2000 and 4000 mg/kg diet, administered for a period of 2 weeks, 4'-BF significantly decreased tumour incidence from 89.5% to 30% and 20%, and multiplicity from 2.63 to 0.65 and 0.20 tumours per rat, respectively. Tumour latency was also greatly enhanced by administration of either dose of 4'-BF and dietary supplementation improved survival. Since DMBA requires activation by P4501A1, the potent chemopreventive effect mediated by 4'-BF may result from modified carcinogen metabolism (inhibition of P4501A1) and excretion (induction of phase II detoxification enzymes). Under the auspices of the RAPID program of the U.S. National Cancer Institute (http://www.cancer.gov/prevention/rapid/), 4'-BF is currently being produced on a large scale and undergoing preclinical development.

Conclusion

At the present time, there are a large number of people who have an increased risk of developing cancer. One major group includes individuals who have had cancer and survived. In these cases, it would be highly desirable to provide therapeutic options that should help diminish the chance of recurrence. Cancer chemoprevention seems ideal and standard risk/benefit analyses can be performed. More generally, as the armamentarium of cancer chemopreventive agents continues to expand, it is reasonable to create a cancer chemoprevention drug formulation for utilization on a widespread basis by the general population. As with other pharmaceutical agents useful for disease prevention, a pharmaco-economic analysis of a cancer chemopreventive formulation would need to be considered and the composition of the formulation should improve over time (Pezzuto, 1997). Safety is of utmost concern when dealing with the general population, and the risk/benefit ratio needs to be extremely good. Nonetheless, it is appropriate to aggressively explore the use of chemoprevention as a means of controlling cancer in the general population. The effect of delaying tumorigenesis beyond the lifespan of a normal human being is equivalent to curing cancer. This type of "cure" can be achieved in our lifetime.

[Supported by P01 CA48112 awarded by the National Cancer Institute].

References

Bhat, K.P.L. & Pezzuto, J.M. (2001) Resveratrol exhibits cytostatic and antiestrogenic properties with human endometrial adenocarcinoma (Ishikawa) cells. *Cancer Res.*, **61**, 6137–6144

Bhat, K.P.L., Lantvit, D., Christov, K., Mehta, R.G., Moon, R.C. & Pezzuto, J.M. (2001a) Estrogenic and antiestrogenic properties of resveratrol in mammary tumor models. *Cancer Res.*, **61**, 7456–7463

Bhat, K.P.L., Kosmeder, J.W. & Pezzuto, J.M. (2001b) Forum review: biological effects of resveratrol. *Antioxid. Redox Signaling*, **3**, 1041–1064

Boone, C.W., Kelloff, G.J. & Malone, W.E. (1990) Identification of candidate cancer chemopreventive agents and their evaluation in animal models and human clinical trials: a review. *Cancer Res.*, **50**, 2–9

Gerhäuser, C., Mar, W., Lee, S.K., Suh, N., Luo, Y., Kosmeder, J., Moriarty, R.M., Luyengi, L., Kinghorn, A.D., Fong, H.H.S., Mehta, R.G., Constantinou, A., Moon, R.C. & Pezzuto, J.M. (1995) Rotenoids mediate potent chemopreventive activity through transcriptional regulation of ornithine decarboxylase. *Nature Med.*, **1**, 260–266

Gerhäuser, C., You, M., Liu, J., Moriarty, R.M., Hawthorne, M., Mehta, R.G., Moon, R.C. & Pezzuto, J.M. (1997) Cancer chemopreventive potential of sulforamate, a novel analog of sulforaphane that induces phase 2 drug-metabolizing enzymes. *Cancer Res.*, **57**, 272–278

Goldberg, D.M., Hahn, S.E & Parkes, J.G. (1995) Beyond alcohol: beverage consumption and cardiovascular mortality. *Clin. Chim. Acta*, **237**, 155–187

Ito, A., Shamon, L.A., Yu, B., Mata-Greenwood, E., Lee, S.K., van Breemen, R.B., Mehta, R.G., Farnsworth, N., Fong, H.H.S., Pezzuto J.M. & Kinghorn, A.D. (1998) Antimutagenic constituents of Casimiroa edulis with potential cancer chemopreventive activity, *J. Agric. Food Chem.*, **46**, 3509–3516

Jang, M., Cai, L., Udeani, G.O., Slowing, K., Thomas, C.F., Beecher, C.W.W., Fong, H.H.S., Farnsworth, N.R., Kinghorn, A.D., Mehta, R.G., Moon, R.C. & Pezzuto, J.M. (1997) Cancer chemopreventive activity of resveratrol, a natural product derived from grapes. *Science*, **275**, 218–220

Kennelly, E.J., Gerhäuser, C., Song, L.L., Graham, J.G., Beecher, C.W.W., Pezzuto, J.M. & Kinghorn, A.D. (1997) Induction of quinone reductase by withanolides isolated from physalis philadelphica (tomatillos), *J. Agric. Food Chem.*, **45**, 3771–3777

Lee, D., Bhat, K.P.L., Fong, H.H.S., Farnsworth, N.R., Pezzuto, J.M. & Kinghorn, A.D. (2001) Aromatase inhibitors from Broussonetia papyrifera. *J. Nat. Prod.*, **64**, 1286–1293

Mehta, R.G., Liu, J., Constantinou, A., Hawthorne, M., Pezzuto, J.M., Moon, R.C. & Moriarty, R.M. (1994) Structure-activity relationships of brassinin in preventing the development of carcinogen-induced mammary lesions in organ culture. *Anticancer Res.*, **14**, 1209–1214

Mehta, R.G., Liu, J., Constantinou, A., Thomas, C.F., Hawthorne, M., You, M., Gerhäuser, C., Pezzuto, J.M., Moon, R.C. & Moriarty, R.M. (1995) Cancer chemopreventive activity of brassinin, a phytoalexin from cabbage. *Carcinogenesis*, **16**, 399–404

Pezzuto, J.M. (1995) Natural product cancer chemopreventive agents. In: Arnason, J.T., Mata, R. & Romeo, J.T., eds, *Recent Advances in Phytochemistry, Vol. 29, Phytochemistry of Medicinal Plants*, New York, Plenum Press, pp. 19–45

Pezzuto, J.M. (1997) Plant-derived anticancer agents. *Biochem. Pharmacol.*, **53**, 121–133

Song, L.L., Kosmeder, J.W. II, Lee, S.K., Gerhäuser, C., Lantvit, D., Moon, R.C., Moriarty, R.M. & Pezzuto, J.M. (1999) Cancer chemopreventive activity mediated by 4'-bromoflavone, a potent inducer of phase II detoxification enzymes. *Cancer Res.*, **59**, 578–585

Song, L.L. (2000) Discovery and mechanistic evaluation of early stage cancer chemopreventive agents. Ph.D. Thesis, University of Illinois at Chicago

Steele, V.E., Wargovich, M.J., McKee, K., Sharma, S., Wilkinson, B.P., Wyatt, G.P., Gao, P. & Kelloff, G.J. (1998) Cancer chemoprevention drug development strategies for resveratrol. *Pharm. Biol.*, **36**, 62–68

Udeani, G.O., Gerhäuser, C., Thomas, C.F., Moon, R.C., Kosmeder, J.W., Kinghorn, A.D., Moriarty, R.M. & Pezzuto, J.M. (1997) Cancer chemopreventive activity mediated by deguelin, a naturally occurring rotenoid. *Cancer Res.*, **57**, 3424–3428

Plant polysaccharides, meat and colorectal cancer

Bingham S.A.[1,2], Luben R.[1], Day N.E.[1], Riboli E.[3]
(for the EPIC working group on dietary patterns)

[1]EPIC Norfolk, Strangeways Research Laboratory, Cambridge, UK. [2]MRC Dunn Human Nutrition Unit, Cambridge, UK. [3]IARC Lyon, France.

Plant polysaccharides and fermentation in the colon

Plant polysaccharides, as dietary fibre (non-starch polysaccharides, NSP), and resistant starch have been associated with lowered risk of colorectal cancer for a number of years. In 1960, Higginson & Oettle attributed low colorectal cancer rates in the Bantu to the fact that 'a large amount of roughage is consumed' (Higginson & Oettle, 1960). Burkitt in 1969 ascribed high rates of bowel cancers in Western countries to 'greatly delayed transit time (most of the delay occurring in the distal colon), which, together with the concentration associated with diminished stool bulk, might enhance the action of any carcinogen by the multiple of these factors' (Burkitt, 1969).

Since that time, mechanisms whereby plant polysaccharides could protect against cancer have been established. Carefully controlled feeding studies have established a linear relationship between NSP consumption and stool weight, and a strong inverse association between high stool weight and colorectal cancer incidence (Cummings *et al.*, 1992). Low stool weight leads to constipation, which together with use of laxatives is a risk factor for colorectal cancer. In one study, odds ratios were 1.48 (1.32–1.66) and 1.46 (1.33–1.61) for constipation and laxative use, respectively, with attributable risks for colon cancer of 4.4% in the US population (Sonnenberg & Muller, 1993). In another study from Seattle, frequent constipation was associated with a relative risk of 4.4 (2.1–8.9) for colon cancer (Jacobs & White, 1998).

However, factors other than stool weight are involved. Carbohydrate entering the large bowel stimulates anaerobic fermentation, leading to the production of short chain fatty acids (SCFAs), acetate, propionate, and butyrate, gas, and an increase in microbial cell mass (biomass). The SCFAs are absorbed by the intestinal mucosa where they stimulate sodium absorption and bicarbonate production (Cummings *et al.*, 1981). The stimulation of bacterial growth, together with water binding to residual unfermented NSP, leads to the increase in stool weight, dilution of colonic contents and faster transit time through the large gut (Cummings *et al.*, 1981). Butyrate is of particular interest because it reduces cell proliferation and induces apoptosis, factors which are associated with inhibition of the transformation of the colonic epithelium to carcinoma (Boffa *et al.*, 1992; Hague *et al.*, 1993). Histone deacetylase is inhibited, leading to hyperacetylation of histones, and caspase activity is induced. Caspase cleaves critical targets such as p21 in the apoptotic process (Chai *et al.*, 2000).

Nitrogen metabolism in the colon

The amount of nitrogen entering the large bowel, mainly in the form of protein, peptides and amino acids, can be increased by increasing protein intake (Silvester & Cummings, 1995). There are many different types of proteolytic bacteria found in the large gut, which, depending on pH and substrate availability, may respond to active carbohydrate fermentation in the right colon or to protein released from bacterial cell lysis in the left colon when readily fermented carbohydrates such as pectin are exhausted (Macfarlane & Cummings, 1991). Some versatile bacteria deaminate to form ammonia, SCFAs and a variety of other products, including phenols and branched chain fatty acids. When carbohydrate fermentation is active, ammonia is assimilated into glutamine or glutamate and the amino group is distributed to other amino acids as required (Macfarlane & Cummings, 1991).

In humans, the increase in nitrogen entering the colon, as a result of consuming high-meat diets, increases faecal ammonia concentration. Ammonia is a promoter of carcinogenesis induced by NOC in rodent models (Clinton *et al.*, 1988) and patients with uterosigmoidostomies who have very high luminal ammonia concentrations have a greatly increased risk of developing tumours distal to the site of ureteric implantation (Tank *et al.*, 1973).

N-nitroso compounds are also found in the colon and are formed endogenously because the amines and amides produced primarily by bacterial decarboxylation of amino acids can be N-nitrosated in the presence of a nitrosating agent. Chemical N-nitrosation may occur in neutral or alkaline conditions (as in the small and large intestine). In the anaerobic large bowel, nitrate, entering the body partly in food and water, is reduced to nitrite in the colon during dissimilatory nitrate metabolism by the colonic flora (Macfarlane & Cummings, 1991). Supplements of nitrate have therefore been shown to elevate faecal NOC levels (Rowland *et al.*, 1991). A number of facultative and anaerobic colonic bacteria are able to catalyse the formation of N-nitroso compounds at an optimum pH of 7.5 (Calmels *et al.*, 1985).

In humans, we have been investigating the hypothesis that high-meat diets increase faecal NOC levels and that an increase in fermentable carbohydrate reaching the colon could be expected to reduce them. All of these studies are carried out in a metabolic suite, where diet can be carefully controlled and all specimens collected over prolonged periods. All diets are isoenergetic and contain equal amounts of fat, and are matched to each individual's energy expenditure. Nitrate-free water is used for drinking and cooking. We first studied the effect of red meat consumption on faecal NOC levels in eight male volunteers who consumed diets low or high in meat (60 or 600 g/day) as beef, lamb or pork. Increased intake of red meat induced a significant (P<0.024) threefold increase from 40 (SE, 7) to an average of 113 (SE, 25) μg per day of NOC, mainly as acidic and basic nitrosamines (Bingham *et al.*, 1996). Subsequent studies have confirmed this effect of red meat and shown that there is a dose response to 0, 60, 240 and 420 g of meat per day (Hughes *et al.*, 2001). Long transit times and low faecal weights are associated with increased NOC formation (Hughes *et al.*, 2001)

In two volunteers, there was no effect of 600 g white meat and fish on faecal NOC: a mean low-white-meat diet, 68 (SE 10) μg per day, high-white-meat diet 56 (SE 6) μg per day (Bingham *et al.*, 1996). This suggests that the increase in faecal NOC and nitrosating products is brought about by a specific effect of red meat not seen with white meat. A major difference between red and white meat is in their content of haem iron, which is poorly absorbed from the small intestine. Subsequent studies have confirmed that the effect of red meat is due to the presence of haem but not inorganic iron (Cross *et al.*, 2002). Under certain conditions, haems are known to be nitrosated and act as nitrosating agents (Bonnett *et al.*, 1975). The formation of N-nitrosoarginine by heme enzymes under anaerobic conditions has also been demonstrated (Hirst & Goodin, 2000). Faecal waters from individuals consuming high-meat low-fibre diets have been reported to be genotoxic, causing DNA strand breakage (Rieger *et al.*, 1999) but it has yet to be established whether the NOC formed in the colon in response to haem consumption as red meat are genotoxic or carcinogenic.

Epidemiology

Despite good mechanisms relating plant polysaccharides to reduced risk of colorectal cancer, recent reports from American prospective studies have suggested that individuals who consume large amounts of either fibre or vegetables are not at reduced risk of colon cancer (Fuchs *et al.*, 1999; Michels *et al.*, 2000). Furthermore, large intervention trials, also in the USA, in which the effect of increased amounts of bran or of vegetables on recurrence rates in patients with adenomatous colorectal polyps has been studied, have failed to reduce polyp recurrence rates (Schatzkin *et al.*, 2000; Alberts *et al.*, 2000).

Analysis of the EPIC results has been complicated by the different food tables in different participating countries; these food tables also incorporate analyses for dietary fibre or plant polysaccharides which are based on different definitions and different analytical techniques (Deharveng *et al.*, 1999). Analyses of preliminary results in EPIC thus have been adjusted by centre to control for this and other centre effects such as follow-up procedures and questionnaire design. As a consequence, preliminary estimates of relative risks do not take into account the dietary heterogeneity of the EPIC cohort and are underestimated in all probability. No estimates of resistant starch are presently available in EPIC.

From 1993 to 1998, 406 323 participants, 122 927 men and 283 396 women, participated in the nine EU countries of EPIC. There were 740 incident cases of colorectal cancer that developed in that time; details of follow-up time are presented elsewhere (Bueno-de-Mesquita *et al.*, 2002). Intakes of dietary fibre were calculated from food frequency questionnaires collected from participants in each centre using local food tables. Data from individuals in

Table 1. Mean and standard deviation of fibre consumption by sex-specific quintile

		1	2	3	4	5
Men	*n*	72	58	51	43	39
	Mean (g/day)	12.8	18.1	22.2	26.9	38.0
	SD (g/day)	2.4	1.2	1.2	1.6	8.3
Women	*n*	104	115	90	83	85
	Mean (g/day)	12.4	17.0	20.4	24.2	32.5
	SD (g/day)	2.2	1.0	1.0	1.3	6.0
All	*n*	176	173	141	126	124
	Mean (g/day)	12.5	17.4	21.0	25.0	34.0
	SD (g/day)	2.3	1.2	1.3	1.8	7.2

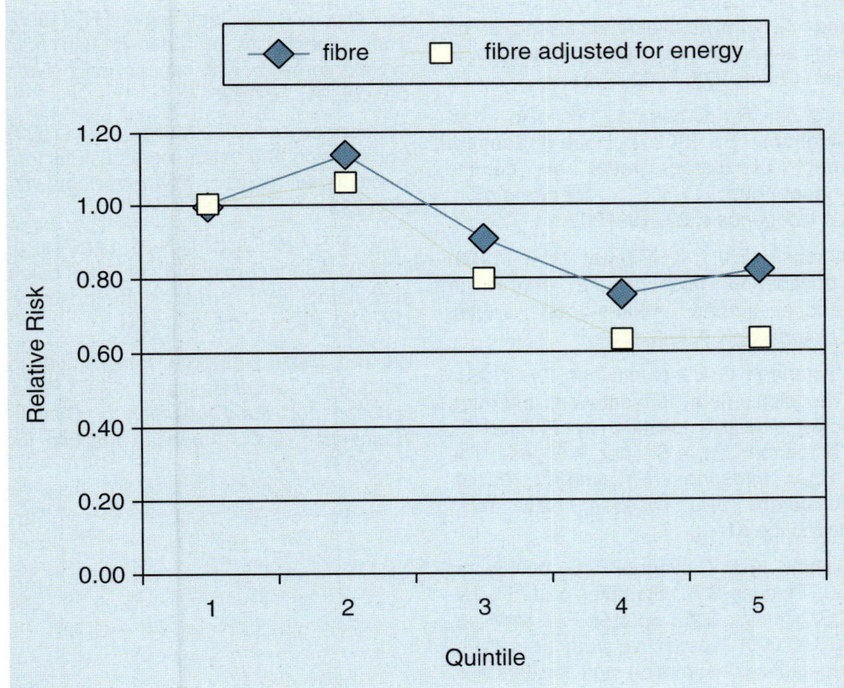

Figure 1
Shows relative risks of colorectal cancer by quintile of fibre intake and for fibre adjusted for total energy intake (g per unit of energy) assessed by questionnaire. In both cases, the relative risk of colorectal cancer was significantly reduced (χ^2 for trend *P*=0.010 and 0.000, respectively). From Table 1 it can be seen that individuals in the top quintile of fibre were consuming about 1.5 times more fibre plant polysaccharides than the average, in line with current recommendations to increase fibre intake by 50% on average (Department of Health, WCRF). These preliminary results from EPIC therefore suggest a protective role for fibre plant polysaccharides in colorectal cancer and support current recommendations to increase intake to prevent this disease

the top and bottom 1% of the ratio of energy intake to estimated energy requirement (calculated from body weight) were excluded from the analysis. Table 1 shows mean intakes of fibre from the 80 000 subjects in each quintile of the distribution and numbers of colorectal cancer cases occurring in each quintile; 124 cases of colorectal cancer had fibre intakes in the top quintile, but 176 cases were placed in the lowest quintile of fibre intake. Table 1 also shows numbers of cases of colorectal cancer by sex-specific quintile of fibre intake.

References

Alberts, D.S., Martinez Roe, D.J., Guillen Rodriguez, J.M., Marshall, J.R., van Leewen, S.B., Reid, M.E., Ritenbaugh, C., Vargas, P.A., Bhattacharryya, A.B., Earnest, D.L. & Sampliner, R.E. (2000) Lack of effect of a high-fiber cereal supplement on the recurrence of colorectal adenomas *N. Eng. J. Med.*, **342**, 1156–1162

Bingham, S.A., Pignatelli, B., Pollock, J., Ellul, A., Mallaveille, C., Gross, G., Runswick, S., Cummings, J.H. & O'Neill, I.K. (1996) Does increased formation of endogenous N nitroso compounds in the human colon explain the association between red meat and colon cancer? *Carcinogenesis*, **17**, 515–523

Boffa, L.C., Luption, J.R., Mariani, M.R., Ceppi, M., Newmark, H., Scalmati, A. & Lipkin, M. (1992) Modulation of colonic cell proliferation, histone acetylation and luminal short chain fatty acids by variation of dietary fibre (wheat bran) in rats. *Cancer Res.*, **52**, 5906–5912

Bonnett, R., Charalambrides, A.A., Martin, R.A., Sales, K.D. & Fitzsimmons, W. (1975) Reactions of nitrous acid and nitric oxide with porphyrins and haem. *J. Chem. Soc. Chem. Comm.*, 884–885

Bueno-de-Mesquita, H.B., Ferrari, P. & Riboli, E. (2002) Plant foods and the risk of colorectal cancer in Europe: preliminary findings. This volume, pp.89–95

Burkitt, D.P. (1969) Related disease-related cause? *Lancet*, **ii**, 1229–1231

Calmels, S., Oshima, H., Vincent, P., Gounot, A. & Bartsch, H. (1985) Screening of micro-organisms for nitrosation catalysis at pH 7. *Carcinogenesis*, **6**, 911–915

Chai, F., Evdoukiou, A., Young, G.P. & Zalewski, P.D. (2000) Involvement of p21 and its cleavage by DEVD-caspase during apoptosis of colorectal cancer cells induced by butyrate. *Carcinogenesis*, **21**, 7–14

Clinton, S.K., Bostwick, D.G., Olson, L.M., Mangian, H.J. & Visek, W.J. (1988) Effects of ammonium acetate and sodium cholate on N-methyl-N'-nitro-N-nitrosoguanidine-induced colon carcinogenesis of rats. *Cancer Res.*, **48**, 3035–3039

Cross, J.A., Pollock, J.R.A. & Bingham, S.A. (2002) Red meat and colorectal cancer risk: the effect of dietary iron and haem on endogenous N-nitrosation. *Cancer and Nutrition.* (IARC Scientific Publication no. 156, Lyon, International Agency on Cancer Research

COMA (Committee on Medical Aspects of Food and Nutrition Policy) (1998) *Nutritional Aspects of the Development of Cancer*, Report on Health and Social Subjects No. 48, Norwich, UK, The Stationery Office

Cummings, J.H., Stephen, A.M. & Branch, W.J. (1981) Implications of dietary fibre breakdown in the human colon. In: Bruce, W.R., Correa, P., Lipkin, M., Tannenbaum, S. & Wilkins, T.D., eds, Banbury Report 7: *Gastrointestinal Cancer*, Cold Spring Harbor, Cold Spring Harbor Laboratory, pp 71–81

Cummings, J.H., Bingham, S.A., Heaton, K.W. & Eastwood, M.A. (1992) Faecal weight, colon cancer and dietary intake of NSP (dietary fibre). *Gastroenterology*, **103**, 1783–1789

Deharveng, G., Charrondière, U.R., Slimani, N., Southgate, D.A.T. & Riboli, E. (1999) Comparison of nutrients in the food composition tables in the nine European countries participating in EPIC. *Eur. J. Clin. Nutr.*, **53**, 60–79

Fuchs, C.S., Giovannucci, E., Colditz, G.A. Hunter, D.J., Stampfer, M.J., Rosner, B., Speizer, F.E. & Willett, W.C. (1999) Dietary fiber and the risk of colorectal cancer and adenoma in women *N. Engl. J. Med.*, **340**, 169–176

Hague, A., Manning, A.M., Hanlon, K.A., Hueschtchav, L., Hart, D. & Paraskeva, C. (1993) Sodium butyrate induces apoptosis in human colonic tumour cell lines. *Int. J. Cancer*, **55**, 498–505

Higginson, J. & Oettle, A.G. (1960) Cancer incidence in the Bantu and Cape coloured race of South Africa. *J. Natl. Cancer Inst.* **24**, 584–671

Hirst, J. & Goodin, D.B. (2000) Unusual oxidative chemistry of N-Hydroxyarginine and H-Hydroyguanidine catalysed at an engineered cavity in heme peroxidase. *J. Biol. Chem.*, **275**, 8582–8591

Hughes, R., Cross, A., Pollock, J. & Bingham, S. (2001) Dose-dependent effect of dietary meat on colonic endogenous N-nitrosation. *Carcinogenesis*, **22**, 199–202

Jacobs, E.J. & White, E. (1998) Constipation, laxative use, and colon cancer among middle-aged adults. *Epidemiology*, **9**, 385–391

Macfarlane, G.T. & Cummings, J.H. (1991) The colonic flora, fermentation, and large bowel digestive function. In: Phillips, S., Pemberton, J.H. & Shorter, R.G., eds, *The Large Intestine: Physiology, Pathophysiology and Disease*. New York, Raven, pp 51–92

Michels, K.B., Giovannucci, E., Joshipura, K.J., Rosner, B.A., Stampfer, M.J., Fuchs, C.S., Colditz, G.A., Speizer, F.E. & Willett, W.C. (2000) Prospective study of fruit and vegetable consumption and incidence of colon and rectal cancers. *J. Natl. Cancer Inst.*, **92**, 1740–1752

Rieger, M.A., Parlesak, A., Pool-Zobel, B.L., Rechkemmer, G. & Bode, C. (1999) A diet high in meat and fat but low in dietary fibre increases the genotoxic potential of faecal water. *Carcinogenesis*, **20**, 2311–2316

Rowland, I.R., Granli, T., Bockman, O.C., Key, P.E. & Massey, R.C. (1991) Endogenous N nitrosation in man assessed by measurement of apparent total N nitroso compounds in faeces. *Carcinogenesis*, **12**, 1359–1401

Schatzkin, A., Lanza, E., Corle, D., Lance, P., Iber, F., Shike, J., Caan, B., Weissfeld, J., Burt, R., Cooper, M.R., Kikendall, J.W. & Cahill, J. (2000) Lack of effect of low-fat high-fiber diet on the recurrence of colorectal adenomas. *N. Engl. J. Med.*, **342**, 1149–1155

Silvester, K.R. & Cummings, J.H. (1995) Does digestibility of meat protein help explain large bowel cancer risk? *Nutr. Cancer*, **24**, 279–288

Sonnenberg, A. & Muller, A. (1993) Constipation and cathartics as risk factors in colorectal cancer. *Pharmacology*, **47**, 224–233

Tank, E.S., Krausch, D.N. & Lapides, J. (1973) Adenocarcinoma of the colon associated with ureterosigmoidoscopy. *Dis. Col. Rectum*, **16**, 300–304

World Cancer Research Fund/American Institute for Cancer Research (1997) *Food, Nutrition and the Prevention of Cancer.* Washington, D.C., American Institute for Cancer Research

Dietary catechins and cancer incidence: the Iowa Women's Health Study

Arts I.C.W.[1,2], Jacobs Jr. D.R.[3], Folsom A.R.[3]

[1]State Institute for Quality Control of Agricultural Products (RIKILT), PO Box 230, 6700 AE Wageningen, The Netherlands. [2]National Institute of Public Health and the Environment (RIVM), Bilthoven, The Netherlands. [3]Division of Epidemiology, University of Minnesota, Minneapolis MN, USA.

Introduction

Catechins are polyphenolic components of plant foods that belong to the family of flavonoids. Due to their strong antioxidant activity and their capacity to influence mammalian enzyme systems, catechins were hypothesized to affect risk of cancer in humans. Tea is a rich source of catechins; they make up about 30% of the dry weight of green tea and 9% of the dry weight of black tea. Epidemiological studies regarding the association between tea and cancer have been inconclusive, but point to the possibility of a lowered risk of digestive tract cancers among tea drinkers (Blot *et al.*, 1996). Because tea is not the sole source of catechins, including other sources of these bioactive components may clarify reported associations. We have determined levels of six major catechins [(+)-catechin, (+)-gallocatechin, (–)-epicatechin, (–)-epigallocatechin, (–)-epicatechin gallate, and (–)-epigallocatechin gallate] in commonly consumed foods and beverages (Arts *et al.*, 2000a; Arts *et al.*, 2000b). The objective of the current study was to explore associations between catechin intake and incidence of cancers of the digestive tract among postmenopausal women in Iowa.

Methods

A cohort of 34 651 postmenopausal cancer-free women aged 55–69 years was followed between 1986 and 1998. At baseline, data on diet (using a 127-item semiquantitative food frequency questionnaire), medical history and lifestyle were collected. In addition to the total catechin intake, the intake of two subgroups of catechins was calculated for each woman, the first reflecting catechins derived mainly or solely from tea (the sum of (+)-gallocatechin, (–)-epigallocatechin, (–)-epicatechin gallate, and (–)-epigallocatechin gallate), and the second reflecting catechins derived mainly from sources other than tea (the sum of (+)-catechin and (–)-epicatechin). Participants were stratified by quintile or quartile, depending on the number of cases of a particular cancer. Incident cancers were obtained through linkage with a cancer registry (SEERCox proportional hazards analysis was used to estimate risk ratios. Multivariate models were adjusted for age, total energy intake, body mass index, waist-to-hip ratio, physical activity, pack-years of smoking, smoking status, number of years since smoking cessation, alcohol intake, and total intake of fruits and vegetables.

Results

The average catechin intake at baseline was 25.4 mg/day (range: 0–278 mg/day). Only 26 participants had an estimated catechin intake of zero. Major contributors to the total intake of catechins were tea (59%) and apples and pears (26%). Chocolate, fruits other than apples and pears, wine, and legumes were minor catechin sources. After 13 years of follow-up, 5038 incident primary cancers were recorded, including cancers of the upper digestive tract (n=176), colon (n=635), and rectum (n=132). After adjustment for potential confounders, only cancer of the rectum showed a statistically significant inverse association with catechin intake (Table 1). After adjustment for confounders and for (+)-catechin and (–)-epicatechin intake, intake of mainly tea-derived catechins was inversely associated with the risk of rectal cancer (P for trend, 0.02), whereas the intake of (+)-catechin and (–)-epicatechin was not (P for trend, 0.75) (Figure 1). There were no clearly distinct associations for the two groups of catechins with other cancers studied.

Discussion and conclusion

In this cohort of postmenopausal women, total catechin intake was inversely associated with rectal cancer incidence, but not with other cancers of the gastrointestinal tract epithelium. Among 728 elderly Dutch men, catechin intake was also not associated with total epithelial cancer incidence, lung cancer or non-lung epithelial cancers (Arts *et al.*, 2001). Our data generally do not support evidence from animal experiments which suggests that catechins may prevent a number of cancers. Proposed anti-cancer mechanisms include inhibition of the metabolic activation of procarcinogens to DNA-reactive species, induction of enzyme systems involved in detoxification, and protection against DNA-damaging free radicals through their antioxidant activity (Middleton & Kandaswami, 1994).

The intake of catechins derived mainly from tea [(+)-gallocatechin, (–)-epigallocatechin, (–)-epicatechin gallate, and (–)-epigallocatechin gallate] was inversely associated with rectal cancer risk. Most literature does not support an inverse association between tea consumption and rectal cancer. Of four prospective cohort studies, one found an increased rectal cancer risk with increasing black tea consumption and three found no association. Of nine case–control studies, only one found an inverse association with rectal cancer and two found a positive association (Blot *et al.*, 1996). A major drawback of all these studies, except for the cohort studies and the one case–control study that reported an inverse association, is that they were conducted in countries where black tea consumption is extremely low (Japan and Italy) and therefore unlikely to exert any physiological effects.

In conclusion, catechins probably do not play a major role in the prevention of gastrointestinal tract cancers. Among several cancers studied, our data suggest that catechins, in particular those derived from tea, may lower the risk of rectal cancer only. Previous studies do not support our findings, but most of these were conducted in countries with a low tea intake. More research is needed to confirm our findings.

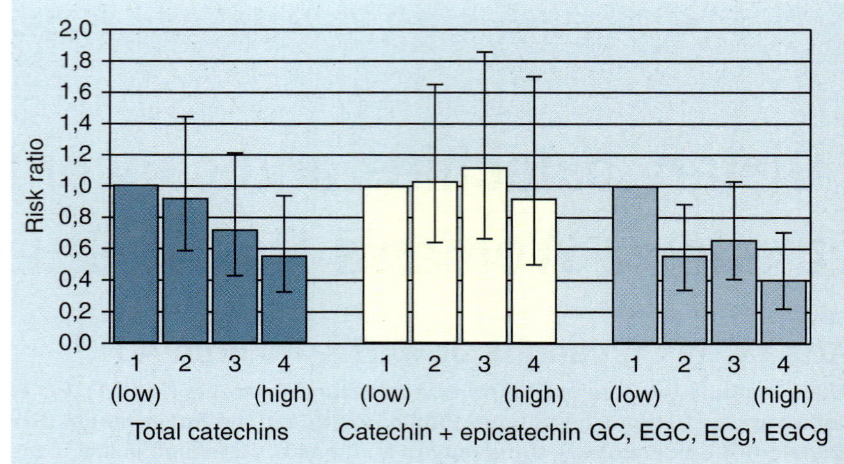

Figure 1
Multivariate adjusted risk ratios and 95% confidence intervals of rectal cancer incidence by quartiles of total catechins, the sum of (+)-catechin and (–)-epicatechin, and the sum of (+)-gallocatechin (GC), (–)-epigallocatechin (EGC), (–)-epicatechin gallate (ECg), and (–)-epigallocatechin gallate (EGCg)

Table 1. Multivariate adjusted risk ratios (RR) and 95% confidence intervals (CI) according to categories of total catechin intake

		Catechin intake category									
		1	2		3		4		5		
Site (ICD-O codes)	n	RR	RR	95% CI	RR	95% CI	RR	95% CI	RR	95% CI	*P* trend
Upper digestive tract (C0-C17)	176	1.00	0.71	0.46–1.09	0.72	0.46–1.12	0.71	0.46–1.11			0.31
Colon (C18)	635	1.00	1.06	0.82–1.37	1.15	0.89–1.50	1.19	0.91–1.55	1.10	0.85–1.44	0.63
Rectum (C20)	132	1.00	0.93	0.59–1.46	0.73	0.44–1.21	0.55	0.32–0.95			0.02

Acknowledgements

This work was supported in part by grant CA-39742 from the National Cancer Institute and by the Commission of the European Community Agriculture and Fisheries (FAIR) specific RTD Programme CT95 0653. ICW Arts was also supported by a grant from the Netherlands Organization for Scientific Research (NWO).

References

Arts, I.C.W., Hollman, P.C.H., Bueno-de-Mesquita, H.B., Feskens, E.J.M. & Kromhout, D. (2001) Dietary catechins and epithelial cancer incidence: The Zutphen elderly study. *Int. J. Cancer*, **92**, 298–302

Arts, I.C.W., van de Putte, B. & Hollman, P.C.H. (2000a) Catechin contents of foods commonly consumed in The Netherlands. 1. Fruits, vegetables, staple foods, and processed foods. *J. Agric. Food Chem.*, **48**, 1746–1751

Arts, I.C.W., van de Putte, B. & Hollman, P.C.H. (2000b) Catechin contents of foods commonly consumed in The Netherlands. 2. Tea, wine, fruit juices, and chocolate milk. *J. Agric. Food Chem.*, **48**, 1752–1757

Blot, W.J., Chow, W.H. & McLaughlin, J.K. (1996) Tea and cancer: a review of the epidemiological evidence. *Eur. J. Cancer Prev.*, **5**, 425–438

Middleton, E. & Kandaswami, C. (1994) The impact of plant flavonoids on mammalian biology: implications for immunity, inflammation and cancer. In: Harborne, J.B., ed, *The Flavonoids: Advances in Research Since 1986*, London, Chapman & Hall, pp. 619–652

Micronutrients and ovarian cancer: an Italian case–control study

Bidoli E.[1], La Vecchia C.[2,3], Talamini R.[1], Negri E.[2], Parpinel M.[1], Conti E.[4], Montella M.[5], Carbone A.[6], Franceschi S.[7]

[1]Servizio di Epidemiologia, Centro di Riferimento Oncologico, via Pedemontana Occ., 33081 Aviano, Italy. [2]Istituto di Ricerche Farmacologiche Mario Negri, via Eritrea 62, 20157 Milan, Italy. [3]Istituto di Statistica Medica e Biometria, Università degli Studi di Milano, via Venezian 1, 20133 Milan, Italy. [4]Servizio di Epidemiologia e Oncogenesi, Istituto Regina Elena, 00161 Rome, Italy. [5]Servizio di Epidemiologia, Istituto Tumori Fondazione Pascale, Cappella dei Cangiani, Naples, Italy. [6]Division of Human Pathology, Centro di Riferimento Oncologico, via Pedemontana Occ., 33081 Aviano, Italy. [7]Field and Intervention Studies Unit, International Agency for Research on Cancer, 150 cours Albert-Thomas, 69732 Lyon Cedex 08, France.

Background

The role of dietary factors on ovarian carcinogenesis was originally suggested on the basis of descriptive epidemiology and correlational studies. Few studies have considered micronutrients and ovarian cancer risk (La Vecchia *et al.*, 1987). Most studies, however, were relatively small in size, not always specifically focused on diet or based on validated food frequency questionnaires that allowed for total energy or other relevant diet-related factors.

The present paper provides further insight on the relation between intakes of several micronutrients, vitamins, and minerals and ovarian cancer using data from a large case–control study conducted in Italy and based on a validated food frequency questionnaire.

Materials and Methods

A case–control study on ovarian cancer was conducted between January 1992 and September 1999 in five Italian areas (Bosetti *et al.*, 2001).

Cases were 1031 patients with a first histologically confirmed epithelial ovarian carcinoma diagnosed 1 year prior to interview, identified in major teaching and general hospitals. Controls were 2411 patients admitted for acute, non-neoplastic diseases to the same network of hospitals. Controls were comparable to cases with reference to age (quinquennia) and study center.

The interviewer-administered food frequency questionnaire assessed the usual diet (including 78 foods, groups or recipes) over the 2 years preceding diagnosis or hospital admission (controls).

To compute micronutrient and energy intake, an Italian food composition database was used (Salvini *et al.*, 1998). Reproducibility and validity of the food frequency questionnaire were satisfactory (Franceschi *et al.*, 1995; Decarli *et al.*, 1996).

Odds ratios (OR) and their corresponding 95% confidence intervals (CI) were obtained by means of unconditional multiple logistic regression models that included eight adjustment terms plus energy according to the residual model. Tests for trend were done between the models with and without a linear term for each nutrient's quintile.

Results

Table 1 gives the distribution of ovarian cancer cases and control subjects according to selected variables. Cases tended to be significantly more educated than controls, to have a lower parity, and to report a family history of ovarian and/or breast cancer more frequently.

Table 2 gives the ORs of ovarian cancer according to subsequent quintiles of intake of various micronutrients compared to the lowest one, together with the tests for linear trend in risk. An inverse association was observed for calcium intake (OR=0.7 for highest versus lowest quintile of intake; 95% CI, 0.6–1.0) and a borderline direct association for zinc

Table 1. Distribution of 1031 cases of epithelial ovarian cancer and 2411 controls, according to age and selected variables. Italy, 1992–1999

	Cases		Controls	
	n	(%)	*n*	(%)
Age (years)				
<45	183	(17.8)	443	(18.4)
45–54	287	(27.8)	615	(25.5)
55–64	325	(31.5)	724	(30.0)
≥ 65	236	(22.9)	629	(26.1)
Education[a] (years)				
<7	577	(56.0)	1442	(59.8)
7–11	227	(22.0)	620	(25.7)
≥ 12	227	(22.0)	349	(14.5)
Parity[a]				
Nulliparous	184	(17.9)	381	(15.8)
1–2	572	(55.5)	1268	(52.6)
3	229	(22.1)	639	(26.5)
≥ 4	46	(4.5)	123	(5.1)
Family history of ovarian and/or breast cancer[a]				
No	902	(87.5)	2291	(95.0)
Yes	129	(12.5)	120	(5.0)

[a]Significant difference between cases and controls adjusted for age and residence (P<0.01).
[b]The sum does not add up to the total because of a few missing values.

(OR=1.4; 95% CI, 1.0–1.8). There was a significant inverse association for vitamin E (OR=0.6; 95% CI, 0.5–0.8), beta-carotene (OR=0.8; 95% CI, 0.6–1.0) and lutein/zeaxanthin (OR=0.6; 95% CI, 0.5–0.8). Most inverse associations were linear across quintiles, with significant trends in risk.

Discussion

Our data support the hypothesis that calcium and selected antioxidant micronutrients are inversely associated with epithelial ovarian cancer.

Vitamin E was mainly derived here from olive oil used in vegetable seasoning. Carotenoids and a fraction of vitamin E are derived from fruits and various vegetables. Calcium has been inversely related to the cancer-promoting effect of high dietary fat intake.

With reference to potential recall and selection bias, awareness of any particular dietary hypothesis in ovarian cancer etiology was very limited since the issue had not received widespread media attention. All diagnoses that might have been associated causally with or have determined special dietary habits of controls were excluded. The comparability of dietary history between cases and controls should have been improved by interviewing subjects in the same hospital setting. Adjustment for total energy intake should have reduced potential bias due to differential over- or underreporting of food intakes.

The major strengths of this study are the large dataset examined, consistency of findings across major categories of controls, reliance on a validated food frequency questionnaire, the nearly complete participation rate of patients, and substantial heterogeneity of the studied populations.

In conclusion, the findings of the present study support the hypothesis that intakes of a few micronutrients are inversely related to epithelial ovarian cancer. Whether this reflects a specific effect of these micronutrients, or the general favourable influence of a diet rich in olive oil and vegetables remains outside the scope of observational epidemiological studies.

Acknowledgements

The authors wish to thank Mrs O. Volpato, Mrs L. Mei and Mrs I. Calderan. The contribution of the Italian Association for Research on Cancer, Milan is gratefully acknowledged.

References

Bosetti, C., Negri, E., Franceschi, S., Pelucchi, C., Talamini, R., Montella, M., Conti, E. & La Vecchia, C. (2001) Diet and ovarian cancer risk: a case–control study in Italy. *Int. J. Cancer*, **93**, 911–915

Decarli, A., Franceschi, S., Ferraroni, M., Gnagnarella, P., Parpinel, M.T., La Vecchia, C., Negri, E., Salvini, S., Falcini, F. & Giacosa, A. (1996) Validation of a food frequency questionnaire to assess dietary intakes in cancer studies in Italy. Results for specific nutrients. *Ann. Epidemiol.*, **6**, 110–118

Franceschi, S., Barbone, F., Negri, E., Decarli, A., Ferraroni, M., Filiberti, R., Giacosa, A., Gnagnarella, P., Nanni, O. & Salvini, S. (1995) Reproducibility of an Italian food frequency questionnaire for cancer studies. Results for specific nutrients. *Ann. Epidemiol.*, **5**, 69–75

La Vecchia, C., Decarli, A., Negri, E., Parazzini, F., Gentile, A., Cecchetti, G., Fasoli, M. & Franceschi, S. (1987) Dietary factors and the risk of epithelial ovarian cancer. *J. Natl. Cancer Inst.*, **79**, 663–669

Table 2. Odds ratios (OR)[a] of ovarian cancer and corresponding 95% confidence intervals (CI) according to intake of selected micronutrients and minerals. Italy, 1992–1999

Micronutrient	Mean[b]	Standard deviation	Quintile, OR (95% CI) 1 (lowest)[c]	2	3	4	5	χ^2
Calcium (g)	1.0	0.4	1	0.9 (0.7–1.2)	0.8 (0.6–1.1)	0.8 (0.6–1.0)	0.7 (0.6–1.0)	6.31[d]
Potassium (g)	3.6	1.1	1	1.0 (0.7–1.3)	0.8 (0.6–1.1)	1.1 (0.9–1.5)	0.8 (0.6–1.1)	0.82
Phosphorus (g)	1.4	0.4	1	1.1 (0.9–1.5)	1.1 (0.8–1.4)	1.1 (0.8–1.5)	0.8 (0.6–1.1)	1.67
Iron (mg)	12.8	4.0	1	1.0 (0.8–1.3)	1.0 (0.7–1.3)	1.0 (0.7–1.3)	1.0 (0.8–1.3)	0.01
Zinc (mg)	11.9	3.5	1	1.1 (0.8–1.4)	1.0 (0.7–1.3)	1.1 (0.8–1.4)	1.4 (1.0–1.8)	3.69
Thiamin (mg)	0.8	0.3	1	1.1 (0.8–1.4)	1.3 (1.0–1.7)	1.2 (0.9–1.6)	1.1 (0.8–1.5)	1.04
Riboflavin (mg)	1.5	0.5	1	1.2 (0.9–1.6)	1.0 (0.8–1.4)	0.9 (0.7–1.2)	1.0 (0.8–1.4)	0.49
Vitamin C (mg)	146.2	78.6	1	1.0 (0.8–1.3)	1.2 (0.9–1.6)	0.9 (0.7–1.2)	1.1 (0.8–1.4)	0.10
Vitamin B6 (mg)	1.8	0.5	1	0.9 (0.6–1.1)	0.9 (0.7–1.2)	1.1 (0.8–1.4)	1.1 (0.8–1.4)	1.79
Folic acid (mcg)	256.0	83.5	1	1.0 (0.7–1.3)	1.1 (0.8–1.4)	1.0 (0.7–1.3)	1.0 (0.7–1.3)	0.07
Niacin (mg)	16.4	4.9	1	1.1 (0.9–1.5)	1.2 (0.9–1.5)	0.9 (0.7–1.2)	0.9 (0.7–1.2)	1.89
Retinol (mg)	0.7	0.9	1	0.9 (0.6–1.1)	0.9 (0.6–1.2)	0.8 (0.6–1.0)	1.1 (0.8–1.4)	0.15
Carotene (mg)	4.3	2.2	1	1.0 (0.8–1.3)	0.9 (0.7–1.1)	0.8 (0.6–1.1)	0.8 (0.6–1.1)	4.43[d]
α-carotene (mg)	0.8	0.7	1	0.9 (0.7–1.1)	0.8 (0.6–1.0)	0.7 (0.5–0.9)	0.9 (0.7–1.2)	2.62
β-carotene (mg)	4.9	2.5	1	0.9 (0.7–1.2)	0.8 (0.6–1.0)	0.6 (0.5–0.8)	0.8 (0.6–1.0)	7.63[e]
β-cryptoxanthin (mg)	0.4	0.4	1	1.1 (0.8–1.4)	1.1 (0.8–1.4)	1.0 (0.7–1.3)	1.2 (0.9–1.6)	1.06
Lutein/zeaxanthin (mg)	4.8	2.6	1	1.1 (0.8–1.4)	0.9 (0.7–1.2)	0.8 (0.6–1.0)	0.6 (0.5–0.8)	14.71[e]
Lycopene (mg)	6.3	3.7	1	1.0 (0.7–1.3)	1.0 (0.7–1.3)	1.1 (0.8–1.4)	1.1 (0.9–1.5)	1.35
Vitamin D (mcg)	2.9	1.3	1	0.8 (0.6–1.1)	0.9 (0.7–1.2)	0.9 (0.7–1.2)	0.7 (0.6–1.0)	2.28
Vitamin E (mg)	14.0	6.0	1	0.8 (0.6–1.1)	0.6 (0.4–0.7)	0.7 (0.5–0.9)	0.6 (0.5–0.8)	13.30[e]

[a]Estimates from multiple logistic regression models including terms for age (quinquennia), study center, year of interview, education, body mass index, parity, oral contraceptive use, occupational physical activity, and energy intake, according to the residual model.

[b]Among controls, per day.

[c]Reference category.

[d]$P<0.05$.

[e]$P<0.01$.

Salvini, S., Parpinel, M., Gnagnarella, P., Maisonneuve, P. & Turrini, A. (1998) *Banca Dati di Composizione Degli Alimenti per Studi Epidemiologici in Italia*. Milan, Istituto Europeo di Oncologia

Micronutrients and the risk of colorectal adenomas: a case–control study in São Paulo, Brazil

Cardoso M.A.[1,2], Maruta L.M.[3], Kida A.A.[3], Hashimoto C.[3], Cordeiro J.A.[2], Iriya K.[4]

[1]Department of Epidemiology, School of Medicine of São José do Rio Preto. [2]Department of Nutrition, School of Public Health, São Paulo University. [3]Santa Cruz Hospital, São Paulo. [4]Department of Pathology, School of Medicine, São Paulo University.

Introduction

There is evidence that colorectal cancers usually arise from adenomatous polyps. For this reason, studying risk factors for adenomas is important in the research of primary prevention of colorectal cancer.

Previous observational studies found lower risk of colorectal cancer among populations with high intakes of fruits and vegetables, the main dietary sources of micronutrients (World Cancer Research Fund, 1997). Some case–control studies suggest that micronutrients, especially folate, calcium, iron and antioxidant vitamins are protective against adenomas (Tseng *et al.*, 1996), whereas iron can also increase risk (Nelson *et al.*, 1994).

This report presents the preliminary analysis of a case–control study on micronutrient intake and colorectal adenomas in Brazilian-Japanese patients in São Paulo in south-eastern Brazil.

Methods

Subject selection

The study was made up of 115 incident cases of adenomatous polyps and 202 controls, aged 40–79 years. Cases and controls were colonoscopy patients admitted to the Santa Cruz Hospital, São Paulo city, between October 1997 and October 2000.

Identification of cases and controls

Exclusion criteria for cases and controls were: a) age under 30 years; b) polyposis; c) colitis of any type; d) previous colon resection; e) previous colon cancer; f) unsatisfactory colon preparation or incomplete examination (i.e., cecum not reached); g) previous diagnosis of adenoma. Case subjects were defined as patients with one or more adenomatous polyps confirmed by histopathology. Control subjects were defined as individuals with no adenomatous polyps.

Measurements

The interview itself consisted of a general questionnaire on medical and family histories, demographic characteristics, lifestyle, smoking and drinking habits. Dietary information was collected using a validated food frequency questionnaire (FFQ) for assessment of usual food and nutrient intakes for a period of 1 year before the colonoscopy (Cardoso *et al.* 2001).

Analysis

Nutrient calculations of the diets were performed using Dietsys 4.01 software (Block *et al.*, 1994). The nutrient database used was based primarily on US Department of Agriculture publications supplied by Dietsys, supplemented by the most recent edition of Standard Food Composition Tables of Brazil and Japan.

The odds ratio (OR) relative to the lowest quartile of intake for iron, folate, calcium, and antioxidant vitamins (C, A, E) were determined using unconditional logistic regression while adjusting for age, sex, body mass index, smoking, total energy and ethnicity (Japanese and non-Japanese). All statistical analyses were performed using the Minitab software, version 12.2.

Table 1. Descriptive characteristics of study groups, Santa Cruz Hospital, São Paulo, Brazil, 1997–2000

	Cases	Controls
Mean age in years (SD)	57 (10)	51 (13)
Gender (%)		
Female	42 (24.6)	129 (75.4)
Male	75 (47.5)	83 (52.5)
Ethnicity (%)		
Japanese	76 (46.1)	89 (53.9)
Non-Japanese	41 (25.0)	123 (75.0)
Smoking (%)		
Never	55 (29.1)	134 (70.9)
Former	42 (44.7)	52 (55.3)
Current	20 (43.5)	26 (56.5)
Ever married (%)	108 (37.6)	179 (62.4)
Educational level attained (%)		
8 years	43 (40.2)	64 (59.8)
15 years	43 (39.1)	67 (60.9)
Alcohol drinkers (%)		
Never	57 (31.3)	125 (68.7)
Former	9 (50.0)	9 (50.0)
Current	47 (38.5)	75 (61.5)
Physical activity (%)		
Vigorous activity (<3 times a week)	89 (35.2)	164 (64.8)
Vigorous activity (3 times a week)	28 (36.8)	48 (63.2)
Mean BMI	24.7 (4.9)	24.1 (6.1)
Mean daily nutrient intakes (SD)		
Total energy (kcal)	1877.11 (690.99)	2022.90 (749.88)
Total fat (g)	58.86 (29.38)	64.00 (29.14)
Saturated fat (g)	16.99 (8.47)	18.69 (9.79)
Dietary fibre (g)	16.40 (6.68)	18.42 (8.44)

SD, standard deviation; BMI, body mass index (kg/m^2).

Results

Table 1 shows the descriptive characteristics of the study groups. There were more female controls among the participants. Regular use of vitamin and mineral supplements was infrequent (less than 12%).

Preliminary analysis can be observed in Table 2. A protective effect was found for total iron and vitamin E intakes against the risk of colorectal adenomas. The strongest inverse association was observed for iron: the adjusted OR comparing the highest with the lowest quartile of intake was 0.18 (95% CI, 0.05–0.72).

Conclusion

In our study, iron intake was inversely related to the risk of adenoma. Why this micronutrient appears to have different effects in previous studies is not yet clear. This contradictory result may be due to differences in bioavailability and the range of the iron consumed across populations.

Acknowledgements

This study was supported by grants from FAPESP (99/01862-7) and CNPq (300167/97-0, 521475/97-0).

References

Block, G., Coyle, L.M., Hartman, A.M. & Scoppa, S.M. (1994) Revision of dietary analysis software for the Health Habits and History Questionnaire. *Am. J. Epidemiol.*, **139**, 1190–1196

Cardoso, M.A., Kida, A.A., Tomita, L.Y. & Stocco, P.R. (2001) Reproducibility and validity of a food frequency questionnaire among women of Japanese ancestry living in Brazil. *Nutr. Res.*, **21**, 725–733

Nelson, R.L., Davis, F.G., Sutter, E., Sobin, L.H., Kikendall, J.W., Bowen, P. (1994) Body iron stores and risk of colonic neoplasia. *J. Natl. Cancer Inst.*, **86**, 455–460

Tseng, M., Murray, S.C., Kupper, L.L. & Sandler, R.S. (1996) Micronutrients and the risk of colorectal adenomas. *Am. J. Epidemiol.*, **144**, 1005–1014

World Cancer Research Fund (1997) *Food, Nutrition and the Prevention of Cancer: A Global Perspective.* Washington, D.C., American Institute for Cancer Research

Table 2. Adjusted odds ration estimates and 95% confidence intervals by quartile of micronutrient intake, Santa Cruz Hospital, São Paulo, Brazil, 1997–2000

Quartile of micronutrient intake	Range	OR[a]	95% CI	*P* value
Total iron (mg)				
1	2.5–10.7	1		
2	10.7–14.5	0.42	0.17–1.00	0.051
3	14.5–20.8	0.17	0.05–0.57	0.004
4	20.9–89.4	0.18	0.05–0.72	0.015
P for trend		0.035		
Folate (μg)				
1	46.5–175.2	1		
2	175.3–248.8	1.18	0.43–3.26	0.752
3	248.9–365.9	1.76	0.52–5.96	0.366
4	366.0–1457.9	1.49	0.31–7.09	0.613
P for trend		0.788		
Calcium (mg)				
1	157.6–550.1	1		
2	550.2–772.7	2.89	1.20–6.99	0.18
3	772.8–1021.9	1.34	0.49–3.67	0.574
4	1022.0–2815.6	1.59	0.49–5.12	0.435
P for trend		0.073		
Vitamin C (mg)				
1	23.6–137.3	1		
2	137.4–207.4	1.3	0.56–3.03	0.545
3	207.5–316.3	1.24	0.46–3.33	0.671
4	316.4–1131.3	0.98	0.30–3.19	0.973
P for trend		0.887		
Vitamin A (IU)				
1	1259–6196	1		
2	6197–9952	0.49	0.21–1.16	0.106
3	9953–15 767	1.43	0.54–3.76	0.470
4	15 768–72 921	0.77	0.28–2.15	0.621
P for trend		0.078		
Vitamin E (K-TE)				
1	1480–4915	1		
2	4916–7040	0.34	0.14–087	0.024
3	7041–9530	0.41	0.13–1.28	0.125
4	9531–76 430	0.30	0.08–1.15	0.079
P for trend		0.138		

[a]Data adjusted for age, sex, body mass index, smoking, total energy and ethnicity.
OR, odds ratio; CI, confidence interval.

Biocide residues in healthy food as risk factors

Frentzel-Beyme R.[1], Helmert U.[2]

[1]Bremer Institut für Präventionsforschung und Sozialmedizin (BIPS), Linzerstr. 8, D-28359 Bremen, Germany.
[2]Zentrum für Sozialpolitik (ZeS), University of Bremen, Bremen, Germany.

Toxic effect of residues acting as depressants

Evidence favouring a protective effect of healthy food and nutrients contained in fruit and vegetables has led to a change in dietary habits in households, particularly in the younger generation. Neurotoxic effects of agrochemicals from residues on highly contaminated vegetables have been associated with depression and reduction of bodily functions.

The promoting effect of long-lasting depressiveness on clinical manifestation of cancer has been demonstrated in more than five recent publications (Knekt, 1996; Penninx, 1998; Friedman, 1999), but the pathogenesis has not been clarified.

Nevertheless, although in general, studies on vegetarians have shown a positive effect not only on specific causes of death but on longevity and balanced health, decreasing cost for medical care and protective effects of vegetable intake may have been confounded by unknown quantities of toxic and cancer-promoting factors, resulting in equivocal results of overviews on so-called protective vegetables and cancer risk, because specific types of cancer were found to have a higher than expected incidence rate.

Although provisions of fresh vegetables and exotic fruits perannually also led to new habits with increasing consumption of imported food, the assessment of regions of origin of samples with residues caused suspicion as to the misuse of biocides, both by overdosing and violating prescribed time until consumption. Therefore, the safety of vegetables such as tomatoes and red peppers has to be established.

How much tomato is healthy?

In a case–control study on risk factors for cancer of the thyroid gland, the consumption of protective vegetables among 174 cases diagnosed in the 1986–1991 period and two control groups of equal size was assessed, including the frequency of vitamin carriers such as tomatoes and peppers and other vegetables such as cruciferous plants as anti-goitrogens (e.g. broccoli and cauliflower), and Brassica vegetables. Whereas the cruciferous vegetables and coffee drinking showed a protective effect, which was consistent with previous findings from other groups, the consumers of more than 200 servings of tomatoes or more than 50 servings of red peppers during all seasons of the year showed an increased risk for thyroid cancer when compared not only with population controls, but also with patients diagnosed with benign adenomas of the thyroid gland (second control group).

The risk increase was not a chance finding in that the association was robust when stable for both sexes alone, and comparing cases with two instead of one non-cancer control group, because the increased risk remained consistent in all comparisons.

This result appears to be consistent with the role of a promotor rather than a carcinogenic effect of these vegetables if organophosphates were involved. Because the regional iodine deficiency of the study population appears to be the environmental risk factor, a promoting role is likely.

Evidence for a promoting effect is indirect in that in the years before diagnosis of the cases, increasing amounts of tomatoes were imported from southern Europe and the Netherlands. In some areas, a well-documented problem of exaggerated applications of organophosphates such as nematocides and fungicides in newly cultivated areas is known. The relatively short time span between consumption of increasing numbers of imported tomatoes from Almeria, Spain and the incidence of adenoma cases favours a promoting effect.

Toxicological evidence

Experimental evidence from two major animal studies has also shown a direct tumorigenic effect on the thyroid gland in male rats (Reuber, 1985). A rat tumour model induced the risk of mammary carcinogenesis by organophosphorous pesticides (Cabello *et al.*, 2001).

Conclusion

Residues of biocides repeatedly found in samples of tomatoes and peppers imported to the USA, the UK and Germany have increased the risk of a substantial contamination if people consume these vegetables during the season in which no regional production prevails. In an iodine-deprived region with an increased risk of malignant thyroid neoplasias, the additional unnecessary exposure to neurotoxic or endocrine-disruptive chemicals may enhance the risk and precocious incidence. The thyroid function in the protection against other cancer localisation and the indication of a strong endocrine disruption through biocides point to the need for further study of other hormone-dependent tumour types.

Even if the association is reason for concern, increased preventive measures and the well-founded advice to increase the consumption of fresh vegetables should not be revised.

The trend of residues on southern European vegetables has decreased but remains a matter of dispute (e.g. in connection with out-of-season strawberries). Further study into the cancer risk of nutritional components ought to include questions about seasonal versus all-year-round consumption as well as on biodynamic growing versus unknown origins of the vegetables and fruit that are the main sources of nutrition, with item-related

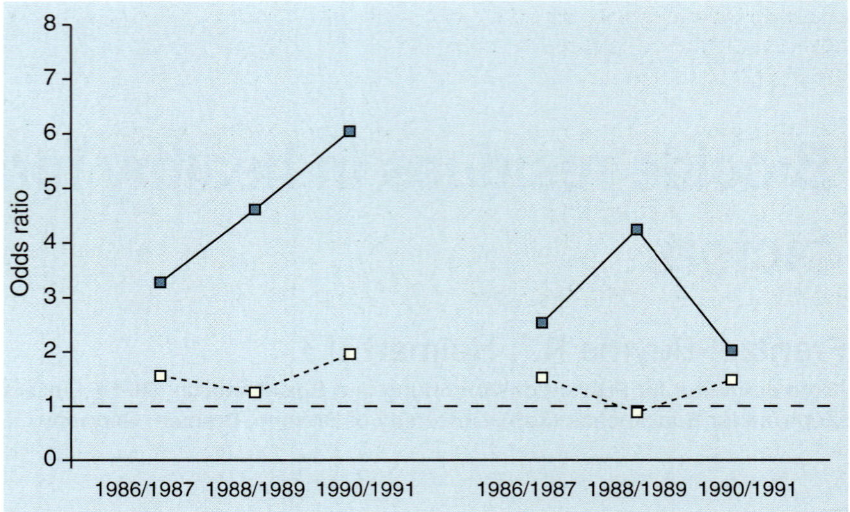

Figure 1
Odds ratios for high (broken line) and very high tomato consumption by year of diagnosis

Table 1. Odds ratios (OR) and 95% confidence intervals (CI) of thyroid cancer by education, consumption of tomatoes and broccoli, amount of decaffeinated coffee and alcoholic beverages for adenoma and population controls – multivariate analysis[a]

	Adenoma		Population controls	
	OR	95% CI	OR	95% CI
Education				
Medium	0.49	0.22–1.08	0.80	0.38–1.68
Low	0.61	0.29–1.26	0.88	0.44–1.76
Very low	0.80	0.35–1.82	0.84	0.39–1.81
Consumption of tomatoes				
50–199 times per year	1.33	0.73–2.43	1.07	0.56–2.05
200 or more times per year	3.79	1.79–8.04	2.64	1.25–5.50
Consumption of broccoli				
50 or more times per year	0.39	0.12–1.28	0.91	0.29–2.87
High consumption of decaffeinated coffee	4.21	0.89–19.9	2.73	0.71–10.6
High consumption of alcoholic beverages	1.16	0.45–3.00	1.48	0.68–3.23

[a]Reference categories, education high, tomatoes less than 50 times per year, broccoli less than 50 times per year.

and specific assessments, especially for fresh vegetables as opposed to deep-frozen food.

References

Cabello, G., Valenzuela, M., Vilaxa, A., Duran, V., Rudolph, I., Hrepic, N. & Calaf, G. (2001) A rat mammary tumor model induced by the organophosphorous pesticides parathion and malathion, possibly through acetylcholinesterase inhibition. *Environ. Health Perspect.*, **109**, 471–479

Friedman, L., Magaziner, J., Hebel, R., Hawkes, W. & Zimmermann, S.I. (1999) Depressive symptoms and 6-year mortality among elderly community-dwelling women. *Epidemiology*, **10**, 54–59

Knekt, P., Raitsalo, R. & Heliövaara, M. (1996) Elevated lung cancer risk among persons with depressed mood. *Am. J. Epidemiol.* **144**, 1096–1103

Penninx, B.W., Guralnick, J.M., Pahor, M., Ferrucci, L., Cerhan, J.R. & Wallace, R.B. (1998) Chronically depressed mood and cancer risk in older persons. *J. Natl. Cancer Inst.*, **90**, 1888–1893

Reuber, M.D. (1985) Carcinogenicity and toxicity of malathion and malaoxon. *Environ. Res.*, **37**, 119–153

Daidzein and genistein intakes in England (the EPIC Norfolk cohort)

Mulligan A.A.[1,2], Luben R.N.[1], Welch A.A.[1], Bingham S.A.[2]

[1]Department of Public Health and Primary Care, University of Cambridge, UK. [2]MRC Dunn Human Nutrition Unit, Cambridge, UK.

Purpose

To estimate the intakes of the isoflavones, daidzein (Da), and genistein (Ge) in a random sample of the UK population using 7-day food diaries.

Introduction

Heart disease, osteoporosis, menopausal symptoms, breast cancer and prostate cancer are rare in Asian populations consuming traditional diets containing soya foods compared with Western populations. Epidemiological studies suggest that consumption of a phytoestrogen-rich diet is associated with a lower risk of the so-called Western diseases.

The information on current intake of soya foods and phytoestrogens is limited in Western populations. Many Asian populations consume 20–80 mg/day of Ge, almost entirely from traditional soya foods, whereas the dietary intake of Ge in the United States has been estimated at 1–3 mg/day.

Methods

The food diaries of a subsample of 335 subjects (167 men, 168 women) aged 45–64 (mean age of 55 years), from the EPIC Norfolk cohort were analysed for Da and Ge intakes. This involved estimating the content of these two isoflavones in approximately 1000 foods thought to be important sources. A literature search on published data and some unpublished in-house values were used to carry out this task.

Results

The average combined daily intakes of Da and Ge were low with a large standard deviation. Even those subjects at the 95th percentile only consumed approximately 1.5 mg per day (Table 1). The contribution made by Ge (55%) was higher than Da (45%) in all cases. All subjects were found to be consumers of both isoflavones even though the frequency distributions were skewed to the right. Men had a higher intake of Da and Ge than women, which is most likely due to the fact that they generally consume more food.

Table 1. Average daily Da + Ge intake (μg) in a random sample of the EPIC Norfolk cohort

Group	*n*	Da + Ge (μg)	SD	P5	P95
Men + women	335	680	687	155	1510
Men	167	761	612	271	1539
Women	168	598	746	98	1327

Table 2. Average daily Da + Ge intake (μg) in a random sample of the EPIC Norfolk cohort, excluding consumers of soya foods

Group	*n*	Da + Ge (μg)	SD	P5	P95
Men + women	321	600	360	155	1327
Men	162	714	393	271	1464
Women	159	484	280	95	1022

Only 14 subjects were found to have consumed traditional soya foods – soya milk, soya-based burgers and sausages, tofu burgers, soya/textured vegetable protein (TVP) granules, and soya yogurt. The analysis of Da and Ge intakes when these 14 subjects were excluded are shown in Table 2. Exclusion of these subjects has resulted in a slight lowering of the average values but a more pronounced change is evident in the standard deviation values. Changes in the values for women are more apparent than for men.

Conclusion

These data illustrate that the intakes of Da and Ge in the UK are extremely low and that traditional soya foods are only consumed by a small percentage of the EPIC Norfolk cohort (4%). The soya foods consumed by this subsample are easily accessible and consist almost entirely of prepared commercial products. Increased consumption of soya foods will be necessary to increase intakes to significant quantities.

Reference

Barnes, S., Peterson, T.G. & Coward, L. (1995) Rationale for the use of genistein-containing soy matrices in chemoprevention trials for breast and prostate cancer. *J. Cell Biochem.*, **22**, 181–187

Sources of selected vitamins in a sample of the Italian population

Parpinel M.[1], Bidoli E.[1], Talamini R.[1], Dal Maso L.[1], Franceschi S.[2]

[1]Epidemiology Unit, Centro di Riferimento Oncologico – Aviano, Pordenone, Italy. [2]Field and Intervention Studies Unit, International Agency for Research on Cancer, Lyon Cedex, France.

Introduction

The knowledge of the contribution of a particular food source to nutrient intake in a population is very important in explaining the discrepancies among the results of nutritional epidemiological investigations in the dietary etiology of cancer.

The aim of this paper is to assess major sources of selected vitamins among Italian men and women by means of the dietary records of 2811 male and 3290 female control subjects included in a large multicentre case–control study on digestive tract, gynaecological and urinary tract cancer.

Subjects and methods

Between 1991 and 1997, a multicentre case–control study on digestive tract, gynaecological and urinary tract cancer was carried out in six Italian areas: the provinces of Pordenone, Gorizia and Forlì and greater Milan and Genoa, in northern Italy; Latina, in central Italy; and Naples in southern Italy. Control subjects considered in this work were patients with no history of cancer, admitted to major teaching and general hospitals for acute, non-neoplastic, non-gynaecological conditions, unrelated to hormonal or digestive tract diseases, or to long-term modifications of diet.

Overall, there were 2811 males aged 19–79 years (median age, 57) and 3290 females aged 20–74 years (median age, 56). Dietary habits were elicited by means of an interviewer-administered food frequency questionnaire (FFQ). The FFQ was developed in order to assess subjects' habitual diet, i.e. macro- and micronutrient intakes. Average weekly frequency of consumption of various foods during the 2 years prior to hospitalization was elicited. The FFQ included 78 questions: 25 inquired about simple food items, 22 about combined food items, and 31 about the consumption of complex dishes. Several questions aimed at assessing fat consumption, i.e. the kind of fat used in different dishes.

Satisfactory reproducibility (Franceschi *et al.*, 1993, 1995) and validity (Decarli *et al.*, 1996) of the FFQ have been reported. Spearman correlation coefficients for intake frequency of various foods ranged from 0.35 (chicken or turkey, boiled) to 0.80 (table sugar). Most coefficients ranged between 0.60 and 0.80 (mean r=0.59).

The Italian Food Composition Database was used to compute vitamin intake (Salvini *et al.*, 1998). Losses due to cooking were subtracted from the computation of vitamin contents when appropriate.

For total carotene, vitamin D, vitamin E and folate, the percentage of consumption contributed by every single food, food group or recipe was calculated as the proportion of nutrient derived from each food, with respect to total intake of that nutrient in the entire sample. Then, an ordered list was created sorting all foods by percent contribution to intake for males and females.

Results

Tables 1 and 2 give the 10 major sources of vitamins for males and females. Fish was the major contributor of vitamin D in males (47.3%) and in females (51.4%). Raw and cooked carrots were the highest source of total carotene in both males (27%) and females (32%). Raw vegetables were the major source of vitamin E in females (24%) and in males (23%).

Bread was the first contributor of folate (16.7%) in males and green salad (12.8%) in females. The sum of contributors of folate from vegetables and fruits was 27.5% in males and 39% in females. Cereals, i.e. bread and pasta with tomato sauce or with ragù, contributed to the intake of folate for 22.1% in males and 12.8% in females. Pasta with tomato sauce contributed to

Table 1. Total carotene, vitamin E, vitamin D, and folate: major sources and percent contribution to intake in males. Italy 1991–1999

Total carotene	%	Cum %	Vitamin E	%	Cum%	Vitamin D	%	Cum %	Folate	%	Cum %
Raw carrots	14.3	14.3	Green and red salads	13.3	13.3	Fish/molluscs, boiled or broiled	36.8	36.8	Bread	16.7	16.7
Cooked carrots	12.7	27.0	Tomatoes	9.7	22.9	Tuna/sardines packed in oil	10.5	47.3	Green and red salads	11.9	28.6
Green and red salads	12.0	39.0	Pasta/rice with tomato sauce	9.1	32.1	Steak/roast beef/lean ground beef, veal or horse meat	7.8	55.1	Citrus fruits	7.1	35.7
Spinach/other greens	9.8	48.9	Apples and pears	5.7	37.8	Chicken/turkey, rabbit roasted, fried or stewed	4.5	59.6	Spinach/other greens	5.6	41.3
Pasta with beans/vegetable soup with noodles	7.5	56.3	Pasta with beans/vegetable soup with noodles	4.5	42.3	Beef or veal stew/meatballs, etc.	4.1	63.7	Pasta with beans/vegetable soup with noodles	5.3	46.7
Salad with carrots, cucumbers, peppers	6.4	62.7	Boiled potatoes	4.2	46.5	Pasta/rice with ragù sauce	2.8	66.5	Light soup with noodles	4.1	50.7
Pasta/rice with tomato sauce	6.0	68.8	Spinach/other greens	3.5	50.0	Boiled/poached or raw eggs	2.8	69.3	Liver	3.0	53.8
Peaches, apricots and prunes	5.1	73.9	Pasta/rice with ragù sauce	3.4	53.4	Lasagne/cannelloni/ tortellini with meat filling	2.7	71.9	Pasta/rice with tomato sauce	2.9	56.7
Citrus fruits	4.3	78.1	Salad with carrots, cucumbers, peppers	3.3	56.7	Raw ham/breasaola/ speck[a]	2.6	47.6	Tomatoes	2.9	59.5
Pasta/rice with ragù sauce	3.6	81.7	Zucchini/eggplants/ peppers, cooked	3.3	60.0	Fish/molluscs, fried	2.6	77.2	Pasta/rice with ragù sauce	2.5	62.0

[a]bresaola and speck are traditional salted meats
Cum %, cumulative frequency.

Table 2. Total carotene, vitamin E, vitamin D, and folate: major sources and percent contribution to intake in females. Italy 1991–1999

Total carotene	%	Cum %	Vitamin E	%	Cum%	Vitamin D	%	Cum %	Folate	%	Cum %
Raw carrots	17.7	17.7	Green and red salads	14.1	14.1	Fish/molluscs, boiled or broiled	41.9	41.9	Green salad	12.8	12.8
Cooked carrots	14.3	32.0	Tomatoes	9.9	24.0	Tuna/sardines packed in oil	9.5	51.4	Bread	10.3	23.1
Green and red salads	11.6	43.6	Pasta/rice with tomato sauce	7.7	31.7	Steak/roast beef/lean ground beef, veal or horse meat	7.7	59.1	Citrus fruits	8.8	31.9
Spinach/other greens	10.4	53.6	Apples and pears	5.8	37.5	Chicken/turkey, rabbit roasted, fried or stewed	4.2	63.3	Spinach/other greens	6.6	38.5
Salad with carrots, cucumbers, peppers	6.5	60.5	Pasta with beans/vegetable soup with noodles	4.3	41.8	Beef or veal stew/meat balls, etc	3.7	67.0	Pasta with beans/vegetable soup with noodles	5.1	43.6
Pasta with beans/vegetable soup with noodles	6.4	66.9	Boiled potatoes	4.2	46.0	Chicken/turkey, broiled or boiled	3.1	70.2	Light soup with noodles	4.6	48.2
Peaches, apricots and prunes	5.5	72.4	Spinach/other greens	4.1	50.1	Boiled/poached or raw eggs	2.9	73.1	Tomatoes	3.0	51.2
Citrus fruits	4.7	77.1	Zucchini/eggplants/ peppers cooked	4.0	54.0	Pound cake, plain cakes, Christmas and Easter cakes	2.7	75.7	Kiwi fruit	2.7	53.8
Pasta/rice with tomato sauce	4.6	81.7	Salad with carrots, cucumbers, peppers	3.7	57.8	Raw ham/breasaola/ speck[a]	2.5	78.2	Liver	2.6	56.5
Tomatoes	3.0	84.7	Raw carrots	2.9	60.7	Wiener schnitzel	2.2	80.4	Pasta/rice with tomato sauce	2.5	59.0

[a]bresaola and speck are traditional salted meats.
Cum %, cumulative frequency.

the intake of vitamin E: 9.1% in males and 7.7% in females.

Discussion

A better understanding of the diet in the target population would help interpret the results of epidemiological studies. Although our sample was not fully representative of the Italian population, a high number of subjects were involved and they resided in various areas of the country and belonged to different socio-economic strata.

Our study shows that major sources of vitamins were similar for vitamin D, vitamin E and total carotene: substantial differences between males and females were observed for folate sources. As also reported by Turrini *et al.* (2001), men consume a higher quantity of starch, particularly bread, than women. Often, then, the major contributors to the intake of specific components were foods with a relatively low content of such nutrients, but eaten in large quantities. The folate quantity in a serving of bread is lower (14.5 μg) than in a serving of spinach/other greens (141.64 μg) (Salvini *et al.*, 1998), but bread was consumed much more often (weekly mean among users: males, 24.6%; females, 12.8%) than spinach/other greens (weekly mean among users: males, 0.66%; females, 0.75%) (data not shown).

As expected, pasta with tomato sauce, a typical Italian dish, contributed significantly to the intake of vitamin E, folate and total carotene; its ingredients, especially tomatoes and vegetable oil used as dressing, are rich in vitamins.

This study shows that the intake of certain vitamins could vary substantially between men and women in relation to frequency and quantity of foods consumed. Our work highlights possible relations between various vitamins and food frequency intake, which may help in interpreting some discrepant findings in epidemiological studies on diet and cancer in different parts of the world.

References

Decarli, A., Franceschi, S., Ferraroni, M., Gnagnarella, P., Parpinel, M.T., La Vecchia, C., Negri, E., Salvini, S., Falcini, F. & Giacosa, A. (1996) Validation of a food frequency questionnaire to assess dietary intakes in cancer studies in Italy. Results for specific nutrients. *Ann. Epidemiol.*, **6**, 110–118

Franceschi, S., Barbone, F., Negri, E., Decarli, A., Ferraroni, M., Filiberti, R., Giacosa, A., Gnagnarella, P., Nanni, O., Salvini, S. & La Vecchia, C. (1995) Reproducibility of an Italian food frequency questionnaire for cancer studies. Results for specific nutrients. *Ann. Epidemiol.*, **5**, 69–75

Franceschi, S., Negri, E., Salvini, S., Decarli, A., Ferraroni, M., Filiberti, R., Giacosa, A., Talamini, R., Nanni, O., Panarello, G. & La Vecchia, C. (1993). Reproducibility of an Italian food frequency questionnaire for cancer studies: results for specific food items. *Eur. J. Cancer*, **29A**, 2298–2305

Salvini, S., Parpinel, M., Gnagnarella, P., Maisonneuve, P. & Turrini, A. (1998) *Banca Dati di Composizione Degli Alimenti per Studi Epidemiologici in Italia*. Milan, Istituto Europeo di Oncologia

Turrini, A., Saba, A., Perrone, D., Cialda, E. & D'Amicis, A. (2001) Food consumption patterns in Italy: the INN-CA study 1994–1996. *Eur. J. Clin. Nutr.*, **55**, 571–588

The effects of an isoflavone intervention on the urinary excretion of hormone metabolites in premenopausal women

Maskarinec G.[1], Franke A.A.[1], Williams A.E.[1], Stanczyk F.C.[2]

[1]Cancer Research Center of Hawaii, Honolulu, HI. [2]University of Southern California, Los Angeles, CA, USA.

Purpose

Low breast cancer incidence in Asian countries with high soy consumption and structural similarities between estrogens and isoflavones, which are phytoestrogens contained in soy foods, have led to the hypothesis that isoflavones may affect breast cancer risk. This randomized double-blind trial with 34 premenopausal women investigated whether 100 mg of soy isoflavones per day versus placebo affects the levels of estrogen metabolites excreted in urine over a period of 1 year. Estrone-3-glucuronide (E1-3-G), a principal urinary metabolite of estradiol, is thought to reflect serum estradiol levels in premenopausal women (Adlercreutz *et al.*, 1982). The metabolite, 16α-hydroxyestrone (16α-OH E1), is considered to be more genotoxic, whereas 2-hydroxyestrone (2-OH E1) appears to inhibit breast cell proliferation (Yager & Liehr, 1996). A higher ratio of 2-OH E1 to 16α-OH E1 has been proposed as a risk factor for the development of breast cancer (Kabat *et al.*, 1997).

Methods

The study was approved by the Committee on Human Studies at the University of Hawaii. All women signed informed consent forms before the beginning of the study and completed a food frequency questionnaire. Potential participants had to be 35–46 years of age, report a low soy intake during the last year, have an intact uterus and ovaries as well as regular menstrual periods, and successfully complete a 2-week run-in period. Women reporting a previous history of cancer, hormone medication, plans of becoming pregnant and serious medical conditions were excluded. The study tablets contained 38 mg aglycone equivalents, with an isoflavone pattern similar to that in soy foods. Urine samples were taken approximately 5 days after ovulation, as determined by an ovulation kit at months 0, 1, 3, 6, and 12. Urinary isoflavone excretion was assessed using high-pressure liquid chromatography (Franke & Custer, 1994). E1-3-G was measured directly in urine by enzyme immunoassay. Commercially available competitive immunoassay kits (Estramet: Immuna Care Corporation, Bethlehem, PA) were used to determine levels of 16α-OH E1 and 2-OH E1 in urine (Bradlow *et al.*, 1998). All estrogen metabolites were expressed in relation to creatinine concentration. After log transformation, we applied a mixed linear model (PROC MIXED, SAS version 8, SAS Institute Inc., Cary, NC, 1999) to test for an intervention effect.

Results

Except for a small difference in age, the two groups were similar in demographic, anthropometric, and dietary characteristics at baseline (Table 1). Compliance as measured by tablet count was slightly higher in the control than in the intervention group. The urinary isoflavone excretion increased more than 10 times in the intervention group and remained high throughout the study. The number of self-reported health effects was low and did not differ by group. Over the 1-year period, we found no significant differences in the levels of any of the measured metabolites by treatment group (Figure 1). The test statistics for a treatment effect were as follows: $F(1,32) = 0.14$, P=0.71 for E1-3-G; $F(1,32) = 1.32$, P=0.26 for 16α-OH E1; and $F(1,32) = 0.46$, P=0.50 for 2-OH E1. No effect was found for the 2-OH E1/16α-OH E1 ratio ($F(1,32) = 0.10$, P=0.75). Controlling for age, excluding cycles without ovulation, restricting the analysis to compliant subjects (urinary isoflavone excretion >412 nmol/h) did not change the results.

Table 1. Characteristics of the study population and compliance with the study regimen

Characteristic	Time of assessment	Control group[a] Mean	SD	Intervention group[a] Mean	SD	P value of difference between groups
Age (years)	Baseline	43.2	1.8	41.5	3.1	0.05
Asian ethnicity	Baseline	5.0		6		0.33
Weight (lbs)	Baseline	145.0	24.0	144.3	32.5	0.94
	12 months	144.8	24.0	145.8	32.8	0.93
Energy intake (kcal/d)	Baseline	1775	544	1795	696	0.93
	12 months	1705	475	1758	960	0.85
Tablets taken (%)						
	1 month	93.9	4.9	83.9	13.7	0.01
	3 months	92.6	8.2	85.3	18.3	0.15
	6 months	91.2	7.7	92.0	15.3	0.87
	12 months	92.6	9.1	87.7	18.6	0.40
Total urinary isoflavones (nmol/h)						
	Baseline	200	349	213	488	0.53
	1 month	227	398	3054	2409	<0.001
	3 months	565	1826	2876	1892	<0.001
	6 months	401	817	3771	2658	<0.001
	12 months	367	911	4757	7001	<0.001

[a] n=17 per group at baseline and n=14 per group for follow-up questionnaire.

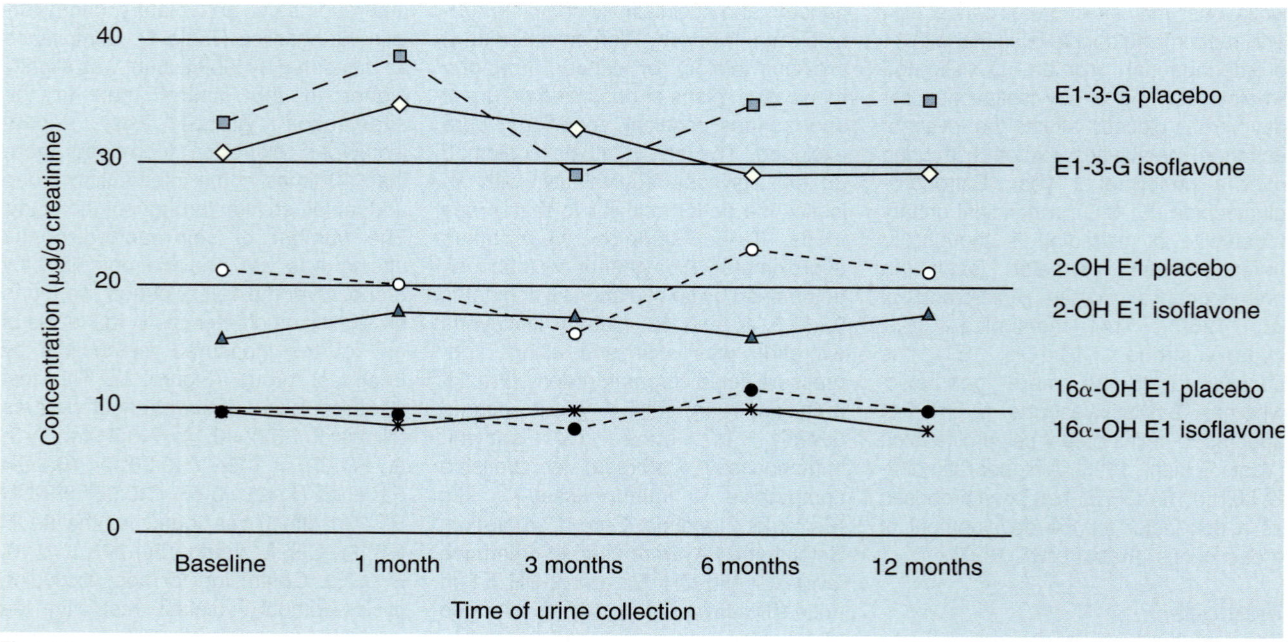

Figure 1
Urinary estrogen metabolites by group and time of urine collection All metabolites are adjusted for creatinine excretion. Dotted lines, placebo group. E1-3-G, estrone-3-glucuronide; 2-OH E1, 2-hydroxyestrone; 16α-OH E1, 16α-hydroxyestrone

Conclusions

Our findings disagree with the findings of two previous interventions using soy protein isolate that described an increase in the ratio of 2-OH E1/16α-OH E1, one based on an increase in 2-OH E1 (Lu *et al.*, 2000), the other one on a decrease in 16α-OH E1 (Xu *et al.*, 1998). The latter study also observed a decrease in other urinary estrogens, which disagrees with our lack of change in E1-3-G levels. The findings of the current study which, in comparison to the two previous reports, was randomized, had more study subjects, and lasted considerably longer, do not support the hypothesis that isoflavone intake changes the patterns of urinary estrogen metabolites in premenopausal women. It remains possible, however, that isoflavones alone may have different effects from isoflavones present in soy foods.

Acknowledgements

We are grateful to the women who donated their time and effort to participate in this study. The project was funded by a contract from the Pharmavite Corporation in San Fernando, California and by a Developmental Funds award from the Cancer Center Support grant to the Cancer Research Center of Hawaii (P30CA071789).

References

Adlercreutz, H., Brown, J., Collins, W., Goebelsman, U., Kellie, A., Campbell, H., Spieler, J. & Braissand, G. (1982) The measurement of urinary steroid glucuronides as indices of the fertile period in women. World Health Organization, Task Force on Methods for the Determination of the Fertile Period, special programme of research, development and research training in human reproduction. *J. Steroid. Biochem.*, **17**, 695–702

Bradlow, H.L., Sepkovic, D.W., Klug, T. & Osborne, M.P. (1998) Application of an improved ELISA assay to the analysis of urinary estrogen metabolites. *Steroids*, **63**, 406–413

Franke, A.A. & Custer, L.J. (1994) High-performance liquid chromatographic assay of isoflavonoids and coumestrol from human urine. *J. Chromotography B, Biomed. Appl.*, **662**, 47–60

Kabat, G.C., Chang, C.J., Sparano, J.A., Sepkovie, D.W., Hu, X.P., Khalil, A., Rosenblatt, R. & Bradlow, H.L. (1997) Urinary estrogen metabolites and breast cancer: a case–control study. *Cancer Epidemiol. Biomarkers Prev.*, **6**, 505–509

Lu, L.J., Cree, M., Josyula, S., Nagamani, M., Grady, J.J., & Anderson, K.E. (2000) Increased urinary excretion of 2-hydroxyestrone but not 16alpha-hydroxyestrone in premenopausal women during a soya diet containing isoflavones. *Cancer Res.*, **60**, 1299–1305

Xu, X., Duncan, A.M., Merz, B.E., & Kurzer, M.S. (1998) Effects of soy isoflavones on estrogen and phytoestrogen metabolism in premenopausal women. *Cancer Epidemiol. Biomarkers Prev.*, **7**, 1101–1108

Yager, J.D. & Liehr, J.G. (1996) Molecular mechanisms of estrogen carcinogenesis. *Annu. Rev. Pharmacol. Toxicol.*, **36**, 203–232

Bracken fern (*Pteridium aquilinum*) ingestion and oesophageal and stomach cancer

Marliére C.A.[1,2], Wathern P.[1], Castro M.C.F.M.[2], O'Connor, P.[3], Galvao, M.A.[2]

[1]University of Wales, UK. [2]Federal University of Ouro Preto, Brazil. [3]CRC Carcinogenesis Group, Paterson Institute for Cancer Research, Christie Hospital, UK.

Purpose

The results of the study by Galvão *et al.* (1992) showed that the proportional mortality from oesophageal and stomach cancer for the period 1979–1987 in Ouro Preto and Mariana, Brazil were 43.45% of all deaths by cancer and 56.55% for all other cancers. The morbidity and mortality due to oesophageal and stomach cancer are 15.02 and 15.78, respectively, for these two towns. Each value is higher than the average cancer rate for the Minas Gerais, for the south-eastern region and for Brazil as a whole. In this region, *Pteridium aquilinum*, subsp *caudatum* var. *arachnoideum*, is habitually eaten as a typical dish. This plant has been associated as a possible risk factor to oesophageal and stomach cancer as reported by Hirayama (1979) and Galpin *et al.* (1990), leading us to investigate a possible association between bracken consumption and cancer of the upper digestive tract.

Methods

A retrospective case–control study of the risk factors for oesophageal and stomach cancer was performed in the Ouro Preto region based on an epidemiological surveillance system established at the only two endoscopy departments available in the region. From March 1991 to March 1995, all patients with suspected oesophageal and stomach cancer admitted to the two main hospitals in the region (86 cases and controls in all) were considered for entry into the study. A group of 39 controls (aged 40–95 years) was also selected. A standardized interview was conducted using the same questionnaire for all cases and controls. The cause–effect relationship between bracken fern ingestion and oesophageal and stomach cancer, the role of socio-economic and demographic factors and life style, such as diet, smoking and alcohol consumption, and the protective effect of micro- and macronutrients in the diet on the upper digestive tract were factors in this investigation. The analysis was by univariate and multivariate methods.

Results

In relation to oesophageal cancer, the findings indicate that bracken fern is a

Table 1. Relative risk of oesophageal cancer associated with bracken intake[a]

			1[b]			2[c]			3[d]		
Bracken	Control	Case	OR	CI	*P* value	OR	CI	*P* value	OR	CI	*P* value
Not eaten	7	3									
Eaten	6	17	6.61	(1.28–34.14)	0.0241	7.03	(1.17–42.36)	0.0334	8.12	(1.33–49.41)	0.0230
Total	13	20									

[a]OR, odds ratio; CI, confidence interval.
[b]Value not adjusted.
[c]Value adjusted for sex, age, smoking and alcohol consumption.
[d]Value adjusted for residence.

Table 2. Relative risk of stomach cancer associated with bracken intake[a]

			1[b]			2[c]			3[d]		
Bracken	**Control**	**Case**	**OR**	**CI**	***P* value**	**OR**	**CI**	***P* value**	**OR**	**CI**	***P* value**
Not eaten	7	4									
Eaten	19	23	2.12	(0.54–8.34)	0.2831	2.09	(0.50–8.74)	0.3126	2.98	(0.58–15.44)	0.1928
Total	26	27									

[a]OR, odds ratio; CI, confidence interval.
[b]Value not adjusted.
[c]Value adjusted for sex, age, smoking and alcohol consumption.
[d]Value adjusted for residence.

strong risk factor, in that those who eat bracken have an 8.12-fold greater chance of developing cancer compared to those who do not eat it (Table 1). In addition, a diet poor in vitamin C shows an association with oesophageal cancer (OR, 4.80; 95% IC, 1.03–7.66; P=0.0414). On the other hand, bracken fern did not show a risk factor for stomach cancer (Table 2).

Discussion

A prospective epidemiological study in Japan (Hirayama, 1979) found that the combined intake of bracken and hot gruel increased the risk of oesophageal cancer of inhabitants in mountainous districts, especially when nutritional deficiencies were present. In this study, an increased risk of oesophageal cancer was associated with bracken fern ingestion and a diet poor in vitamin C. According to Alonso-Amelot *et al.* (1996), in a study with cows, 8.6% of the total ptaquiloside eaten by the bracken-fed animal was present in its milk and that the quantity of ptaquiloside present in milk was linearly dependent on the amount of bracken fern ingested. In another study, any association of the incidence of *Helicobacter pylori* in the nonendemic bracken areas and the presence of ptaquiloside in milk led to the conclusion that the consumption of patquiloside-contaminated milk may contribute to gastric cancer rates in this Andean country of Venezuela (Alonso-Amelot, 2001). In this study, no association was found between bracken fern ingestion and stomach cancer. Therefore, it would not be reasonable to investigate the role of this bacterium, *Helicobacter pylori,* in the etiology of stomach cancer in the Ouro Peto region given the methodology employed. This led to the conclusion that although this bacterium is an important risk factor for stomach cancer, bracken fern ingestion in this region was not sufficient to explain the development of stomach cancer in persons who eat it.

Acknowledgements

Research supported by CAPES, Brazil.
Universidade Federal de Ouro Preto
Escola de Nutrição
Campus Universitário, s/n
Ouro Preto, MG
35400000 – Brazil

References

Alonso-Amelot, M.E. & Avandano, M. (2001) Possible association between gastric cancer and bracken fern in Venezuela: an epidemiologic study. *Int. J. Cancer*, **91**, 252–259

Alonso-Amelot, M.E., Castillo, U. & De Jongh, F. (1996) Bracken ptaquiloside in milk. *Nature*, **382**, 587–588

Galpin, O.P., Whitaker, C.J., Whitaker, R. & Kassab, J.Y. (1990) Gastric cancer in Gwynedd. Possible links with bracken. *Br. J. Cancer*, **61**, 737–740

Galvão, M.A.M., Marliére, C.A. & Coimbra, M.B. (1992) Mortalidade por câncer de esôfago e estômago em Minas Gerais e na região de Ouro Preto, Minas Gerais. In: Abrasco, ed. *Congresso Brasileiro de Epidemiologia*, Belo Horizonte, Minas Gerais, Brazil, 108–109

Hirayama, T. (1979) Diet and Cancer. *Nutr. Cancer*, **1**, 67–81

Ranking chemopreventive agents on rat colon carcinogenesis

Corpet D.E., Taché S.

UMR Xénobiotiques, Institut National de la Recherche Agronomique, Ecole Nationale Vétérinaire de Toulouse, 23 ch. Capelles, 31076 Toulouse, France.

Introduction

In the study of colon carcinogenesis, more than 500 potential chemopreventive agents have been tested in rodents. The aim of animal studies is to find potent agents that might be given to people to reduce their risk of colorectal cancer. The standard endpoint for chemoprevention in rodents is the incidence of macroscopic tumours induced by a chemical carcinogen. Aberrant crypt foci (ACF), putative precursors of colon cancer, were recently proposed as a simple tool for screening potential chemopreventive agents (Bird, 1987). The major goal of this study was to find the most potent chemopreventive agents already published. To reach this goal, we had three aims:

1. Gather published studies on the effect of dietary chemopreventive agents against colon carcinogenesis in rodents after carcinogen injection.
2. Rank the agents, according to their potency in inhibiting colon ACF and colon tumours.
3. Test the hypothesis that ACF and tumour data are correlated.

Materials and methods

A total of 259 publications on the effect of dietary chemopreventive agents against colon carcinogenesis in rodents was gathered in March 2001. Since our goal was to point out the most potent agents, we kept only the single most potent agent and dose from each article. However, we kept several agents from the articles dealing with more than seven agents (e.g. Wargovich *et al.*, 2000).

Data were gathered from 122 articles with the ACF endpoint, yielding 171 ACF preventive agents. A primary ACF table was constructed containing the mean number of total ACF per colon, of large ACF per colon, and of crypts per ACF in each group of rats (control and treated). Data were also gathered from 137 articles with the tumour endpoint, yielding 151 tumour preventive agents or diets. A primary tumour table was constructed with the incidence of tumours, the incidence of invasive carcinomas, and the mean tumour multiplicity in each group of rats (control and treated).

The potency of each agent was then estimated by the ratio of value in control rats divided by value in treated rats (Tables 1 and 2). Thus, potency tells the time-fold reduction in carcinogenesis endpoint due to the agent. The correlation between ACF and tumour endpoints was calculated for the 54 agents that were present in both ACF and tumour tables.

Results

Table 1 shows the efficacy of chemopreventive agents on ACF endpoints. The agents were ranked according to their potency in reducing the number of ACFs per rat. The most potent agents are thus placed on the top of the table; 10 articles report agents that reduce the ACF number by more than 80% (potency higher than 5). Among the 171 agents in the ACF table, the median agent halved the number of ACF (median potency, 2). To save space, Table 1 displays only the top 27 agents out of 171, but the full table is shown on a website with sorting abilities (http://www.inra.fr/reseau-nacre/corpet).

Table 2 shows the efficacy of chemopreventive agents on tumour endpoints. The agents were ranked according to their potency in reducing the incidence of tumours in the colon and rectum. Sixteen articles report agents that reduce the tumour incidence by more than 80% (potency higher than 5). Among the 151 agents in Table 2, the median agent halved the tumour incidence (median potency, 2). To save space, Table 2 displays only the top 27 agents out of 151, but the full table is shown on a website with sorting abilities (http://www.inra.fr/reseau-nacre/sci-memb/corpet).

Table 1. Ranking chemopreventive potencies of agents to reduce the aberrant crypt foci in the colon of rats and mice after initiation with a chemical carcinogen: top 27 agents out of 171

Agent name and dose; carcinogen (when not AOM or DMH); mice (when not rats)[a]	Reference	Potency on ACF[b]	Percent inhibition of ACF[c]	Potency on large of ACF[d]	Potency on ACF size[e]	Protocol[e]
PEG-like pluronic F68 5%	Parnaud, 2001	76	99	85	1.5	Post
PEG 8000 5%; MNU	Corpet, 2000	56	98	58	2.0	Post
PEG 8000 5%	Corpet, 1999	18	94	104	2.3	Post
PEG 8000 5%	Parnaud, 2001	14	93	14	1.1	Post
Perilla oil 12% + β-carotene	Komaki, 1996	11	91		1.2	Init
Indole-3-carbinol 0.1%; PhIP	Guo, 1995	11	91	14	2.0	Init
PEG 8000 5%	Parnaud, 1999	8	87	30	1.3	Post
Sulindac sulfide 0.2%	Wargovich, 2000	7	85	10		Post
Caffeate PEMC 500 ppm	Rao, 1993	6	82	21	1.0	Both
PEG 8000 5%	Naigamalla, 2000	6	82	36	1.4	Post
Linolenic CLA 0.5%; IQ	Liew, 1995	4	74	–	0.9	Init
Cooking salt 4.4%	Masaoka, 2000	4	74	–	1.0	Init
Perilla oil 12% vs olive oil	Onogi, 1996	4	74	–	1.1	Init
Bifidobacteria 1.7%+ inulin 5%	Rowland, 1998	4	73	2		Post
Butylhydroxyanisole 0.56%	Wargovich, 1992	4	71	–	–	Init
DFMO 0.4%	Wargovich, 1992	4	71	–	–	Init
DFMO 0.4%	Wargovich, 1996	4	71	–	–	Init
Piroxicam 400 ppm	Wargovich, 2000	3	70	–	–	Post
Sphingomyelin diOH 0.1%; mice	Schmelz, 1997	3	70	–	1.2	Post
Sanshishi 2%	Fukutake, 2000	3	70	–	1.5	Both
Sphingomyelin 0.1%; mice	Schmelz, 1996	3	69	–	1.5	Post
Rutin 3%	Wargovich, 2000	3	69	–	–	Post
TGF-β1 2 ng/day	Mikhailowsli, 1998	3	69	–	1.2	Both
Piroxicam 400 ppm	Wargovich, 2000	3	67	–	–	Init
Retinoic acid all trans 190 ppm	Wargovich, 2000	3	67	3	–	Post
Wheat bran 20% vs no fibre	Ishizuka, 1996	3	67	0.6	–	Init
Glucose vs sucrose bolus	Stamp, 1993	3	67		–	Init

[a]Doses are reported as percent of the diet (w/w), or ppm (1000 ppm = 0.1%).
[b]The potency of each agent was estimated by the ratio of the value in control rats divided by the value in treated rats.
[c]The percent inhibition afforded by the agent is equal to 100 x (1–1/potency) e.g., a potency of 5 corresponds to a 80% inhibition.
[d]Most articles report ACF of 4 crypts or more as large ACF. Values missing in original article are not reported here.
[e]ACF size measured as the mean number of aberrant crypts per ACF.
[e]The animals were given the agent during the initiation with chemical carcinogen (init) or after the end of initiation (post) or during both periods (both).
AOM, azoxymethane; BB, Bowman-Birk; CLA, conjugated linoleic acid; DFMO, difluoromethylornithine; DMH, dimethylhydrazine; IQ, 2-amino-3-methylimidazo[4,5-f]quinoline; MMTS, S-methyl methane thiosulfonate; MNU, methyl nitroso urea; PEG, polyethylene glycol; PEMC, phenylethyl-3-methylcaffeate; PhIP, 2-amino-1-methyl-6-phenylimidazo[4,5-b] pyridine; TGF-β1, transforming growth factor beta1.

Table 2. Ranking chemopreventive potencies of agents to reduce the tumours in the colon of rats and mice after initiation with a chemical carcinogen: top 27 agents out of 151

Agent name and dose; carcinogen (when not AOM or DMH); mice (when not rats)	Reference	Potency reduce T. incid.[a]	Percent inhib. T. incid.[b]	T. incid. in each group[c]		Percent inhib. Cancer incid	Potency reduce tumour multiple	Protocol[d]
				Control	Treated			
Celecoxib 0.15%	Kawamori, 1998	15.4	93	29/34	2/36	96	32	Both
Bifidobacteria longum 0.5%; IQ	Reddy,1993	14.0	93	*7/30	0/30	–	26	Both
BB protease inh. 0.5%; mice	St Clair, 1990	10.4	90	*7/62	1/92	87	10	Both
DFMO 0.2% + pirox. 200 ppm	Rao, 1991	9.0	89	27/36	3/36	88	16	Both
PEG 8000 5%	Corpet, 2000	8.6	88	22/27	2/21	100	10	Post
MMTS 100 ppm	Kawamori, 1995	7.9	87	17/30	2/28	100		Post
BB protease inh. 0.5%; mice	Weed, 1985	7.3	86	*7/46	0/24		11	Both
PEG 8000 5%	Parnaud, 1999	7.0	86	14/20	1/10	100	21	Post
Folate 8 ppm	Kim, 1996	7.0	86	*7/10	1/10	–	11	Both
Piroxicam 200 ppm	Li, 1999	6.5	85	100 %	15 %	63	3	Post
Pectin 15% vs cellulose 5%	Reddy, 1987	5.7	82	57 %	10 %			Both
Obacunone 500 ppm	Tanaka, 2001	5.5	82	18/25	2/16	82	6	Post
DFMO 0.1% + aspirin 0.06%	Li, 1999	5.3	81	71 %	13.3 %	38	6	Both
$Mg(OH)_2$ 500 ppm	Mori, 1993	5.3	81	17/32	3/30	77	7	Post
Copper 8 ppm vs 0.2 ppm	DiSilvestro, 1992	5.0	80	*5/11	1/11	–	3	Both
Glucarate calcium 0.1 mol/kg	Dwivedi, 1989	5.0	80	*5/18	1/18	–		Post
Tetracycline 10 mg/day in meat	Goldin,1981	4.8	79	15/31	3/30	–	5	Both
Hesperidin 0.1%	Tanaka,1997	4.7	79	12/17	3/20	79	6	Post
DFMO 0.2%	Rao,1991	4.5	78	75 %	16.6 %	77	6	Both
Germfree vs normal flora	Reddy, 1975	4.5	78	14/15	5/24	91	10	Both
Celecoxib 0.15%	Reddy, 2000	4.5	78	76 %	17 %	77	6	Both
Quercetin 2%; mice	Deschner, 1991	4.3	76	*8/32	2/34	–	6	Both
Beef vs milk protein; mice	Nutter, 1983	4.2	76	61/91	15/95	–	6	Both
Wheat bran +caloric Restriction (–10%)	Kritchevsky, 1997	4.2	76	16/23	4/24	–	–	Post
Aspirin 60 mg/kg/day	Davis, 1994	4.0	75	*8/8	2/8	–	8	Both
Olive vs corn oil 23.5%	Reddy, 1984	3.5	72	46 %	13 %	–	–	Post
Acetoxychavicol 500 ppm	Tanaka, 1997	3.5	72	12/17	4/20	93	3	Post

[a]The potency of each agent was estimated by the ratio of the value in control rats divided by the value in treated rats. We used tumour data confirmed by histology when available.

[b]The percent inhibition afforded by the agent is equal to 100 x (1– 1/potency) e.g., a potency of 5 corresponds to a 80% inhibition.

[c]Data are number of tumour-bearing rats/number of rats, or percent tumour incidences (indictated by a %) in both control and treated groups. Potency based on small numbers of tumour-bearing rats are not accurate, thus numbers smaller than 10 are labeled with an asterisk. When no tumour was seen, potency calculation was arbitrarily based on 0.5 tumour.

[d]The animals were given the agent during the initiation with chemical carcinogen (init) or after the end of initiation (post) or during both periods (both).

Fifty-four agents were found in both Tables 1 and 2. A significant correlation was found between the potencies in the ACF assay and in the tumour assay (r=0.45, n=54, P=0.001). A marked outlier was celecoxib, very potent in one tumour study (Kawamori *et al.*, 1998), but not in one ACF study. When this point was dropped, the correlation increased to r=0.68 (n=53, P<0.001).

Discussion

By combining six carcinogenesis endpoints from Tables 1 and 2, this review suggests that the most potent agents are polyethylene glycol (Corpet *et al.*, 2000), Bowman-Birk protease inhibitor, difluoromethylornithine alone or with piroxicam or aspirin, hesperidin, celecoxib, sulindac sulfone or sulfide, and *Bifidobacteria* strains. We think these agents should be tested in people at risk, provided they are not toxic.

A significant correlation was found between the potencies in the ACF assay and in the tumour assay. Out of 40 agents, Steele *et al.* (1999) also showed that of the 30 agents tested as positive in the aberrant crypt foci assay, 21 prevented colon cancer in rats. The present study does not prove that ACF are true preneoplastic lesions, but suggests that ACF may be used as a surrogate endpoint for tumours in rats.

Finally, we propose that the potency of each new agent should be compared with previously published agents. According to this review, the median potency of effective agents published so far is 2. An agent that leads to a twofold reduction in ACF or tumour is thus an average one. In contrast, an agent that reduces the ACF number or the tumour incidence more than fivefold is of outstanding potency.

References

Bird, R.P. (1987) Observation and quantification of aberrant crypts in murine colon treated with a colon carcinogen: preliminary findings. *Cancer Lett.*, **37**, 147–151

Corpet, D.E., Parnaud, G., Delverdier, M., Peiffer, G. & Tache, S. (2000) Consistent and fast inhibition of colon carcinogenesis by polyethylene glycol in mice and rats given various carcinogens. *Cancer Res.*, **60**, 3160–3164

Kawamori, T., Rao, C.V., Seibert, K. & Reddy, B.S. (1998) Chemopreventive activity of celecoxib, a specific cyclooxygenase-2 inhibitor, against colon carcinogenesis. *Cancer Res.*, **58**, 409–412

Steele, V.A., Wargovich, M.J., Pereira, M.A., Rao, C.V., Lubet, R.A., Reddy, B.S. & Kelloff, G.J. (1999) Comparison of the azoxymethane AOM-induced rat colon crypt assay with the rat colon tumor assay for cancer chemopreventive agents. *Proc. Am. Assoc. Cancer Res.*, **40**, 57 (A377)

Wargovich, M.J., Jimenez, A., Mckee, K., Steele, V.E., Velasco, M., Woods, J., Price, R., Gray, K. & Kelloff, G.J. (2000) Efficacy of potential chemopreventive agents on rat colon aberrant crypt formation and progression. *Carcinogenesis (Lond.)*, **21**, 1149–1155

Anti-tumour-promoting action of *Allium* constituents

Le Bon A.M.[1], Guyonnet D.[1], Chaumontet C.[2], Bergès R.[1], Pinnert M.F.[1], Martel P.[2]

[1]Unité Mixte de Recherche Toxicologie Alimentaire, Institut National de la Recherche Agronomique, Université de Bourgogne, 17 rue Sully, 21065 Dijon cedex, France. [2]Laboratoire Nutrition et Sécurité Alimentaire, Institut National de la Recherche Agronomique, Domaine de Vilvert, 78352 Jouy-en-Josas, France.

Introduction

Many epidemiological studies suggest that *Allium* vegetable intake is associated with a reduced risk of cancer in humans. Some organosulfur compounds present in these vegetables have been demonstrated to inhibit chemical initiation of carcinogenesis but their effects on the promotion phase have been less thoroughly investigated (Le Bon and Siess, 2000). This study was designed to evaluate the effects of two garlic compounds, diallyl disulfide (DADS) and diallyl sulfide (DAS), on the development of liver preneoplastic foci in rats, when administered during the promotion phase induced by phenobarbital (PB). To investigate the mechanisms which might be involved, we studied the *in vitro* action of these organosulfur compounds on gap junctional intercellular communications (GJIC) in a rat liver epithelial (REL) cell line. GJIC is a reliable endpoint for the detection of tumour-promoting or anti-tumour-promoting agents. We investigated the ability of DAS and DADS to counteract the GJIC inhibition induced by a tumour promoter, 3,5-ditertiobutyl-4-hydroxytoluene (BHT). In addition, we measured the effects of these molecules on REL proliferation.

Methods

Hepatocarcinogenesis protocol: a medium-term liver assay (Ito assay) was performed on 5-week-old male Wistar rats (Ito *et al.*, 1988). Initiation was accomplished with a single intraperitoneal injection of diethylnitrosamine (200 mg/kg b.w.). Animals were subjected to partial hepatectomy at the beginning of the third week. From the second week onwards till the 18th week, rats were given a diet containing either 0.05% PB or PB plus DAS (0.05%) or PB plus DADS (0.05%). Placental glutathione-S-transferase-positive foci were used as end-point markers. They were detected by immunohistochemistry and quantified by image analysis.

In vitro studies were performed on REL cells which had been isolated previously as described by Carrera *et al.* (1992). For GJIC determination, cells (400×10^3) were plated in duplicate in 35-mm petri dishes. Two days after plating, confluent cells were treated by organosulfur compounds for 1 h followed by organosulfur compounds plus BHT for 10 min. Then the cells were microinjected with lucifer yellow as described by Chaumontet *et al.* (1994) and the intercellular transfer of the dye was determined by counting the number of fluorescent cells surrounding the microinjected cell. For each treatment, 10–20 microinjection trials were counted.

In the cell proliferation assay, cells (150×10^3) were plated in triplicate in 60-mm petri dishes. Twenty-four hours after plating, cells were treated with organosulfur compounds (10–100 µM) for 1–8 days. At the end of the incubation period, cells were counted with a Coulter counter-channelizer (Coultronics).

Results

In vivo study

Co-administration of DADS with PB during the promotion phase reduced the total area of preneoplastic foci by 35% with respect to phenobarbital group (Figure 1). DADS did not affect the number of foci but induced a shift in the size distribution of foci towards smaller-size foci. DAS did not modify the effect of phenobarbital.

In vitro studies.

BHT reduced the number of dye-coupled cells by half (Figure 2). The incubation of REL cells with DADS partially counteracted the inhibition of

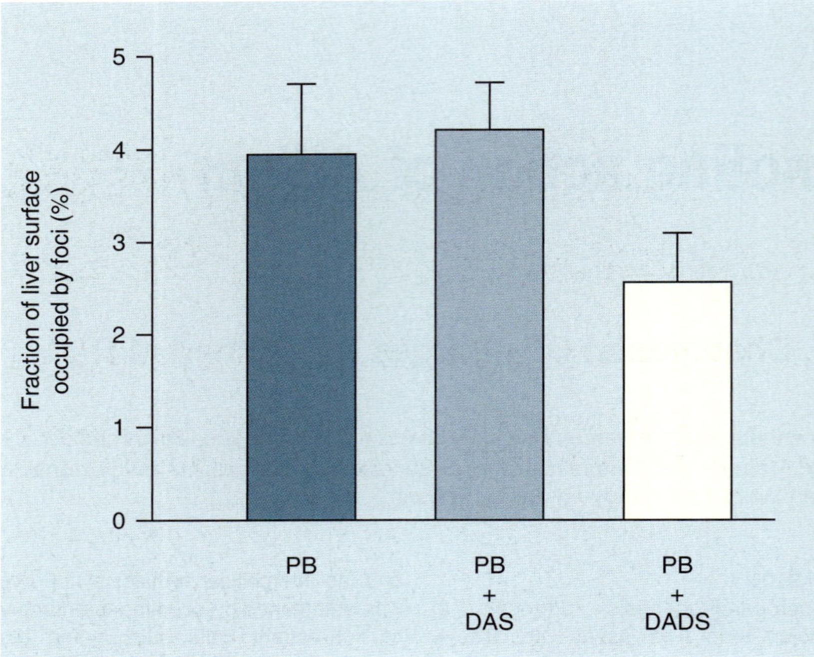

Figure 1
Effects of diallyl sulfide (DAS) and diallyl disulfide (DADS) on the promotion phase induced by phenobarbital (PB) in rat liver

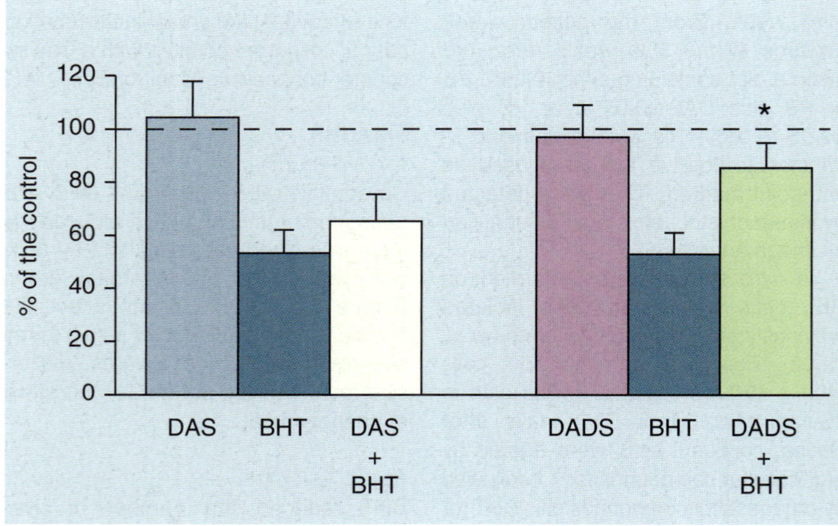

Figure 2
Effects of 3,5-ditertiobutyl-4-hydroxytoluene(BHT), diallyl sulfide (DAS) and diallyl disulfide (DADS) on gap junctional intercellular communication in REL cells.

GJIC induced by BHT and reduced cell proliferation at the concentrations higher than 25μM (data not shown). In contrast, DAS neither altered GJIC inhibition induced by BHT (Figure 2) nor REL proliferation (data not shown).

Conclusion

The enhancement of GJIC and the inhibition of cell proliferation induced by DADS could be the major mechanisms responsible for the anti-tumour-promoting action of DADS *in vivo*. Conversely, DAS neither affects hepatocarcinogenesis nor *in vitro* cellular communication and proliferation. DADS can therefore be regarded as a promising natural chemopreventive agent as it has the capacity to prevent both the initiation and the promotion phases of carcinogenesis. This suggests that consumption of garlic with a high DADS content could offer protection against carcinogenesis.

References

Carrera, G., Melgar, J., Alary, J., Lamboeuf, Y. & Martel, P. (1992) Cadmium accumulation and cytotoxicity in rat hepatocytes co-cultured with a liver epithelial cell line. *Toxicol. In Vitro*, **6**, 201–206

Chaumontet, C., Bex, V., Gaillard-Sanchez, I., Seillan-Heberden, C., Suschetet, M. & Martel, P. (1994) Apigenin and tangeretin enhance gap junctional intercellular communication in rat liver epithelial cells. *Carcinogenesis*, **15**, 2325–2330

Ito, N., Tsuda, H., Tatematsu, M., Inoue, T., Tagawa, Y., Aoki, T., Uwagawa, S., Kagawa, M., Ogiso, T., Masui, T., Imaida, K., Fukushima, S. & Asamoto, M. (1988) Enhancing effect of various hepatocarcinogens on induction of preneoplastic glutathione S-transferase placental form positive foci in rats – an approach for a new medium-term bioassay system. *Carcinogenesis*, **9**, 387–394

Le Bon, A.M. & Siess, M.H. (2000) Organosulfur compounds from Allium and the chemoprevention of cancer. *Drug Metab. Drug Interact.*, **17**, 51–79

Purified and endogenous phytic acid in wheat bran affects early biomarkers of colon cancer risk

Jenab M., Thompson L.U.

Department of Nutritional Sciences, Faculty of Medicine, University of Toronto, Toronto, ON, Canada M5S 3E2.

Introduction

Wheat bran has consistently been shown to have a colon cancer protective effect at early and late stages of tumorigenesis (Jenab and Thompson, 1998; Alabaster *et al.*, 1995), possibly due to its high dietary fiber and/or phytic acid (myo-inositol-hexa phosphate) content (Jenab & Thompson, 1998). Pure, exogenous phytic acid, provided in the drinking water, has been shown to be protective of colon cancer in rats, probably due to its ability to regulate colonic cellular proliferation (Shamsuddin *et al.*, 1997). However, it is unknown whether phytic acid found within the matrix of wheat bran (endogenous phytic acid) contributes to the colon cancer protective effects of wheat bran observed in previous studies. It is also unclear whether a diet rich in wheat bran affects other important processes involved in the maintenance of the colonic epithelium, i.e. cell proliferation, differentiation and apoptosis, which also need to be considered in the evaluation of colon cancer risk. In addition, to date, very little work has focused on the effects of phytic acid or wheat bran on aberrant crypt (AC) and foci (ACF) formation and characteristics. ACF are known to be valid preneoplastic markers of colon carcinogenesis. However, the particular ACF parameters or types of ACF that may be more or less reflective of this risk are largely unknown. Recently it has been observed that ACF may differ in their type of mucin production, with some producing sialomucins (SIM; found in high proportions in colon cancer) and others producing sulphomucins (SUM; the normal type of mucin present in human and rat colons) (Caderni *et al.*, 1995). It has been suggested that SIM-ACF are at a more advanced stage of carcinogenesis, along the stepwise sequence of colon carcinogenesis, than SUM-ACF.

Thus, the objectives of this study were to determine whether:

1. Wheat bran is protective of colon cancer using ACF characteristics and indices of colonic cell proliferation as early risk markers.
2. Phytic acid is the component responsible for these changes.
3. Endogenous and exogenous phytic acids are equally effective.
4. SIM-ACF are at a more advanced stage of carcinogenesis than other types of ACF.

Methods

Five groups of azoxymethane (AOM)-treated male F344 rats were fed a low-fiber basal diet (control), a basal diet supplemented with either 25% wheat bran, 25% dephytinized wheat bran, 25% dephytinized wheat bran plus 1.0% phytic acid or 1.0% phytic acid until sacrifice 100 days after AOM injection. Early biomarkers of colon cancer risk such as the colon total number of ACF and SIM-ACF, rate of cell proliferation, differentiation and apoptosis were then measured as previously described (Jenab & Thompson, 1998, 2000).

Results and discussion

The number of ACF was reduced by all treatment groups versus the basal diet, but it only reached significance in the phytic acid group (Table 1), suggesting that the exogenous phytic acid may have a stronger colon cancer protective effect than endogenous phytic acid or wheat bran. There were no differences between endogenous and exogenous phytic acid or between the dietary fiber and phytic acid components of wheat bran. If phytic acid was the only active component in wheat bran, it would be expected that the dephytinization of wheat bran would cause an increase in

Table 1. ACF parameters, apoptotic index, degree of differentiation, rate of cell proliferation for the various dietary groups in the distal or whole colon

Biomarkers	Dietary groups BD	WB	DWB	DWBPA	PA
Number of ACF	64.67 ± 4.59[a]	51.09 ± 2.37[ab]	54.55 ± 3.28[ab]	54.82 ± 3.46[ab]	44.93 ± 4.10[b]
Number of SIM -ACF	34.33 ± 3.58[a]	15.64 ± 1.83[b]	18.64 ± 2.16[b]	18.55 ± 3.64[b]	12.57 ± 3.13[b]
Degree of luminal alterations	2.57 ± 0.07[a]	2.27 ± 0.04[b]	2.21 ± 0.06[b]	2.32 ± 0.05[b]	2.29 ± 0.05[b]
Apoptotic index	1.84 ± 0.24[b]	5.84 ± 0.54[a]	5.44 ± 0.69[a]	4.34 ± 0.46[ab]	6.59 ± 0.54[a]
Lectin scores	0.94 ± 0.12[b]	2.52 ± 0.20[a]	2.30 ± 0.21[a]	2.59 ± 0.15[a]	2.62 ± 0.19[a]
Labelling index (top 40% of crypt)	18.45 ± 1.38[a]	7.97 ± 0.99[d]	13.71 ± 1.48[bc]	9.69 ± 0.91[cd]	12.69 ± 1.19[bc]

Values are means ± SEM. BD = control group fed the AIN 93G diet; WB = AIN93G diet supplemented with 25% wheat bran diet; DWB = AIN 93G diet supplemented with 25% dephytinized wheat bran diet; DWBPA = AIN 93G diet supplemented with 25% dephytinized wheat bran plus 1.0% exogenous PA; PA = AIN 93 G diet supplemented with 1.0% exogenous PA. Number of ACF, Number of SIM- ACF and Degree of LA data are for the whole colon; For the determination of the degree of luminal alterations, each AC was given a grade from 1 to 3 based on whether the luminal shape was mildly altered (enlarged and round; 1), moderately altered (elliptical; 2), or severely altered (slit-like; 3); n=14 rats per group. Apoptotic index = (no. of apoptotic cells / total no. of cells) x 100; n=10 per group. Lectin Scores range from 0 to 4 and are calculated depending on percentage of cells stained and staining intensity. A higher score indicates greater degree of differentiation; n=10 rats per group. LI in the top 40% of the crypt is on a sample size of 24 crypts from the distal colon, per rat with 6 rats per group. Values with different superscripts within a row are significantly different by one way ANOVA followed by a multiple groups comparisons test, $P < 0.05$.

Table 2. Type of mucin production in ACF and relationship to ACF size, degree of dysplasia and rate of cell proliferation

Type of mucin production in ACF	Size of ACF ($x10^{-2}mm^2$)	Degree of dysplasia	ACF labelling index (top 40% of crypt)[a]
SUM	2.78 ± 0.29[b]	1.60 ± 0.31[b]	25.01 ± 8.74[b]
SUM + SIM	4.68 ± 0.42[a]	2.12 ± 0.15[ab]	50.54 ± 6.49[a]
SIM	5.16 ± 0.40[a]	2.32 ± 0.10[a]	49.50 ± 3.47[a]

Comparison of type of mucin production in ACF based on 77 ACF; SUM=ACF producing only sulfomucins, SUM+SIM= ACF producing sulfomucins and sialomucins, SIM=ACF producing only sialomucins. Values with different superscripts within a column are significantly different by one way ANOVA followed by a multiple groups comparisons test, $P < 0.05$.

[a] Labelling index values represent absolute difference of the labelling index in ACF and the labelling index of normal tissue surrounding the ACF.

ACF parameters. Thus, components other than phytic acid likely also contribute to the potential colon cancer protective effects of wheat bran.

SIM-ACF are thought to be more advanced towards tumorigenesis and hence better markers of colon cancer risk than other ACF. This is highlighted by the increased size, dysplasia and labelling index of SIM-ACF versus SUM-ACF (Table 2). Using SIM-ACF as an early biomarker, their number was significantly reduced by all treatment groups compared to the basal diet, indicating that the treatment diets were protective of colon carcinogenesis (Table 1). There were no differences between endogenous versus exogenous phytic acid. There were also no differences among wheat bran, dephytinized wheat bran, and phytic acid groups, indicating that both the fiber and phytic acid components of wheat bran may be equally protective.

The degree of luminal alterations may reflect the degree of dysplasia within each ACF. It was significantly reduced for all treatment groups compared to the basal diet, indicating that the treatment diets likely slowed the development of dysplasia and consequently the advancement towards neoplasticity for the ACF observed.

Increased cell proliferation and decreased cellular apoptosis and differentiation affect the growth kinetics of cells and are thought to be valid biomarkers of colon carcinogenesis. In this study, the labelling index was significantly reduced by all treatment groups versus the basal diet (Table 1). In addition, the wheat bran group had significantly lower values than the dephytinized wheat bran and phytic acid groups, suggesting that the endogenous phytic acid is better at reducing the labelling index than the wheat bran fiber or exogenous phytic acid.

All the dietary treatment groups had significantly higher lectin scores (a marker of differentiation) in the entire crypt than the basal diet group. Similarly, compared to the basal diet, a significant increase in apoptosis in the whole crypt was observed in the wheat bran, dephytinized wheat bran and phytic acid groups, suggesting a mechanism along with altering cell proliferation rate whereby wheat bran and phytic acid may exert colon cancer protective effects.

Wheat bran is thought to exert its colon cancer protective effect by several mechanisms including physical dilution of gut contents, shortening transit times, alterations in the mutagenicity of intestinal contents, alterations in mucosal kinetics, increased fermentation producing butyrate, and an effect on the production, absorption and excretion of putative carcinogens. Many of these mechanisms appear to be analogous to those suggested for the protective effects of phytic acid, suggesting that phytic acid may be one of the components of wheat bran contributing to its colon cancer protective effects.

It is concluded that wheat bran significantly reduced early biomarkers of colon cancer risk due, in part, to its phytic acid and dietary fiber. Exogenous and endogenous phytic acid in wheat bran are both effective, but exogenous phytic acid is more effective in a low-fibre diet. SIM-ACF are more advanced along the stepwise sequence of colon carcinogenesis than other ACF and may be a better biomarker of colon cancer risk.

References

Alabaster, O., Tang, Z.C., Frost, A. & Shivapurkar, N. (1995) Effect of β-carotene and wheat bran fiber on colonic aberrant crypt and tumour formation in rats exposed to azoxymethane and high dietary fat. *Carcinogenesis*, **16**, 127–132

Caderni, G., Giannini, A., Lancioni, L., Luceri, C., Biggeri, A. & Dolara, P. (1995) Characterisation of aberrant crypt foci in carcinogen-treated rats: association with intestinal carcinogenesis. *Br. J. Cancer*, **71**, 763–769

Jenab, M. & Thompson, L.U. (1998) The influence of phytic acid in wheat bran on early biomarkers of colon carcinogenesis. *Carcinogenesis*, **19**, 1087–1092

Jenab, M. & Thompson, L.U. (2000) Phytic acid in wheat bran affects colon morphology, cell differentiation and apoptosis. *Carcinogenesis*, **21**, 1547–1552

Shamsuddin, A.M., Vucenik, I. & Cole, K.E. (1997) IP6: a novel anti-cancer agent. *Life Sci.*, **61**, 343–354

Indigestible carbohydrates which reduce colon tumour incidence in Min mice may interfere with the local immune response

Menanteau J.[1], Pierre F.[1], Bassonga E.[1], Forest V.[1], Bornet F.[2], Perrin P.[1], Meflah K.[1]

[1]Human Nutrition Research Center of Nantes, U419 INSERM, Institut de Biologie, 9, Quai Moncousu, 44035 Nantes Cedex 01, France. [2]Eridania Beghin-Say, Vilvoorde Research and Development Center, Nutrition and Health Service, Havenstraat 84, B-1800 Vilvoorde, Belgium.

Introduction

Colorectal cancer is one of the most common cancers in the developed world. A cause and effect relationship between dietary or lifestyle factors and colorectal cancer is difficult to establish. Red meat, saturated fat, refined carbohydrates and alcohol are believed to be positively related. Dietary fiber, vegetables, fruits, calcium and folate are frequently negatively associated with the development of colorectal cancer. Recent epidemiological and human intervention studies with fibres have been unsuccessful and disappointing. On the other hand, continuing low cancer incidence in African populations, despite considerable lifestyle changes (with increased obesity, diabetes and hypertension) should encourage a new look at Burkitt's original observation linking fibre consumption to low colon cancer incidence. In a recent editorial, Segel *et al.* (2000) put forward a fairly convincing hypothesis based on data obtained in humans and published in the same journal. Persistent consumption of a high amount of resistant starch (a fibre-like compound generated by certain cooking methods) would establish a butyrogenic microflora early in life (as early as the age of 3 years). These people would benefit from two synergistic mechanisms: the consumption of high amounts of nondigestible carbohydrates and the presence of a colon microflora with high fermentation capabilities, leading to the production of very high amounts of short-chain fatty acids (especially butyrate) in the lumen. In good agreement with previous epidemiological and experimental studies, we recently provided data showing that only fibres promoting a stable butyrate-producing colonic ecosystem (a resistant starch and fructo-oligosaccharides) decrease the rate of precancerous lesions (aberrant crypt foci) in rats (Perrin *et al.*, 2001). In another model, which also concerns later stages of carcinogenesis (the genetic Min mice model), only one butyrogenic diet, fructo-oligosaccharides (FOS), lowered the number of colon tumours (but not of small intestine tumours) and developed gut-associated lymphoid tissue (GALT) (Pierre *et al.*, 1997). FOS are documented as prebiotic (able to favour the growth of lactic-acid-producing bacteria). Prebiotics have been shown to stimulate the GALT and to inhibit the growth of transplantable tumors. We examined these results in light of our previous experience in using butyrate in dual therapies in an experimental model of intraperitoneal carcinomatosis initiated with colon cancer cells. A combination of butyrate and interleukin-2 (stimulator of the immune system) was shown to cure the rats, whereas either compound alone was ineffective (Perrin *et al.*, 1994). We postulated that butyrate would increase the immunogenicity of viable or apoptotic colonocytes, allowing rejection by the immune system. Transposed to the preventive studies where butyrate is locally generated by fermentation, the flora would be the stimulator of the immune response, operating in the Min mice model in addition to butyrate. Our objective was to document if the effect of indigestible carbohydrates on the course of colon carcinogenesis involves the local immune system.

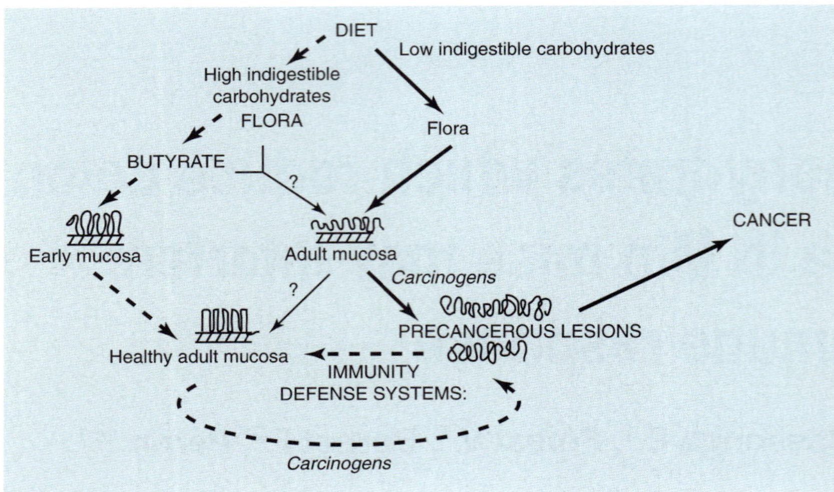

Figure 1
Indigestible carbohydrates may contribute to development of colon cancer immunoprophylaxis

Methods

Immunocompetent and immunodeficient (depleted of CD4+ and CD8+ T lymphocytes with antibodies) Min mice (a strain bearing a mutation on the *Apc* gene, an antioncogene gate-keeper of intestinal carcinogenesis) were fed an energy-balanced diet enriched (5.8%) with short-chain FOS (Actilight P, Beghin-Meiji) for 42 days. The mice were killed and the number of large intestine tumours were scored. Total RNAs were prepared from colon portions of the immunocompetent mice and cytokines were analysed by multiprobe ribonuclease protection assays with the mCK1 matrix (Pharmingen, USA).

Results and discussion

The immunodeficient mice developed twice as many tumours as the immunocompetent mice (0.8 as compared with 0.4, P=0.02) (Pierre *et al.*, 1999). IL-4, IL-5, IL-13, IL-15 and INFγ were detected in the colon of the Min mice, but only IL-15 mRNA expression was significantly amplified (more than twofold) (Bassonga *et al.*, 2001).

It is concluded that T-cells participate in a mechanism of colon cancer surveillance in Min mice fed indigestible carbohydrates exhibiting a probiotic activity. That IL-15 was amplified is of interest, since this cytokine is a key regulator of cellular homeostasis, supporting the lymphocytes that persist in the mucosa, cells which modulate the turnover of epithelial intestinal cells. In addition, IL-15 has been shown to exert antitumoral activity.

As a whole, our recent and previous studies suggest, as a novel working hypothesis, that some indigestible carbohydrates may generate or amplify a mechanism of immunoprophylaxis that can contribute to anticancer properties exhibited by specific fibres under certain conditions. This hypothesis appears consistent with both reported positive and negative data (epidemiological, interventional and experimental) as concerns fibres and colon cancer and is depicted in Figure 1. Early in life, indigestible carbohydrates may generate a colonic ecosystem able to generate large amounts of butyrate and a competent immune system, both acting in synergy to eliminate precancerous cells (thick dashed lines) a mechanism otherwise inefficient (thick lines). It is probably more difficult to generate such a response when targeting adults bearing a stable and previously equilibrated colonic ecosystem (light dashed lines). This kind of biological response, together with others, may account for the discrepancies appearing between some epidemiological and interventional studies.

References

Bassonga, E., Forest, V., Pierre, F., Bornet, F., Perrin, P., Meflah, K., & Menanteau, J. (2001) Cytokine mRNA expression in mouse colon: IL-15 mRNA is overexpressed and is highly sensitive to a fiber-like dietary component (short-chain fructo-oligosaccharides) in an *Apc* gene manner. *Cytokine,* **14**, 243–246

Perrin, P., Cassagnau, E., Burg, C., Patry, Y., Vavasseur, F., Harb, J., Le Pendu, J., Douillard, J.Y., Galmiche, J.P., Bornet, F. & Meflah, K. (1994) An interleukin-2/sodium butyrate combination as immunotherapy for rat colon cancer peritoneal carcinomatosis. *Gastroenterology*, **107**, 1697–1708

Perrin, P., Pierre, F., Patry, Y., Champ, M., Berreur, M., Pradal, G., Bornet, F., Meflah, K. & Menanteau, J. (2001) Only fibers promoting a stable butyrate-producing colonic ecosystem decrease the rate of aberrant crypt foci in rats. *Gut*, **48**, 53–61

Pierre, F., Perrin, P., Champ, M., Bornet, F., Meflah, K. & Menanteau J. (1997) Short chain fructo-oligosaccharides reduce colonic tumor occurrence and develop the GALT in Min mice. *Cancer Res.*, **57**, 225–228

Pierre, F., Perrin, P., Bassonga, E., Bornet, F., Meflah, K. & Menanteau, J. (1999) T-cell status influences colon tumor occurrence in Min mice fed short-chain fructo-oligosaccharides as a diet supplement. *Carcinogenesis*, **10**, 1953–1956

Segal, I., Edwards, C.A. & Walker, A.R.P. (2000) Continuing low colon cancer incidence in African populations. *Am. J. Gastroenterol.*, **95**, 859–860

Analysis of oxidized and nitrated proteins in plasma and tissues as biomarkers for exposure to reactive oxygen and nitrogen species

Ohshima H., Pignatelli B., Li C.-Q., Baflast S., Gilibert I., Boffetta P.
International Agency for Research on Cancer, Lyon, France.

Oxidative stress contributes to cancer, ageing and various pathophysiological disorders. Upon exposure to infectious agents and other carcinogenic foreign substances and also during chronic inflammation, mammalian cells produce a variety of reactive oxygen and nitrogen species such as nitric oxide (NO), superoxide (O_2^-) and hypochlorous acid (HOCl). These oxidants contribute to oxidative stress by damaging proteins, lipids and nucleosides (Ohshima *et al.*, 2000). Dietary antioxidants can inhibit such damage. In order to study the roles of oxidative stress in human carcinogenesis, we have developed a new simple and sensitive method, requiring very small amounts of plasma or tissue biopsies, to measure the extent of oxidative and nitrative damage in humans. The method has been successfully applied to molecular epidemiological studies.

Materials and methods

Free and protein-bound nitrotyrosine (NTYR) have been measured as markers of protein damage induced by peroxynitrite and other reactive nitrogen species. Similarly, carbonyl groups in proteins, determined as 2,4-dinitrophenylhydrazine (DNPH) derivatives, have been analyzed as a marker of oxidative damage of proteins. New methods to measure oxidized (carbonyl-containing) and nitrated (NTYR-containing) proteins in plasma or tissues have been developed using immunodot and Western blot assays. The methods require only 20 μg of protein (Li *et al.*, 2001; Pignatelli *et al.*, 2001).

Human plasma proteins (albumin, transferrin and fibrinogen) were incubated at 1 mg/mL with 1 μM authentic peroxynitrite in 0.5 M phosphate buffer (pH 7.4). Concentrations of NTYR in proteins were measured by high-performance liquid chromatography using a postseparation on-line reduction column and an electrochemical detector (Ohshima *et al.*, 1999). The concentrations of protein carbonyls were determined spectrophotometrically after formation of the DNPH derivative (Levin *et al.*, 1990).

For immunodot blot analysis, 20 μg of proteins either from plasma or tissue extracts were used either directly for NTYR analysis or after DNPH-derivatization for analysis of oxidized proteins (Li *et al.*, 2001; Pignatelli *et al.*, 2001). Proteins were diluted in 200 mL of PBS and dotted onto a Millipore Immobilon-P membrane using a Bio-Dot SF microfiltration apparatus (Bio-Rad, Hercules, California, USA). NTYR and carbonyls in proteins were measured using a mouse anti-NTYR monoclonal IgG antibody (Upstate Biotechnology, Lake Placid, NY, USA) or a rabbit anti-DNP antibody (Oxyblot; Oncor, Gaithersburg, MD, USA), respectively. Western blot analysis was also carried out to obtain information on number and molecular weights of modified proteins.

Results and discussion

We have applied immunodot and Western blot analyses to measure nitrated and oxidized proteins in plasma samples collected from 52 lung cancer patients and 43 healthy controls (heavy and light smokers, non-smokers with or without exposure to environmental tobacco smoke). The levels of nitrated proteins were significantly higher in lung cancer patients than in healthy controls (P=0.003). On the other hand, the levels of oxidized proteins were significantly higher in smokers than non-smokers (P<0.001). Western blot analyses showed the presence of two to five nitrated proteins and one oxidized

Table 1. Possible biomarkers (protein damage) in cancer molecular epidemiology

Oxidized (carbonyls) proteins: reactive oxygen species
Nitrated (NTYR) proteins: reactive nitrogen species
4-Hydroxynonenal (HNE)-adduct: lipid peroxidation
Malondialdehyde (MDA)-adduct: lipid peroxidation
Acetaldehyde-adduct: alcohol intake/aldehyde damage
Carcinogen (e.g. aflatoxin) adduct: exposure to carcinogen

protein. Using immunoprecipitation and Western blot analyses with eight different antibodies against human plasma proteins, we identified fibrinogen, transferrin, plasminogen and ceruloplasmin as nitrated proteins and fibrinogen as only one oxidized protein present in human plasma of lung cancer patients and smokers. Our results clearly indicate that cigarette smoking increases oxidative stress and that during lung cancer development reactive nitrogen species are formed, nitrating plasma proteins (Pignatelli *et al.*, 2001).

We have also measured levels of nitrated and oxidized proteins in 216 human gastric biopsies in order to study the role of *Helicobacter pylori* infection in gastric carcinogenesis. Significantly higher levels of both oxidized and nitrated proteins were found in patients with either chronic gastritis or duodenal ulcer than in those with normal mucosa ($P<0.05$ and $P<0.01$, respectively). The levels of modified proteins were significantly higher in inflamed samples with *H. pylori*, especially cagA+ strains, and in those with expression of interleukin-8 and inducible nitric oxide synthase mRNAs than in those negative for these parameters. These results indicate that infection with cagA+ *H. pylori* induces significant oxidative and nitrative stress in stomach mucosa, contributing to the pathogenesis of *H. pylori*-associated gastroduodenal diseases (Li *et al.*, 2001.

Modified proteins could be measured as better biomarkers than modified DNA bases because target proteins occur at higher concentrations than DNA and they may exist for a longer period than modified DNA bases, as they are possibly not repaired efficiently. Depending upon availability of antibodies, the immunoassays described in this study can be applied to analyze other types of protein modifications which would be useful for future studies, especially to investigate the effects of human nutrition, disease status, life style and antioxidants on oxidative stress and carcinogen exposure (Table 1).

References

Levine, R.L, Garland, D., Oliver, C.N., Amici, A., Climent, I., Lenz, A.G., Ahn, B.W., Shaltiel, S. & Stadtman, E.R. (1990) Determination of carbonyl content in oxidatively modified proteins. *Methods Enzymol.*, **168**, 464–478

Li, C.Q., Pignatelli, B. & Ohshima, H. (2001) Increased oxidative and nitrative stress in human stomach associated with cagA+ *Helicobacter pylori* infection and inflammation. *Dig. Dis. Sci.*, **46**, 836-844

Ohshima, H., Celan, I., Chazotte, L., Pignatelli, B. & Mower, H.F. (1999) Analysis of 3-nitrotyrosine in biological fluids and protein hydrolyzates by high-performance liquid chromatography using a postseparation, on-line reduction column and electrochemical detection: results with various nitrating agents. *Nitric Oxide*, **3**, 132–141

Ohshima, H., Chazotte-Aubert, L., Li, C.-Q., Masuda, M. & Pignatelli, B. (2000) Modifications of DNA, RNA and proteins by interactions of nitric oxide, superoxide and hypochlorous acid: implications for inflammation-associated carcinogenesis. In: Yoshikawa, T., Toyokuni, S., Yamamoto, Y. & Naito, Y., eds, *Free Radicals in Chemistry, Biology and Medicine*. London, Oica International, pp. 90–101

Pignatelli, B., Li, C.-Q., Boffetta, P., Chen, Q., Ahrens, W., Nyberg, F., Mukeria, A., Bruske-Hohlfeld, I., Fortes, C., Constantinescu, V., Ischiropoulos, H. & Ohshima, H. (2001) Nitrated and oxidized plasma proteins in smokers and lung cancer patients. *Cancer Res.*, **61**, 778–784

Beneficial effect of an antioxidant micronutrient-enriched food on DNA damage: experimental study in rats using a modified comet assay in total blood

Hininger I., Chollat-Namy A., Osman M., Arnaud J., Ducros V., Favier A., Roussel A.M.

L.B.S.O. UFR Pharmacie, 38700 La Tronche, France.

Introduction

Diet is an important determinant for cancer incidence (Byers & Perry, 1992) and cardiovascular disease but the mechanisms by which dietary components might affect these pathologies are not fully understood. Antioxidant micronutrients could be involved. However, data from interventional studies are scarce and controversial (Huttunen, 1996). Oxidative damage to DNA, caused by reactive oxygen species (ROS) and their cellular consequences have been implicated in the etiology of cancers. We carried out a study in rats receiving a diet containing low, adequate or high levels of antioxidant micronutrients (vitamin E, Zn and Se) for three months, to compare the effects of such diets on DNA oxidative damage. A modified comet assay was used in total blood for detecting DNA strand breaks and not in isolated cells as usually described, in order to simplify the sampling.

Materials and methods

Male Sprague-Dawley rats (54 ± 6 g) were fed with a standard laboratory diet (Iffa-Credo, U.A.R., France). Rats were randomly divided into three groups and for 3 months received three different diets according to dietary Zn, Se and vitamin E contents as follows: group 0, low: (Zn, 0.89 mg/100 g; Se, 0.01 mg/100 g; E, 68 mg/100 g); group 1, adequate, (Zn, 3.72 mg/100 g; Se, 0.02 mg/100 g; E, 87 mg/100 g); group 2, high, (Zn, 6.12 mg/100 g; Se, 0.035 mg/100 g; E 110 mg/100 g). Fasting rats were killed and oxidative biological parameters measured. A modification of the assay described by Singh *et al.* (1988) detects single-strand break DNA on total blood. Total blood (500 μL) was mixed with 500 μL DMSO/RPMI (20/80) and stored at −140°C until analysis. Frozen blood samples were treated in a water bath (37°C), washed by PBS and spun twice for 10 min at room temperature before analysis. Quantification was achieved by visual scoring based on fluorimetric measurement of DNA intensities in the head and tail of cells from total blood. The arbitrary units were tail moment extent (TME), reflecting percentage of DNA damage in the tail. Plasma Zn, Se, lipid peroxidation products (plasma TBARs) and vitamin E concentrations and erythrocyte GPx activity were determined using routine laboratory methods as described (Hininger *et al.*, 1997). Data were statistically analysed using the non-parametric Kruskall-Wallis test and the Mann and Whitney test. Statistical significance was set at $P<0.05$.

Results

Changes in antioxidant status were significant depending on the diets (Table I). A low-micronutrient diet resulted in significantly lower levels of femoral Zn, plasma Se, vitamin E and GPX activity. We did not observe any changes in TBAR concentrations depending on the diets. In contrast, oxidative DNA

Table 1. Variation of the antioxidant status after 3 months of diet

	G0	G1	G2
Zn femoral µg/g	68 ± 7.32[a]	98 ± 12[b]	101 ± 16[b]
Se pl (µmol/L)	5.07 ± 0.33[a]	5.71 ± 0.60[b]	5.67 ± 0.32[b]
Vitamin E pl (µmol/L)	10.46 ± 5.02[a]	13.79 ± 5.89[b]	17.67 ± 6.43[b]
GPx (U/gHb)	386 ± 41[a]	541 ± 42[b]	502.22 ± 63[b]
TBARs/PUFA	1.29 ± 0.52	1.10 ± 0.20	1.14 ± 0.15

Means ± SD.
Means within a row, not sharing a common superscript are significantly different ($P<0.05$).

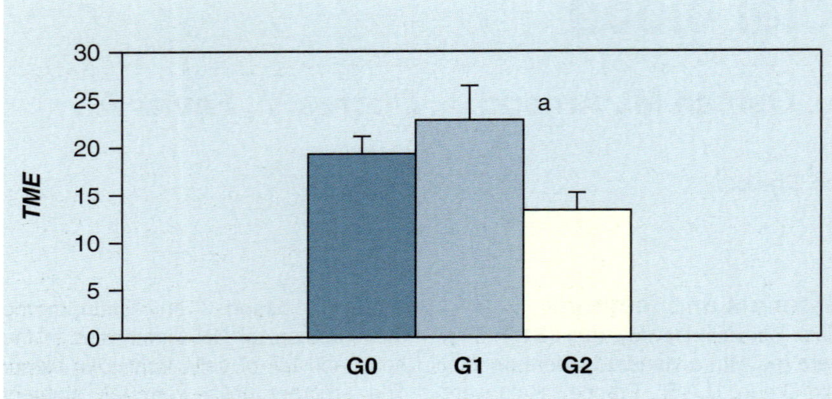

Figure 1
Comparison of oxidative DNA damage (expressed as TME) in rats fed with antioxidant Zn, Se, vitamin E in a low (G0), adequate(G1), or high (G2) diet

damage was significantly less ($P<0.01$) in the high-micronutient diet (G2) than in the adequate or low diet (Fig. 1).

Discussion

Using an original method of measurement of DNA damage on total blood, we observed a significant protecting effect of the enriched (G2) food compared to a normal (G1) or subdeficient (G0) diet. In contrast, we failed to observe changes in lipid peroxidation. These data suggest that the comet assay could be a more sensitive method for detecting oxidative damage than biological markers of lipid peroxidation in plasma. Similar to our results, Duthie *et al.* (1996) reported a beneficial effect of antioxidant supplementation on oxidative damage in lymphocytes, supporting the hypothesis that dietary antioxidants might protect against cancer. The comet assay was usually performed in freshly isolated blood cells or cultured cells. Our results obtained in frozen blood samples offer a simplified way to detect DNA damage, which could be proposed in a future epidemiological approach.

References

Byers, T. & Perry, G. (1992) Dietary carotenes, vitamin C, and vitamin E as protective antioxidants in human cancers. *Ann. Rev. Nutr.*, **12**, 139–159

Duthie, S.J., Ma, A., Ross, A.A. & Collins, A.R. (1996) Antioxidant supplementation decreases oxidative DNA damage in human lymphocytes. *Cancer Res.*, **56**, 1291–1295

Hininger, I., Chopra, M., Thurnham, D., Laporte, F., Richard, M.-J., Favier, A. & Roussel A.M. (1997) Effect of increased fruit and vegetable intake on the susceptibility of lipoprotein to oxidation in smokers. *Eur. J. Clin. Nutr.*, **51**, 601–606

Huttunen, J.K. (1996) Why did antioxidants not protect against lung cancer in the alpha-tocopherol, beta-carotene cancer prevention study? In: Hakama, M., Beral, V., Buiatti, E., Faivre, J. & Parkin, D.M. (eds), *Chemoprevention in Cancer Control* (IARC Scientific Publications No. 136), Lyon, IARC, pp. 63–65

Singh, N.P., McCoy, M.T., Tice, R.R. & Schneider, E.L. (1988) A simple technique for quantification of low levels of DNA damage in individual cells. *Exp. Cell Res.*, **175**, 184–191

Peroxyl radical-scavenging activity of beverages *in vitro*, especially of tea, coffee and wine

Maeda H.[1], Kanazawa A.[2]

[1]Kumamoto University Medical School, Kumamoto, Japan. [2]Faculty of Education, Kumamoto University, Kumamoto, Japan.

Purpose

Epidemiological evidence suggests a correlation between high intake of red meat and fat and cancer incidence of the colon, the prostate and the breast. On the other hand, it is suggested that some beverages have an effect on preventing cancer and other diseases. We (Sawa *et al.*, 1998; Sawa *et al.*, 1999; Kanazawa *et al.*, 2000) previously found that oxidized lipid (lipid hydroperoxide, LOOH) and haem-iron, e.g. myoglobin in red meat, produce lipid peroxyl radicals (LOO•), which damage DNA *in vitro*. LOO• has a long half-life (Akaike *et al.*, 1992) and induces chain propagation reactions generating LOO• quickly; it also has a potential to harm organelles, cells and tissues at a local site and may be capable of damaging a distant site due to its long half-life. This LOO•-forming mechanism is likely to occur with daily dietary components. However, it can be scavenged by coexisting dietary components. Therefore, we examined the LOO•-scavenging activity of the anti-oxidative ability of various beverages.

Methods

Linoleic acid hydroperoxide was purified from air-oxidized linoleic acid by fractionating using a column chromatography technique. The purity of linoleic acid hydroperoxide was checked by thin-layer chromatography and then used for the chemiluminescence assay as a source of LOOH (Kanazawa *et al.*, 2001). Tea and coffee were prepared as practiced in routine drinking. The amount of tea leaves and ground coffee beans and extraction time were as follows: Sencha (green tea, 5 g/dL in water at 75°C, 2 min and 3 min; roasted green tea, 5 g/dl in boiling water, 0.5 min; Darjeeling tea, 1.67 g/dL in boiling water, 3 min; coffee, 5 g/dL in boiling water, 1.5 min. An aliquot of diluted beverage was added to a reaction mixture of luminol and LOOH in 0.01 M phosphate buffered 0.15 M saline containing 0.5% Tween 20. After adding hemoglobin, chemiluminescence was determined using the chemiluminescence multichannel analyzer (Berthold Model LB9505 AT, Wildbad, Germany). The potency to inhibit the luminol-enhanced chemiluminescence induced by LOO• was estimated by potency relative to that of 1 mM quercetin.

Results

The most popular type of Japanese green tea is Sencha, which varies widely in both quality and price. Among the Sencha products manufactured in the same estate (Kawane, Shizuoka Prefecture, Japan), the LOO•-scavenging activity was highest in the product of leaves harvested in early May, and it lowers as the picking time of tea leaves progresses thereafter. The LOO•-scavenging activity shows a linear increase parallel to price (Figure 1). In the case of Japanese green tea, the price and quality of tea are strongly influenced by picking time. On the other hand, there were no differences in the LOO•-scavenging activity among the first, the second, and the autumnal flushes of Darjeeling tea. The quality of Japanese green tea appears to retain the LOO•-scavenging activity after roasting because the high-grade green tea showed higher activity than the low-grade green tea after roasting. In red wines, pinot noir showed higher activity than merlot, shiraz, and cabernet sauvignon. With the exception of pinot noir, they seemed almost equal to green tea but less than coffee. Coffee showed the highest LOO•-scavenging activity among teas, coffee, and red wine. Coffee prepared from freeze-dried powder (12.5 mg/mL)

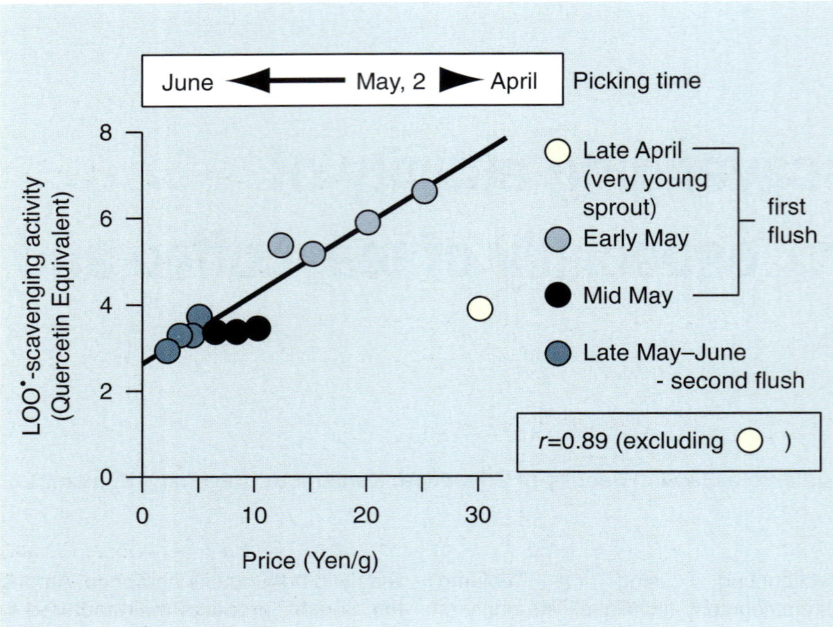

Figure 1
The LOO•-scavenging activity of Sencha, the most popular type of Japanese green tea, manufactured in the estate located in Kawane, Japan

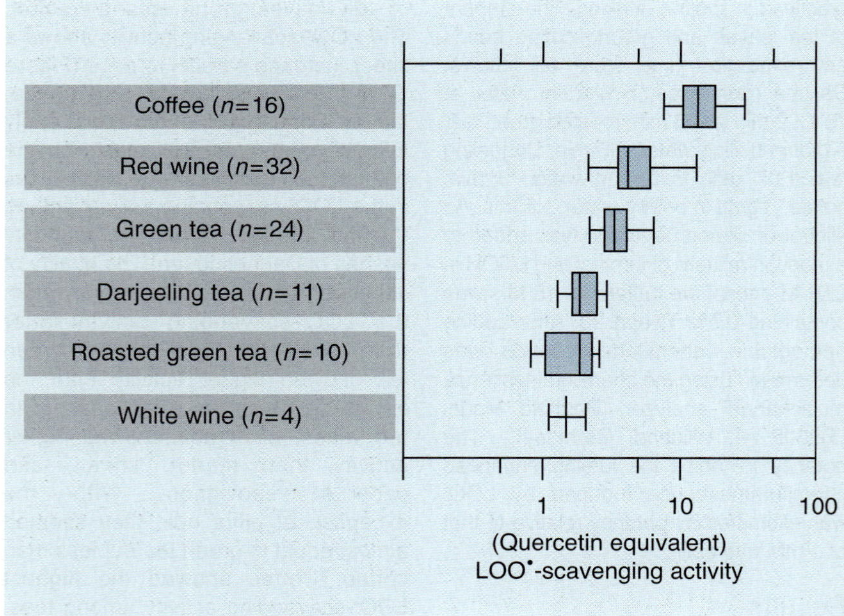

Figure 2
Comparison of LOO•-scavenging activity among beverages.

exhibited an activity as high as coffees brewed from ground coffee beans.

Conclusion

Most of the tested beverages showed high anti-oxidative activity in terms of scavenging LOO•. These findings are consistent with many epidemiological studies, suggesting that these beverages may be effective for preventing cardiovascular disease and cancer. Among the samples tested, the order of anti-LOO• capacity is as follows: coffee > red wine ≥ green tea ≥ Darjeeling tea = roasted green tea ≥ white wine (Figure 2).

References

Akaike, T., Sato, K., Ijiri, S., Miyamoto, Y., Kohno, M., Ando, M., & Maeda, H. (1992) Bactericidal activity of alkyl peroxyl radicals generated by heme-iron-catalyzed decomposition of organic peroxides. *Arch. Biochem. Biophys.*, **294**, 55–63.

Kanazawa, A., Sawa, T., Akaike, T. & Maeda, H. (2000) Formation of abasic sites in DNA by t-butyl peroxyl radicals: implication for potent genotoxicity of lipid peroxyl radicals. *Cancer Lett.*, **156**, 51–55

Kanazawa, A., Sawa, T., Akaike, T. & Maeda, H. (2001) Generation of lipid peroxyl radicals from edible oils and heme-iron: suppression of DNA damage by unrefined oils and vegetable extracts. In: Morello, M. & Shahidi, F., eds, *Free Radicals in Foods: Chemistry, Nutrition and Health* (in press), Washington D.C., American Chemical Society

Sawa, T., Akaike, T., Kida, K., Fukushima, Y., Takagi, K. & Maeda, H. (1998) Lipid peroxyl radicals from oxidized oils and heme-iron: implication of a high-fat diet in colon carcinogenesis. *Cancer Epidemiol. Biomarkers Prev.*, **7**, 1007–1012

Sawa, T., Nakao, M., Akaike, T., Ono, K., & Maeda, H. (1999) Alkylperoxyl radical-scavenging activity of various flavonoids and other phenolic compounds: implications for the anti-tumor-promoter effect of vegetables. *J. Agric. Food Chem.* **47**, 397–402

Micronutrients and the regulation of cancerous cell growth and death: effect of sulforaphane, an isothiocyanate from broccoli

Rouimi P., Assoumaya C., Tulliez J., Gamet-Payrastre L.

UMR 1089 Xénobiotiques, INRA, 180 Chemin de Tournefeuille, BP3, 31931 Toulouse Cedex 9, France.

Introduction

Isothiocyanates occur as conjugates in a variety of cruciferous vegetables. Normal consumption of these vegetables results in the uptake of substantial amounts of isothiocyanates. These compounds are effective inhibitors of chemical carcinogenesis in a wide variety of animal models, which, at least in part due to their effect on enzymes involved in carcinogen metabolic activation such as cytochrome P450 enzymes, has led to the proposal that they be used in the chemoprevention of cancer (Hecht, 1995). The ubiquitous enzymes glutathione S-transferases (GSTs), which have been described as also being involved in isothiocyanate metabolism (Zhang *et al.*, 1995) and in the regulation of stress-activated protein kinases (Adler *et al.*, 1999), may also play a role in the chemoprotective effects of these compounds. We have recently demonstrated the induction of apoptosis in cultured human colon cancerous cells by sulforaphane (Gamet-Payrastre, 2000), the major isothiocyanate in broccoli. Here we have investigated the effect of this compound on both GST and mitogen-activated protein kinases (MAPK) involved in the early events of apoptosis expression, in the human carcinoma colonic cells Caco2.

Methods

Exponentially growing cells were treated with 15 μM of sulforaphane with a short time exposure. Cells were rapidly lysed in Laemly buffer and boiled 1 min at 100°C for analysis by Western blot. Equal amounts (20–50 μg) of total proteins were separated by SDS-PAGE (10% or 12.5% acrylamide) and transferred on a nitrocellulose sheet. Expression of GSTs, activated MAPKs and P38 was analysed using specific antibodies. Additional treatment with 25 μM PD 098059 (PD), 5 μM SB 203580 (SB) and 5 μM curcuma, which are kinase inhibitors specific for ERKs (extracellular signal regulated kinase), P38 and JNK (cJUN N-terminal kinase), respectively, was performed for 1 h before sulforaphane exposure. Floating cells were counted in the culture supernatant 48 h after treatment in order to evaluate the percentage of sulforaphane-induced cell death.

Results and discussion

Our results (Figs. 1 and 2) clearly show a sustained induction of the MAP kinase ERK-1 and ERK-2 by sulforaphane in exponentially growing Caco-2 cells (Fig. 2). Moreover, sulforaphane-induced apoptosis was diminished by interfering with the ERK pathways. Indeed, SB and to a lesser extent PD, but not the curcuma treatment, induce a significant decrease in the apoptotic effect of sulforaphane ($P<0.001$ and $P<0.01$, respectively; $n=5$). These results suggest that beneficial properties of isothiocyanates may be effective prior to acting favourably on carcinogen metabolism. In Caco-2 cells, sulforaphane also strongly induces GSTa, (Fig. 1) a class of enzyme which has been shown to be associated with intestinal cell differentiation (Vecchini *et al.*, 1997). In conclusion, our results suggest that anticarcinogenic properties of sulforaphane *in vitro* may be related to both changes in the early signal of the apoptotic cascade and the induction of GSTα, a class of GSTs whose expression is associated with the endogenous mechanism of intestinal differentiation.

References

Adler, V., Yin, Z., Fuchs, S.Y., Benezra, M., Rosario, L., Tew, K., Pincus, M.R., Sardana, M., Henderson, C.J., Wolf, C.R., Davis, R.J. & Ronai, Z. (1999) Regulation of JNK signaling by GSTp, *EMBO J.*, **18**, 1321–1334

Gamet-Payrastre, L., Li, P., Lumeau, S., Cassar, G., Dupont, M.-A., Chevolleau, S., Gasc, N., Tulliez, J. & Tercé, F. (2000)

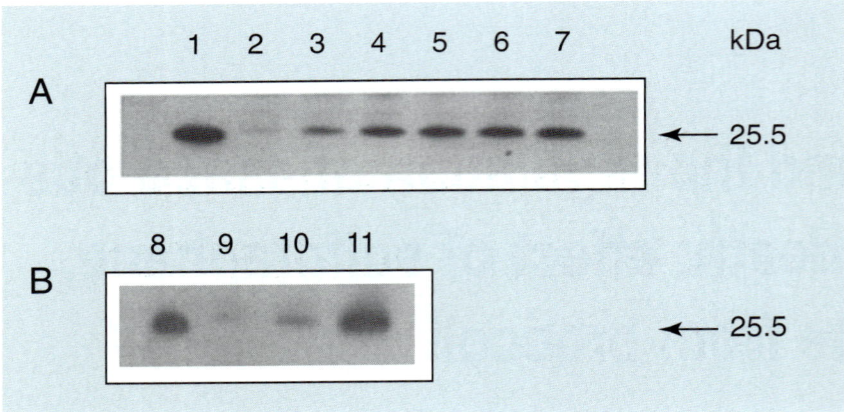

Figure 1
Western blot analysis of GSTα expression in subconfluent, confluent and postconfluent Caco-2 cells. Effect of sulforaphane exposure.
(A) Proliferating cells were exposed to various concentrations of sulforaphane for 48 h in conditions described in the methods. From left to right, lanes 2–7: 0, 5, 10, 15, 20 and 25 μM sulforaphane. (B) Effect of confluence on untreated cells grown for 3 days (lane 9), 7 days (lane 10) and 15 days (lane 11). Confluence occurs at about 7 days. Lanes 1 and 8 are HPLC-purified with rGSTA1 subunit as control. Equal amounts of cytosolic proteins were loaded for each lane. Primary antibody anti-hGSTA1-2 diluted to 1/250, secondary antibody (goat anti rabbit antisera) diluted to 1/500. Revelation by ECL

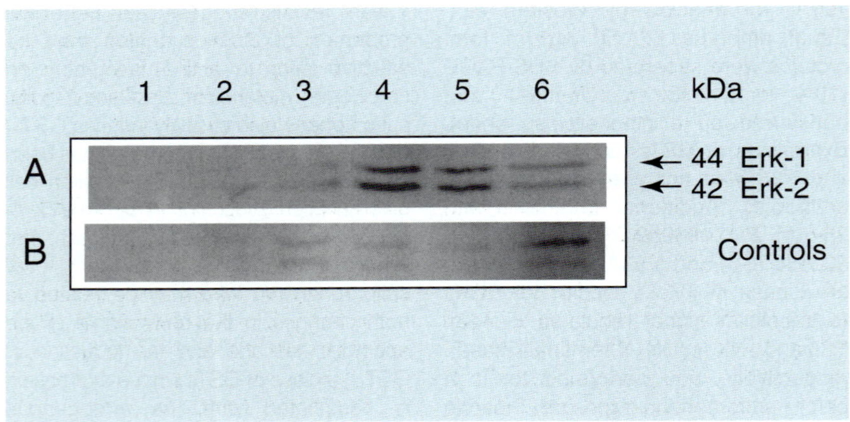

Figure 2
Western blot analysis of ERK-1 and ERK-2 expression in exponentially growing Caco-2 cells and under sulforaphane exposure.
(A) Lanes 1–6 correspond to Caco-2 cell extracts after 0, 5, 20, 40, 60, 240 min of treatment with 15 μM sulforaphane. At the indicated time, cells were lysed and total proteins were loaded on the corresponding lane. (B) Control untreated cells. Primary antibody directed against activated ERK-1 and ERK-2 diluted to 1/5000, secondary antibody (goat ant rabbit antisera) diluted to 1/500. Revelation by ECL

Sulforaphane, a naturally occurring isothiocyanate, induces cell cycle arrest and apoptosis in HT29 human colon cancer cells, *Cancer Res.*, **60**, 1426–1433

Hecht, S.S. (1995) Chemoprevention by isothiocyanates. *J. Cell Biochem.*, **22**, 195–209

Vecchini, F., Pringault, E., Billar, T.R., Geller, D.A., Hausel, P. & Felley-Bosco, E. (1997) Decreased activity of inducible nitric oxide synthase type 2 and modulation of the expression of glutathione S-transferase alpha, bcl-2, and metallothioneins during the differentiation of Caco-2 cells, *Cell Growth Differ.*, **8**, 261–268

Zhang, Y., Kolm, R.H., Mannervik, B. & Talalay, P. (1995) Reversible conjugation of isothiocyanates with glutathione catalyzed by human glutathione transferases. *Biochem. Biophys. Res. Commun.*, **206**, 748–755

Lack of chemoprevention of indole-3-carbinol in *N*-methyl-*N*-nitrosourea-induced mammary carcinogenesis in rats

Kang, J.K.

National Institute of Toxicology Research, Korea Food and Drug Administration, Nokbun-dong, Eunpyung-ku, Seoul 122-704, South Korea.

Introduction

It has been reported (Dashwood *et al.*, 1998) that indole-3-carbinol (I3C) exerts a cancer chemopreventive action in liver, colon and mammary tissue when applied before or concurrent with exposure to a carcinogen, but consumption of I3C after carcinogen treatment may be associated with tumour promotion in some organs. Although Grubbs *et al.* (1995) showed that preinitiation administration of I3C proved effective for chemoprevention of DMBA or MNU-induced mammary tumours, Malejka-Giganti *et al.* (2000) reported that I3C treatment after DMBA exposure did not suppress mammary tumour development. This contradictory modifying effect of I3C led us to focus on the postinitiation action. We therefore investigated the effects of I3C on mammary carcinogenesis after treatment with *N*-methyl-*N*-nitrosourea (MNU).

Material and methods

Treatments

Ninety-six 4-week-old female Sprague-Dawley rats were randomly divided into five groups. Animals in groups 1, 2 and 3 (24, 24 and 34 rats, respectively) were intraperitoneally injected with MNU (50 mg/kg b.w.) dissolved in saline (pH 4.0 adjusted with acetic acid) at the age of 50 days, while those in groups 4 and 5 received saline alone as vehicle controls. Animals in groups 1 and 2 were then given a diet containing 100 and 300 ppm I3C (group 1, MNU+I3C 100 ppm; group 2, MNU+I3C 300 ppm) for 24 weeks starting 1 week after the MNU treatment. Animals in group 3 (MNU alone) served as the carcinogen alone controls. Animals in group 4 (I3C 300 ppm alone) also received I3C 300 ppm without prior initiation. Animals in group 5 (basal diet) were maintained on CRF-1 basal diets throughout the experimental period. Pellet diets containing I3C should be kept in cold room before use within 2 weeks of production. Body weights, food consumption and palpable tumours of all animals were measured every other week after MNU treatment and animals were sacrificed at 32 weeks of age. After histopathological examination, tumour incidence and multiplicity values were calculated for all the groups.

Statistical analysis

Body weight and food consumption were compared with the ANOVA test. Mammary tumour incidences were compared with the Mantel-Haenszel χ^2 test and tumour multiplicities were compared with the Kruskal-Wallis test. Duncan's multiple range *t* test was applied as a post hoc test. For all comparisons, probability values less than 5% ($P<0.05$) were considered to be statistically significant.

Results

Changes in body weight and food consumption

There were no differences in body weight among the groups, but food consumption of groups 1, 2 and 4 showed a higher value than that of groups 3 and 5.

Incidence and multiplicity for mammary tumours

The incidences of the mammary tumours in groups 1, 2 and 3 were 95.8%, 83.3% and 82.4%, respectively, and tumour multiplicities of groups 1, 2 and 3 were 2.21±0.37, 3.21±0.61 and 2.03±0.30, respectively (Table 1). The numbers of tumours in group 2 continued to be greater than in group 3 (Fig. 1). Histopathological examination of tumours demonstrated most of them were adenocarcinomas.

Table 1. Incidences and multiplicities of mammary tumours of rats treated with MNU followed by I3C

Treatments	No. of rats	No. of tumour-bearing rats (percent incidence)	Tumour multiplicity (no. of tumours/rat)	No. of tumours in tumour-bearing rat
MNU[a]+I3C[b] 100 ppm	24	23 (95.8)	2.21 ± 0.37[c]	2.30 ± 0.37
MNU+I3C 300 ppm	24	20 (83.3)	3.21 ± 0.61	3.85 ± 0.63
MNU alone	34	28 (82.4)	2.03 ± 0.30	2.46 ± 0.31
I3C 300 ppm alone	7	0 (0)	0	0
Basal diet	7	0 (0)	0	0

[a]MNU, *N*-methyl-*N*-nitrosourea (50 mg/kg b.w., single i.p. injection).
[b]I3C, indole-3-carbinol (100 or 300 ppm in CRF-1 basal diet).
[c]Data represent mean ± SE.

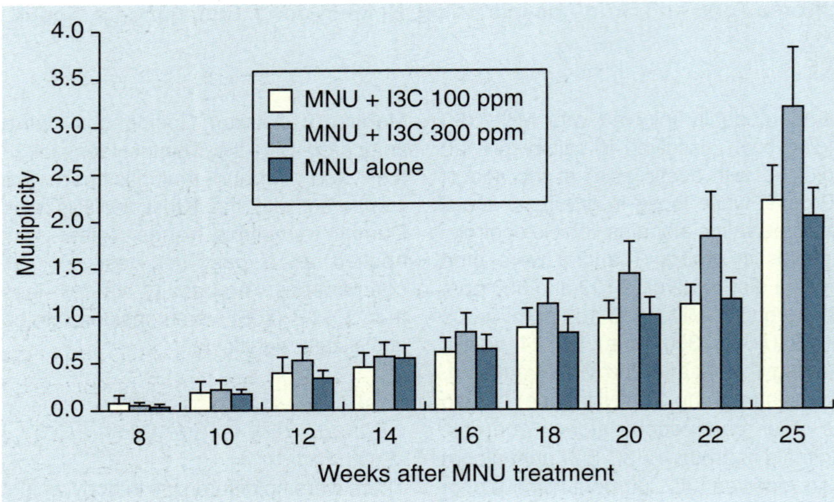

Figure 1
Multiplicities of mammary tumours of rats treated with MNU followed by I3C

Discussion

The primary cause of the loss of suppressing the mammary carcinogenesis might be associated with food consumption. An increase in food consumption after exposure to a carcinogen would be a risk factor. An alternative explanation was that metabolites produced from I3C could have estrogenic actions, as Liu *et al.* (1994) and Riby *et al.* (2000) have reported. Given that Blum *et al.* (2001) recently reported that postinitiation treatment of I3C could influence the pattern of β-catenin mutations in colon tumours, it would be interesting to elucidate the genetic alterations in mammary tumours caused by dietary factors with relevant parameters in further study.

References

Blum, C.A., Xu, M., Orner, G.A., Fong, A.T., Bailey, G.S., Stoner, G.D., Horio, D.T., & Dashwood, R.H. (2001) Beta-catenin mutation in rat colon tumors initiated by 1,2- dimethylhydrazine and 2-amino-3-methylimidazo. *Carcinogenesis*, **22**, 315–320

Dashwood, R.H. (1998) Indole-3-carbinol: anticarcinogen or tumor promoter in brassica vegetables? *Chem. Biol. Interact.*, **110**, 1–5

Grubbs, C.J., Steele, V.E., Casebolt, T., Juliana, M.M., Eto, I., Whitaker, L.M., Dragnev, K.H., Kelloff, G.J., & Lubet, R.L. (1995). Chemoprevention of chemically induced mammary carcinogenesis by indole-3-carbinol. *Anticancer Res.*, **15**, 709–716

Liu, H., Wormke, M., Safe, S.H., & Bjeldanes, L.F. (1994) Indolo[3,2-b]carbazole: a dietary-derived factor that exhibits both antiestrogenic and estrogenic activity. *J. Natl. Cancer Inst.*, **86**, 1758–1765

Malejka-Giganti, D., Niehans, G.A., Reichert, M.A., & Bliss, R.L. (2000) Post-initiation treatment of rats with indole-3-carbinol or beta-naphthoflavone does not suppress 7, 12-dimethylbenz [a]anthracene-induced mammary gland carcinogenesis. *Cancer Lett.*, **160**, 209–218

Riby, J.E., Feng, C., Chang, Y.C., Schaldach, C.M., Firestone, G.L., & Bjeldanes, L.F. (2000) The major cyclic trimeric product of indole-3-carbinol is a strong agonist of the estrogen receptor signaling pathway. *Biochemistry*, **39**, 910–918

Interaction of dietary beta-carotene and alpha-linolenic acid: effect on promotion of experimental mammary tumours

Maillard V.[1], Hoinard C.[1], Steghens J.P.[2], Jourdan M.L.[1], Pinault M.[1], Bougnoux P.[1], Chajès V.[1]

[1]Nutrition, Croissance et Cancer, UPRES-EA 2103, Université François Rabelais, Tours. [2]Laboratoire de Biochimie, Hôpital E. Herriot, Lyon, France.

Several epidemiological studies, based on adipose tissue fatty acid composition as a biomarker of past dietary intake of fatty acids, reported an inverse association between n-3 to n-6 polyunsaturated fatty acids (PUFA) ratio and the risk of breast cancer, suggesting a protective effect of n-3 PUFA on breast cancer risk, dependent on n-6 PUFA levels (Maillard *et al.*, 2002; Simonsen *et al.*, 1998). Before n-3 PUFA can be considered as a target for breast cancer prevention in intervention trials, experimental data are needed to document the effect of n-3 PUFA on mammary tumour growth. Recent studies performed on an experimental model of chemically induced mammary tumours in rats showed that the antioxidant vitamin E, when added to a high-n-3-PUFA diet, suppressed the inhibitory effect of n-3 PUFA on tumour growth and even led to an increase in tumour growth (Cognault *et al.*, 2000). These data suggested that the inhibitory effect of n-3 PUFA on tumour growth might be mediated by an increased formation of lipid peroxidation products and indicated that the interaction between dietary antioxidants and PUFA plays an important role on tumour growth. Other nutritional compounds act as antioxidants and thus may interact with n-3 PUFA on tumour growth. Among dietary antioxidants, beta-carotene, one of the main carotenoids, is of particular interest because of its potential protective effect on breast cancer risk reported in some recent epidemiological studies (Kim *et al.*, 2001; Toniolo *et al.*, 2001). No data is yet available on the role of the interaction between beta-carotene and n-3 PUFA on tumour growth. The aim of this study was to document the role of the interaction between beta-carotene and alpha-linolenic acid, the essential fatty acid of the n-3 family, on mammary tumour growth in a rodent model of chemically-induced mammary tumours.

Ninety female Sprague-Dawley rats were randomly assigned to cages housing three rats per cage in a room maintained at constant temperature (24°C) and humidity with a 12-h light:dark cycle. At 47 days of age, all rats received a single subcutaneous injection of N-nitroso-N-methylurea (25 mg/kg of animal body weight) to initiate mammary tumours.

The experimental diets were prepared by adding fat (15 w% fat) to basal diet with a normal amount of vitamin E for rat diet (50 IU/kg of diet). They contained either a low or a high alpha-linolenic acid level (4% or 17% of total fatty acids, obtained by using either a peanut oil/rapeseed oil or a peanut oil/linseed oil mixture). The levels of beta-carotene used were 0, 10 or 200 mg/kg diet/day. Rats were separated into three groups according to dietary beta-carotene level. Each group was divided into two subgroups (15 rats per subgroup) receiving either a low or a high content of alpha-linolenic acid. Experimental diets were given to rats from initiation to sacrifice. Rat weight gain was measured every week. The appearance and measurement of each mammary tumour were checked by weekly palpation of animals and recorded. Incidence (percentage of tumour-bearing rats), latency (delay in weeks of the first tumour appearance) and multiplicity (number of tumours per tumour-bearing rat) were assessed in each dietary group.

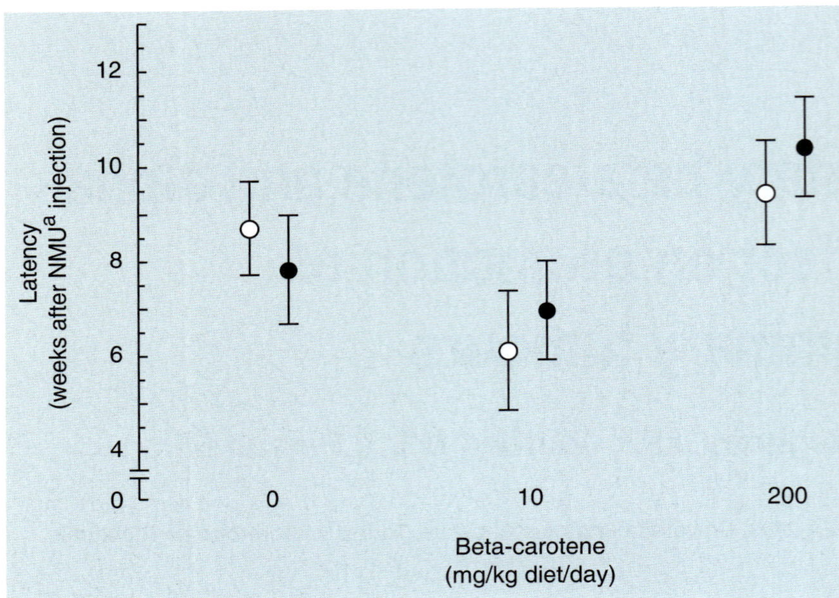

Figure 1
Effect of beta-carotene on mammary tumour latency in rats fed a low or high alpha-linolenic acid content

Values are means ± standard error for each group.
○ Rats fed the low alpha-linolenic acid content; ● rats fed the high alpha-linolenic acid content.
[a]NMU, N-nitroso-N-methylurea.
Significantly different effects of beta-carotene levels on tumour latency, as evaluated by the factorial ANOVA test (P=0.016).

Rat growth was not affected by the different dietary conditions. With respect to incidence, no significant difference was found between the different diets (Table 1). In contrast, tumour latency and multiplicity were influenced. We observed that beta-carotene, at the pharmacological dose of 10 mg/kg diet/day, led to a reduced latency compared to no beta-carotene or to very high beta-carotene (200 mg/kg diet/day) (Fig. 1). This effect on latency was found whatever the alpha-linolenic acid level in diets (Fig. 1). In rats fed a low alpha-linolenic acid content, 10 mg of beta-carotene led to increased multiplicity, compared to no beta-carotene supplementation (Table 1). At a very high dose, beta-carotene had no effect on multiplicity, whatever the level of alpha-linolenic acid (Table 1).

In conclusion, in our rodent model of autochthonous mammary tumours, beta-carotene used at a pharmacological level (10 mg/kg diet/day) did not have the expected protective effect on tumour growth, but rather may have acted as a tumour promoter as evidenced by its effects on tumour latency. The combined effects of alpha-linolenic acid and beta-carotene on multiplicity documents the importance of their interaction. These data show that beta-carotene influences mammary carcinogenesis in a way dependent on the presence of other lipid components such as alpha-linolenic acid.

Acknowledgements

This work was supported in part by grants from the French Ministry of Research (Nutrialis), La Ligue Nationale Contre le Cancer (Comités d'Indre et Loire, Indre, Loire-et-Cher and Charente). V. Chajès is the recipient of a grant from the Agence Régionale d'Hospitalisation, Région Centre, France. V. Maillard is a recipient of a fellowship from the French Ministry of Research.

References

Cognault, S., Jourdan, M.L., Germain, E., Pitavy, R., Morel, E., Durand, G., Bougnoux, P. & Lhuillery, C. (2000) Effect of an alpha-linolenic acid-rich diet on rat mammary tumor growth depends on the dietary oxidative status. *Nutr. Cancer*, **36**, 33–41

Kim, M.K., Ahn, S.H. & Lee-Kim, Y.C. (2001) Relationship of serum α-tocopherol, carotenoids and retinol with the risk of breast cancer. *Nutr. Res.*, **21**, 797–809

Maillard, V., Bougnoux, P., Ferrari, P., Jourdan, M.L., Pinault, M., Lavillonnière, F., Body, G., Le Floch, O. & Chajès, V. (2002) N-3 and n-6 fatty acids in breast adipose tissue and relative risk of breast cancer in a case–control study in Tours, France. *Int. J. Cancer*, **98**, 78–83

Simonsen, N., Van't Veer, P., Strain, J.J., Martin-Moreno, J.M., Huttunen, J.K., Navajas, J.F., Martin, B.C., Thamm, M., Kardinaal, A.F., Kok, F.J. & Kohlmeier, L. (1998) Adipose tissue omega-3 and omega-6 fatty acid content and breast cancer in the EURAMIC study. *Am. J. Epidemiol.*, **147**, 342–352

Toniolo, P., Van Kappel, A.L., Akhmedkhanov, A., Ferrari, P., Kato, I., Shore, R.E. & Riboli, E. (2001) Serum carotenoids and breast cancer. *Am. J. Epidemiol.*, **153**, 1142–1147

Effects of conjugated linoleic acid on adenoma formation in the *Apc*Min mouse

Rajakangas J.[1], Turpeinen A.M.[1], Salminen I.[2], Mutanen M.[1]

[1]Department of Applied Chemistry and Microbiology, Division of Nutrition, P.O. Box 27, FIN-00014 University of Helsinki, Helsinki, Finland. [2]Department of Nutrition, National Public Health Institute, Helsinki, Finland.

Introduction

Conjugated linoleic acid (CLA) is a term used for the different conjugated isomers of linoleic acid (C18:2). The most common forms are the *cis*-9, *trans*-11-, and *trans*-10, *cis*-12 isomers. The naturally occurring *cis*-9, *trans*-11 isomer is found in milk and dairy products and in the meat of ruminants.

In 1987 Ha *et al.* found CLA to be anticarcinogenic in chemically induced epidermal carcinogenesis in mice. Since then, several studies have supported this theory by showing that CLA inhibits tumour formation and growth in different animal models as well as in cell cultures. The most convincing results on the anticarcinogenic effects of CLA have been obtained from studies on mammary tumour inhibition. Ip *et al.* (1994) showed in the rat that the anticarcinogenic effect of CLA in DMBA-induced mammary carcinogenesis was dose-dependent.

The multiple intestinal neoplasia (Min) mouse is an animal model for intestinal carcinogenesis. The mice have a heterozygous mutation in their adenomatous polyposis coli (*APC*) gene, and as a consequence they develop sporadic tumours in their intestine. The human *Apc* gene is closely related to the murine *APC* and a mutation in the *Apc* gene is found in up to 80% of colon cancer cases (Kinzler & Vogelstein, 1996). Thus the *Apc*Min mouse provides a suitable model to investigate the effects of diet on the formation of colorectal cancer.

So far, only one study has been published on the effects of CLA on intestinal tumour formation in the *Apc*Min mice (Hansen-Petrik *et al.*, 2000). The aim of the present study was to confirm the results of Hansen-Petrik and to examine more closely the effect of CLA on tumour growth in the *Apc*Min mouse.

Materials and methods

The male mice were obtained from Jackson laboratories (Bar Harbour, ME, USA) at 7 weeks of age. The control group (n=10) was kept on an AIN-93G-based diet for 8 weeks, while the experimental group (n=10) had a diet containing 1% CLA (Natural Lipids, Hovdebygda, Norway), also for 8 weeks. The CLA used contained 48.2% *trans*-10, *cis*-12 CLA, 48% *cis*-9, *trans*-11 CLA and small amounts of *cis*-9, *cis*-11, *cis*-10, *cis*-12 , *trans*-9, *trans*-11, *trans*-10, *trans*-12 isomers. The animals were weighed weekly to follow their weight development. At the end of the feeding period, the adenomas developed in the intestine of the animals were counted and their sizes measured by light microscopy.

The plasma fatty acid composition of the animals was analysed to test the compliance of the diets. Serum total lipids were determined as described earlier (Salminen *et al.*, 1998). *Cis*-9, *trans*-11 and *trans*-10, *cis*-12 CLA isomers were identified with a standard mixture (Nu chek prep). The results were expressed as normalized percentage fatty acid composition.

Results

The control animals had only small amounts of the *cis*-9, *trans*-11 isomer in their plasma, and no *trans*-10, *cis*-12 isomer was found (Fig. 1). The animals in the CLA group had a 20-fold increase in their plasma *cis*-9, *trans*-11 isomer compared to the controls, and the amounts of the *trans*-10, *cis*-12 isomer were significant. The ratio of the *trans*-10, *cis*-12:*cis*-9, *trans*-11 isomers in the plasma of the CLA animals was approximately 3:5 compared to the ratio in the diet a(1:1).

The water consumption of the two groups varied significantly. The weekly water consumption in the control and the CLA group was 174 ± 19.0 mL (mean ± SD) and 270 ± 23.9 mL, respectively (P<0.001).

The number of adenomas developed in the intestine did not differ between the two groups. The control mice developed

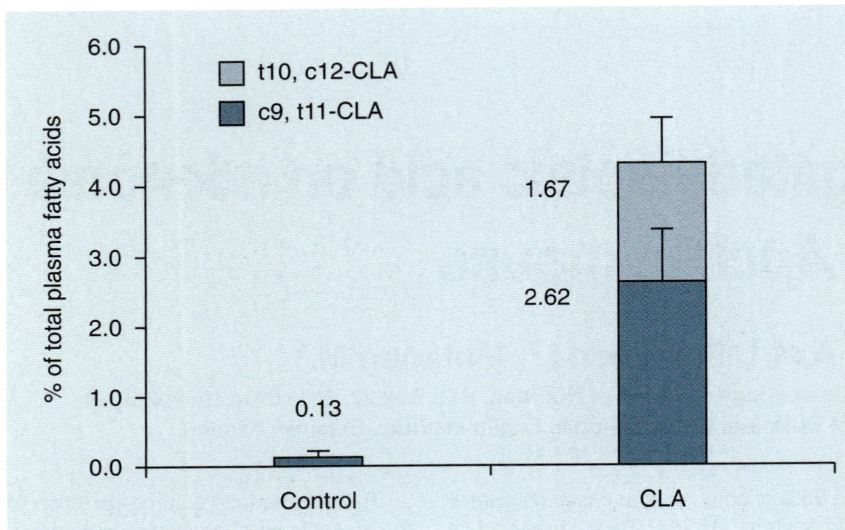

Figure 1
The normalized percentage of *trans*,10, *cis*-12 and *cis*-9, *trans*-11 isomers of conjugated linoleic acid (CLA) found in the plasma of the control and CLA group.

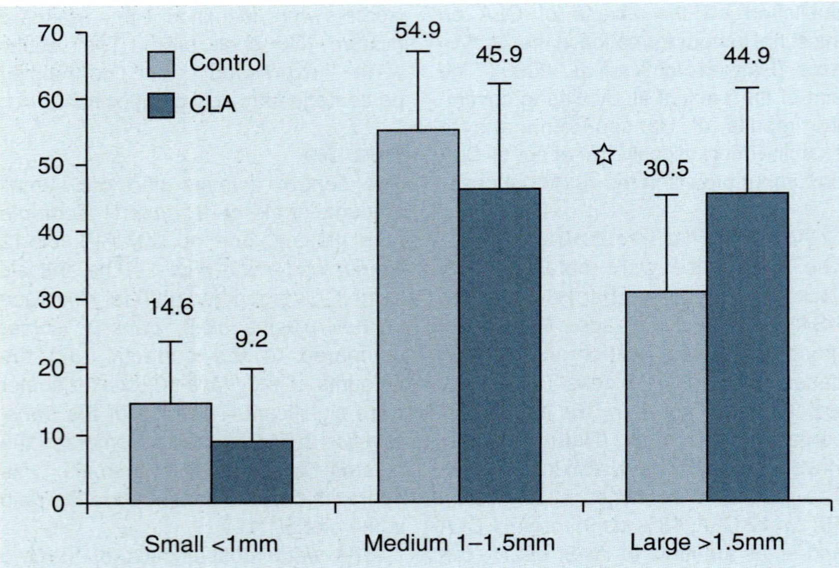

Figure 1
The percent distribution of small, medium and large adenomas. (*P<0.05). CLA, conjugated linoleic acid

34.1 ± 16.4 (mean ± SD) adenomas and the CLA mice 32.9 ± 20.0 adenomas. There was no difference in the number or size of the adenomas developed in the colon. However, the adenomas in the small intestine were larger in the CLA group than in the control group (1.51 ± 0.58 mm vs 1.38 ± 0.56 mm, P<0.01). When comparing the percent distribution of the small (<1 mm), medium (1–1.5 mm) and large (>1.5 mm) adenomas, the CLA group had more large adenomas than the control group (P<0.05) (Fig. 2).

Discussion

The results of this study suggest that CLA has no chemopreventive effect on adenoma formation in the *Apc*Min mouse. This is in accordance with the results earlier published by Hansen-Petrik *et al.* (2000). It seems that in the intestine, CLA enhances the growth of the adenomas, as the adenomas were larger in the CLA group. Clearly, CLA acts differently in the intestine than in other tissues, where it has been shown to prevent tumour growth. The reason for this difference will hopefully become clear when the mechanism of action of CLA is established. The effects of the two major isomers, the *cis*-9, *trans*-11 and *trans*-10, *cis*-12 isomers in the *Apc*Min mouse will be separately examined in our forthcoming studies.

References

Ha, Y.L., Grimm, N.K. & Pariza, M.W. (1987) Anticarcinogens from fried ground beef: heat altered derivates of conjugated linoleic acid. *Carcinogenesis*, **8**, 1881–1887

Hansen-Petrik, M.B., McEntee, M.F., Johnson, B.T., Obucowicz, M.G. & Whelean, J. (2000) Highly unsaturated (n-3) fatty acids, but not alfa-linoleic, conjugated linoleic or gamma-linoleic acids, reduce tumorigenesis in *Apc*Min mice. *J. Nutr.*, **130**, 2434–2443

Ip, C., Singh, M., Thompson, H.J. & Scimeca, J.A. (1994) Conjugated linoleic acid suppresses mammary carcinogenesis and proliferative activity of the mammary gland in the rat. *Cancer Res.*, **54**, 1212–1215

Kinzler, K.W. & Vogelstein, B. (1996) Lessons from hereditary colorectal cancer. *Cell*, **87**, 159–170

Salminen, I., Mutanen, M., Jauhiainen, M. & Aro, A. (1998) Dietary trans fatty acids increase conjugated linoleic acid levels in human serum. *J. Nutr. Biochem.*, **9**, 93–98

Geraniol, a component of plant essential oils, sensitizes human colon cancer cells to 5-fluorouracil treatment

Carnesecchi S.[1], Langley K.[2], Exinger F.[3], Gosse F.[1], Raul F.[1]

[1]Laboratory of Nutritional Chemoprevention in Digestive Oncology, Institut de Recherche contre les Cancers de l'Appareil Digestif (IRCAD). [2]Laboratory of Biological Cellular Communication, INSERM U338. [3]Laboratory of Carcinogenesis, UPR 9003 CNRS; Strasbourg, France.

Clusters of cells expressing differentiation characteristics of enterocytes are present in all colon cancers and have been proposed as a factor responsible for the resistance of colon cancer to anti-neoplastic agents. It has been shown that resistance to high concentrations of chemotherapeutic agents seems to be restricted to cells of the enterocytic phenotype (Lesuffleur *et al.*, 1998).

The human colon cancer cell line Caco-2 spontaneously undergoes structural and functional enterocytic differentiation at late confluence. Phenotypic changes after confluence include formation of brush border membranes and expression of intestinal hydrolases which are markers of the functional differentiation also found in enterocytes and human fetal colonocytes (Rousset, 1986). Since prevention of colon cancer cell differentiation might be an important feature in the treatment of colon cancer, the purpose of this work was to determine whether the inhibition of Caco-2 cell differentiation by geraniol could sensitize Caco-2 cells to 5-fluorouracil (5-FU) treatment.

Methods

We investigated the effects of geraniol on cell morphology, and on several differentiation markers which are normally expressed in Caco-2 cells after confluence. We also evaluated the effects 5-FU on cancer cell growth and cytotoxicity in the presence of geraniol.

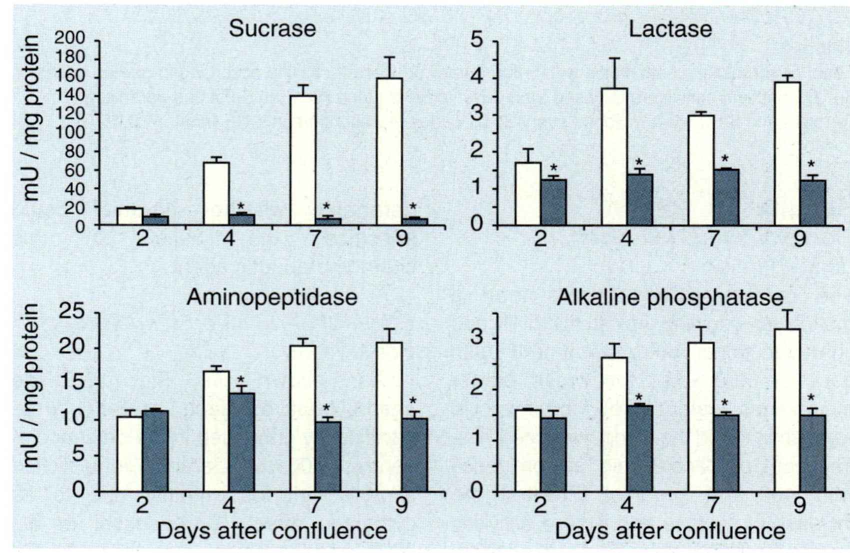

Figure 1

Specific activity (mU/mg protein) of sucrase, lactase, alkaline phosphatase and L-aminopeptidase in the brush border membranes isolated from Caco-2 cells. Confluent cells (7 days after plating) were maintained for 2, 4, 7 and 9 days in culture in the absence (open columns) or in the presence (hatched-line columns) of 400 μM geraniol. The culture medium was replaced every 24 h. Results are means ± SE of three separate experiments. For each column, $P<0.05$ (Student's *t* test)

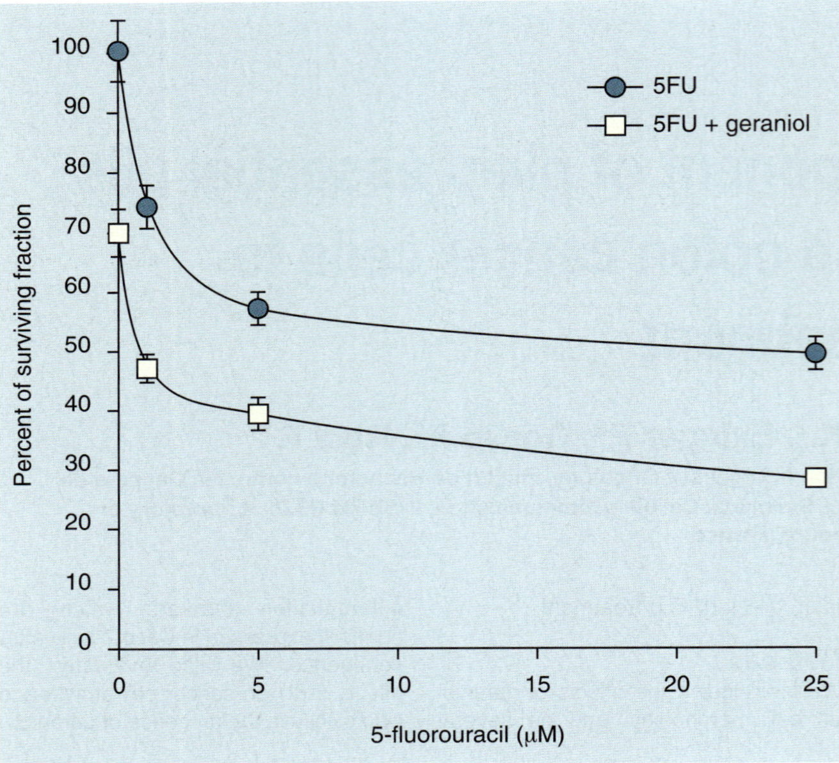

Figure 2
Effect of geraniol in combination with 5-fluorouracil on Caco-2 cell line according to graded doses of 5-FU. Confluent cells were exposed for 8 days, to 5-FU alone (●) or to 5-FU and geraniol (□). Geraniol and 5-FU were replaced every 24 h. Values represent mean ± SE (n=8), P<0.05.

Results

Geraniol and Caco-2 cell differentiation

The confluent Caco-2 cells form a monolayer showing apical microvilli and tight junctions. After treatment with geraniol (400 μM), the brush border membranes were altered, the microvilli were scarce and their length reduced. The treatment of Caco-2 cells at confluence with 400 μM geraniol inhibited the increase of sucrase and lactase activities by 90% and 70%, respectively. In addition, geraniol also inhibited the increase of alkaline phosphatase and aminopeptidase activities by 50% (Fig. 1).

The effects of 5-FU were then evaluated on cell growth in order to determine whether geraniol could sensitize the cells to this chemotherapeutic agent.

Effect of geraniol on 5-fluorouracil-treated Caco-2 cells

As shown in Fig. 2, the antiproliferative effects of 5-FU were significantly enhanced in the presence of geraniol (400 μM). Geraniol alone elicited a 30% cell loss mainly due to its cytostatic effect (Carnesecchi *et al.*, 2001) and the treatment with 5 μM 5-FU alone caused a 50% cell loss. When combined with geraniol, 5-FU (5 μM) caused a 75% cell loss. Similarly, at higher concentrations of 5-FU, the number of surviving cells was reduced by twofold in the presence of geraniol. The effect of geraniol on 5-FU cytotoxicity was assessed after confluence by measuring LDH (lactate dehydrogenase) release in the culture medium. Geraniol, which alone showed no cytotoxic effect, doubled the cytotoxic effect of 5-FU (5 μM). Intracellular accumulation of 5-[6-3H] FU was determined in the presence or absence of geraniol after 9 h of treatment. We show that the uptake of 5-FU by Caco-2 cells was doubled in the presence of geraniol.

Conclusions

Our data show that geraniol, a component of vegetable essential oil, sensitizes human colon cancer cell lines to 5-fluorouracil treatment. This effect is related to the disturbance of cellular morphological and functional differentiation. Geraniol may act on two major targets involved in the resistance of colon cancer cells to chemotherapeutic agents: the process of cell differentiation and the membrane permeability to the chemotherapeutic agent.

We show that interactions of geraniol with cell membrane prevent the differentiation process and facilitate the uptake of the chemotherapeutic agent by cancer cells. Recent studies have shown that geraniol interferes with membrane function of Candida Saccharomyces and increases membrane fluidity on liposomal membranes (Tsuchiya, 2001). Changes in membrane fluidity induced by heptacain, a component of Capsicum fruit (pepper), have been related to the insertion of the lipophilic fragment into phospholipid acyl chains to create a free volume in the hydrophobic membrane region (Gallova *et al.*, 1995). Phospholipid acyl chains band cooperatively and fill the free volume to fluidize membrane. A similar mechanism of action may be proposed for geraniol.

By fluidizing the membrane, geraniol may favour the uptake of anticancer drugs by the cancer cells. This could decrease the concentration of drugs used during chemotherapy and, at the same time, lower their secondary effects. Therefore, the combination of geraniol and 5-FU might be a promising approach for optimizing colorectal cancer therapy.

References

Carnesecchi, S., Schneider, Y., Ceraline, J., Duranton, B., Gosse, F., Seiler, N. & Raul, F. (2001) Geraniol, a component of plant essential oils, inhibits growth and polyamine biosynthesis in human colon cancer cells. *J. Pharma. Exp. Therapeutics*, **298**, 197–200

Gollava, J., Cizzmarik, J. & Balgavy, P. (1995) Biphasic effect of local anesthetic and β-blocker heptacaine on fluidity of phosphatidyl-choline bilayers as detected by ESR spin probe method. *Pharmazie*, **50**, 486–488

Lesuffleur, T., Violette, S., Vasile-Pandrea, I., Dussaulx, E., Barbat, A., Muleris, M. & Zweibaum, A. (1998) Resistance to high concentrations of methotrexate and 5-fluorouracil of differentiated HT-29 colon-cancer cells is restricted to cells of enterocytic phenotype. *Int. J. Cancer*, **76**, 383–392

Rousset, M. (1986) The human colon carcinoma cell lines HT-29 and Caco-2: two *in vitro* models for the study of intestinal differentiation. *Biochimie*, **68**, 1035–1040

Tsuchiya, H. (2001) Biphasic membrane effects of capsaicin, an active component in capsicum species. *J. Ethnopharmacol.*, **75**, 295–299

Could apigenin metabolism explain the estrogenic effect of this flavonoid in the female immature rat?

Gradolatto A., Teyssier C., Stroheker T., Chagnon M.-C., Canivenc-Lavier M.-C.
UMR 0938 de Toxicologie Alimentaire, INRA-ENSBANA, 17 rue Sully, BP 86510, 21065 Dijon Cedex, France.

Purpose

Flavonoids are polyphenolic compounds present throughout the plant kingdom. Some of them, such as isoflavonoids (genistein), lignans, coumestrans and a few flavones (apigenin, kaempferol) are described as phytoestrogens, as they can mimic or influence estrogen effects in the body. They have been investigated by many researchers and they are thought to have beneficial effects on human health.

Apigenin, which is present in our daily diet (1 mg/day), has anti-carcinogenic properties (Boyong & Birt, 1996; Suschetet *et al.*, 1998) and can influence enzymes required for the synthesis of estradiol (Santti *et al.*, 1998).

The purpose of this work was to assess the estrogenic effects of apigenin in female Wistar rats and to study its metabolism (blood kinetics, elimination and *in vitro* metabolites) for a better comprehension of its mode of action.

Methods

Estrogenic effects are determined using the uterotrophic test. Immature female Wistar rats are fed *ad libitum* with the AO4C diet. The animals received either apigenin (25–200 mg/kg b.w.), genistein (100 mg/kg b.w.) or estradiol (45 μg/kg b.w.) orally. Other groups received either apigenin or genistein (100 mg/kg) with estradiol. The control group was given corn oil orally. All the groups received the treatment for 4 days. Then animals were killed and the uterus was removed, dried and weighed.

Blood kinetics and elimination of apigenin were assessed in female Wistar rats fed ad libitum with a flavonoid-free semi-synthetic diet. For both experiments, a single oral dose [^{3}H]apigenin (10 mg/kg b.w. and 10 μCi/kg b.w.) was given to animals. The control group received corn oil.

For kinetics studies, blood samples were collected at different time points for 15 days and radioactivity was counted after digestion of the samples. Elimination of radioactivity was assessed by collecting urine and faeces samples daily for 10 days. Radioactivity was counted directly for urine samples and after digestion for faecal samples.

Primary metabolites of apigenin were investigated *in vitro* by incubating aroclor-induced rat microsomes, apigenin and NADPH for 10 min at 37°C. After addition of cold methanol and centrifugation, metabolites were separated by HPLC. They were identified by comparison of their retention time and their UV spectra with those of standards, and by mass spectrometry (determination of molecular weight and fragmentation).

Results

The results of the uterotrophic test indicate that apigenin alone had no effect on uterine weight as compared to controls. Co-treatment of apigenin (100 mg/kg b.w.) and estradiol increased the weight of the uterus significantly (Fig. 1). This estrogenic effect was more significant than the effect observed with genistein or estradiol alone or co-administration of these two molecules.

Radioactivity recovered in blood after ingestion of [^{3}H]apigenin showed a peak at 24 h, followed by a gradual decrease. Fifteen days after ingestion, radioactivity was still detected in blood. The half-life and distribution volume were 95.2 h and 4938 L, respectively.

Radioactivity in urine and faecal samples was mainly detected within the first 3 days, with a peak at 24 h. After 10 days, 37.53% of radioactivity was eliminated, which is less than that observed by Ueno *et al.* (1983) for [^{14}C]quercetin.

The *in vitro* assay revealed the presence of three hydroxylated

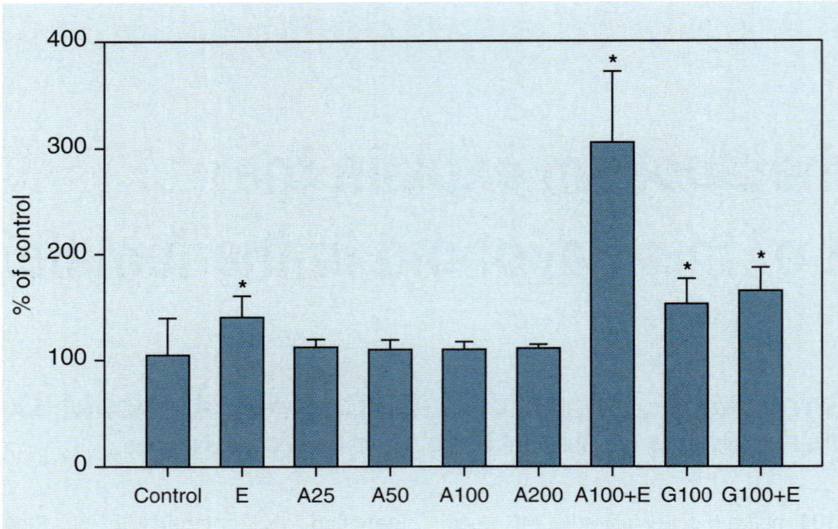

Figure 1
Effect of oral administration of phytoestrogens on uterus weight. Animals were administered 45 μg estradiol/kg b.w. (E), 25, 50, 100, 200 mg apigenin/kg b.w. (A25, 50, 100, 200), A100+E or 100 mg genistein/kg b.w. (G100), or G100+E.
*Significantly different from control (Dunnett's test, $P \leq 0.05$).

metabolites: scutellarein, iso-scutellarein and luteolin (Fig. 2). The cytochrome P450 1A1 seems to be the major isoform involved in the reaction.

Conclusion

The estrogenic effect of apigenin was revealed only in the presence of estradiol and this effect was more significant than the effect observed for the reference phytoestrogen, genistein. These results suggest that these molecules have a different estrogenic effect.

The metabolism of apigenin can explain this effect. First, this molecule is poorly eliminated (less than 40% after 10 days) as compared to other flavonoids, and parameters of blood kinetics underline this fact. Second, hydroxylation of apigenin leads to the formation of three metabolites including luteolin, which does have estrogenic effects (Hiremath *et al.* 2000).

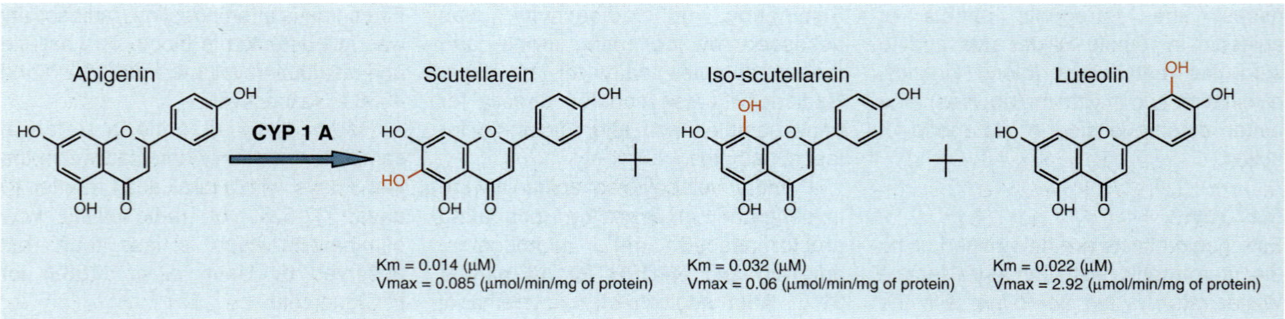

References

Boyong, L. & Birt, D.-F. (1996) *In vivo* and *in vitro* percutaneous absorption of cancer preventive flavonoid apigenin in different vehicles in mouse skin. *Pharm. Res.*, **13**, 1710–1715

Hiremath, S.P., Badami, S., Hunasagatta, S.K. & Patil, S.B. (2000) Antifertility and hormonal properties of flavones of Striga orabanchioides. *Eur. J. Pharmacol.*, **391**, 193–197

Santti, R., Makela, S., Strauss, L., Korkman, J. & Kostian, M.L. (1998) Phytoestrogens: potential endocrine disruptors in males. *Toxicol. Ind. Health*, **14**, 223–237

Suschetet, M., Siess, M.-H., Le Bon, A.-M. & Canivenc-Lavier, M.-C. (1998) Anticarcinogenic properties of some flavonoids. *Polyphenols*, **87**, 165–204

Ueno, I., Nakano, N. & Hirono, I. (1983) Metabolic fate of [^{14}C]quercetin in the ACI rat. *Jpn. J. Exp. Med.*, **53**, 41–50

Apigenin — CYP 1 A → Scutellarein + Iso-scutellarein + Luteolin

Scutellarein: Km = 0.014 (μM), Vmax = 0.085 (μmol/min/mg of protein)

Iso-scutellarein: Km = 0.032 (μM), Vmax = 0.06 (μmol/min/mg of protein)

Luteolin: Km = 0.022 (μM), Vmax = 2.92 (μmol/min/mg of protein)

Figure 2
Hydroxylated derivatives of apigenin obtained by in vitro incubation with rat liver microsomes

Estrogenic effects of apigenin, kaempferol and bisphenol A in immature Wistar female rats and in MCF-7 cells

Stroheker T., Pinnert M.F., Picard K., Chagnon M.C., Canivenc-Lavier M.C.
UMR 0938 de Toxicologie Alimentaire, INRA/ENSBANA, 17 rue Sully, BP 86510, 21065 Dijon Cedex, France.

Introduction

Over the last 50 years, the reproductive capacity of humans and wildlife has been declining, with a decrease in sperm quality and an increase in reproductive tract abnormalities. Hormone-dependent cancers are also increasing in industrial countries. Molecules called endocrine disrupters are suspected of inducing these malformations. Among them, natural (phytoestrogens) and environmental (xenoestrogens) compounds could disrupt the endocrine system via an estrogenic mechanism.

The aim of this study was to evaluate estrogenic potentials of two natural compounds and one xenoestrogen. We chose two flavonoids commonly present in the western diet: apigenin present in parsley, celery, wheat germ and honey and kaempferol found in cabbage and cruciferous vegetables, and a xenoestrogen, bisphenol A, used for tin coating, which can migrate into the food. Two reference compounds were used as positive controls in order to assess our study: estradiol and genistein, a phytoestrogen found in soya.

Materials and methods

The e-screen test *in vitro* and the uterotrophic test *in vivo* were used to identify estrogenic activities.

In vitro: an e-screen assay was performed with human breast cancer cell lines (MCF-7) which possess the estrogen receptor (ER+). Each well of 24-well plates was seeded with 30 000 cells. Tested molecules were dissolved in dimethylsulfoxide (DMSO) at a non-cytotoxic concentration (0.1%) in medium DMEM/F12 (1:1) without phenol red, with 10% desteroided fetal calf serum, which was changed every 48 hours for 6 days. The e-screen test was also assessed on MDA-MB-231 and (ER–) was used to eliminate false-positives. The cytotoxicity of each compound was tested using the neutral red method (Rat *et al.*, 1994). The DABA test was used for proliferation studies (Kissane and Robins, 1958).

In vivo: We chose immature female Wistar rats for their sensitivity (Zacharewski, 1998) on the uterotrophic assay and on the vaginal cornification test (Allen and Doisy, 1923). Animals were fed *ad libitum* with the AO4C diet, which contains low phytoestrogens, and water was applied *ad libitum.* Tested compounds were dissolved in corn oil for the phytoestrogens and in polyethylene glycol (PEG) for bisphenol A and administered daily at 100 mg/kg per day by gavage (5 mL/kg) for 3 days. Estradiol was administered at 45μg/kg per day, at a low estrogenic dose. Control rats received vehicle alone. Harris-Shorr coloration was used for staining vaginal smears (Clark and Mani, 1994).

Results and discussion

In vitro: The most active molecule was genistein, then apigenin and bisphenol A showed similar estrogenic activity (Fig. 1). Kaempferol seemed to be a relatively poor estrogenic compound.

In vivo: There was no difference between control with corn oil as vehicle and control with PEG as vehicle. Administered alone, only genistein was significantly active on the uterotrophic assay (Fig. 2). Apigenin and kaempferol associated with estradiol (45 μg/kg per day) had a synergic effect on the uterotrophic test whereas genistein and bisphenol A did not.

Genistein is the most potent endocrine disrupter tested in this study in both *in vitro* and *in vivo* assays.

Xenoestrogen (bisphenol A) and phytoestrogen (apigenin and kaempferol) showed similar estrogenic activity *in vitro* (Fig. 1) but no significant estrogenic activity has been

Table 1. E-screen assay performed on MCF-7 cell line

Compounds	Maximal activity vs E_2[a] (10^{-8}M)	PS_{50}[b] (M)
Estradiol	100%	$0.00013.10^{-7}$
Genistein	85%	$0.097.10^{-7}$
Bisphenol A	75%	$4.1.10^{-7}$
Apigenin	73%	$4.1.10^{-7}$
Kaempferol	58%	$8.3.10^{-7}$

[a]E_2 (10^{-8}M) was chosen as 100% reference.
[b]PS_{50} = xenobiotic concentration leading to 50% of the proliferation observed with E_2.

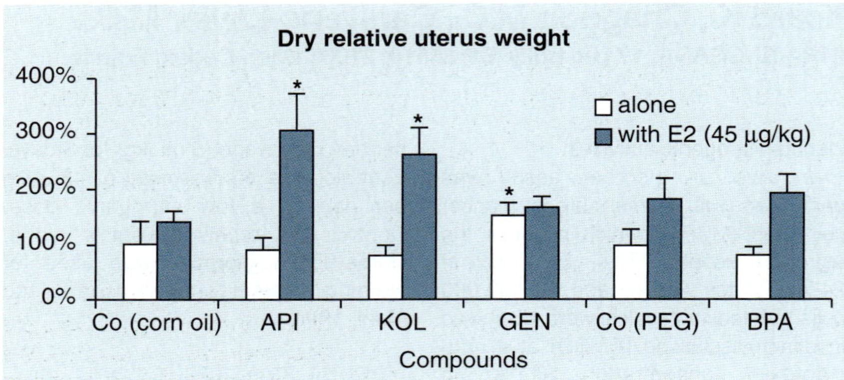

Figure 1
Effects of API, KOL, GEN and BPA (100 mg/kg per day) administered with or without E2 at 45 µg/kg per day on the dry uterus weight relative to the body weight

observed on the dry uterus relative weight (Fig. 2).

All the tested compounds showed estrogenic potencies *in vitro* and induced cornification in vaginal smears (data not shown) but only estradiol and genistein had a significant effect with the uterotrophic test. Vaginal cornification appeared to be more sensitive than uterotrophy.

Whereas apigenin and kaempferol seemed to be poor estrogenic compounds, they induced a strong synergic effect administered with estradiol in the uterotrophic test (Fig. 2). These results could be explained by the properties of the flavonoids, which could interact with multiple mechanisms of the endocrine system like steroid biosynthesis and metabolism.

Conclusion

In vitro assays are useful to identify intrinsic activity of compounds and *in vivo* tests are a realistic representative model to assess exposure.

In vivo, vaginal cornification appears to be a sensitive complementary test to the uterotrophic assay commonly used.

Some endocrine disrupters with poor estrogenic activity could induce a strong synergic effect in the presence of estradiol. These results raise the question: what is the risk of multi-exposure to environmental endocrine disrupters combined with hormonal treatments?

References

Allen, E. & Doisy, E.A. (1923) An ovarian hormone: preliminary report on its localization, extraction and partial purification, and action in test animals. *JAMA*, **81**, 819–821

Clark, J.H. & Mani, S.K. (1994). Actions of ovarian steroid hormones. In: Knobil, E. & Neill, J.D., eds, *The Physiology of Reproduction*, New York, Raven Press, pp. 1011–1059

Kissane, J.M., & Robins, E. (1958) The fluorometric measurement of deoxyribonucleic acid in animal tissues with special reference to the central nervous system. *J. Biol. Chem.*, **233**, 184–188

Rat, P., Korwin-Zmijowska, C., Warnet, J.M., & Adolphe, M. (1994) New *in vitro* fluorometric microtitration assays for toxicological screening of drugs. *Cell Biol. Toxicol.*, **10**, 329–337

Zacharewski, T. (1998) Identification and assessment of endocrine disruptors: limitations of *in vivo* and *in vitro* assays. *Environ. Health Perspect.*, **106**, 577–582

Animal tissue components may be anticarcinogenic

Griciute L., Uleckiene S., Domkiene V.
Lithuanian Oncology Center.

Various compounds are being investigated for possible anticarcinogenic activity. However, extractions from animal tissues have so far been neglected by researchers. Therefore, the publications on this problem are quite rare. Norwegian researchers have investigated pentapeptides extracted from mice liver, intestine and skin epidermis as well as synthetic peptides. These compounds inhibited tumour growth both *in vivo* and *in vitro* (Watt *et al.*, 1989; Paulsen *et al.*, 1992).

Russian investigators have studied the anticarcinogenic effect of cytomedines – peptides of low molecular weight. Some of them inhibited the growth of experimental tumours (Sinakewich, 1991).

We tested the original peptide-like substances Ventriculine and Duodenin derived from gastrointestinal tissues of pigs not yet fully identified (Griciute, 1997). The rationale of the study was that in the tissues of the gastrointestinal tract there must be factors which prevent a deteriorating action of substances in food (personal communication, 1987; Raffes, 2001).

Purpose

The search for the new anticarcinogenic substances.

Material and methods

We used 635 Wistar rats and 550 mice of different lines. Carcinogenesis in different groups of animals was induced with the chemical carcinogens organotropic dimethylhydrazine, N-nitrosodimethy-lamine, N-nitrosodiethylamine, urethane

Table 1. Inhibition of tumour morbidity

Animals	Carcinogenic compound used	Kind of tumour	Anticarcinogen used	Inhibition (%)
Rats	Dimethylhydrazine	Colon cancer	Ventriculine	Up to 30
			Duodenin	50
Rats	N-nitrosodiethylamine	Kidney cancer	Ventriculine	35
			Duodenin	66
Rats	N-nitrosodimethylamine	Different tumours	Ventriculine	0
			Duodenin	50
Mice	Urethane	Pulmonary adenomas	Ventriculine	43
			Duodenin	37
Mice	Benz(a)pyrene (subcutaneous administration)	Subcutaneous sarcomas	Ventriculine	24
			Duodenin	37
Mice	Benz(a)pyrene (skin painting)	Skin cancer	Duodenin	56
Rats	All body ionizing radiation	Different tumours	Ventriculine	0
			Duodenin	0

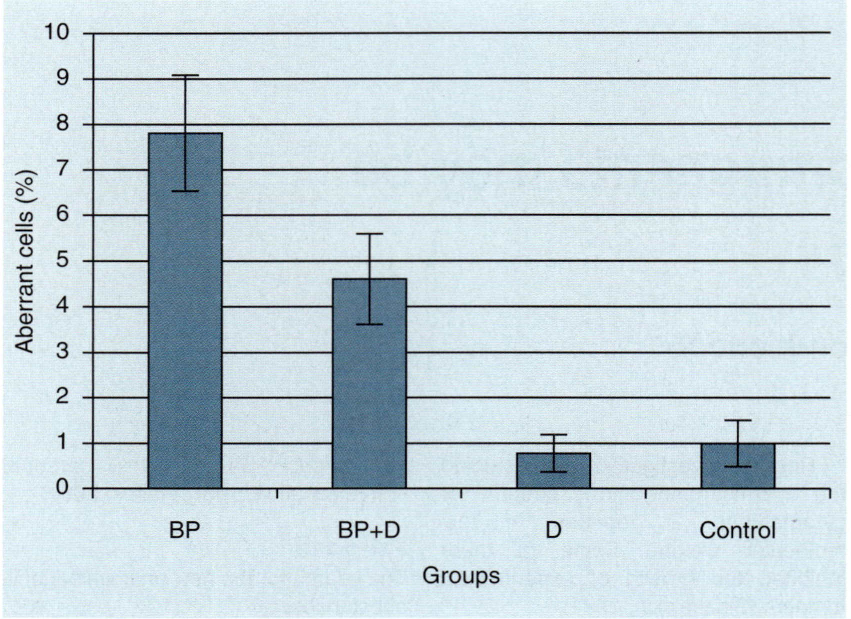

Figure 1
Chromosomal aberrations in mice bone marrow 24h after treatment with benz(a)pyrene (BP) and Duodenin (D)

and directly acting benz(a)pyrene. Ionizing radiation for the entire body was used as well. Ventriculine and Duodenin were administered by gavage starting the day before the first administration of the carcinogenic factor and for the following 6 months at doses of 50 or 200 mg/kg body weight.

Results and discussion

Malignant tumour morbidity in animals given Ventriculine and Duodenin was diminished in comparison with the tumour morbidity in control animals given only a carcinogenic substance (Table 1). The inhibition was dose-dependent.

The Norwegian researchers as well as the Russian authors presumed that the effect of peptides on the tumour cells had a direct inhibitory effect, not involving cells belonging to the immunological system.

The underlying mechanisms of action of Ventriculine and Duodenin has not been determined. It is known that both of them are antistressors; they inhibit no antioxidative potency. Ventriculine is a weak inductor of interferon and TNF. Duodenin inhibits chromosome aberrations induced with benz(a)pyrene in mice bone marrow cells (Fig. 1).

This suggests that these preparations inhibit chemical carcinogenesis acting directly on the cells as do the other peptides studied.

Conclusions

Ventriculine and Duodenin inhibited chemical carcinogenesis. The use of animal tissue components may be promising in cancer chemoprevention.

References

Griciute, L. (1997) Anticancerogenic activity of animal tissue components. *Theory and Practice of Cancer Prevention* (Conference materials, UICC, Lithuanian Oncology Center), Vilnius, Lithuanian Cancer Society, pp. 79–80

Paulsen, J.E., Hall, K.S., Rugstad, H.E., Reichelt, K.L., & Elgjo, K. (1992) The synthetic hepatic peptides pyroglutamylglutamylglycylserylaspargine and pyroglutamylglutamylglycylserylaspartic acid inhibit growth of MH1C1 rat hepatoma cells transplanted into Buffalo rats or athymic mice. *Cancer Res.* **52**, 1218–1221

Raffes, J. (2001) *Duodenal Antifatigue Hormonal Factor Origin and Treatment of Digestive Fatigue Syndrome and Other Food-Related Disorders.* New York, Begell House, Inc.

Sinakewich, N. (1991) Peptide bioregulators – cytomedines. Introduction in the problem [in Russian], *Vrach*, **3**, 36–38

Watt, F.M., Reichelt, K.L., & Elgjo, K. (1989) Pentapeptide inhibitor of epidermal mitosis: production and responsiveness in cultures of normal transformed and neoplastic human keratinocytes. *Carcinogenesis*, **10**, 2249–2253

Diet modulates the genotoxicity of IQ (2-amino-3-methylimidazo[4,5-f]quinoline) in rats associated with a human faecal flora

Humblot C.[1], Kassie F.[2], Nugon-Baudon L.[1], Knäsmuller K.[2], Lhoste E.F.[1]

[1]Unité d'Ecologie et de Physiologie du Système Digestif, INRA, 78350 Jouy-en-Josas, France. [2]Institute of Cancer Research, 1090 Vienna, Austria.

According to numerous epidemiological studies, the development of colorectal cancer is associated with the consumption of a western-style diet low in fruits and vegetables and high in meat. The promoting effect of meat may be related to the nature of the fat or to the presence of high amounts of genotoxic substances such as heterocyclic amines. Heterocyclic amines are pyrolysis products formed during broiling or smoking meat and fish. They are potent mutagens and carcinogens. Both the endogenous detoxication system and the bacterial enzymes of the colic flora are involved in their metabolism *in vivo* (King *et al.* 2000). Therefore, their genotoxic effects may be modulated by diets influencing both systems. Dietary constituents such as glucosinolates (present in cruciferous vegetables) induce the phase II enzymes while others such as pre- and probiotics[1] orient the functions of the bacterial flora towards beneficial effects (Wollowski *et al.*, 2001). Since the properties of the rat gut microflora are rather different from that of humans, we evaluated the genotoxic effect of a heterocyclic amine (2-amino-3-methyl-3H-imidazo[4-5-f]quinoline: IQ) in rats harbouring a human flora and fed experimental diets enriched in one of three candidate ingredients for a cancer-protective effect: Brussels sprouts (rich in glucosinolates), a prebiotic (RAFTILOSE, synergy 1, a long-chain inulin) or a commercially available fermented milk (probiotic).

Experimental design

Thirty-two germ-free F344 adult male rats (UEPSD-INRA breeding unit) were inoculated with the flora of a human donor (Roland *et al.*, 1996). After a 1-week adaptation to the control diet and the flora, the rats were divided into four groups and fed the experimental diets (human-type diets enriched with one ingredient (Table 1). After 4 weeks, the rats were killed by CO_2 inhalation. In each group, four rats were used for the comet assay: they received a 90-mg/kg gavage of IQ 3 h prior to sacrifice. The genotoxicity of IQ was detected in the liver and colon by the modified alkaline single-cell gel electrophoresis assay (Miyamae *et al.*, 1998). The remaining rats were used to determine:

1. The specific activities of the detoxication enzymes (glutathion-S-transferase: GST and UDP-glucuronosyl transferase: UGT) in the liver and of the β-glucuronidase
2. Bacterial metabolites in the caecal contents (Lhoste *et al.* in press).

The activity of β-glucuronidase was measured with *p*-nitrophenol as a substrate. The activities of GST and UGT were assayed spectrophotometrically using, respectively, 1-chloro-2,4-dinitrobenzene and 4-methyl umbelliferone as substrates. Short-chain fatty acids were analysed by gas chromatography and ammonia by spectrophotometry. The data were compared by an analysis of variance followed by a Neumann-Keuls test.

Results and discussion

The genotoxic effects of IQ on the liver and colon were decreased by the chronic consumption of the three experimental diets since the length of the tail comets was smaller in the experimental groups than in the control group (Brussels sprouts, 0.47-fold,

[1] Prebiotics beneficially influence the equilibrium of the gut microflora and its metabolism. Probiotics are living bacteria incorporated in food.

Table 1. Composition of the experimental diets (g/kg dry matter)[a]

	Control	Inulin	Brussels sprouts
Cornstarch	290	240	250
Mashed potatoes	290	290	290
Saccharose	50	0	50
Casein	50	50	50
Soybean isolate	120	120	100
RAFTILOSE, synergy 1	0	100	0
Brussels sprouts	0	0	100
Corn oil	30	30	30
Lard	30	30	30
Cholesterol	0.15	0.15	0.15
Cellulose	60	60	60
Minerals, vitamins	80	80	80

[a]The diets were provided as powder. The fermented milk was mixed with the control diet.

P<0.05; inulin, 0.39-fold, *P*<0.05; fermented milk, 0.55-fold in the colon). All three diets acted through different mechanisms. Indeed, Brussels sprouts increased the specific activities of GST and UGT (respectively 1.5- and 1.8-fold, *P*<0.05) in the liver; UGT is involved in the detoxication of IQ. Inulin did not alter the phase II enzymes but decreased the specific activities of bacterial β-glucuronidase (0.5-fold, *P*<0.05). The deconjugation of the glucuronide from hydroxy-IQ releases a metabolite that is highly genotoxic. In addition to their effects on the metabolism of IQ, both diets decreased the caecal content of ammonia (respectively, 0.41- and 0.59-fold, *P*<0.05) while that of short-chain fatty acids was not modified. Since the production of ammonia is considered as negative for the gut mucosa, a decrease may be protective. The consumption of the fermented milk altered the specific activities of neither GST or UGT nor b-glucuronidase but significantly decreased the production of ammonia (0.47-fold, *P*<0.05).

Since the three protective diets decreased the genotoxicity of IQ via different mechanisms, their synergic effects should be tested. In addition, it would be interesting to determine whether the function of different floras, chosen, for example, for their β-glucuronidase activity, can be modulated to the same extent by these protective foods.

References

King, R.S., Kadlubar, F.F. & Turesky, R.J. (2000) *In vivo* metabolism. In: Nagao, M. & Sugimura, T., eds, *Food-Borne Carcinogens: Heterocyclic Amines*. Chichester, Wiley, pp. 90–111

Lhoste, E.F., Andrieux, C., Lory, S., Meslin, J.C., & Nugon-Baudon, L. The fermentation of lactulose in rats inoculated with clostridium paraputrificum influences the activities of liver and intestinal xenobiotic-metabolizing enzymes. *J. Sci. Food Agric.* (in press)

Miyamae, Y., Yamamoto, M., Sasaki, Y.F., Kobayashi, H., Igarashi, S.M., Shimoi, K. & Hayashi, M. (1998) Evaluation of a tissue homogenization technique that isolates nuclei for the *in vivo* single cell gel electrophoresis (comet) assay: a collaborative study by five laboratories. *Mutat. Res.*, **418**, 131–140

Roland, N., Rabot, S. & Nugon-Baudon, L. (1996) Modulation of the biological effects of glucosinolates by inulin and oat fibre in gnotobiotic rats inoculated with a human whole faecal flora. *Food Chem. Toxicol.*, **34**, 671–677

Wollowski, I., Rechkemmer, G. & Pool-Zobel, B.L. (2001) Protective role of probiotics and prebiotics in colon cancer. *Am. J. Clin. Nutr.*, **73**, 451–455

IQ (2-amino-3-methylimidazo[4,5-f]quinoline)-induced aberrant crypt foci and colorectal tumour development in rats fed two different carbohydrate diets

Mølck A.-M., Thorup I., Kristiansen E., Meyer O.

Institute of Food Safety and Toxicology, Danish Veterinary and Food Administration, Mørkhøj Bygade 19, DK-2860 Søborg, Denmark.

Introduction

Aberrant crypt foci (ACF) are considered as possible preneoplastic lesions in the colorectal mucosa indicative of later development of colorectal tumours (Bird *et al.*, 1989). Therefore, the ACF assay in rodents has been extensively used to study the modifying effect of different dietary components on colorectal carcinogenesis. In most of the published ACF studies, the colon carcinogen 1,2-dimethylhydrazine dihydrochloride (DMH) or its metabolite azoxymethane (AOM), not naturally present in the human diet, have been used as initiators. The use of food-borne initiators, such as the heterocyclic amines formed during the cooking of fish and meat enhances the relevance of the assay to the human situation. A diet high in refined carbohydrates has been suggested as a risk factor for ACF and colorectal cancer development (Caderni *et al.*, 1994; Kristiansen *et al.*, 1996). The purpose of the present study was to investigate the effect of a refined carbohydrate-rich diet on the development of IQ-induced ACF over time.

Methods

Two groups of 26 male F344 rats were each fed continuous doses of 0.03% IQ in a purified diet for 10 or 14 weeks followed by 32 weeks without IQ in the latter case. Group I was fed a diet high in cornstarch and potato starch whereas group II was fed a diet high in sucrose and dextrin (Table 1). Ten animals from each group were sacrificed after 10 weeks (published earlier by Kristiansen *et al.*, 1996) and the remaining after 46 weeks. Complete gross necropsy was performed on all animals and macroscopically visible lesions were recorded. To visualize the ACF, the colon/rectum was processed and the ACF enumerated according to Kristiansen *et al.* (1996).

Results

Nine animals were euthanized during week 25–44 of the study due to tumours of the skin, mucous membranes, Zymbal gland or liver.

The total number and distribution of ACF are presented in Table 2. For the categories small and total ACF, the sucrose-rich diet as well as the time period led to a statistically significant increase in number. However, as no statistically significant interaction between diet and time was seen, sucrose had no intensifying effect over time. With respect to the number of medium-sized ACF, sucrose had an intensifying effect over time as a statistical interaction between time and diet was observed. A nonparametric pairwise comparison revealed that the number of large ACF increased over time, whereas feeding the sucrose-rich diet had no effect. The number of extra-large ACF was not affected by the type of diet or time period.

At the scheduled necropsy, a few tumours in the large intestine were observed. In group I, two animals carried tumours in the colon whereas one animal from group II carried a colonic tumour (Table 2).

The autopsy revealed a 100% incidence of liver tumours, including the euthanized animals. Occurrence of a liver tumour was first observed after 25 weeks in an animal harbouring a Zymbal

Table 1. Composition of diets

	Group I	Group II
Ingredients[a]		
Na-caseinate	20	20
Carbohydrate mix[b]	67.3	0
Carbohydrate mix[c]	0	67.3
Soy bean oil (with vitamins A, D and E)	4	4
Mineral mixture	3.3	3.3
Vitamins B and K, choline chloride,		
inositol and methionine	1.4	1.4
Cellulose	4	4
IQ	0.03	0.03

[a]All data are percentages.
[b]Carbohydrate mix: 45% cornstarch, 45% potato starch, 5% sucrose, 5% dextrin.
[c]Carbohydrate mix: 5% cornstarch, 5% potato starch, 45% sucrose, 45% dextrin.

gland tumour. In addition, the autopsy revealed tumours in the skin, mucous membranes and the Zymbal gland in some animals.

Discussion

IQ was shown to induce tumours in the colon, cecum, liver, Zymbal gland and skin, which are known target organs. The incidence of liver tumours, however, was surprising, as Ohgaki *et al.* (1991) found lower incidences ranging from 19% to 68%. It cannot be ruled out that the presence of liver tumours may have influenced the metabolism of sucrose. IQ shares this problem with DMH, which causes liver toxicity and induces preneoplastic lesions in the liver.

The present data demonstrate that a sucrose-rich diet enhances the outcome of total and small IQ-induced ACF and thereby support our previous results (Kristiansen *et al.*,1996). Further, after

Table 2. Influence of different diets and time periods on the number of IQ-induced ACF, the distribution of ACF according to the number of crypts in the focus and colorectal tumour development

ACF/Colon[a]

Group[b]	Diet[c]	Weeks[d]	*N*[e]	Total	Small 1–3 crypts/ACF	Medium[f] 4–6 crypts/ACF	Large[g] 7–9 crypts/ACF	Extra-large[g] ≥ 10 crypts/ACF	Animals with colorectal tumours
I_{10}	BD	10	10	6.0±1.0	5.3±0.9 (88)	0.7±0.4 (12)[1]	0[x]	0[x]	0
II_{10}	SD	10	10	10.6±1.9	10.3±1.9 (97)	0.3±0.2 (3)[1]	0[x]	0[x]	0
I_{14}	BD	46	11	11.8±1.9	7.8±1.1 (66)	3.1±0.8 (26)[2]	0.8±0.3 (7)[y]	0.1±0.1 (1)[x]	2[h]
II_{14}	SD	46	12	21.8±2.3	14.4±1.7(66)	5.3±0.8(24)[3]	1.8±0.5(8)[y]	0.3±0.2 (1)[x]	1
Statistical significance (2-way analysis of variance, *P* values)									
Diet				0.0004	0.0003	–	Not calculated	Not calculated	
Weeks				0.0001	0.0278	–	Not calculated	Not calculated	
Diet x weeks				0.1633	0.5851	0.0439	Not calculated	Not calculated	

[a]Values are means ± SE; numbers in parentheses represent percentage of total.
[b]Rats initiated with IQ for 10 ($_{10}$) and 14 ($_{14}$) weeks, respectively.
[c]BD, basic diet; SD, sucrose-rich diet.
[d]Number of weeks on test after commencement of IQ feeding.
[e]*N*, effective number of rats as animals euthanized before terminal sacrifice are excluded. All rats harboured ACF.
[f]Groups not sharing a common superscript (1, 2, 3) differ significantly when pairwise comparisons by least square means (general linear models procedure) were performed.
[g]Groups not sharing a common superscript (x, y) differ significantly when pairwise comparisons (Wilcoxon) were made.
[h]In addition, caecal tumours were seen in two animals. One of these also had colorectal tumours.

46 weeks, an intensifying effect of the sucrose-rich diet was seen for the medium-sized ACF. In the sucrose-rich diet, part of the cornstarch and potato starch was replaced considerably lowering the content of resistant starch, as potato starch contains 57% resistant starch. Therefore, it could be speculated that the enhancing effect of the sucrose-rich diet is caused by a lack of resistant starch reaching the colon, leading to a lower concentration of short-chain fatty acids (SCFAs). SCFAs are suggested as being important modulators of cell proliferation, differentiation and apoptosis (Johnson, 1995). However, when sucrose replaced cornstarch containing 5%–10% resistant starch, only a similar enhancing effect on ACF and tumour development was observed (Caderni *et al.*, 1994). Comparison over time shows a statistically significant increase in all ACF categories, except for the category of extra-large ACF from week 10 to 46. Thus, the data indicate that although the IQ exposure was ceased 32 weeks before sacrifice, progression in ACF development has taken place. Early and late ACF development is correlated, as the result obtained after 46 weeks parallels the ACF pattern seen after 10 weeks. In contrast, due to the low colorectal tumour incidence, it was not possible to correlate it with the development of ACF.

Acknowledgements

The authors wish to thank the publisher of the European Journal of Cancer Prevention for allowing us to present these data, which are part of a study accepted for publication. Additionally, we wish to thank Merete Lykkegaard, Heidi Rokkedahl, and Bo Herbst for excellent technical assistance.

References

Bird, R.P., McLellan, E.A. & Bruce, W.R. (1989) Aberrant crypts, putative precancerous lesions, in the study of the role of diet in the aetiology of colon cancer. *Cancer Surv.* **8**, 189–200

Caderni, G., Luceri, C., Spagnesi, M.T., Giannini, A., Biggeri, A. & Dolara, P. (1994) Dietary carbohydrates modify azoxymethane-induced intestinal carcinogenesis in rats. *J. Nutr.* **124**, 517–523

Johnson, I.T. (1995) Butyrate and markers of neoplastic change in the colon. *Eur. J. Cancer Prevent.*, **4**, 365–371

Kristiansen, E., Meyer, O. & Thorup, I. (1996) Refined carbohydrate enhancement of aberrant crypt foci (ACF) in rat colon induced by the food-borne carcinogen 2-amino-3-methyl-imidazo[4,5-f]quinoline (IQ). *Cancer Lett.*, **105**, 147–151

Ohgaki, H., Takayama, S. & Sugimura, T. (1991) Carcinogenicities of heterocyclic amines in cooked food. *Mutat. Res.*, **259**, 399–410

L-Methionine supplementation accelerates tumour growth and shifts the phospholipid derivative pattern in a murine model of malignant melanoma. A proton HRMAS NMR spectroscopy study

Demidem A.[1], Morvan D.[2,3], Papon J.[1], Madelmont J.C.[1]

[1]UMR 484 INSERM, [2]UMR 484 Université d'Auvergne, [3]Centre de Lutte Contre le Cancer, 63005 Clermond-Ferrand, France.

Introduction

Methionine (Met) is a nutriment of concern in tumour cell proliferation (Judde *et al.*, 1989). Among its fates are protein synthesis, polyamine synthesis and phospholipid (PL) metabolism in which it is a substrate for phosphatidylcholine (PtdCho) synthesis from phosphatidylethanolamine (PtdEth). The PL metabolism plays an important role in tumour cell proliferation and cell signalling (Podo, 1999). PtdCho, the main PL, is tightly regulated in cancer cells (Baburina & Jacowski, 1999). Its biosynthesis involves two pathways: the cytidine diphosphate choline (CDP-choline) pathway mainly, and the PtdEth methylation pathway. On the other hand, PtdCho is catabolized by phospholipases (Plases): Plases-A2 generate glycerophosphocholine (GPC) and glycerophosphoethanolamine (GPE) (Baburina & Jackowski, 1999), and Plases-C generate phosphocholine (PC) and phosphoethanolamine (PE). PC and PE increases may also result from an activation of choline- and ethanolamine-kinases (Podo, 1999).

We recently developed a proton NMR spectroscopy technique to follow PL derivative metabolites in tumour tissue samples. Here we investigated the relationship between Met supplementation, tumour growth and PL metabolism in a model of murine malignant melanoma.

Materials and methods

Six-week-old male C57BL6/6J mice were injected subcutaneously with 5 x 10^5 B16 melanoma cells. Two groups of mice were experimented: a control (CT) group and an L-Methionine-supplemented group. L-Methionine (L-Met) was administrated intraperitoneally at 10 mg/g daily from day 10 to day 24 after B16 cell inoculation. The Met group could not be followed later since animals died. Half of the animals in both groups served to determine tumour growth curves and the remaining animals were sacrificed at several moments of evolution, with tumour removal for NMR spectroscopy analysis. Each data point of growth and PL derivative curves were the average of measurements on three recipients. Tumour growth curves were fitted to a Gompertz model.

Proton NMR spectroscopy was carried out in high-resolution conditions at 500 MHz (Bruker DRX 500) using a magic angle spinning accessory. Fresh *ex-vivo* tumour samples were deposited into rotor tubes spun at 4 kHz at a temperature of 20°C. Measurement of PtdCho used a saturation recovery sequence (repetition time: 10 s, duration: 5 min 20 s). Other PL derivatives (PC, PE, GPC, GPE) were determined using an editing Tocsy sequence (mixing time, 75 ms; repetition time, 2 s; sampling, 4 K x 256; duration, 1 h 30 min). The mixing time and the sequence duration were optimized for PL derivative signal-to-noise and sample preservation considerations. Quantification was performed using the Bruker Xwinnmr software. Internal standardization of PL derivative signals was done on the glycine signal which was previously verified to vary poorly in comparison with that of PL derivatives.

Results and discussion

The analysis of growth curves showed that, in the Met group, growth was accelerated with a growth rate peak occurring 4 days earlier than in the CT group (Fig. 1).

The analysis of NMR spectroscopy data revealed that in the Met group:

1. PtdCho levels were quite elevated, especially during early growth (Fig. 2a), likely indicating increased biosynthesis. A decreased demand for PtdCho was unlikely since the growth rate at that time was increased.
2. PC and PE levels reached their maximum during early growth (Fig. 2b, c), accompanying the shift to the left of growth curves, consistent with a role of PC and PE as promoters of mitogenesis (Kiss, 1999). PC and PE waves could result from an activation of Plases C, or choline- and ethanolamine-kinases. In addition, the PC wave may be associated with increased activation of the CDP-choline pathway and explain contemporary elevated PtdCho levels.
3. Between days 15 and 21, GPC and mainly GPE transiently increased, reflecting the activation of Plases-A2 (Fig. 2d, e), possibly in relation with increased PtdCho levels (Baburina & Jackowski, 1999).
4. During delayed growth (day 24), PE was still elevated despite a return to baseline of other PL derivatives (Fig. 2c). This pattern may have a role in stimulating proliferation or represent a regulatory mechanism due to persistent Met administration.

Our data show that Met supplementation shifts to the left growth curves of melanoma and important PL derivatives (PtdCho, PC and PE). However, the putative role of an increased methylation of PtdEth in these changes remains unelucidated. This study provides new data on some of the events triggered by Met and allows inferring some of the consequences of Met deprivation in cancer treatment protocols. The role of an increased methylation of PtdEth due to increased Met availability remains to be established. The activity of PtdEth N-methyl transferases is low in most tissues except the liver and a large enhancement of PtdEth methylation in our model is unlikely. Most probably, increased PtdCho levels originated from increased CDP-choline pathway activation. However, some papers have shown that an increased amount of PtdEth methylation paradoxically enhanced the CDP-choline pathway in non-liver tumour cells (Lee *et al.*, 1996). We plan further investigation using 13C-labelled substrates (choline, ethanolamine, Met) and molecular biology to enlighten some of the hypotheses raised.

References

Baburina, I. & Jackowski, S. (1999) Cellular responses to excess phospholipid *J. Biol. Chem.*, **274**, 9400–9408

Judde, J.G., Ellis, M., & Frost, P. (1989) Biochemical analysis of the role of transmethylation in the methionine dependence of tumor cells. *Cancer Res.*, **49**, 4859–4865

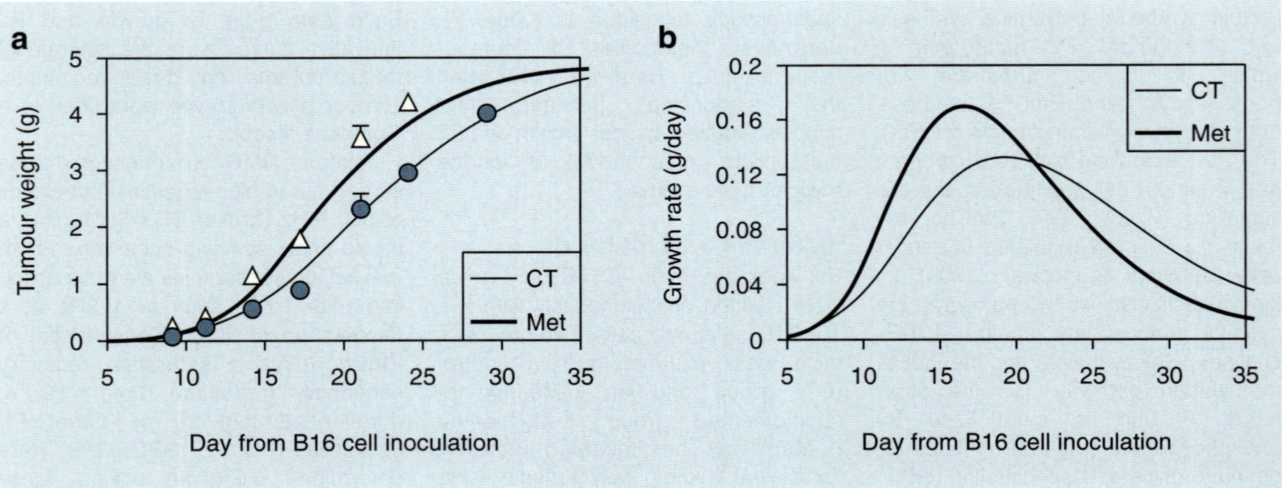

Figure 1
Tumour growth curves (a) and growth curve first derivatives (b) showing growth acceleration in the Met group. Circles and thin lines, Control (CT) group; triangles and bold lines, L-methionine-supplemented group

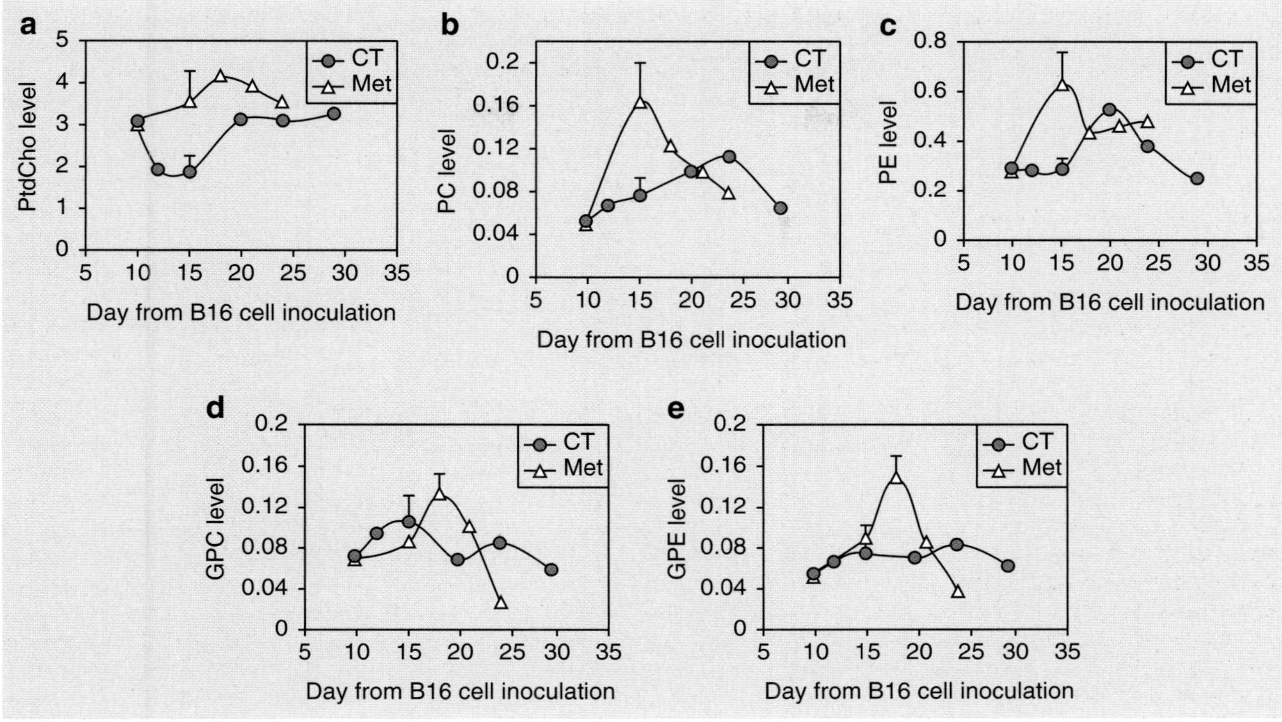

Figure 2
Proton NMR spectroscopy data. Time course of PtdCho (a), PC (b), PE (c), GPC (d), and GPE (e) in the CT group (circles) and in the Met group (triangles). Error bars were obtained from variance analysis of the time series. The PtdCho level was the concentration of PtdCho relative to that of glycine. Other PL derivative levels were concentrations relative to that of glycine and to a factor depending on NMR properties. These levels can be compared between one another and, to a proportionality factor, with the PtdCho level

Kiss, Z. (1999) Regulation of mitogenesis by water-soluble phospholipid intermediates. *Cell Signal.*, **11**, 149–157

Lee, M.W., Bakovic, M. & Vance, D.E. (1996) Overexpression of phosphatidylethanolamine N methyl transferase 2 in CHO K1 cells does not attenuate the activity of the CDP-choline pathway for phosphatidylcholine biosynthesis. *Biochem. J.*, **320**, 905–910

Podo, F. (1999) Tumor phospholipid metabolism. *N. M. R. Biomed.*, **12**, 413–439

Simple sugars modulate the development of aberrant crypt foci in rat colon during post-initiation

Poulsen M., Mølck A.-M., Thorup I., Breinholt V., Meyer O.

Institute of Food Safety and Toxicology, Danish Veterinary and Food Administration, Mørkhøj Bygade 19, DK-2860 Søborg, Denmark.

Introduction

The intake of dietary sugar in humans has been suggested as a risk factor in the development of colorectal cancer in humans (Burley, 1997; Potter, 1999). Similar observations are found in studies with laboratory rodents where sugar in some studies enhanced the development of preneoplastic lesions and colonic tumours. From these studies it is not clear whether sugar acts as a co-initiator, promoter or as a combination of these. Thus, the present study was performed with the objectives of investigating the influence of feeding sucrose and dextrin during the pre-initiation, initiation, and/or the post-initiation period with regard to the development of carcinogen-induced aberrant crypt foci (ACF) in F344 rats. Furthermore, the study was designed to investigate whether colonic cell proliferation, altered redox status or interference with selected detoxification enzymes in the colon could explain the specific mechanisms involved in the suggested effect of sucrose and dextrin on ACF development.

Methods

Male F344 rats were randomly assigned to eight experimental groups of 10 rats each. All groups except the control group were dosed subcutaneously with azoxymethane at 15 mg/kg body weight twice, 1 week apart. The animals were fed a diet high in sucrose and dextrin (61%) and low in starch (7%) or a diet low in sucrose and dextrin (7%) and high in starch (61%) during the pre-initiation, the initiation, and/or the post-initiation stage of the ACF development (Table 1). Colonic cell proliferation measured as the BrdU-labelling index, activity of phase II enzymes (quinone reductase and glutathione-S-transferase), and malondialdehyde as a biomarker of lipid peroxidation were also examined. Colonic tissue deviations suspected to be tumours were embedded in paraffin, sectioned and stained for histopathological examination.

Results

The number of medium and large AFC, as well as the total number, were statistically significantly increased by feeding sucrose and dextrin in the post-initiation period (Table 2). There was no statistically significant enhancing effect on ACF development when diets high in sucrose and dextrin were given in the pre-initiation period and during initiation (Table 2). Cell proliferation of the entire crypt as well as the bottom third of the crypt was decreased in the mid-colon and unaffected in the distal colon. Thus no positive correlation between colonic cell proliferation and ACF was seen. The level of malondialdehyde, glutathione-S-transferase and quinone reductase in the cytosol from the proximal colon was not affected by the sugar feeding. A few colorectal tumours were induced in the present study but no quantitative difference in tumour incidence could be detected between the groups. Malignant tumours were seen only in the groups given a high-sugar diet during the initiation phase.

Discussion

Based on the observations in the present study, it can be concluded that sucrose and dextrin enhance the number of preneoplastic lesions in AOM-initiated rats and act primarily as a promoter for the development of ACF. As the level of malondialdehyde, quinone reductase and glutathione-S-transferase in the various groups did not differ, a diet high in sucrose and dextrin apparently does not increase the level of oxidative stress in the colon nor affect the detoxification capacity in the colonic tissue. The parameters investigated in

Table 1. Experimental design and feeding scheme

Group	Pre-initiation Week 1–4	AOM[a] initiation Week 5–6	Post-initiation Week 7–24
cHHH	HSD[b]	HSD[c]	HSD
LLL	LSD[d]	LSD	LSD
LLH	LSD	LSD	HSD
HLL	HSD	LSD	LSD
HLH	HSD	LSD	HSD
LHL	LSD	HSD	LSD
LHH	LSD	HSD	HSD
HHH	HSD	HSD	HSD

[a]AOM, azoxymethane.
[b]HSD, high-sugar diet.
[c]Not given AOM.
[d]LSD, low-sugar diet.

the present study did not clarify the mechanisms underlying the effect of sucrose and dextrin on ACF formation. It has been suggested that high blood glucose and insulin levels as seen after intake of a diet with a high glycemic index might be a risk factor for colon cancer (Giovannucci, 1995; McKeown-Eyssen, 1994). This theory is consistent with the findings in our study, as the sugar diet presumably has a higher glycemic index than the starch diet.

Cornstarch and potato starch constitute the starch pool of the diets. In the study, the diet high in sugar and low in starch is compared with the diet low in sugar and high in starch. The enhancing effect on the development of ACF of the diet high in sugars could therefore just as well be a consequence of an inhibiting effect of the starches. In another study, potato starch was found to be protective towards the development of preneoplastic lesions (Thorup *et al.*, 1995).

In the study, three animals from the non-initiated group receiving a diet high in sucrose and dextrin spontaneously developed ACF. This is a rare observation but could, together with the observation of malignant tumours in the groups given a diet high in sugar during initiation, indicate that sucrose and dextrin may act as a weak initiator or co-initiator and enhance the progression towards malignancy.

Acknowledgement

This paper is partly reproduced from Cancer Letters, vol 167, Poulsen *et al.* The influence of simple sugars and starch given during pre- or post-initiation on aberrant crypt foci in rat colon, 135–143, 2001, with permission from Elsevier Science.

References

Burley, V.J. (1997) Sugar consumption and cancers of the digestive tract – review. *Eur. J. Cancer Prev.*, **6**, 422–434

Giovannucci, E. (1995) Insulin and colon cancer. *Cancer Causes Control*, **6**, 164–179

Table 2. Number and multiplicity of aberrant crypt foci (ACF)[a, b] and colorectal tumour development

Group	*N*	Total[c]	Small[c]	Medium[c]	Large[c]	Number of tumour-bearing animals	Total number of tumours
LLL	10	56 ± 10[1, 2]	36 ± 6[1, 2]	18 ± 5[1]	2 ± 1[1]	0	0
LLH	10	108 ± 18[3, 4]	59 ± 11[2, 3]	41 ± 7[2, 3]	8 ± 2[2, 3]	0	0
HLL	10	43 ± 7[1]	27 ± 5[1]	15 ± 3[1]	2 ± 1[1]	2	2
HLH	10	91 ± 10[3]	42 ± 5[2]	38 ± 3[2, 3]	12 ± 4[3]	2	2
LHL	10	74 ± 15[2, 3]	43 ± 8[1, 2]	27 ± 7[1, 2]	4 ± 1[1, 2]	3	5 (1)[d]
LHH	10	171 ± 30[4]	85 ± 12[3]	63 ± 13[3]	23 ± 6[4]	2	3 (3)
HHH	10	94 ± 14[3]	43 ± 8[1, 2]	39 ± 5[2, 3]	12 ± 2[3, 4]	2	4 (3)

[a]Mean ± SE.
[b]Small foci, 1–3 aberrant crypt (AC)/ACF; medium foci, 4–6 AC/ACF; large foci, ≥ 7 AC/ACF.
[c]Groups not sharing a common superscript differed significantly when a least significant difference test was performed ($P \leq 0.05$).
[d]Figures in parentheses indicate carcinomas.

McKeown-Eyssen, G. (1994) Epidemiology of colorectal cancer revisited: are serum triglycerides and/or plasma glucose associated with risk. *Cancer Epidemiol.*, **3**, 687–695

Potter, J.D. (1999) Colorectal cancer: molecules and populations. *J. Natl. Cancer Inst.*, **91**, 916–932

Thorup, I., Meyer, O. & Kristiansen, E. (1995) Effect of potato starch, cornstarch and sucrose on aberrant crypt foci in rats exposed to azoxymethane. *Anticancer Res.*, **15**, 2101–2106

Colonic luminal contents (faecal water) induce *COX-2*

Glinghammar B.

Department of Medical Nutrition, Karolinska Institutet, Novum, S-141 86 Huddinge, Sweden.

Introduction

Cyclooxygenases (COX) catalyze the synthesis of prostaglandins (PGs) from arachidonic acid. There are two isoforms of COX, designated *COX-1* and *COX-2*. *COX-1* is expressed constitutively in most tissues and appears to be responsible for housekeeping functions. In contrast, *COX-2* is not detectable in most normal tissues but is induced by oncogenes, growth factors, carcinogens and tumour promoters. Several lines of evidence support the idea that *COX-2* is important in carcinogenesis: *COX-2* is up-regulated in transformed cells and in malignant tissues; a null mutation for *COX-2* in APC knockout mice, a murine model of familial adenomatous polyposis, markedly reduces the number and size of intestinal tumours; treatment with a selective inhibitor of *COX-2* caused nearly complete suppression of azoxymethane-induced colon cancer. Several different mechanisms could account for the link between the activity of *COX-2* and carcinogenesis. For example, enhanced synthesis of PGs occurs in a variety of tumours; PGs can promote angiogenesis, inhibit immune surveillance and increase cell proliferation. Overexpression of *COX-2* also inhibits apoptosis and increases the invasiveness of malignant cells.

In recent years, there has been considerable interest in the role of the aqueous phase of human faeces (faecal water) in studies examining the mechanisms underlying the dietary etiology of colon cancer, the motivation being that components of this faecal fraction are more likely to be able to exert untoward effects on the cells of the colonic epithelium than components bound to food residues and the bacterial mass. The lipid component of faecal water (e.g. bile acids and fatty acids) has received particular attention, in view of the possible role of dietary fat as a tumour promoter in colon cancer. It was recently demonstrated that dihydroxy bile acids could activate the transcription of *COX-2* in human oesophageal adenocarcinoma cells and it was suggested that this effect was mediated by the activator protein-1 (AP-1) transcription factor complex acting on a cyclic AMP response element in the *COX-2* promoter. In this study we were interested in determining whether the in vivo faecal matrix (human faecal water) which contains a mixture of luminal components and which interact with the epithelial cells in the colon, are also playing a role in the transcriptional regulation of the *COX-2* gene.

Results and discussion

Treatment of the colon carcinoma cells, HCT 116 with bile acids and deoxycholic acid (DCA), resulted in a dose–response induction of *COX-2* promoter activity, with the highest dose (250 μM) yielding the greatest effect (Fig. 1) in the cells surviving bile acid exposure. Dose–response effects were also indicated, with chenodeoxycholic acid (CDCA) while cholic acid (CA) had basically no capacity to induce *COX-2* promoter activity. We confirmed the results from the promoter studies by investigating *COX-2* protein expression using Western blot. Treatment with increasing concentrations of DCA resulted in a dose-dependent induction of *COX-2* protein in HT-29 cells. Interestingly, induction of *COX-2* expression in HT-29 cells by DCA was negatively correlated ($r = -0.99$, $P < 0.01$) with DCA's effects on cell survival over the concentration range studied.

Having confirmed that in the colon cancer cells pure colonic luminal components could increase *COX-2* promoter activity, which led to synthesis of the *COX-2* protein exemplified using DCA, we were interested in investigating whether components of the aqueous phase of human faeces (faecal water), in intimate contact with the colonocytes *in vivo*, could also influence *COX-2* promoter activity. Ten diluted faecal lipid extracts were examined and exhibited significant effects on *COX-2* promoter activity at one of the dilutions tested (Fig. 2). Effects differed markedly

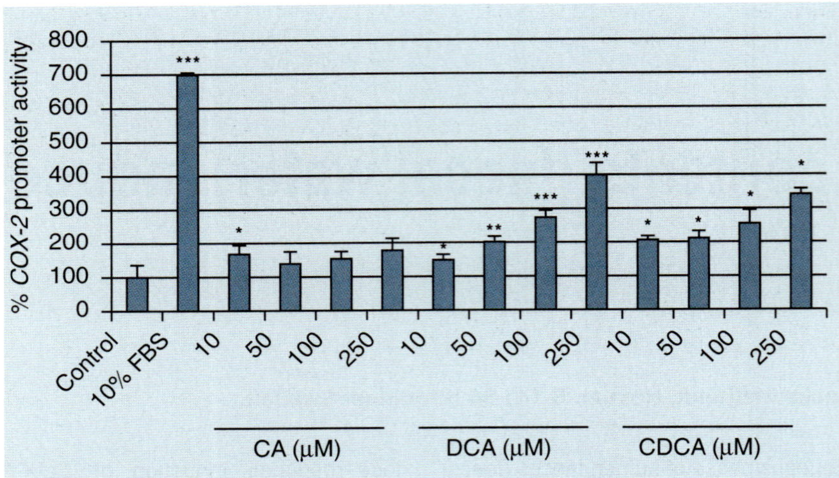

Figure 1
Pure luminal compounds increase *COX-2* promoter activity. HCT 116 cells were transfected with 0.4 μg of human *COX-2* promoter construct (–1432/+59). After transfection, cells were treated with 10% FBS, CA, DCA, CDCA at the concentrations shown. Luciferase activities were measured in cellular extracts 15 h later. Diagram bars represent mean values (SD) (n=4) in relation to the untreated cells (control), which were set to 100%. *, P<0.05, **, P<0.01, ***, P<0.001 compared to control

between lipid fractions from faecal waters from different individuals, with the majority of samples increasing the activity and one sample actually blocking basal *COX-2* promoter activity. Interestingly, with half of the samples, dilution resulted in a decreased effect, while with the other samples dilution resulted in an increased effect.

In conclusion, by using a novel *ex vivo* technique applied to in vivo material, shown to be a promising experimental system to probe the complex relation between diet and colon cancer, we have demonstrated that lipid components of the human faecal fraction in intimate contact with the epithelium can alter the transcription of *COX-2*. Available data supports an influence of diet on the levels of these luminal components. In view of the knowledge that the amount of *COX-2* is important, since there is a correlation between its level of expression and the size of the colorectal tumours and their propensity to invade

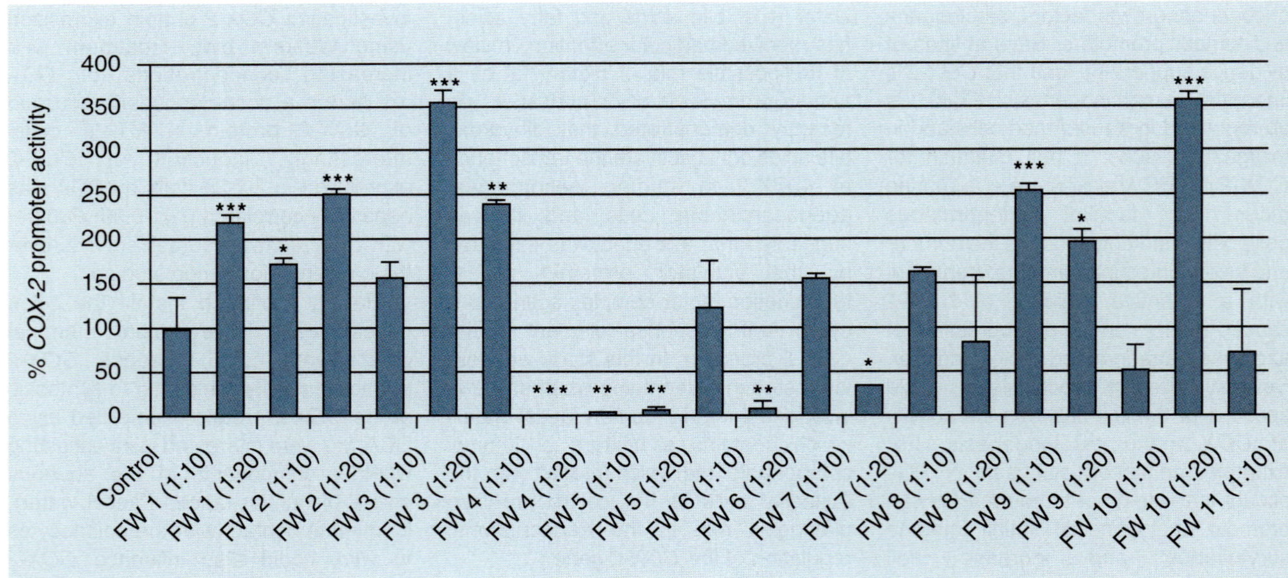

Figure 2
Human faecal water components alter *COX-2* promoter activity. HCT 116 cells were transfected with 0.4 μg of human *COX-2* promoter construct (–1432/+59). After transfection, cells were treated with lipid extracts of 10 human faecal water samples, at 1:10 and 1:20 dilution. Luciferase activities were measured in cellular extracts 15 h later. Diagram bars represent mean values (SD) (n=4) in relation to the untreated cells (control), which were set to 100%. *, P<0.05, **, P<0.01, ***, P<0.001 compared to control

underlying tissue, even small effects over time on the transcriptional regulation of this enzyme by dietary components may be important for tumour development in the colon.

References

Glinghammar, B., Rafter, J. (2001) Colonic luminal contents induce cyclooxygenase-2 transcription in human colon carcinoma cells. *Gastroenterology*, **120**, 401–410

Rafter, J.J., Child, P., Anderson, A.M., Alder, R., Eng, V. & Bruce, W.R. (1987) Cellular toxicity of fecal water depends on diet. *Am. J. Clin. Nutr.*, **45**, 559–563

Subbaramaiah, K., Telang, N., Ramonetti, J.T., Araki, R., DeVito, B., Weksler, B.B. & Dannenberg, A.J. (1996) Transcription of cyclooxygenase-2 is enhanced in transformed mammary epithelial cells. *Cancer Res.*, **56**, 4424–4429

Steinbach, G., Lynch, P.M., Phillips, R.K., Wallace, M.H., Hawk, E., Gordon, G.B., Wakabayashi, N., Saunders, B., Shen, Y., Fujimura, T., Su, L.K. & Levin, B. (2000) The effect of celecoxib, a cyclooxygenase-2 inhibitor, in familial adenomatous polyposis. *N. Engl. J. Med.*, **342**, 1946–1952

Tsujii, M. & DuBois, R.N. (1995) Alterations in cellular adhesion and apoptosis in epithelial cells overexpressing prostaglandin endoperoxide synthase 2. *Cell*, **83**, 493–501

Chapter 8

Trials on the dietary prevention of cancer

Trials on dietary prevention of cancer

Berglund G.
Department of Medicine, University Hospital Malmö, SE 205 02 Malmö, Sweden.

Trials on dietary prevention of cancer have a long way to go before valid scientific grounds for proper design of such trials have been constructed. The reasons are several:

1. The dietary factors that are assumed to be preventive are often linked to other dietary factors with other effects.
2. The means by which diet could be changed over the long term have been less than optimally developed, especially in groups of individuals with dietary problems, as these are often related to socio-economic and lifestyle factors.
3. Proven relations between a dietary factor and risk of disease have often proven to be weak, implying that other factors may be as important for the development of cancer at a specific site.

We will, however, present a few examples of intervention trials that, despite the above-mentioned problems, have been started. Some of them use cancer as their end-point, others use intermediate risk factors such as hormone levels. It is our hope that these examples can be used to stimulate a discussion on the design, feasibility and interpretation of trials studying dietary prevention of cancer.

DIANA trials on diet and endogenous hormones

Berrino F., Bellati C., Ooldani S., Mastroianni A., Allegro G., Berselli E., Venturelli E., Cavalleri A., Cambié M., Pala V., Pasanisi P., Secreto G.
Istituto Nazionale per lo Studio e la Cura dei Tumori, Milan, Italy.

Several prospective studies have shown that, after menopause, high serum levels of steroid sex hormones – both androgens and estrogens – are associated with increased risk of subsequent breast cancer (Endogenous Hormones and Breast Cancer Collaborative Group, in press). Such findings are consistent with the observation that, after menopause, overweight is associated both with increased levels of serum estrogens and with increased risk of breast cancer (IARC, 2002). The role of androgens, on the other hand, is corroborated by the association of breast cancer risk with sebum production and hirsutism, two markers of increased androgenic activity (Muti *et al.*, 2000). A few studies have also shown an association of breast cancer with insulin levels (Kaaks, 1996), possibly mediated by its effects on the ovarian production of androgens and on the liver production of sex hormone-binding globulin (SHBG). The role of insulin is also corroborated by the negative association of breast cancer with physical activity (IARC 2001), that increases insulin sensitivity. Other studies have shown that serum levels of triglycerides (Goodwin *et al.*, 1997), bio-available IGF-I, blood glucose (Muti *et al.*, submitted to publication) and may predict breast cancer risk, suggesting that dietary intake of high glycemic index food, as well as other lifestyle determinants of insulin resistance, may be a key factor in breast cancer promotion.

We hypothesized that these hormonal imbalances associated with breast cancer risk are aspects of a common underlying metabolic syndrome linked to overnutrition and the Western dietary style. To test this hypothesis, we carried out two dietary intervention trials – the DIANA (Diet and Androgens) studies – with hormonal levels as endpoints on postmenopausal women and on postmenopausal patients with a previous diagnosis of breast cancer (DIANA-1 and DIANA-2).

The dietary intervention was the same in both studies. It was designed to 1) reduce the average plasma insulin level first by increasing the consumption of low-glycemic-index food as well as monounsaturated and n-3 polyunsaturated fatty acids, and second by decreasing highly refined carbohydrates and total and saturated fat; and, 2) augment the intake of phytoestrogen-rich foods, including soy products, legumes, flax and other seeds, and cruciferous vegetables. Both studies included intensive dietary counseling with cooking classes and specially prepared group meals, mainly based on Mediterranean and macrobiotic recipes (Berrino *et al.*, 2001).

In the DIANA-1 study, 104 postmenopausal women, healthy but with high serum testosterone level (>0.38 ng/mL), were randomized into intervention and control groups. The diet was *ad libitum* and there was no recommendation to limit the caloric intake. The women of the intervention group, however, consumed about 250 kcal/day less than those of the control group and lost, on average, 4 kg (versus 0.5 kg in the control group). Waist and hip circumferences, as well as waist-to-hip ratio also decreased significantly. SHBG increased (+25%) and serum levels of testosterone decreased (–20%). Estradiol decreased (–18%) but the difference with the control group was not statistically significant. Fasting plasma glycemia, cholesterol levels, and the total area under the insulin curve during oral glucose tolerance test also decreased significantly (Berrino *et al.*, 2001).

A second study was then undertaken to test 1) the effect of the same diet on the bioavailability of sex hormones and on other relevant parameters in breast cancer patients, 2) the long-term effects over 1 year of diet and 3) the interaction with adjuvant hormonal (tamoxifen) treatment. The present paper presents preliminary results of this DIANA-2 study.

Material and methods

Study design

We recruited 114 postmenopausal breast cancer patients, operated on 1 year or more before and without recurrence, with the help of breast cancer patient associations and advertising the study in the oncological units of a few hospitals. Patients had to be postmenopausal for at least 2 years (including menopause induced by treatment), not on a special diet, not on treatment for metabolic or endocrine disease, and have at least one ovary. Of these patients, 41 were on tamoxifen adjuvant treatment. After signing an informed consent, patients were individually randomized into a dietary intervention and a control group. A few close friends, however, were randomly allocated to the same group. Patients randomized in the intervention group were invited twice a week over 3 months for a common dinner preceded by a cooking lesson. In the fourth month, the same teaching was offered twice a week to the control group. In the fifth and sixth months, participants were free for holidays. From the seventh to the twelfth month both groups were invited to a single lesson-dinner per month (Fig. 1). Early morning fasting blood samples were collected at baseline, 3 months, and 12 months. Height, weight, waist and hip circumferences, abdominal and thigh skinfolds were measured by a trained health assistant according to a standardized protocol (Muti *et al.*, 2000). The aim was to compare intervention and control women for changes in hormonal concentrations at 3 months (randomized comparison) and to compare baseline concentrations and 12-month concentrations in the whole group of patients (before–after comparison). The Scientific Review board and Ethical Committee of the Milan National Cancer Institute approved the study.

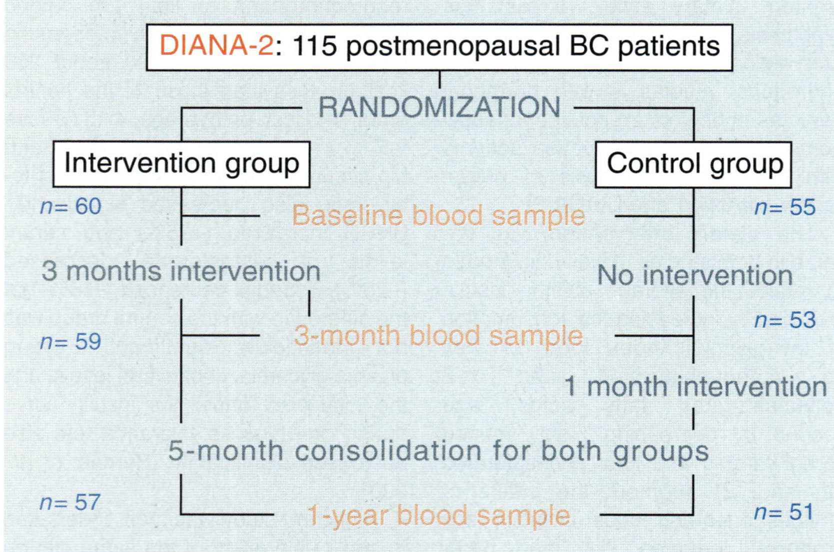

Figure 1
DIANA-2 study design

Dietary intervention

The DIANA diet has been described in detail elsewhere (Berrino *et al.*, 2001). The main teaching and instructions concerned how to prepare dishes based on whole grain cereals (mainly rice, but also millet, oat, barley, buckwheat, spelt); whole wheat flour; sweets with dried fruit or naturally fermented cereal malts as sweeteners and almonds, hazelnuts and oleiferous seeds as fat; traditional Mediterranean dishes based on pasta, cous-cous, broccoli and other cruciferous vegetables, various beans, lentils, chickpeas, fish; and oriental dishes with soy products such as miso, tempeh, tofu and soy milk. Patients were recommended to reduce their consumption of meat, eggs and dairy products to no more than once a week and were instructed to increase the vegetable sources of calcium. Every time they met for a dinner together, participants received a complementary package with some of the recommended food to consume at home and the relevant instructions to repeat the recipes they had learned in the cooking class. To prevent excessive bowel fermentation and swelling, whole grain products and legumes were introduced gradually. Patients randomized in the control group received a general recommendation of increasing the consumption of fruit and vegetables but no specific dietary advice. Dietary consumption was monitored, through 24-h food frequency diaries, twice in the randomized phase of the study and three times in the subsequent phase.

Laboratory measurements

Circulating hormones were measured using commercial kits: RIA kits from Orion Diagnostic (Turku, Finland) for testosterone and estradiol, IRMA kits from Farmos (Oulunsalo, Finland) for SHBG, and MEIA kits from Abbot (Abbot Park, IL) for insulin. Total cholesterol and triglycerides were determined by enzymatic-colorimetric

Table 1. DIANA 2 study: comparison between intervention and control group at 3 months

	Average values Intervention (n=58)[b]		Control (n=52)		*t* test[a]
	Baseline	After 3 months	Baseline	After 3 months	
Body weight (kg)	65.9	62.4	65.0	64.2	0.000
Waist circumference (cm)	84.3	81.7	81.9	81.5	0.000
Hip circumference (cm)	104.3	101.1	102.8	102.0	0.000
Abdominal skinfold (mm)	45.1	38.5	43.8	41.4	0.000
Thigh skin-fold (mm)	45.3	42.1	44.4	43.4	0.009
Glycemia (mg/dL)	92.4	88.4	92.7	91.7	0.058
Total cholesterol (mg/dL)	221	192	228	218	0.000
HDL (mg/dL)	56	49	55	53	0.000
LDL (mg/dL)	141	122	154	144	0.038
Triglycerides (mg/dL)	114	100	101	108	0.028
Insulin (µUI/mL)	8.01	7.23	8.27	7.90	0.489
SHBG (nmol/L)	67.0	76.8	60.1	59.2	0.000
Estradiol (pg/mL)	6.04	6.04	6.53	5.69	0.452
Testosterone (pg/mL)	420	388	418	391	0.702

[a]Of the mean change in the intervention group versus control group.
[b]56 for sex hormones.

Table 2. DIANA 2 study: comparison between baseline and 1-year values (before and after the dietary intervention)

n=107 patients[a]	Baseline		1 year		Difference
	Mean	SD	Mean	SD	
Body weight (kg)	65.4	9.7	62.2	9.5	–3.2[b]
Waist circumference (cm)	83.2	9.3	79.9	9.1	–3.3[b]
Hip circumference (cm)	103.6	7.0	101.7	12.0	–1.87
Abdominal skinfold (mm)	44.5	11.5	33.8	12.3	–10.7[b]
Thigh skinfold (mm)	44.9	12.5	37.7	12.0	–7.14[b]
Glycemia (mg/dL)	92.6	10.7	88.5	10.8	–4.11[b]
Total cholesterol (mg/dL)	224.1	41.1	199.5	37.8	–24.6[b]
HDL (mg/dL)	55.7	9.5	53.7	8.1	–2.0
LDL (mg/dL)	147	38.6	127.5	34.9	–19.5[b]
Triglycerides (mg/dL)	107.8	60.9	92.7	41.4	–15.1[b,a]
Insulin (µUI/mL)	8.13	4.12	6.77	3.87	–1.36[b]
SHBG (nmol/L)	63.7	29.7	67.6	30.8)	+3.9
Estradiol (pg/mL)	6.28	4.33	5.89	4.36	–0.39
Testosterone (pg/mL)	419	150	380	140	–39[b]

[a]105 for HDL, LDL and hormones, 105 for the other metabolic variables.
[b]$P<0.05$.

Table 3. DIANA 2 study: comparison between baseline and 1-year values in women with and without tamoxifen treatment

	Tamoxifen + (*n*=40)[a]		Tamoxifen – (*n*=67)		*t* test[a]
	Baseline	1 Year	Baseline	1 Year	
Body weight (kg)	64.1	61.4	66.3	62.7[b]	0.031
Waist circumference (cm)	81.4	78.5	84.3	80.7[b*]	0.078
Hip circumference (cm)	103.0	100.9	104.0	102.2	0.901
Abdominal skinfold (mm)	43.3	33.4[b]	45.2	34.0[b]	0.654
Thigh skinfold (mm)	44.7	37.9[b]	45.0	37.6[b]	0.104
Glycemia (mg/dL)	91.5	87.6	93.2	88.9[b]	0.680
Total cholesterol (mg/dL)	203	182[b]	237	210[b]	0.323
HDL (mg/dL)	59	56	54	52	0.878
LDL (mg/dL)	125	106[b]	160	140[b]	0.776
Triglycerides (mg/dL)	105	101	110	88[b]	0.024
Insulin (μUI/mL)	7.14	6.35	8.72	7.00	0.033
SHBG (nmol/L)	83.7	86.2	51.9	57.0	0.208
Estradiol (pg/mL)	4.84	4.41	7.13	6.73	0.941
Testosterone (pg/mL)	410	397	424	371	0.027

[a]38 for HDL, LDL & hormones, 39 for the other metabolic variables.
[b]$P<0.05$ of the mean change in TAM+ versus TAM–.

methods (Roche Diagnostics, Mannheim, Germany), HDL cholesterol was measured by the direct enzimatic assay (Roche Diagnostics), apo A-I immunoturbidometrically with antisera and calibrators from Roche Diagnostics, and LDL was computed with the Friedewald formula. For testosterone, estradiol and SHBG, baseline, 3-month and 12-month samples were preserved at –20°C and analysed in the same batch to reduce the effect of interassay variability. The laboratory was blind to intervention or control status of the samples.

Statistical analysis

The statistical analysis of the randomized component of the study focused on changes in hormonal and other variables, calculated as the difference between third month examination and baseline, respectively in the intervention and control group. For the before–after component of the study, the differences between the average measurements at baseline and 12 months were tested by *t* test for unpaired samples. Hormone values were log transformed to obtain approximately normal frequency distributions. All of the *P* values are two-tailed.

Results

Three patients were excluded because they developed metastasis and/or started hormonal treatment during the study. The final analysis, therefore, was carried out on 111 patients, 44–70 years of age, mean 58 years. Fifty-eight were randomized in the intervention group and 53 in the control group. According to the food frequency diaries filled in during the first 3 months of the study, patients in the intervention group consumed whole grain cereal products 4.5 times more frequently than control patients (3.7 versus 0.8 per day); soy products (either milk, miso, tempeh or tofu) 2.2 times per day versus less than 0.1 among controls; nuts and oleaginous seeds (mainly flax, sesame, and sunflower) 4.2 times per day versus 0.2 times. Only intervention women used seaweeds as ingredients of various dishes (5 times a week). Intervention women also increased the weekly consumption of legumes (3 times versus 1), cruciferous vegetables (8 times versus 1), onions or leeks (4.7 versus 1.5), and fish (3.8 versus 2.4 times per week). On the other hand, controls consumed meat or meat products more frequently (5.6 times a week on average as opposed to twice a week in the intervention group); milk or dairy (11 versus 2 times per week); other vegetables and fruits (4.2 versus 3.3 times per day); sweets and cookies (1.5 versus 0.7 per day); and beverages with added sugar (once a day versus every other day).

Table 1 summarizes the effect of 3 months of diet on anthropometric, metabolic and hormonal parameters in the randomized phase of the study. Body weight decreased in both study groups but intervention patients lost more weight than control patients did (3.51 kg versus 0.77 kg). Waist and hip circumferences decreased significantly in the intervention group only, by a similar magnitude (2.66 and 3.51 cm, respectively). Abdominal skinfold, however, decreased by a greater magnitude than the thigh skinfold (6.6 and 3.2 mm). Triglycerides and total, HDL and LDL cholesterol decreased significantly in the intervention group compared to the control group, but the HDL/LDL ratio did not change. SHBG increased significantly in the intervention group (+15%) and did not change in the control group. Insulin, estradiol and testosterone levels did not show any differential change.

Table 2 shows the comparison between mean values at baseline and at 12 months, i.e. before and after the dietary intervention, in the whole series of patients. Body weight, waist circumference, waist-to-hip ratio, both skinfolds, total and LDL cholesterol, LDL/HDL ratio, glucose, triglycerides, insulin and testosterone decreased significantly. SHBG was slightly higher and estradiol slightly lower than baseline but the differences did not reach statistical significance. There were no major differences between patients originally randomized in the intervention and in the control group.

Table 3 shows the comparison between mean values at baseline and at 12 months separately for patients under tamoxifen treatment and without hormonal treatment. Apart from cholesterol, that decreased by about the same magnitude in the two groups, all the other differences were more marked in the patients without hormonal treatment, the interaction being significant for body weight, triglycerides, insulin and testosterone. In absence of tamoxifen treatment, testosterone decreased by 12.5%, insulin and triglycerides by 20% and fasting glucose by 5%.

Discussion

A comprehensive modification of dietary habits over 1 year, aiming at reducing high-glycemic-index food and total and saturated fats and at increasing unrefined cereals, legumes and other seeds and several vegetables, including phytoestrogen-rich food, caused a significant reduction of body weight, serum testosterone, fasting insulin, fasting glycemia, triglycerides, and total and LDL cholesterol. Serum SHBG increased significantly after 3 months of diet but was only slightly higher than at baseline after 12 months. All such effects were less marked and not statistically significant in the subgroup of women under tamoxifen treatment. The results in patients without tamoxifen treatment were broadly similar to those previously observed in healthy hyperandrogenic women in DIANA-1. Hormonal effects, however, were less marked. After 3 months of diet, SHBG increased only by 15% (while in DIANA-1 increased by 25% in 4.5 months) and sex steroids did not decrease at all. There are a number of potential explanations for these differences, including the physiological differences between women with and without a history of breast cancer, the effect of hormonal treatment, dietary differences between the two studies at baseline and different study design. SHBG was already very high at baseline in patients on tamoxifen treatment (84 nmol/L versus 52 nmol/L in untreated patients). At 12 months it was only 2.6% and 9.8% higher than baseline, respectively, in treated and untreated women (Table 3). One might speculate that SHBG increases during active weight reduction and tends to return towards the original values when body weight no longer decreases. Actually, in DIANA-2, body weight did not further decrease between the third and the twelfth month. Also, the other baseline metabolic and hormonal parameters had a more favourable distribution in patients under tamoxifen treatment than in patients without hormonal treatment (Table 3). This might explain why the overall effect was generally lower in treated than in untreated women and in DIANA-2 than in DIANA-1. Nevertheless, a clear effect on triglycerides was present only in DIANA-2, albeit only in patients without tamoxifen treatment. Usually dietary intervention trials that reduce total and saturated fat consumption observe a decrease in total cholesterol but an increase in triglycerides, especially if the diet is isocaloric (Schaefer *et al.*, 1995). This is likely to be due to the increased consumption of sugars that compensate the decreased consumption of fat. In the DIANA trials, a moderate reduction of total fat consumption was actually accompanied by an increase in carbohydrates, but not in simple sugars (Berrino *et al.*, 2001).

The dietary instructions were exactly the same in the two studies but the usual diet at baseline was different, because breast cancer patients enrolled in the DIANA-2 trial had markedly changed their diet after the diagnosis of breast cancer, reducing the consumption of red meat and increasing fruit and vegetables (data not shown). Baseline total cholesterol levels, in fact, were lower in DIANA-2 than in DIANA-1 in both tamoxifen-treated and untreated women.

DIANA-1 women were selected on the basis of high testosterone levels (above the upper tertile) while no such selection was done in DIANA-2. Baseline testosterone levels in DIANA-2 patients, however, were fairly high, thus confirming the association of testosterone and breast cancer. Actually, the average baseline serum testosterone level was the same in DIANA-1 and -2 (0.42 ng/mL).

In DIANA-2 the randomized dietary intervention study lasted 3 months instead of the 4.5 months of DIANA-1. The reason for this difference was that patients volunteering for the study, when informed of the randomized design, declared that they would not accept to be randomized in the control group. Many of them were aware of the positive results of DIANA-1 and presumed that the diet under study could confer a prognostic advantage. A randomized phase of 3 months was an acceptable compromise. Three months of dietary change, however, may have not been sufficient to obtain the marked effect on sex hormones observed in the first study. Metabolic and anthropometric changes, however, were fairly similar.

In conclusion, the DIANA trials demonstrated that an *ad libitum* diet based on Mediterranean and macrobiotic traditions can favorably modify the hormonal and metabolic pattern at high risk of breast cancer. Lower body weight and lower plasma levels of testosterone, insulin, glucose and triglycerides can be maintained for at least 1 year. Further studies are needed to establish if these effects imply a lower risk of subsequent breast cancer.

References

Berrino, F., Bellati, C., Secreto, G., Camerini, E., Pala, V., Panico, S., Allegro, G. & Kaaks, R. (2001) Reducing bioavailable sex hormones through a comprehensive change in diet: the diet and androgens (DIANA) randomized trial. *Cancer Epidemiol. Biomarkers Prev.*, **10**, 25–33

Endogenous Hormones and Breast Cancer Collaborative Group. Breast cancer and endogenous sex hormones in postmenopausal women: a collaborative re-analysis of data on 650 cases and 1700 controls from nine prospective studies. *J. Natl. Cancer Inst.* (in press)

Goodwin, P.J., Boyd, N.F., Hanna, W., Hartwick, W., Murray, D., Qizilbash, A., Redwood, S., Hood, N., DelGiudice, M.E., Sidlofsky, S., McCready, D., Wilkinson, R., Mahoney, L., Connelly, P. & Page, D.L. (1997) Elevated levels of plasma triglycerides are associated with histologically defined premenopausal breast cancer risk. *Nutr. Cancer*, **27**, 284–292

IARC (2002) *Weight Control and Physical Activity.* IARC Handbooks of Cancer Prevention, vol 6, Lyon, IARC Press

Kaaks, R. (1996) Nutrition, hormones and breast cancer: is insulin the missing link? *Cancer Causes Control*, **7**, 605–625

Muti, P., Stanulla, M., Micheli, A., Krogh, V., Freudenheim, J.L., Yang, J., Schunemann, H.J., Trevisan, M. & Berrino, F. (2000) Markers of insulin resistance and sex steroids activity in relation to risk of breast cancer. A prospective analysis of abdominal adiposity, sebum production, and hirsutism. *Cancer Causes Control*, **11**, 721–730

Schaefer, E.J., Lichtenstein, A.H., Lamon-Fava, S., McNamara, J.R., Schaefer, M.M., Rasmussen, H. & Ordovas, J.M. (1995) Body weight and low-density lipoprotein cholesterol changes after consumption of a low-fat *ad libitum* diet. *JAMA*, **274**, 1450–1455

Lack of effect of a low-fat high-carbohydrate diet on ovarian hormones in premenopausal women: results from a randomized trial

Boyd N.F., Greenberg C., Martin L., Stone J., Hammond G., Minkin S.
(for the Canadian Diet and Breast Cancer Prevention Study Group)

[1]Division of Epidemiology and Statistics, Ontario Cancer Institute, University Health Network, Toronto, Canada.
[2]London Regional Cancer Centre, London, Ontario, Canada.

Introduction

Wide variation in age-specific incidence rates of breast cancer (Parkin *et al.*, 1997) cannot be explained by inherited differences between populations, because migrants from low-risk to high-risk countries show a marked increase in risk (Ziegler *et al.*, 1993; Kelsey & Horn-Ross, 1993; McMichael, 1988). Ecological studies show that breast cancer incidence and mortality, as well as changes in rates in migrants, are strongly and positively correlated with estimates of dietary fat consumption within countries (Prentice *et al.*, 1989), but although dietary fat intake influences breast cancer risk in animals (Welsch, 1992; Freedman *et al.*, 1990; Rogers & Lee, 1986), observational cohort and case–control studies in humans have shown little if any association between fat intake and risk of breast cancer (Hunter *et al.*, 1996; Boyd *et al.*, 1993). These results may indicate a true lack of association between dietary fat and breast cancer, or they may arise because of the difficulty in finding a true effect in the face of the combined effects of measurement error and the limited range of dietary fat intake within countries.

We are carrying out a long-term randomized controlled trial designed to find out if intervention with a low-fat high-carbohydrate diet, which creates a wide range of dietary fat intake, reduces risk of breast cancer. The short-term biological effects of this dietary change may provide information about the potential mechanisms by which diet may influence risk of disease. In previous work we have found evidence that the adoption of a low-fat high-carbohydrate diet may reduce blood levels of estradiol and progesterone (Boyd *et al.*, 1997). The purpose of the present proposal is to determine whether these findings can be replicated in a larger number of subjects.

Methods

General method

We performed hormone assays on blood samples and nutrient analysis on food records collected from subjects taking part in an ongoing dietary intervention trial, designed to determine whether a low-fat high-carbohydrate diet will reduce the incidence of breast cancer among women at increased risk for the disease because of extensive mammographic densities (Boyd *et al.*, 1990).

Here we test the hypothesis that in subjects on a low-fat high-carbohydrate diet who remain premenopausal at 2 years, serum levels of estradiol would fall significantly compared to controls.

Trial procedures

We have recruited subjects aged 30–65 years, with mammographic densities in at least 50% of the breast area (Oza & Boyd, 1993) and enrolled them in a randomized trial of dietary intervention aimed at reducing total dietary fat to a target of 15% of calories. Controls received general advice about diet but were not counselled to change their intake of fat.

Subjects were excluded if they had a previous history of cancer or breast augmentation or reduction, were pregnant (or planning to be) or breast feeding, or were on a medically prescribed diet for any reason. Eligible subjects were randomized by telephone contact with the Department of Biostatistics at the Ontario Cancer Institute. Randomization was stratified according to centre and balanced within each centre. Trial sites are located in Toronto, Hamilton, London, and Windsor, Ontario, and in Vancouver and Surrey, British Columbia. The present study is limited to premenopausal subjects enrolled in sites in Ontario.

Dietary intervention

For subjects randomized to the intervention group, an individual dietary prescription was prepared using a food exchange system, in which calories derived from fat were replaced by isocaloric exchange with carbohydrate. Subjects were also given dietary aids, including dietetic scales, a printed guide containing low-fat recipes, a shopping guide and the individual's diet prescription. After randomization, subjects in the intervention group visited the dietitian once a month for the first 12 months, and subjects in the control group once every 3 months. Both groups were seen once every 3 months for the second year. At each of these visits, subjects were weighed and asked to provide 3 days of food records, kept on nonconsecutive days in the interval before the next clinic visit, which included 2 weekdays and one weekend day, selected by the dietitian. Nutrient analysis of food records was done using the Minnesota Nutrient Data System software, developed by the Nutrition Coordinating Center (NCC), University of Minnesota, Minneapolis, MN.

Selection of subjects for the present study

The 896 subjects whose data were analyzed in the present paper were a consecutive series of subjects who had remained in the trial for at least 2 years after randomization, were premenopausal at entry and at 2 years and were not taking exogenous hormones at entry or at 2 years.

Collection and analysis of blood samples

Blood was taken from subjects in the trial at entry and once a year thereafter. Blood was taken at the time of clinic visits, which were not timed in relation to the menstrual cycle. Although the day of the last menstrual period was recorded at both initial and 2-year clinic visits, blood could be taken at any time during the run-in period that preceded randomization, which lasted several weeks. However, at 2 years, blood was taken on the day of the clinic visit, when the date of the last menstrual period was recorded.

Serum was separated and divided into 2-mL aliquots and stored at –70°C. All assays were performed in Dr Hammond's laboratory at the London Regional Cancer Center. Estradiol and FSH were assayed using a coated tube immunoradiometric assay, and SHBG with an immunoradiometric assay. All assays were performed using kits obtained from Orion Diagnostica, Espoo, Finland. A quality control program was applied to these assays using sera with known concentrations of high, medium and low values for each of the hormones measured and included in each batch of assays run.

Statistical analysis

Distributions of variables were examined and log transformations applied when necessary. Changes in serum levels of hormones, from baseline to 1 year and at 2 years, were compared between intervention and control groups using *t* tests, or if not normally distributed after transformation, by the Wilcoxon 2 sample tests. Regression analysis was carried out with change in hormone levels as the dependent variable and group, age, weight and SHBG as independent variables.

Results

Characteristics of subjects

Table 1 shows selected baseline characteristics of the subjects included in the present study. There were 448 subjects in each group. The mean age at randomization was 43 years. Subjects in intervention and control groups were similar at the time of randomization in height, weight and other risk factors for breast cancer.

Dietary characteristics

Table 2 shows the mean intake of selected nutrients as estimated from food records collected at baseline and at 2

Table 1. Selected baseline demographic characteristics of subjects

Characteristics	Intervention	Control	*P* value
No. of subjects	448	448	
Age (years)	43.53 (4.3)[a]	43.65 (4.5)	0.68[b]
Weight (kg)	62.18 (8.3)	61.86 (7.7)	0.56[b]
Height (cm)	163.3 (6.2)	163.45 (6.3)	0.71[b]
BMI (kg/m^2)	23.29 (2.6)	23.13 (2.4)	0.36[b]
Age at menarche (years)	12.72 (1.4)	12.85 (1.4)	0.17[b]
Parity (% parous)	75.67	77.23	0.64[c]
Age at first live birth (years)	26.61 (4.6)	26.99 (4.9)	0.32[b]
First-degree relative with breast cancer (%)	18.08	21.21	0.27[c]

[a]Mean (standard deviation).
[b]*T* test.
[c]Chi-square.

Table 2. Intake of selected nutrients according to group

Dietary variable	Intervention (*n*=227) Baseline	Intervention (*n*=227) 2 Years	Control (*n*=219) Baseline	Control (*n*=219) 2 Years
Total carbohydrate (g)	200.94 (55.95)	239.84 (66.56)	207.83 (61.56)	215.30 (61.08)
Carbohydrate (%)	49.27 (7.11)	60.61 (8.00)	48.18 (7.93)	49.78 (7.62)
Dietary cholesterol (mg)	231.75 (110.18)	169.90 (83.67)	257.45 (121.58)	237.00 (103.00)
Total fat (g)	61.97 (21.17)	37.81 (13.42)	66.62 (22.44)	63.38 (20.08)
Total fat (%)	33.11 (6.21)	21.50 (6.38)	33.86 (6.05)	32.37 (6.30)
Monounsaturated (%)	12.02 (2.75)	7.72 (2.63)	12.42 (2.60)	11.88 (2.77)
Polyunsaturated (%)	6.43 (2.13)	4.44 (1.63)	6.76 (2.14)	6.32 (1.99)
Saturated (%)	12.03 (3.12)	7.18 (2.61)	12.01 (3.29)	11.54 (3.26)
Total fibre (g)	16.53 (6.05)	19.20 (6.74)	16.72 (5.82)	17.50 (6.50)
Soluble fibre (g)	5.43 (1.96)	6.59 (2.32)	5.52 (2.07)	5.87 (2.31)
Insoluble fibre (g)	10.64 (4.28)	12.35 (4.69)	10.67 (4.05)	11.35 (4.45)
MUFA (g)	22.61 (8.42)	13.63 (5.43)	24.51 (8.74)	23.35 (8.08)
PUFA (g)	11.86 (5.01)	7.76 (3.14)	13.05 (5.08)	12.17 (4.51)
SFA (g)	22.66 (8.91)	12.68 (5.33)	23.91 (10.03)	22.78 (8.92)
Protein (g)	67.13 (16.10)	68.40 (15.18)	69.47 (18.21)	70.69 (16.36)
Protein (%)	16.86 (3.64)	17.68 (3.03)	16.52 (3.40)	16.66 (2.80)
Energy (kcal)	1646.34 (397.40)	1578.77 (345.11)	1739.56 (450.29)	1736.88 (404.46)

MUFA, monounsaturated fatty acids; PUFA, polyunsaturated fatty acids; SFA, saturated fatty acids.

years in a sample of subjects from the intervention (*n*=227) and control (*n*=219) groups. At baseline the nutrient intakes of control and intervention groups were similar. Two years after randomization, the mean total energy intake of the intervention group was approximately 71 kcal per day less than at baseline. The mean daily intake of fat in the intervention group was reduced from an average of 62 g to 38 g, as the result of a reduction in intake of saturated, monounsaturated and polyunsaturated fat, but was unchanged from baseline in controls. Total carbohydrate intake increased in the intervention group from 201 g/day to 239 g/day and intake of total dietary fibre increased from 17 to 19 g/day. All of the differences between intervention and control groups in the intake of fat, type of fat, carbohydrate and fibre were statistically significant (P<0.001).

Body weight at 2 years was unchanged from baseline in the intervention group and had increased by 1.3 kg in the control group (data not shown).

Changes in hormone levels

The median hormone levels at baseline and at 2 years and the median individual changes at 2 years are shown in Table 4. Change in level is calculated for individuals and is thus not the same as the difference between the group median values at baseline and at 2 years. Levels of estradiol were similar in intervention and control groups at baseline and at 2 years. In the intervention group, the median change in estradiol was a 10% (24.5 pmol/L) reduction over 2 years compared to a reduction of 8% (20 pmol/L) in the control group. Levels of progesterone, FSH, and SHBG were also similar in intervention and control groups at baseline and at 2 years and changes in levels of these hormones between these times were also similar.

Analysis of 2-year hormone levels according to day since last menstrual period

At their 2-year visit, the date of last menstrual period on the day of blood collection for 820 of the 898 subjects (intervention group, *n*=403; control group, *n*=417) was recorded. The blood sample was taken a median of 24 days after the last period in the intervention group and 22 days in controls (Wilcoxon test: P=0.12). Table 4 shows the 2-year hormone levels, according to the day of the menstrual cycle on which blood was taken, and the progesterone level (as an indicator of ovulation). A similar number in the intervention and control groups was sampled at each of the intervals examined and a similar number in each group had progesterone levels above and below 5 nmol/L.

In those with blood taken 15–30 days after the last period, only progesterone levels in those with levels below

Table 3. Median hormone levels and changes according to group and time of collection

Hormone	Intervention	Control	*P* value[a]
Estradiol			
Baseline (*n*=437, 442)[b]	240 (140, 410)[c]	250 (145, 400)	0.92
Two years (*n*=441, 443)	220 (105, 360)	225 (110, 370)	0.48
Change at 2 years[d] (*n*=430, 437)	−24.5 (−200, 133)	−20 (−190, 106)	0.84
Progesterone			
Baseline (*n*=437, 442)	3.0 (1.2, 19.5)	3.1 (1.3, 17.0)	0.89
Two years (*n*=440, 443)	2.1 (1.1, 14.0)	2.3 (1.1, 16.0)	0.64
Change at 2 years (*n*=430, 437)	−0.2 (−10.1, 5.4)	−0.1 (−10.0, 7.0)	0.63
FSH			
Baseline (*n*=437, 442)	6.8 (4.6, 10.0)	6.8 (4.6, 9.9)	0.98
Two years (*n*=441, 442)	8.0 (4.8, 15.0)	7.8 (5.2, 15.0)	0.80
Change at 2 years (*n*=430, 436)	1.3 (−1.4, 6.6)	1.2 (−1.8, 7.8)	0.54
SHBG			
Baseline (*n*=446, 447)	49.0 (38.0, 63.0)	50.0 (38.0, 64.0)	0.90
Two years (*n*=447, 448)	47.0 (35.0, 63.0)	45.0 (36.0, 60.0)	0.47
Change at 2 years (*n*=445, 447)	−2.0 (−10.0, 6.0)	−3.0 (−10.0, 5.0)	0.40

[a]Wilcoxon two-sample test.
[b]Sample size for intervention and control respectively.
[c]Median (first quartile, third quartile).

5 nmol/L and SHBG levels in those with progesterone over 5 nmol/L were significantly different between intervention and control groups. All other comparisons between intervention and control subjects did not show a statistically significant difference.

We also carried out a series of regression analyses, in which we examined log-transformed hormone levels between intervention and control groups at 2 years, controlling for age, weight at 2 years, and length of time between the blood sample date and date of the start of the last menstrual period. As expected, serum levels of estradiol, progesterone and FSH, but not SHBG, were strongly influenced by the day of the menstrual cycle, and by age. Weight was significantly associated with SHBG, but not with any of the other measures. After adjusting for the effects of day of the menstrual cycle, age and weight, there were no statistically significant effects of group membership on serum levels of any of the hormones measured (data not shown).

Discussion

These results show that after 2 years in a randomized trail of dietary intervention aimed at substantially reducing dietary intake of total fat, there was no difference between intervention and control subjects in the blood levels of estradiol, progesterone, follicle-stimulating hormone or sex hormone-binding globulin. All subjects in the present study had been carefully selected and those in the intervention group had been given intensive individual dietary counselling. Nutrient analysis of food records collected at baseline and at 2 years in a sample of subjects shows a substantial reduction in intake of total dietary fat, accompanied by stabilization of weight, and by changes in total cholesterol and HDL-C (data not shown). Controls, by contrast, did not change intake of dietary fat, gained weight over 2 years, and showed changes in total cholesterol and HDL-C that were opposite in direction to those seen in intervention subjects (data not shown). Further, measurements of hormones were all made in a single laboratory, using radioimmunoassay and rigorous quality control standards.

In previous work, based upon a smaller number of subjects than in the present study, we reported that estradiol levels were lower after 2 years in women in the intervention group (Boyd *et al.*, 1997). However, this finding was based entirely upon observations made in a small group of women whose blood at 2 years was taken more than 30 days after the last menstrual period. No statistically significant differences were seen in previous work between the blood estradiol levels in women in the intervention and control groups when blood was taken less than 30 days after the last period. The findings of the present study are thus similar to our previous work for those sampled less than 30 days after the last period. The present findings, like the previous ones, do show lower levels of estradiol in the intervention group in those whose blood was taken more than 30 days after the last period, but in the larger number of subjects in the present study, this difference is no longer statistically significant.

Wu *et al.* have reviewed and examined by meta-analysis the effect of dietary fat reduction on estradiol levels observed in intervention studies, including 10 studies in premenopausal women of which only one (our own) had a control group and lasted longer than 3 months (Wu *et al.*, 1999). Estradiol levels after dietary intervention fell in

Table 4. Median serum hormone levels according to day of blood collection and serum progesterone level

	Intervention			Control		
Day of cycle	Progesterone Day 5	Progesterone Day > 5	All	Progesterone Day 5	Progesterone Day > 5	All
Estradiol						
1–15	193 (90, 430)[a]	225 (160, 290)	200 (98, 370)	220 (105, 450)	235 (175, 350)	223 (110, 410)
16–30	230 (56, 490)	255 (190, 345)	255 (155, 360)	190 (52, 380)	240 (185, 340)	233 (150, 350)
>30	100 (20, 185)	200 (120, 270)	128 (46, 240)	130 (28, 420)	210 (110, 270)	170 (35, 350)
Progesterone						
1–15	1.3 (0.9, 1.8)	16.0 (10.5, 26.0)	1.5 (0.9, 2.7)	1.2 (0.9, 1.6)	19.0 (11.5, 34.0)	1.5 (0.9, 2.9)
16–30	1.5 (1.0, 1.8)[b]	21.0 (13.0, 38.0)	14.5 (3.5, 30.0)	2.0 (1.3, 3.4)	23.0 (13.0, 33.0)	15.5 (3.9, 29.0)
>30	1.2 (0.8, 1.8)	10.5 (7.2, 21.0)	2.1 (1.0, 7.8)	1.1 (0.9, 1.5)	11.3 (7.0, 31.0)	1.7 (1.0, 8.0)
FSH						
1–15	8.8 (6.0, 14.8)	8.4 (5.4, 9.4)	8.5 (6.0, 14.0)	8.6 (6.3, 15.0)	6.8 (4.9, 9.3)	8.4 (6.0, 13.5)
16–30	11 (6, 36)	4.5 (3.4, 7.0)	5.5 (3.8, 9.8)	13.3 (6.8, 24.0)	4.5 (3.3, 6.8)	5.9 (3.5, 11.0)
>30	60 (20, 98)	5.6 (4.4, 7.4)	19.5 (5.4, 77.0)	40 (21, 72)	5.4 (3.0, 8.8)	21.0 (5.7, 58.0)
SHBG						
1–15	44 (34, 58)	52 (38, 77)	46 (35, 60)	45 (36, 57)	50 (38, 67)	46 (36, 59)
16–30	44 (28, 60)	40 (41, 66)[b]	48 (37, 65)	47 (40, 66)	44 (34, 60)	45 (36, 62)
>30	48 (39, 63)	39 (29, 60)	47 (38, 62)	43 (35, 58)	42 (36, 69)	42 (35, 59)
Number						
1–15	168	37	205	169	41	210
16–30	42	104	146	46	110	156
>30	33	19	52	33	18	51

[a]Median (first quartile, third quartile); Wilcoxon tests compare intervention and control groups overall and within each of the categories of progesterone level.
[b]$0.01<P<0.05$.

eight of these studies and increased in two. The pooled estimate from these 10 studies of the change in estradiol level in premenopausal women following dietary intervention was a reduction of 7.4%. A change of this magnitude corresponds to a reduction from baseline levels of 18.5 pmol/L in the subjects in the intervention group of our study. A greater reduction in estradiol, of 25 pmol/L, was observed in our intervention group, which contains more than twice the total number of subjects in all previous studies combined, but a reduction of similar magnitude also occurred in the controls.

Seven other studies in premenopausal women included in the meta-analysis of Wu *et al.* showed a reduction in estradiol levels following reduction of dietary fat intake, of which six employed metabolic diets. It is possible that the greater control of intakes associated with metabolic diets reduces estradiol, while our dietary intervention does not. None of these studies lasted longer than 3 months; it is also possible that effects of dietary fat reduction on estradiol levels are seen only in the short term.

Lower blood levels of estradiol have been found in Asian women than in Caucasians (Key *et al.*, 1990) and estradiol levels have been shown in large prospective studies to be related to risk of breast cancer. However, differences in age-specific breast cancer rates between countries are most marked after about the age of 50 and it is in postmenopausal women that differences in estrogen levels have most consistently been found to be associated with risk of breast cancer. Further, the analysis of Wu *et al.* (1999) showed an average reduction in estradiol levels of 23% in postmenopausal women following dietary fat reduction, compared to an average 7% reduction in the premenopausal women. Thus, both the international epidemiological data and the results of intervention studies are most consistent, with an effect of diet on estrogen levels in postmenopausal women.

The present results suggest that, if a reduction in dietary fat intake does reduce risk of breast cancer, it is unlikely to do so through an effect on blood estradiol levels in premenopausal women. These results do not, of course, exclude effects of dietary fat reduction on other aspects of estrogen such as effects on estrogen metabolism and other potential effects of diet that may be relevant to breast cancer risk in premenopausal women, e.g. effects on insulin-like growth factor, have not yet been examined (Hankinson *et al.*, 1998).

Acknowledgements

Supported by grants from the American Institute for Cancer Research, the Ontario Ministry of Health, and the Canadian Breast Cancer Research Initiative.

References

Boyd, N.F., Cousins, M., Lockwood, G. & Tritchler, D. (1990) The feasibility of testing experimentally the dietary fat-breast cancer hypothesis. *Br. J. Cancer*, **62**, 878–881

Boyd, N.F., Martin, L.J., Noffel, M. & Lockwood, G.A., Tritchler, D.L. (1993) A meta-analysis of studies of dietary fat and breast cancer risk. *Br. J. Cancer*, **68**, 627–636

Boyd, N.F., Lockwood, G.A., Greenberg, C.V., Martin, L.J. & Tritchler, D.L. (1997) Effects of a low-fat high-carbohydrate diet on plasma sex hormones in premenopausal women: results from a randomized controlled trial. *Br. J. Cancer*, **76**, 127–135

Freedman, L.S., Clifford, C. & Messina, M. (1990) Analysis of dietary fat, calories, body weight and the development of mammary tumours in rats and mice: a review. *Cancer Res.*, **150**, 5710–5719

Hankinson, S.E., Willet, W.C., Colditz, G.A., Hunter, D.J., Michaud, D.S., Deroo, B., Rosner, B., Speizer, F.E. & Pollak, M. (1998) Circulating concentrations of insulin-like growth factor-I and risk of breast cancer. *Lancet*, **351**, 1393–1396

Hunter, D.J., Spiegelman, D., Adami, H.O., Beeson, L., van den Brandt, P.A., Folsom, A.R., Fraser, G.E., Goldbohm, R.A., Graham, S. & Howe, G.R. (1996) Cohort studies of fat intake and the risk of breast cancer – a pooled analysis. *N. Engl. J. Med.*, **334**, 356–361

Kelsey, J.L. & Horn-Ross, P.L. (1993) Breast cancer: magnitude of the problem and descriptive data. *Epidemiol. Rev.*, **15**, 7–16

Key, T.J.A., Chen, J., Wang, D.Y., Pike, M.C. & Borcham, J. (1990) Sex hormones in women in rural China and in Britain. *Br. J. Cancer*, **62**, 631–636

McMichael, A.J. (1988) Cancer in migrants to Australia: extending descriptive epidemiological data. *Cancer Res.*, **48**, 751–756

Oza, A.M., Boyd, N.F. (1993) Mammographic parenchymal patterns: a marker of breast cancer risk. *Epidemiol. Rev.*, **15**, 196–208

Parkin, D., Whelan, S., Ferlay, J., Raymond, L. & Young, J. (1997) *Cancer incidence in five continents*, Vol VII. (IARC Scientific Publications No. 143), Lyon, IARC

Prentice, R.L., Pepe, M. & Self, S.G. (1989) Dietary fat and breast cancer: a quantitative assessment of the epidemiological literature and a discussion of methodologic issues. *Cancer Res.*, **49**, 3147–3156

Rogers, A.E. & Lee, S.Y. (1986) Chemically induced mammary gland tumors in rats: modulation by dietary fat. In: Ip, C., Birt, D.F., Rogers, A.E. & Mettlin, C., eds. *Dietary Fat and Cancer. Progress in Clinical and Biological Research, Vol.* **222**, 255–282, New York, Alan R Liss Inc.

Welsch, C.W. (1992) Relationship between dietary fat and experimental mammary tumorigenesis – a review and critique. *Cancer Res.*, **52**, S2040–S2048

Wu, A.H., Pike, M.C. & Stram, D.O. (1999) Meta-analysis: dietary fat Intake, serum estrogen levels, and the risk of breast cancer. *J. Natl. Cancer Inst.*, **91**, 529–534

Ziegler, R.G., Hoover, R.N., Pike, M.C., Hildesheim, A., Nomura, A.M., West, D.W., Wu-Williams, A.H., Kolonel, L.N., Horn-Ross, P.L. & Rosenthal, J.F. (1993) Migration patterns and breast cancer risk in Asian-American women. *J. Natl. Cancer Inst.*, **85**, 1819–1827

The SU.VI.MAX trial on antioxidants

Hercberg S.[1], Galan P.[1], Preziosi P.[1], Malvy M.[2], Briançon S.[3], Ait Hadad M.[1], Rahim B.[1], Favier A.[4]

[1]U557 INSERM/U1125 INRA, ISTNA-CNAM, 5, rue Vertbois, 75003 Paris. [2]INSERM U330, Université de Bordeaux. [3]Faculté de Médecine, Nancy. [4]Laboratoire de Biochimie, CHU de Grenoble, France.

Introduction

There is a large body of evidence indicating that free radical production can directly or indirectly play a major role in cellular processes implicated in atherosclerosis and carcinogenesis (Ames, 1987; Halliwell & Gutteridge, 1989). Many basic and clinical research investigations have pointed out the protective effect of antioxidant nutrients such as beta-carotene, vitamin C, vitamin E, selenium and zinc (Sies *et al.*, 1992; Niki, 1987; Diplock, 1991). Epidemiological data obtained by cross-sectional, case–control and prospective studies have also raised strong supportive arguments for an inverse relationship between the intake of antioxidant vitamins and trace elements and the risk of cancer, cardiovascular disease, cataracts and infectious diseases (Byers & Pery, 1992; Block *et al.*, 1992; Stampfer & Rimm, 1993; Kohlmeier & Hastings,1995; Stampfer & Rimm, 1995; Taylor *et al.*,1995; Meydani *et al.*, 1995; Hercberg *et al.*, 1998); however, the observational nature of these studies did not enable establishment of a causal relationship. Few randomized placebo-controlled trials testing different antioxidants on different target populations are available and results appear to be conflicting (Blot *et al.*, 1993; ATBC, 1994; Omenn *et al.*, 1996; Hennekens *et al.*, 1996). Most of these interventional studies involved higher levels of antioxidants than the dietary intake found in observational studies to be associated with the lowest risk of cancer and cardiovascular disease.

The SUpplementation en VItamines et Minéraux AntioXydants (SU.VI.MAX) Study is a randomized double-blind, placebo-controlled, primary-prevention trial designed to test the efficacy of a supplementation with antioxidant vitamins (vitamin C, vitamin E and beta-carotene) and minerals (selenium and zinc) at nutritional doses (one to three times the daily recommended dietary allowances) in reducing several major health problems in industrialized countries, and especially the main causes of premature death.

The design, background and rationale behind the SU.VI.MAX study, and especially the advantage of using a combination of antioxidant vitamins and minerals at low nutritional doses, has been described previously (Hercberg *et al.*, 1997). Many reasons support the hypothesis of the particular efficacy of a combination of antioxidants. Some metabolic inter-relationships exist between antioxidant nutrients with beneficial mutual protection and regeneration. Moreover, antioxidant nutrients have a complementary scavenging capacity toward free radicals. Accumulation of mechanistic data suggests that antioxidants act not only individually but also cooperatively and, in some cases, synergistically. The intrinsic chemical reactivity of each antioxidant, their different locations in the membrane and lipoproteins, their additive or synergistic effects, their multiple interactions and their cooperative action led us to test, in the SU.VI.MAX study, not a single antioxidant nutrient, but rather a balanced combination of antioxidants which might provide maximal efficacy associated with maximal safety.

The primary objective of this experimental epidemiological study is to substantiate and quantify, in a general population of adults, the preventive effect of a combination of antioxidant vitamins and minerals, namely beta-carotene, vitamin C, vitamin E, selenium and zinc, at doses considered to be nutritional and non-pharmacological, on the incidence of cancers (all sites) and ischemic heart diseases. Secondary objectives are to assess the effect of the supplementation on the incidence of the main localizations of cancers and infectious diseases, overall and cause-specific mortality, and perceived health and health care consumption.

This brief presentation will mainly describe the design, implementation and preliminary results of baseline characteristics of participants in this 8-year cohort study, which started in 1994 in France.

Materials and methods

Population, sampling

The study cohort consists of French adult women in the age range of 35–60 years and men in the age range of 45–60 years. The trial includes more women than men (sex ratio, 0.60) because of the lower incidence of main outcomes among women. The complete design of the SU.VI.MAX study has been described previously (Hercberg *et al.*, 1998).

Recruitment

A total of 79 976 subjects sought to participate in the study after a 5-month (March–July 1994) national multimedia campaign that included television, radio, and newspapers. Subjects received detailed information about the study and 15 capsules as a self-test of acceptability of daily supplement. They were also requested to fill in and return a comprehensive questionnaire meant to provide demographic, lifestyle, nutritional, and present and past health information.

Among the information sheets and informed consent returned to us, 21 481 were complete enough to be assessed. To be definitively eligible, the subjects had to:

- Provide complete data.
- Fall into the selected age range.
- Declare themselves free of any severe pathology that might limit participation for 8 years.
- Not be taking supplements containing any of the studied vitamins or minerals.
- Manifest no qualms about complying with protocol constraints, especially that of receiving a placebo.
- Express no ambiguous motivations or obsessional behavior concerning diet and health.

In all, 14 412 subjects were selected.

Enrollment of 12 735 participants began on October 12, 1994 and ended on April 30, 1995. This difference from the selected population was due to late refusals, postal problems, and the impossibility for some potential subjects to be present on the day of the inclusion visit.

Supplementation

Enrolled subjects were randomly assigned to receive either multivitamin and mineral supplement or a placebo. The daily multi-vitamin and mineral supplement contains beta-carotene, 6000 μg, which is equivalent to 1000 retinol equivalents; vitamin C, 120 mg; vitamin E, 30 mg; selenium, 100 μg (as selenium-enriched yeast); and zinc 20 mg (as gluconate).

Follow-up examination and review

Biological, clinical and dietary data are regularly collected in order to assess compliance with supplementation, evaluate changes in behavior, provide individual benefit to participants, and permit refined statistical analysis.

Each subject undergoes a yearly visit alternating between biological sampling and a clinical examination. On the first sample, before the start of supplementation, buffy coat and plasma samples were saved and stored in plastic straws at –196 °C to constitute a frozen sample bank.

Using the Minitel Telematic Network, participants can connect to the main computer SU.VI.MAX server to provide and receive information. The minitel is a small terminal widely used in France as an adjunct to the telephone. At the beginning of the study, participants received free-of-charge a tiny central processing unit specifically developed for the study and loaded with specialized software. This allows subjects to fill out computerized questionnaires off-line and to transmit data during a brief telephone connection. Each month, participants declare any health events, consultations, and hospitalizations that occurred during the current month, as well as medication intake, perceived health, and compliance with supplementation.

Subjects keep a total of six 24-h dietary records per year. They are helped in this task by the conversational features of the software and an instruction manual for codification of foods, including photographs showing portions in three sizes.

Results

Participant characteristics at baseline

A total of 7679 women and 5056 men were included in the SU.VI.MAX cohort during the first recruitment period. Mean age was 46.4±6.7 years for women and 51.1±4.7 years for men. Table 1 shows principal characteristics of participants at the start of intervention for multivitamin and mineral supplement or placebo groups. Groups are comparable for all studied characteristics.

Antioxidant vitamin and trace element status at baseline

Mean values (±SD) for markers of antioxidant vitamin and trace element according to gender are presented in Table 2. Serum concentrations of beta-carotene and vitamin C were significantly higher in women than in men. No difference was found betwen men and women for plasma vitamin E, zinc and selenium concentrations.

Antioxidant vitamin and trace element status after 2 years of supplementation

Table 3 shows laboratory variables in a representative subsample of 1000 subjects after 2 years of supplementation in the supplemented group and in the placebo group.

Table 1. Principal characteristics of participants at the start of the trial, for multivitamin and mineral supplement and placebo groups

	Placebo group Women	Men	Supplemented group Women	Men
No. of subjects	3859	2531	3820	2525
Age (years)	46.4±6.6	51.2± 4.7	46.4±6.6	51.1±4.6
Socioprofessional categories				
Farmers, self employed	4.7%	9.2%	5.0%	8.7%
Managerial staff, intermediate professions	52.6%	60.3%	54.1%	62.9%
Employed, workers	21.0%	13.9%	18.2%	12.5%
Nonactive subjects	21.7%	16.6%	22.7%	15.9%
Level of education				
Elementary school	19.6%	25.0%	19.0%	23.0%
Secondary school	40.6%	35.4%	38.5%	36.5%
University or equivalent	39.8%	39.6%	42.5%	40.5%
Family situation				
Living alone	22.3%	11.3%	21.8%	12.4%
Co-habitating	77.7%	88.7%	78.2%	87.6%
Tobacco habits				
Non-smokers	54.1%	32.3%	54.0%	31.6%
Former smokers	28.9%	46.2%	28.6%	47.3%
Current smokers	17.0%	21.5%	17.4%	21.1%
Contraceptive habits				
No contraception	58.7%	–	58.9%	–
Oral contraception	15.9%	–	14.8%	–
Intrauterine device	25.4%	–	26.3%	–
Percent postmenopausal	26.9%	–	26.2%	–
BMI (kg/m^2)	23.10±3.77	25.23±3.09	23.02±3.95	25.21±3.07
Serum cholesterol (μmol/L)	5.81±1.02	6.14±0.97	5.86±1.02	6.14±1.02
Glycemia (g/L)	0.99±0.13	1.08±0.18	0.99±0.14	1.08±0.20

Table 2. Mean values (±SD) for markers of antioxidant vitamin and trace element status at baseline

	Women	Men
Beta-carotene (μmol/L)	0.71±0.43	0.51±0.32
Alpha-tocopherol (μmol/L)	31.2±7.0	31.9±7.4
Vitamin C (μg/mL)	10.51±5.29	8.85±5.38
Selenium (μmol/L)	1.07±0.18	1.11±0.19
Zinc (μmol/L)	12.89±1.88	13.54±1.84

At baseline, mean values for biochemical markers of vitamin and trace element status did not differ between the two groups for any of the parameters tested. After 2 years, serum concentrations were significantly higher in the supplemented group for beta-carotene, vitamins C and E, zinc and selenium.

Discussion

The SU.VI.MAX Study was designed and initiated to test the hypothesis that a combination of antioxidant and trace elements, given at nutritional doses, in a general population of adults, may reduce the incidence of cancer and cardiovascular disease, thereby decreasing premature mortality. The antioxidant agents tested are at a nonpharmacological level that may be reached by dietary intake of natural sources of these micronutrients and/or possible enriched foods.

The SU.VI.MAX study is founded upon different types of arguments. First, experimental work has supported the possible role of oxidative stress in the determinism of pathological processes and protection against oxidative damage by antioxidant nutrients such as vitamins E and C, beta-carotene, selenium and zinc. Second, many epidemiological studies have suggested that the low dietary intake or borderline biochemical status of some antioxidant trace-elements and vitamins may be an important risk factor for various diseases. Third, a significant percentage of the affluent world population has a relatively low intake or borderline vitamin and/or mineral status, considered to be a high risk factor for developing such diseases of "affluence" as cancers and cardiovascular diseases.

Although the results of many epidemiological studies converge in suggesting a relationship between antioxidant micronutrient status and risk of cancer or cardiovascular diseases, most of these are observational studies.

Table 3. Serum vitamin levels (mean ± SD) after 2 years of supplementation in the supplemented group and in the placebo group

	Men Placebo	Intervention	Women Placebo	Intervention
Beta-carotene (μmol/L)	0.56±0.5	0.86±0.7	0.76±0.6	1.25±0.9
Alpha-tocopherol, (μmol/L)	31.7±7.9	35.3±9.3	31.7±7.8	34.9±8.4
Vitamin C (μg/mL)	9.3±4.2	11.5±4.7	10.8±4.3	12.6±4.0

The few recently reported randomized placebo-controlled trials, which tested different antioxidants on different target populations, reached different conclusions. Randomized controlled trials on populations at high risk, in which single nutrients are given in high doses over short periods, have not yet shown any substantial benefits. Indeed, the Alpha Tocopherol and Beta Carotene (ATBC) Study, which studied male heavy smokers in Finland, observed a significantly higher lung cancer incidence rate in a group receiving relatively high levels of beta-carotene alone or associated with vitamin E. In the same study, subjects receiving vitamin E had significantly more hemorrhagic strokes than controls. These conclusions were supported by the recently published results of the Carotene and Retinol Efficacy Trial (CARET), a study in the United States on asbestos-exposed workers and heavy smokers who are at high risk for lung cancer. Cases of lung cancer were significantly more frequent in the group receiving relatively high levels of beta-carotene associated with vitamin A than in the placebo group. Finally, the Physicians' Health Study in the USA did not demonstrate any positive or negative effects of long-term supplementation with quite similar doses of beta-carotene. The only intervention study demonstrating a positive effect was the Nutritional Intervention Trial in Linxian (China). This study showed, in a general population, a beneficial effect of nutritional doses of an association of beta-carotene, vitamin E and selenium on total mortality and the incidence of cancer, particularly oesophagal cancer.

These apparent discrepancies may be explained by the choice of the study population (general or high-risk subjects), the different doses of supplementation (nutritional or higher), the number of antioxidants tested (one, two, or more) and the type of administration (alone or in a balanced association). Moreover, in high-risk populations receiving high doses of antoxidants, some of these intervention studies have reported a greater relative risk of some pathologies. Therefore, randomized, controlled trials were needed on average or low-risk individuals given combination multiple nutrients. The advantage lies in testing a combination of nutrients at levels similar to those contained in a healthy diet associated, in observational study, with the lowest risk of disease.

In the SU.VI.MAX study, mean values observed for initial serum vitamin and trace element concentrations were similar to those previously described for French adult populations. The effect of supplementation by antioxidant micronutrients over a 2-year period on serum concentrations of biochemical markers assessing vitamin and trace element status was significant for all of the studied nutrients: vitamin C, E, beta-carotene, zinc and selenium. In CARET, as in ATBC, the relatively high levels of supplementation were associated with a substantial increase in the plasma concentrations of beta-carotene. For example, the initial concentrations of plasma carotene were multiplied by 18 in ATBC and by 12 in CARET. The final concentrations were higher than those associated, in observational studies, with the lower risk of diseases. They were also higher than those observed in the SU.VI.MAX study.

These preliminary data thus indicate that a 2-year supplementation with moderate doses of antioxidant vitamins and trace elements, in presumaly healthy subjects, clearly though moderately alter vitamin and mineral status, with blood concentrations reaching concentrations consistent with a positive effect.

Our study demonstrates the efficacy of an intake of antioxidant vitamins and trace elements, given at nutritional doses, on biochemical indicators of vitamin and trace element status. After 2 years of supplementation, these indicators reached a reasonable level without reaching concentrations as high as those observed in the Finnish and American intervention studies, which tested relatively high doses of antioxidants and resulted in with higher risk of pathology.

As the trial is not finished and the double-blind not opened, no data are available concerning the main results of the intervention on cancers and cardiovascular diseases. Opening of the blinding code is planned for spring 2003.

Acknowledgements

The project SU.VI..M.AX has support from public and private sectors. Special thanks are adressed to Fruit d'Or Recherche, Candia, Lipton, Kellogg's, Centre d'Information sur Canderel, Orangina, Estée Lauder, Cereal, Grands Moulins de Paris, CERIN, L'Oréal,

Peugeot, Jet Service, RP Scherer, Sodexho, France Telecom, Santogen, Becton Dickinson, Fould Springer, Boehringer Diagnostic, Seppic Givaudan Lavirotte, Le Grand Canal.

References

Ames, B.N. (1987) Dietary carcinogens and anticarcinogens. *Science*, **221**, 1256–1264

Block, G., Patterson, B. & Subar, A. (1992) Fruit, vegetables, and cancer prevention, a review of the epidemiological evidence. *Nutr. Cancer*, **18**, 1–29

Blot, W.J., Li, J.Y., Taylo, P.R., Guo, W., Dawsey, S., Wang, G.Q., Yang, C.S., Zhang, S.F., Gail, M., Li, G.Y., Yu, Y., Liu, B.Q., Tangrea, J., Sun, Y.H., Liu, F., Fraumeni, J.F., Zhang, Y.H. & Li, B. (1993) Nutrition intervention trials in Linxian, China: supplementation with specific vitamin/mineral combinations, cancer incidence, and disease-specific mortality in the general population. *J. Natl. Cancer Inst.*, **85**, 1483–1492

Byers, T. & Perry, G. (1992) Dietary carotenes, vitamin C, and vitamin E as protective antioxidants in human cancers. *Annu. Rev. Nutr.*, **12**, 139–159

Diplock, A.T. (1991) Antioxidant nutrients and disease prevention: an overview. *Am. J. Clin. Nutr.*, **53** (1 Suppl),189S–193S

Halliwell, B. & Gutteridge, J.M.C. (1989) *Free Radicals in Biology and Medicine.* 2nd ed. Oxford, Clarendon Press

Hennekens, C.H., Buring, J.E., Manson, J.E., Stampfer, M., Rosner, B., Cook, N.R., Belanger, C., LaMotte, F., Gaziano, J.M., Ridke, P.M., Willett, W. & Peto, R. (1996) Lack of effect of long-term supplementation with beta-carotene on the incidence of malignant neoplasms and cardiovascular disease. *N. Eng. J. Med.*, **334**, 1145–1149

Hercberg, S., Galan, P., Preziosi, P., Alfarez, M.J. & Vazquez, C. (1998) The potential role of antioxidant vitamins in preventing cardiovascular diseases and cancers. *Nutrition*, **14**, 513–520

Hercberg S., Galan, P., Preziosi, P., Roussel, A.-M., Arnaud, J., Richard, M.-J., Malvy, D., Paul-Dauphin, A., Briançon, S. & Favier, A. (1997) Background and rationale behind the SU.VI.MAX Study, a prevention trial using nutritional doses of a combination of antioxidant vitamins and minerals to reduce cardiovascular diseases and cancers. *Int. J. Vit. Nutr. Res.*, **68**, 3–20

Hercberg, S., Preziosi, P., Briançon, S., Galan, P., Paul-Dauphin, A., Malvy, D., Roussel, A.-M. & Favier, A. (1998) A primary prevention trial of nutritional doses of antioxidant vitamins and minerals on cardiovascular diseases and cancers in general population: the SU.VI.MAX Study. Design, methods and participant characteristics. *Control Clin. Trial.* **19**, 336–351

Kohlmeier, L. & Hastings, S.B. (1995) Epidemiologic evidence of a role of carotenoids in cardiovascular disease prevention. *Am. J. Clin. Nutr.*, **62**, 1370S–1376S

Meydani, S.N., Wu, D., Santos, M.S. & Hayek, M.G. (1995) Antioxidants and immune response in aged persons: overview of present evidence. *Am. J. Clin. Nutr.*, **62**, 1462S–1476S

Niki, E. (1987) Antioxidants in relation to lipid peroxidation. *Chem. Phys. Lip.*, **44**, 227–253

Omenn, G.S., Goodman, G.E., Thorquis, M.D., Balmes, J., Cullen, M.R., Glass, A., Keogh, J.P., Meyskens, F.L., Valaxis, B., James, P.H., Williams, J.H. & Barnhart, S. (1996) Effects of a combination of beta-carotene and vitamin A on lung cancer and cardiovascular disease. *N. Eng. J. Med.*, **334**, 1150–1155

Sies, H., Staahl, W. & Sundqquist, A.R. (1992) Antioxidant functions of vitamins: vitamin E and C, beta-carotene, and other carotenoids. *Ann. N.Y. Acad. Sci.*, **669**, 7–20

Stampfer, M.J. & Rimm, B. (1993) A review of the epidemiology of dietary antioxidants and risk of coronary heart disease. *Can. J. Cardiol.*, **19**, 14B–18B

Stampfer, M.J. & Rimm, B. (1995) Epidemiologic evidence for vitamin E in prevention of cardiovascular disease. *Am. J. Clin. Nutr.*, **62**, 1365S–1369S

Taylor, A., Jacques, P.F. & Epstein, E.M. (1995) Relations among aging, antioxidant status, and cataract. *Am. J. Clin. Nutr.*, **62**, 1439S–1447S

The Alpha-Tocopherol, Beta Carotene Cancer Prevention Study Group (1994) The effect of vitamin E and beta carotene on the incidence of lung cancer and other cancers in male smokers. *N. Eng. J. Med.*, **330**, 1029–1035

Effect of fibre and calcium supplementation on adenoma recurrence and growth

Faivre J., Bonithon-Kopp C.

Registre des Cancers, INSERM EPI 0106, Registre associé INSERM-InVS, Faculté de Médecine, BP 87900, 21079 Dijon Cedex, France.

Colorectal cancer is a major public health problem in all developed countries (Parkin *et al.*, 1997). Despite advances in diagnostic techniques and treatment, the 5-year survival rates remain poor. Strong evidence indicates that a high proportion of colorectal cancers arises in adenomas. These lesions could be a potential target for secondary prevention as well as for primary prevention. Several arguments maintain that the adenoma-carcinoma sequence is a multistep process (Hill *et al.*, 1978). Cancer can be prevented by intervention either at the step of adenoma occurrence and growth or of transformation into carcinoma.

Many case–control studies, along with some cohort studies, have provided substantial epidemiological evidence for the overwhelming role of diet in the occurrence of the disease (World Cancer Research Fund, 1997). However, analytical studies have led to equivocal findings. Available data are not sufficient to serve as a basis for firm specific dietary advice, but they provide attractive hypotheses, which in turn suggest a rational basis for a preventive approach. Faced with this situation, it is important to test them within the framework of intervention studies in order to evaluate the possibilities of primary prevention. The objective of this report is to review the design, along with the available results, of randomized colorectal cancer intervention trials with fibre or calcium supplementation.

Fibre trials

The results of analytical studies on dietary fibre are rather contradictory. It must be emphasized that dietary fibre is not a homogeneous entity and that different components may have different physiological effects. Food composition tables lack data on the different types of dietary fibre. In this context, studies examining the effect of a single source of fibre on experimental carcinogenesis in rodents are of interest. Pectin, cellulose, lignin, guargum, alfalfa, carrageen and cutin seem to have little effect (Faivre *et al.*, 1991). However, a protective effect has been observed in most studies for wheat bran and mucilaginous substances (such as ispaghula husk), particularly during the promoting phase. The relevance of these data to human cancer has to be evaluated by means of intervention studies. Wheat bran supplementation was proposed in three studies, a diet high in fibre in two studies, and a supplementation with a mucilaginous substance in one study (Table 1). The effect of wheat bran at the dose of 22.5 g/day, together with vitamin C (4 g/day) and vitamin E (400 mg/day) has been evaluated in patients with familial polyposis and with the rectum left in place (De Cosse *et al.*, 1989). The ratio between the number of adenomas at the time of the follow-up examination and the number of adenomas at base line was the main trial outcome. Altogether, 58 subjects were randomized and followed up by rigid proctosigmoidoscopy every 6 months. The overall compliance to treatment was 74%. Intent-to-treat analysis suggested a limited effect of the treatment in the group receiving wheat bran, vitamin C and vitamin E compared with the group receiving vitamins alone or a placebo. There were significant differences only at 33 and 39 months. When compliance was taken into account, there was a stronger benefit in the combined fibre–vitamin group, particularly at the 2-year midpoint of the study.

In the Toronto study, the intervention group received counselling on diet high in fibre (50 g/day) and low in fat (20% of energy from fat). The control group continued with its usual diet (McKeown-Eyssen *et al.*, 1994). Overall, 201 subjects were randomized and the compliance to treatment rate was 71%. Compliance to the final colonoscopy was 82%. After 12 months of counselling, fibre consumption was 35 g in the intervention group and 16 g in the control group and fat consumption was 25% and 33% of energy, respectively.

Table 1. Study design, endpoints and results of chemoprevention trials with fibre on colorectal cancer carcinogenesis

Study	Subjects	Intervention	Number of subjects	Duration	Endpoint results
De Cosse *et al.*, New York, 1989	Familial polyposis	Wheat bran 22.5 g/d + vitamin C 4 g/d + vitamin E 400 mg/d	58	4 years	Nonsignificant reduction in the number of rectal adenomas
MacKeown-Eyssen *et al.*, Canada, 1994	Previous adenoma	Diet high in fibre and low in fat	201	2 years	No effect of adenoma recurrence
Mac Lennan *et al.*, Australia, 1995	Previous adenoma	Wheat bran 11 g/d	378	4 years	No effect on adenoma recurrence
Alberts *et al.*, Arizona, 2000	Previous adenoma	Wheat bran 13.5 g/d	1400	5 years	No effect on adenoma recurrence
Bonithon-Kopp *et al.*, Europe, 2000	Previous adenoma	Ispaghula husk	656	3 years	Significant increase in adenoma recurrence
Schatzkin *et al.*, USA, 2000	Previous adenoma	Diet high in fibre, fruits, vegetables, low in fat	2079	4 years	No effect on adenoma recurrence

After two years, the relative risk (RR) for adenoma recurrence was 1.2 (CI, 0.6–2.8). There was a reduced risk of adenoma recurrence in women (RR, 0.7) and an increased risk in men (RR, 1.7), which did not reach the significant level because of the small sample size. Thus the issue of a gender effect related to adenoma recurrence remains a definite question to be addressed by much larger studies.

The effect of wheat bran (25 g/day) on adenoma recurrence was considered in the Australian study (MacLennan *et al.*, 1995). The effect of a low-fat diet (<25% of calories from fat) and of β-carotene (20 mg/day) were also tested using a 2 x 2 factorial design. It has the advantage of allowing the effect of the combination of two treatments to be evaluated and of giving more power to the study compared with a parallel scheme with the same number of participants. In this study, 411 subjects were randomized. The compliance rate to treatment was 74% and compliance to coloscopy was 95% at 2 years and 74% at 4 years. There was no evidence that any intervention reduced the recurrence rate of adenomas at 2 or 4 years. A significant reduction in the recurrence rate of large adenomas (>1 cm) was found only when the low-fat diet was combined with wheat bran supplementation. However, these results must be interpreted cautiously because of the small number of patients with large adenoma at the follow-up colonoscopy. It has not been confirmed by the other studies (Bonithon-Kopp *et al.*, 2000; Alberts *et al.*, 2000; Schatzkin *et al.*, 2000).

A trial was performed in Arizona to determine whether wheat bran can prevent the recurrence of colorectal adenoma (Alberts *et al.*, 2000). Altogether, 1429 patients with previous adenomas received a dietary supplementation of either 13.5 g or 2 g per day of wheat bran for 3 years. Compliance by the third year was 74% in the high-fibre group and 84% in the low-fibre group; 91% had a 3-year colonoscopy. The relative risk of recurrence of adenomas in the high-fibre group was 0.88 (CI, 0.70–1.11). There was no evidence of an effect of the supplementation regarding the size of the adenomas or their histological appearance. However, there was a significantly higher proportion of subjects with 3 or more recurrent adenomas in the high-fibre group.

We will just mention the large US Study (2079 subjects) which evaluated the effect of a diet low in fat (20% of calories), high in fibre (18 g per 1000 kcal), fruits and vegetables (3.5 servings for 1000 kcal) on adenoma recurrence

(Schatzkin *et al.*, 2000). It will be presented in another paper. This diet did not influence the risk of recurrence of colorectal adenomas which was similar to the no intervention group (OR, 1.0; CI, 0.90–1.12). The rate of recurrence of large adenomas (≥ 1 cm), of advanced adenomas, or of multiple adenomas did not differ significantly between the two groups.

A multicentre European study performed within the European Cancer Prevention Organisation (ECP) has been assessing a mucilaginous substance in the form of ispaghula husk (3.8 g/day) (Bonithon-Kopp *et al.*, 2000). This dose was recommended by the manufacturer to obtain stool bulking. In this study, a second group received calcium (2 g/day) and a third group a placebo. The duration of the study was 3 years and 665 subjects were randomized. The final colonoscopy was performed in 87% of the subjects. The compliance for supplements was obtained in 83% of the subjects. The results suggest a deleterious effect of fibre on the recurrence of colorectal adenoma (OR adjusted,1.63; 95% CI, 1.01–2.69). We chose ispaghula husk because it is known to have stool bulking properties and to decrease faecal pH. Furthermore, it is widely used as a laxative agent and only negligible side effects have been reported. In animal models of colon carcinogenesis, this agent has been one of the most effective soluble fibres in tumour prevention (Jacobs 1990; Wilpart & Robertfroid, 1987). The detrimental effects of soluble fibre could be due to an increasing production of short chain fatty acids by bacterial fermentation and an excessive acidification which may stimulate proliferation of epithelial cells. However, the significance of hyperproliferation in relation to the carcinogenesis process is unclear.

Calcium trials

The role of dietary calcium intake in the prevention of colorectal cancer and adenomas is debated (Bergsma-Kadjik *et al.*, 1996; Martinez & Willett, 1998). Support for this hypothesis was obtained from cohort studies and from the fact that oral intake of calcium may induce a more quiescent equilibrium of epithelial cell proliferation in the colonic mucosa of subjects at high risk of colorectal cancer.

Three intervention studies aimed at evaluating the possibility of primary prevention of colorectal cancer with calcium supplements have been carried out (Table 2). All these studies investigated subjects with a previous history of colorectal adenoma and used adenoma recurrence as the primary outcome measure. One study also evaluated the effect of calcium supplementation on adenoma growth.

In the Oslo study, the intervention group received calcium carbonate at the dose of 1.6 g/day together with a mixture of antioxydants: selenium, 101 μg/day; β-carotene, 15 mg/day; vitamin E, 75 mg/day; and vitamin C, 150 mg /day for 3 years (Hofstad *et al.*, 1998). The compliance with the supplements (5 tablets per day) was 81% and compliance to the final colonoscopy was 87%. All adenomas less than 1 cm in diameter were left unresected for 3 years. A yearly colonoscopy was performed for 3 years by the same endoscopist, to measure the left-in adenomas (which had

Table 2. Study design, endpoints and results of chemoprevention trials with fibre on colorectal cancer carcinogenesis

Study	Subjects	Intervention	Number of subjects	Duration	Endpoint results
Hofstad *et al.*, Oslo, 1998	Previous adenoma	Calcium 1.6 g/d + b carotene 15 mg/d + vitamin E 75 mg/d + vitamin C 150 mg/d + selenium 101 mg/d	116	3 years	No effect on adenoma growth Significant decrease in adenoma recurrence
Baron *et al.*, USA, 1999	Previous adenoma	Calcium 1.2 g/d	930	4 years	Significant decrease in adenoma recurrence
Bonithon-Kopp *et al.*, Europe, 2000	Previous adenoma	Calcium 2.0 g/d	656	3 years	Decrease in adenoma recurrence

to be removed if they reached 1 cm in diameter) and detect new adenomas. On completion of the study, all adenomas were removed. Altogether, 116 subjects were randomized. There was a significantly higher number of patients free of new adenomas in the active medication group compared to those in the placebo group (OR, 0.31; CI, 0.11–0.84). No difference was detected in growth of adenomas between the active and the placebo group from year to year and for the total study period. Moreover, there was no effect on the polyps less than 5 mm or 5–9 mm or on the polyps in the different colonic segments analysed separately.

In a study in the US, the effect of calcium 1.2 g/day as calcium carbonate was tested on adenoma recurrence (Baron *et al.*, 1999). A total of 930 patients were randomized and the duration of the study was 4 years. During the fourth year of the study, 79% of the subjects took the study agents 90%–100% of the time and the compliance to the final colonoscopy was 89%. The adjusted risk ratio for having at least one adenoma in the calcium group as compared with the placebo group was 0.81 (CI, 0.67–0.99) and the adjusted risk ratio of the average number of adenomas in the calcium group to that in the placebo group was 0.76 (CI, 0.60–0.96). The risk ratio for having at least an adenoma over 0.5 cm in diameter was 0.87 (CI, 0.63–1.21). The effect of calcium was independent of initial dietary fat and calcium intake.

In the European study (ECP study), one arm evaluated the effect of calcium gluconolactate carbonate, corresponding to 2 g elemental calcium daily, in the prevention of adenoma recurrence over 3 years. The compliance rate to treatment was 80%. Side effects were more often reported in the calcium group (15%) than in the fibre group (10%) or the placebo group (7%) ($P<0.04$). There was a reduction in the risk of adenoma recurrence (OR, 0.66; CI, 0.38–1.17). Calcium may protect against colon carcinogenesis by binding secondary bile acids and fatty acids to form insoluble soaps in the bowel lumen, thus reducing their proliferative effect on colonic cells. Changes in bile acid metabolism could selectively increase the risk of right colon cancer. Interestingly, our results suggest that calcium supplementation may be particularly beneficial in patients with low dietary calcium intake (OR, 0.51; CI, 0.22–1.18) and in those who initially had adenomas on the right colon (OR, 0.26; CI, 0.08–0.84). Our study was not designed to examine the interaction between calcium and fibre supplementation. We have no evidence that dietary fibre intake may interfere with the effects of calcium supplementation. On the other hand, we found that the adverse effect of ispaghula fibre supplementation was significantly stronger in patients with a high dietary calcium intake than in those with a low calcium intake (OR, 2.81; CI, 1.33–5.92). This finding was unexpected and we cannot rule out that it was due to chance alone.

Conclusion

Available data do not support a protective effect of fibre supplementation with wheat bran or mucilagenous substance on adenoma recurrence. They even suggest that they can have a deleterious effect. There are not enough arguments to suggest a protective effect on adenoma growth. We cannot draw any conclusions about the effect of fibre supplementation on the latter stages of carcinogenesis. In contrast, there are strong arguments for a moderate protective effect of calcium on adenoma recurrence, but not on adenoma growth.

References

Alberts, D.S., Ritenbaugh, C., Story, J.A., Aickin, M., Rees-McGee, S., Buller, M.K., Martinez, M.E., Roe, D.J. Guillen-Rodriguez, J.M., Marshall, J.R., van Leeuwen, J.B., Reid, M.E., Ritenbaugh, C., Vargas, P.A., Bhattacharyya, A.B., Earnest, D.L. & Sampliner, R.E. (2000) Lack of effect of a high-fiber cereal supplement on the recurrence of colorectal adenomas. *N. Engl. J. Med.*, **342S**, 1156–1162

Baron, J.A., Beach, M., Mandel, J.S., Van Stolk, R.U., Haile, R.W. & Sandler, R.S. (1999) Calcium supplements for the prevention of colorectal adenomas. *N. Engl. J. Med.*, **340**, 101–117

Bergsma-Kadijk, J.A. Van't Veer, P., Kampman, E. & Burema, J. (1996) Calcium does not protect against colorectal neoplasia. *Epidemiology*, **7**, 590–597

Bonithon-Kopp, C., Kronborg, O., Giacosa, A., Räth, U., Faivre, J. & the European Cancer Prevention Organisation Study Group (2000) Calcium and fiber supplementation in prevention of colorectal adenoma recurrence: a randomised intervention trial. *Lancet*, **356**, 1300–1336

De Cosse, J.J., Miller, H.H. & Lesser, M.L. (1989) Effect of wheat fiber and vitamin C and E on rectal polyps in patients with familial adenomatous polyposis. *J. Natl. Cancer Inst.*, **81**, 1290–1297

Faivre, J., Wilpart, M. & Boutron, M.C. (1991) Primary prevention of colorectal cancer. *Recent Results Cancer Res.*, **122**, 85–89

Hill, M.J., Morson, B.C. & Bussey, H.J.R. (1978) Aetiology of adenoma-carcinoma sequence in the large bowel. *Lancet*, **i**, 245–247

Hofstad, B., Almendingen, K., Vatn, M., Andersen, S.N., Owen, R.W. & Larsen, S. (1998) Growth and recurrence of colorectal polyps: a double-blind 3-year intervention with calcium and antioxidants. *Digestion*, **5**, 148–156

Jacobs, L.R. (1990) Influence of soluble fibers on experimental colon carcinogenesis In: Kritchevsky, D. Bonfield, C. & Anderson, J.W. (eds) *Dietary Fiber Chemistry, Physiology and Health Effects*, New York, Plenum, pp. 389–401

MacKeown-Eyssen, G., Bright-See, E., Dion, P., Bruce, W.R. & Jazmaji, V. (1994) A randomized trial of a low-fat high-fibre diet in the recurrence of colorectal polyps. *J. Clin. Epidemiol.*, **47**, 525–536

MacLennan, R., Macrae, F.A., Bain, C., Battistutta, D., Chapuis, P. & Gratten, H. (1995) Randomized trial of intake of fat, fiber and beta carotene to prevent colorectal adenomas. *J. Natl. Cancer Inst.*, **87**, 1760–1766

Martinez, M.E. & Willett, W.C. (1998) Calcium, vitamin D and colorectal cancer: a review of the epidemiologic evidence. *Cancer Epidemiol. Biomarkers Prev.*, **7**, 163–168

Parkin, D., Whelan, S., Ferlay, J., Raymond, L. & Young, J. (1997) *Cancer incidence in five continents*, Vol VII. (IARC Scientific Publications No. 143), Lyon, IARC

Schatzkin, A., Lanza, E., Corle, D., Lance, P., Iber, F., Caan, B., Shike, M., Weissfeld, J., Burt, R., Cooper, M.R., Kikendall, J.W. & Cahill, J. (2000) Lack of effect of a low-fat high-fiber diet on the recurrence of colorectal adenomas. *N. Engl. J. Med.*, **342S**, 1149–1155

Wilpart, M. & Roberfroid, M. (1987) Intestinal carcinogenesis and dietary fibers: the influence of cellullose and fybogel chronically given after exposure to DMH. *Nutr. Cancer*, **10**, 39–51

World Cancer Research Fund/American Institute for Cancer Research (1997) *Food, Nutrition and the Prevention of Cancer: A Global Perspective*. Washington D.C., WCRF/AICR.

Polyps and vegetables (and fat, fibre): the polyp prevention trial

Schatzkin A., Lanza E. and the Polyp Prevention Trial Study Group.
National Cancer Institute, Bethesda MD 20814, USA.

Diet has long been regarded as the most important environmental influence on colorectal cancer. Animal experiments have shown conclusively that nutritional modulation can alter colorectal carcinogenesis (Zhao *et al.*, 1991; Kritchevsky, 1999). Epidemiological studies have implicated a variety of dietary factors in the etiology of this disease (Potter *et al.*, 1993).

Because the generalizability of animal experiments to humans is problematic and confounding of modest epidemiological associations is difficult to rule out, the clinical trial design offers a valuable alternative approach to advancing our understanding of the role of diet in large bowel cancer. In that light, we conceived and conducted the Polyp Prevention Trial (PPT), an experimental epidemiological study of the effect of a low-fat, high-fibre, fruit- and vegetable-enriched diet on the recurrence of colorectal adenomas (Schatzhin *et al.*, 2000).

At the time we initiated this trial, the fat, fibre, and fruit and vegetable hypotheses were all considered promising. Data from the prospective study of diet and colorectal adenomas in the Health Professionals Follow-up Study were particularly compelling (Giovannucci *et al.*, 1992). As Table 1 shows, this study found that dietary fat doubled adenoma risk whereas dietary fibre as well as fruit and vegetable intake halved that risk. In the PPT, we elected to intervene with a multifactorial rather than a single-nutrient-oriented eating plan in order to capture potential joint effects of nutrients and foods, incorporate the effects of unknown nutrients or nonnutritive food constituents and maximize the likelihood of observing a treatment effect.

If we are interested in the relation of diet and invasive colorectal cancer, why carry out a trial with adenoma endpoints? The polyp trial model is attractive for three reasons. First, the recurrence rate for colorectal adenomas is approximately two orders of magnitude greater than the incidence rate for invasive cancer. (Recurrence is defined as the development of a new adenoma anywhere in the large bowel after identification and removal of one or more adenomas.) Therefore, an adenoma recurrence trial can be substantially smaller, faster, and less costly than a trial with cancer endpoints. Second, it is possible to integrate a polyp trial with standard post-polypectomy endoscopic surveillance practice. This provides a convenient means for ascertaining endpoints. Finally, the concept of the adenoma–carcinoma sequence reflects the fact that the large majority of invasive colorectal cancers develop through a polypoid phase. In other words, because colorectal adenomas are necessary precursor lesions for most invasive cancers, an intervention that reduces adenoma recurrence will likely reduce cancer incidence.

The PPT design is depicted in Fig. 1. Following a run-in phase, which consisted of the satisfactory completion of dietary assessment instruments, 2079 eligible participants were randomized to either the low-fat, high-fibre, high-fruit and -vegetable or the usual diet arm.

Table 1. Prospective study of diet and colorectal adenoma in male health professionals

	RR (95% CI) for quintile 5 versus quintile 1
Total fat	2.3 (1.4–3.9)
Total fibre	0.4 (0.2–0.6)
Vegetables	0.5 (0.3–0.9)

Table 2. PPT: changes in reported dietary intake

Variable	Intervention group		Control group		Net change
	Baseline	Year 4	Baseline	Year 4	
Fat (% kcal)	35.6	23.8	36.0	33.9	–9.7
Fibre (g/1000 kcal)	10.0	17.4	9.5	10.0	6.9
Fruit/vegetable (servings/1000 kcal)	2.05	3.41	2.00	2.23	1.13

Table 3. PPT: risk of adenoma recurrence among participants completing the study

	Intervention group (*n*=958)		Control group (*n*=947)		Risk ratio (95% CI)
	No.	%	No.	%	
≥ 1 adenoma	380	39.7	374	39.5	1.00 (0.90–1.12)
Largest adenoma ≥ 1 cm	47	4.9	53	5.6	0.88 (0.60–1.28)
Advanced adenoma	60	6.3	66	7.0	0.90 (0.64–1.26)

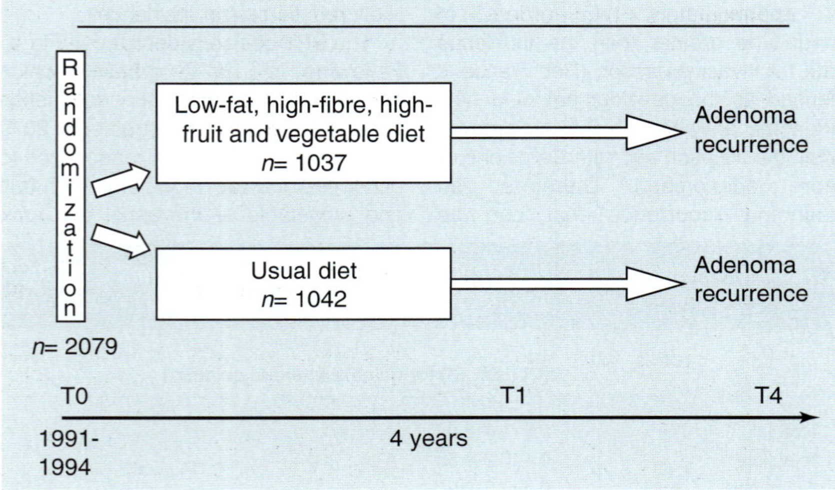

Figure 1
PPT design

Recruitment at eight clinical centres in the United States took place between 1991 and 1994. Within 6 months of randomization, all participants had to have had at least one adenoma removed and pathologically confirmed at the clinical centre.

The dietary intervention was complex and intensive. For participants in the intervention group, the dietary goals were to provide 20% of total calories from fat, 18 g of dietary fibre per 1000 kcal, and 3.5 servings of fruits and vegetables per 1000 kcal (range, 5–8 daily servings, depending on total energy intake). The intervention program included nutritional information and behavior-modification techniques. An extensive series of training modules was specifically developed for intervention participants and nutritionists. We offered each participant more than 50 h of counseling sessions during the 4-year intervention period, including 20 h in the first year. Each subject in the intervention group was assigned to one nutritionist for counseling and another for dietary assessment. We provided participants in the control group with general dietary guidelines from the National Dairy Council but gave them no additional nutritional or behavioral information.

Each year all participants completed a 4-day food record followed by a food-frequency questionnaire, the Block Health Habits and History Questionnaire, which was modified slightly to reflect the intake of low-fat and high-fibre foods. In addition, participants in the intervention group completed a 4-day food record 6 months after randomization. Each year we administered unscheduled 24-h dietary recall questionnaires to a newly selected random sample of 10% of participants.

The trial protocol required participants to return to their usual endoscopist for colonoscopy 1 and 4 years after randomization. The 1-year colonoscopy, performed at least 180 days after randomization but less than 2 years afterward, was considered a 'clearing' procedure to detect and remove any adenomas that had been missed at the qualifying colonoscopy. We obtained data on any unscheduled endoscopic procedure carried out in addition to the follow-up procedures at 1 and 4 years. We asked all investigators and subjects not to discuss a subject's randomization status with the endoscopists.

Two central pathologists, who were unaware of the subjects' group assignment, determined the histological features and degree of atypia (low-grade versus high-grade) of all lesions. The endoscopists' reports provided information on the size, number, and location of all polyps. We defined an adenoma as recurrent if it was found during any endoscopic procedure after the 1-year colonoscopy or, for subjects who missed the 1-year colonoscopy, during any endoscopic procedure performed at least 2 years after randomization. Adenomas found during the 1-year colonoscopy were not considered recurrent. The few colorectal cancers diagnosed after the 1-year colonoscopy were counted as recurrent lesions.

The primary endpoint was the recurrence of adenomas during the interval from the 1-year to the 4-year colonoscopy. Secondary endpoints were the number, size, location, and histological features of the adenomas that were found. We used the intention-to-treat principle to compare the intervention and control groups, defining groups according to the initial random assignment rather than according to actual or reported compliance with the protocol.

The trial was logistically quite successful. Over 90% of study participants completed the trial: 958 (92.4%) and 947 (90.9%) participants, respectively, in the intervention and control arms. The average follow-up time and mean number of procedures were virtually identical in the two groups.

Table 2 shows the changes in reported dietary intake for fat, fibre, and fruits and vegetables. Fat intake was reduced by about one-third; fibre increased by about 75%; fruit and vegetable intake increased by about two-thirds. As we expected, other dietary factors changed as well. For example, intake of red meat dropped by about 25%; consumption of whole grains increased by about 40%. Although we did not observe a statistically significant drop in serum cholesterol (the polyunsaturated saturated fat ratio, not a focus of this study, was essentially unchanged), there was, in the intervention compared to control arm participants, a statistically significant increase in serum carotenoids as well as a significant reduction in body weight. (Changes at 4 years were somewhat less than those observed at the end of the first year.)

The disappointing results of the PPT are reflected in Table 3. Adenoma recurrence proportions were virtually identical in the intervention and control arms. Nor was there any significant difference in recurrence of large or advanced (defined as 1 cm or more in size, having high-grade dysplasia or having at least 25% villous elements).

The straightforward interpretation of these PPT results is that dietary change has no effect on colorectal neoplasia and, by inference, on colorectal cancer. It is important, however, to recognize the limitations of the PPT polyp trial model. First, the intervention and follow-up lasted only 4 years. It is possible that the intervention needs to occur over a longer period of time. It is also possible, particularly if diet affects early events in the neoplastic process, that participants need to be followed for a longer period of time before treatment differences in adenoma recurrence emerge. In that regard, we are continuing to follow PPT participants, without active intervention, for an additional 5 years.

The polyp trial model involves only a limited segment of neoplasia history: all participants have already had one or more adenomas and most recurrent lesions are small. Therefore this model cannot evaluate the effect of diet on either the pre-adenoma state or the progression of small adenomas to large adenomas or invasive cancer.

Finally, we may not have intervened with the optimum diet. It is conceivable that more extreme changes (in, say, fat intake or fruit and vegetable intake) are necessary before an effect is observed. Changes in other dietary factors may be required. Perhaps more than a 25% reduction in red meat is necessary before adenoma recurrence is affected. Finally, although modest changes in 'hard' endpoints such as blood carotenoids and body weight were observed, we cannot completely rule out the possibility that intervention participants did not truly make all the reported dietary changes.

Thus, the results of this study should not be taken as proving that dietary change is ineffective in reducing the risk of colorectal cancer. Nor do the findings mean that the fat, fibre, and fruit and vegetable hypotheses are dead. Nevertheless, the PPT did not provide evidence that a low fat, high-fibre, fruit- and vegetable-enhanced diet can reduce the risk of large bowel cancer. We clearly have not yet resolved the diet–colorectal cancer question.

References

Giovannucci, E., Stampfer, M.J., Colditz, G., Rimm, E.B. & Willett, W.C. (1992) Relationship of diet to risk of colorectal adenoma in men. *J. Natl. Cancer Inst.*, **84**, 91–98

Kritchevsky, D. (1999) Protective role of wheat bran fiber: preclinical data. *Am. J. Med.*, **106**, Suppl 1A, 28S–31S

Potter, J.D., Slattery, M.L., Bostick, R.M. & Gapstur, S.M. (1993) Colon cancer: a review of the epidemiology. *Epidemiol. Rev.*, **15**, 499–545

Schatzkin, A., Lanza, E., Corle, D., Lance, P., Iber, F., Caan, B., Shike, M., Weissfeld, J., Burt, R., Cooper, M.R., Kikendall, J.W., Cahill, J. & Polyp Prevention Trial Study Group. (2000) Lack of effect of a low-fat, high-fiber diet on the recurrence of colorectal adenomas. *N. Engl. J. Med.*, **342**, 1149–1155

Zhao, L.P., Kushi, L.H., Klein, R.D. & Prentice, R.L. (1991) Quantitative review of studies of dietary fat and rat colon carcinoma. *Nutr. Cancer*, **15**, 169–177

Chapter 9

Gene–nutrient interactions

DNA adducts and the protective role of fruits and vegetables

Vineis P.

University of Torino and CPO-Piemonte, via Santena 7, Torino, Italy and ISI Foundation, Institute for Scientific Interchange, viale Settimio Severo 65, Torino, Italy.

A Darwinian model of carcinogenesis

Breivik (2001) has suggested that cancer can arise as a consequence of a Darwinian selection process related to genetic instability, i.e. genome-wide elevation of mutation rate in cancer cells. Such cells would not repair DNA damage and tend to substitute normal cells. According to Breivik, a combination of epidemiology, mutagenic fingerprints, and DNA repair mechanisms points to a miscellaneous group of agents that cause large alterations in the structure of DNA. Such bulky-adduct-forming (BAF) mutagens, comprising dietary components, pollutants, and intrinsic metabolites, appear as primary candidates for a selection pressure that promotes CIN (chromosomal instability). Two different phenotypes in cancer are chromosome instability (CIN), which is the dominating phenotype of cancer cells and is recognized as numerical and structural aberrations of the genome, and microsatellite instability (MIN), which involves slippage of the repeat number at microsatellite loci. A relationship between the CIN phenotype and BAF mutagens has now been demonstrated in a model system, i.e. an experiment conducted by Bardelli and colleagues (2001) with the food-borne carcinogen PhIP. Since it has been proposed that the type of genetic instability in cancer cells reflects the selection pressures exerted by specific carcinogens, Bardelli and colleagues have tested this hypothesis by treating immortal, genetically stable human cells with different carcinogens. They found that cells resistant to 2-amino-1-methyl-6-phenylimidazo[4,5-b]pyridine (PhIP) exhibited CIN, whereas cells resistant to the methylating agent N-methyl-N'-nitro-N-nitrosoguanidine (MNNG) exhibited MIN associated with mismatch repair defects. Conversely, they found that cells purposely made into CIN cells were resistant to PhIP, whereas MIN cells were resistant to MNNG. Interestingly, PhIP is a diet-borne carcinogen that causes the formation of bulky adducts and induces colon and breast cancer in rats and mice (Table 1).

According to Breivik, cancer can be compared to the “cell cycle Grand Prix” in the following scenario: “Team I always stops for repairs when a problem is indicated, whereas team II ignores all warning lights. Team I wins under ordinary conditions because it always has a faultless vehicle, whereas team II accumulates errors. In the harsher environment the vehicles accumulate damage more quickly than can be repaired, and team I gets trapped in the

Table 1. Results of experiments in animals orally treated with selected heterocyclic amines (From Bogen, 1994)

Compound	Species	Dose (mg/kg/day)	Incidence of colon cancer[a] Exposed	Controls
Glu-P-1	Rats M	3.8	19/42	0/50
Glu-P-1	Rats F	3.8	7/42	0/50
Glu-P-1	Mice M	17	6/42	0/50
Glu-P-1	Mice F	16	8/42	0/50
IQ	Rats M	1.4	25/40	0/50
IQ	Rats F	3.3	9/40	0/50
MeIQ	Rats M	0.71	7/20	0/20
MeIQ	Rats F	0.72	5/20	0/20
PhIP	Rats M	2.1	16/29	0/40

[a]No. animals with tumours / total number of animals alive at the time of first death.
M, male; F, female.

checkpoint. Team II, on the other hand, jerks along in its faulty vehicle with a fair chance of making the finish line. This simple assessment of repair strategies thereby provides an explanation for the paradox that mutagenic environments favor repair deficiency." (Breivik, 2001).

The role of bulky adducts in carcinogenesis

If we accept the carcinogenesis model proposed by Breivik, we can understand some epidemiological observations concerning DNA adducts, which we briefly summarize in the following. Bulky DNA adducts (those that seem to be a prelude to CIN) share a number of properties: (a) they tend to be associated with exposures to aromatic compounds including PhIP; (b) their level is influenced by metabolic polymorphisms and their susceptibility is related to DNA repair; (c) their level is influenced by components of fruit and vegetables (possibly folic acid); (d) they are predictive of the risk of cancer. I will mainly refer to bulky adducts measured by ^{32}P-postlabelling in white blood cells (WBC), although evidence on other types of adducts is also relevant.

Concerning point (a), WBC bulky adducts have not been generally associated with known exposures, including smoking, whereas a clearcut association has been found in target organs such as the lung (Hemminki *et al.*, 2000). For example, Alexandrov *et al.*, (1992) found an association between the number of cigarettes smoked and the level of aromatic adducts in the lung biopsies of lung cancer patients.

A particularly interesting adduct-forming agent is PhIP, which is formed in fried or charbroiled meat and fish. Oral administration of PhIP to hamsters resulted in DNA adducts in the pancreas, bladder and colon (Fretland *et al.*, 2001). PhIP adducts are partly repaired by the XPA repair system and mice deficient in the XPA gene had twice as high levels of adducts in the liver, colon and lung as wild type mice (Imaida *et al.*, 2000). XPA has an essential role in the damage recognition step of nucleotide excision repair (NER), a crucial pathway in the maintenance of genome stability.

As regards point (b), there is a fair amount of literature on gene–environment interactions, that I will not summarize here; I refer the reader to a recent review on adduct levels and metabolic polymorphisms (Bartsch, 2000). In addition to metabolic susceptibility, susceptibility based on DNA repair is also involved. For example, we have shown in the context of the EPIC investigation that DNA repair polymorphisms, and more specifically XRCC3 polymorphisms, are associated with variable levels of bulky adducts, after adjustment for relevant exposures (Table 2). XRCC3 participates in DNA double-strand break-recombination repair and is a member of an emerging family of proteins that likely participate in homologous recombination to maintain chromosome stability and repair DNA. Therefore, adducts seem to integrate not only external exposure, but also individual susceptibility related to carcinogen metabolism and DNA repair.

With reference to point (c), in the same Italian EPIC population, we have demonstrated that the levels of adducts are negatively correlated with the consumption of fruit and vegetables (Palli *et al.*, 2000). This observation is not new; in particular, experimental studies have shown that eating fruit and vegetables decreased the levels of oxidative damage to DNA. For example, Thompson *et al.* (1999) tailored a special cuisine in order to increase the intake of fruit and vegetables from about 5 portions per day to 12 after intervention. The level of 8-OhdG adducts in lymphocytes decreased by 32% and in the urine it decreased by 57%. In another study, Verhagen *et al.* (1997) fed Brussels sprouts to healthy non-smoking volunteers, leading to a statistically significant 28% reduction in 8-OhdG adducts. Also, rats treated with freeze-dried strawberries and a carcinogen (NMBA) developed fewer oesophageal tumours and had fewer O6-methylguanine adducts in the oesophageal mucosa than rats treated with NMBA alone (Carlton *et al.*, 2001)

Although it is not directly related to DNA adducts, an interesting observation has been made by Nyberg *et al.* (2001) among 158 lung cancer patients and 154 controls. Significantly decreased HPRT mutation frequency in lymphocytes was demonstrated in relation to intake of vegetables, citrus fruit and berries, suggesting that components of such dietary items can directly or indirectly modulate somatic mutagenesis (hypoxanthine-guanine phosphoribosyl-transferase, HPRT, is a reporter gene used to study mutagenesis *in vivo*). Previous studies had shown a good correlation between the level of aromatic DNA adducts and HPRT mutation frequency (Beland, 1995; Chen *et al.*, 2001).

With regard to point (d), bulky adducts seem to predict the occurrence of cancer, at least in the lung and the bladder (Vineis & Perera, 2000). In brief, a number of case–control studies of lung cancer and one on bladder cancer show that a high level of adducts is associated with statistically significant relative risks in the order of 5 to 7 (Peluso *et al.*, 2000; Vulimiri *et al.*, 2000; Li *et al.*, 1996; Tang *et al.*, 1995; Cheng *et al.*, 2001), with one exception (Hou *et al.*, 1999). Interestingly, such estimates persist after adjustment for the relevant risk factors such as smoking, indicating that DNA bulky adducts are independently predictive of risk. The study by Cheng *et al.* (2001) was conducted among non-smokers and showed both that DNA adducts were higher in cases than in controls (P=0.0001) and that they were higher in women than in men. One might object that such observations have been made in the context of cross-sectional studies, i.e. adducts were measured in cases when cancer was already present and their level could be influenced by metabolic impairment associated with cancer. However, such criticism is now overcome by a prospective study on lung cancer (Tang *et al.*, 2001), reporting a relative risk of about 3 in smokers with high levels of adducts, after adjustment for smoking levels; the relative risk increased when only subjects whose blood was drawn more than 5 years before cancer diagnosis were considered. In the study by Peluso (2000) on bladder cancer, the relative risks were 3.0 (95% confidence interval, 1.45–6.1), 5.4 (CI, 2.5–11.7) and 7.9 (CI, 3.4–18.4) in the three highest quartiles of adducts, compared with the lowest quartile, clearly suggesting a dose–response relationship (estimates adjusted by smoking).

Mechanisms for the modulation of DNA adducts

Which are the mechanisms that are hypothesized to explain the positive effect of fruit and vegetables on DNA adducts? At least three have been proposed. One is the hypothesis of the role of antioxidants, which is still alive but would explain only the inhibition of oxidative damage. In addition, it is well known that randomized trials in smokers based on the administration of vitamins failed: two of them were even characterized by an increase in lung cancer (Omenn *et al.*, 1996; Rautalahti *et al.*, 1997). DNA oxidation was not modified by antioxidant administration in a number of experimental studies (Prieme *et al.*, 1998; Collins *et al.*, 1998; Van Poppel *et al.*, 1995).

A second potential mechanism is related to induction of metabolic enzymes by constituents of fruit and vegetables: for example, cruciferous vegetables induce CYP1A2, an enzyme involved in the metabolism of aromatic amines and other dietary carcinogens (Kall *et al.*, 1996). Lin *et al.* (1998) have shown a protective effect of broccoli for colorectal adenomas that was present only in GSTM1 null subjects. Isothiocyanates are potent anticarcinogens that induce metabolic enzymes, and are eliminated through conjugation by glutathione-*S*-transferases μ and τ (GSTM1 and GSTT1). In a nicely designed prospective study, London *et al.* (2000) demonstrated that isothiocyanates measured in the urine decreased the risk of lung cancer, particularly in subjects deficient in GSTM1 and GSTT1.

In addition to cruciferous vegetables and isothiocyanates, other chemicals have also been implicated in protecting from adduct formation, possibly via metabolic induction. Phenolics are the most investigated class of compounds. Green tea and black tea, which are rich in phenolics, strongly reduced the formation of PhIP-DNA adducts in the colon, breast and liver of rats (Hirose *et al.*, 1999; Schut & Yao, 2000). Lycopene, a compound that abounds in tomatoes, is a powerful inducer of quinone reductase, GSTs and superoxide dismutase (Breinholt *et al.*, 2000).

A third mechanism is DNA repair. DNA repair enzymes are involved in repairing bulky adducts by the nucleotide excision repair or the double-strand break repair systems. One study shows that the levels of DNA adducts in the EPIC population varies according to the *XRCC3* genotype (Matullo *et al.*, 2001); subjects with the *Met/Met* genotype had a relative risk of 2.7 (95% CI, 1.1–6.7) for having detectable levels of adducts (Table 2). In another study, reduced expression of NER repair genes was associated with an increased risk of lung cancer (Cheng *et al.*, 2001). In addition to such evidence, many phenotypic tests have been conducted, showing that cancer cases have impaired DNA repair as measured by indirect tests, compared with healthy controls (mutagen sensitivity tests; for a review see Berwick & Vineis, 2000). It is likely that such greater sensitivity of cancer cases to the induction of DNA damage by mutagens (including chromosome breaks and carcinogen-DNA adducts) reflects an inherited or acquired susceptibility related to DNA repair systems.

It has been suggested that fruit and vegetables might influence the function of DNA repair genes. Kucuk *et al.* (1995) found a strong inverse relationship between plasma nutrients and the mutagen sensitivity assay (correlation coefficient, –0.76 for beta-carotene and –0.72 for total carotenoids). However, in randomized double-blind trials, Hu *et al.* (1996) and Goodman *et al.* (1998) found no association between supplementation and DNA repair activity.

Rather strong experimental evidence has been provided in studies by Fenech and collaborators, suggesting that folic acid interferes with DNA repair. According to such studies, folic acid plays a critical role in the prevention of chromosome breakage and hypomethylation of DNA. The most plausible explanation for the chromosome-breaking effect of low folate is excessive uracil misincorporation into DNA, a mutagenic lesion that leads to strand breaks in DNA during repair. *In vitro* experiments indicate that genomic instability in human cells is minimized when the folic acid concentration in culture medium is greater than 227 nmol/L, while intervention studies in humans show that DNA hypomethylation, chromosome breaks, uracil misincorporation and micronucleus formation are minimized when red cell folate concentration is greater than 700 nmol/L folate (Fenech, 2001).

Conclusions

The relationships between dietary patterns, adduct formation, individual susceptibility and the risk of cancer are extremely complex. Diet is a particularly interesting field, since much of the metabolic interindividual variation is likely to have originated from the so-called animal–plant warfare, i.e. the elaboration of defensive metabolic responses by animals who ate toxic components of plants. Drug-metabolizing enzymes such as those encoded by the cytochrome *P450* genes have a high degree of interspecies and intraspecies variability. It

Table 2. Distribution of 308 Italian EPIC individuals according to detectable/nondetectable levels of DNA adducts, for three DNA repair genotypes, and for the wild allele homozygotes vs subjects with at least a variant allele (From Matullo *et al.*, 2001)

	All subjects (308) *n*(%)	Nondetectable adducts (83) *n*(%)	Detectable adducts (224) *n*(%)	Crude OR (95% CI)	Adjusted OR[b] (95% CI)	Above[a] (155) *n*(%)	Crude OR (95% CI)	Adjusted OR[b] (95% CI)
XRCC1 exon 10								
Codon 399								
Arg/Arg	134 (43.6)	37 (44.6)	97 (43.3)	1	1	68 (43.9)	1	1
Arg/Gln	139 (45.3)	40 (48.2)	99 (44.2)	0.94 (0.55–1.60)	0.95 (0.53–1.70)	68 (43.9)	0.92 (0.57–1.49)	0.90 (0.53–1.53)
Gln/Gln	34 (11.1)	6 (7.2)	28 (12.5)	1.78 (0.68–4.65)	1.87 (0.69–5.07)	19 (12.3)	1.22 (0.57–2.62)	1.45 (0.64–3.31)
Gln/Gln + Arg/Gln	173 (56.4)	46 (55.4)	127 (56.7)	1.05 (0.63–1.75)	1.08 (0.63–1.87)	87 (56.2)	0.98 (0.62–1.54)	1.02 (0.62–1.67)
		χ^2=1.755[c]	*P*=0.416			*P*=0.765		
XRCC3 exon 7								
Codon 241								
Thr/Thr	104 (33.8)	33 (39.8)	71 (31.6)	1	1	45 (29)	1	1
Thr/Met	149 (48.4)	42 (50.6)	107 (47.6)	1.18 (0.68–2.04)	1.33 (0.73–2.41)	71 (45.8)	1.19 (0.72–1.97)	1.31 (0.75–2.30)
Met/Met	55 (17.9)	8 (9.6)	47 (20.8)	2.73 (1.16–6.42)[a]	2.68 (1.07–6.68)	39 (25.2)	3.19 (1.58–6.42)[a]	4.01 (1.82–8.83)[a]
Met/Met + Thr/Met	204 (66.3)	50 (60.2)	154 (68.4)	1.43 (0.85–2.41)	1.54 (0.87–2.72)	110 (71.0)	1.53 (0.95–2.47)	1.70 (1.00–2.89)[a]
		χ^2=5.622[c]	*P*=0.060			*P*=0.003[a]		
XPD Exon 23								
Codon 751								
Lys/Lys	102 (33.1)	28 (33.7)	74 (32.9)	1	1	48 (31)	1	1
Lys/Gln	157 (51)	42 (50.6)	115 (51.1)	1.04 (0.59–1.81)	1.06 (0.58–1.94)	80 (51.6)	1.16 (0.71–1.92)	1.19 (0.68–2.08)
Gln/Gln	49 (15.9)	13 (15.7)	36 (16.0)	1.05 (0.49–2.26)	1.25 (0.54–2.88)	27 (17.4)	1.38 (0.70–2.73)	1.53 (0.71–3.27)
Gln/Gln + Lys/Gln	206 (66.9)	55 (66.3)	151 (67.1)	1.04 (0.61–1.77)	1.11 (0.63–1.97)	107 (69.0)	1.21 (0.75–1.95)	1.25 (0.74–2.10)
		χ^2=0.021[c]	*P*=0.990			*P*=0.635		

[a]Statistically significant comparison.

[b]Below and above 4.9 per 10^9 RAL (relative adduct labeling x 10^9) median value.

[c]Multivariate logistic regression: OR adjusted by age, sex, BMI, centres, month and year of blood drawing, repair genes and smoking status.

[d]3 x 2 contingency table χ^2 test for the three different genotypes above/below RAL median value and between detectable/nondetectable groups.

OR, odds ratio; CI, confidence interval.

is generally believed that such diversity is the result of coevolution of plants producing toxic compounds and animals responding with new enzymes to detoxify these chemicals (Gonzales & Nebert, 1990). The evolutionary meaning of DNA repair genes is less clear (Eisen & Hanawalt, 1999).

This is the context in which the meaning of genetically based susceptibility to disease must be understood. According to the interpretation put forward by Manfred Eigen (1992), different individuals belonging to a species carry variants of each gene, which allow them to find better adaptation to the environmental changes: "Functionally competent mutants, whose *selection values* come close to that of the wild type (though remaining below it), reach far higher population numbers than those that are functionally ineffective. An asymmetric spectrum of mutants builds up, in which mutants far removed from the wild type arise successively from intermediates. The population in such a chain of mutants is influenced decisively by the structure of the *value landscape*. The value landscape consists of connected plains, hills and mountain ranges. In the mountain ranges, the mutant spectrum is widely scattered, and along ridges even distant relatives of the wild type appear with finite frequency. It is precisely in the mountainous region that further selectively superior mutants can be expected. As soon as one of these turns up on the periphery of the mutation spectrum the established ensemble collapses. A new ensemble builds up around the superior mutant, which thus takes over the role of the wild type... This causal chain results in a kind of 'mass action', by which the superior mutants are tested with much higher probability than inferior mutants, even if the latter are an equal distance away from the wild type" (Eigen, 1992). This description can be used both to understand how so-called superior mutant individuals are selected to adapt to particular external environments (including metabolic variants in the animal–plant warfare) and to understand the cancer process, i.e. how mutant cells are selected because of a proliferative advantage in a changing internal environment. In this context, the study of the relationships between DNA adducts, dietary components and the risk of cancer is likely to be crucial.

Acknowledgements

This study has been made possible by grants from the European Commission (V Network Programme, Quality of Life Contract No. QLK4-CT-1999-00927), by the Associazione Italiana per le Ricerche sul Cancro, by the Compagnia San Paolo (Torino), and by the World Cancer Research Fund.

References

Alexandrov, K., Rojas, M., Geneste, O., Castegnaro, M., Camus, A.M., Petruzzelli, S., Giuntini, C. & Bartsch, H. (1992) An improved fluorometric assay for dosimetry of benzo(a)pyrene diol-epoxide-DNA adducts in smokers' lung: comparisons with total bulky adducts and aryl hydrocarbon hydroxylase activity. *Cancer Res.*, **52**, 6248–6253

Bardelli, A., Cahill, D.P., Lederer, G., Speicher, M.R., Kinzler, K.W., Vogelstein, B. & Lengauer, C. (2001) Carcinogen-specific induction of genetic instability. *Proc. Natl. Acad. Sci. U S A*, **98**, 5770–5775

Bartsch, H. (2000) Studies on biomarkers in cancer etiology and prevention: a summary and challenge of 20 years of interdisciplinary research. *Mutat. Res.*, **462**, 255–279

Beland, F.A. (1995) DNA adduct formation and T lymphocyte mutation induction in F344 rats implanted with tumorigenic doses of 1,6-dinitropyrene. *Res. Rep. Health Eff. Inst.*, **72**, 1–27

Berwick, M. & Vineis, P. (2000) Markers of DNA repair and susceptibility to cancer in humans: an epidemiologic review. *J. Natl. Cancer Inst.*, **92**, 874–897

Bogen, K.T. (1994) Cancer potencies of heterocyclic amines found in cooked foods. *Food Chem. Toxic.*, **32**, 505–515

Breinholt, V., Lauridsen, S.T., Daneshvar, B. & Jakobsen, J. (2000) Dose-response effects of lycopene on selected drug-metabolizing and antioxidant enzymes in the rat. *Cancer Lett.*, **154**, 201–210

Breivik, J. (2001) Don't stop for repairs in a war zone: Darwinian evolution unites genes and environment in cancer development. *Proc. Natl. Acad. Sci. U S A*, **98**, 5379–5381

Carlton, P.S., Kresty, L.A., Siglin, J.C., Morse, M.A., Lu, J., Morgan, C. & Stoner, G.D. (2001) Inhibition of N-nitrosomethyl-benzylamine-induced tumorigenesis in the rat esophagus by dietary freeze-dried strawberries. *Carcinogenesis*, **22**, 441–446

Chen, T., Mittelstaedt, R.A., Aidoo, A., Hamilton, L.P., Beland, F.A., Casciano, D.A. & Heflich, R.H. (2001) Comparison of hprt and lacI mutant frequency with DNA adduct formation in N-hydroxy-2-acetylaminofluorene-treated Big Blue rats. *Environ. Mol. Mutagen.*, **37**, 195–202

Cheng, Y.W., Hsieh, L.L., Lin, P.P., Chen, C.P., Chen, C.Y., Lin, T.S., Su, J.M. & Lee, H. (2001) Gender difference in DNA adduct levels among nonsmoking lung cancer patients. *Environ. Mol. Mutagen.*, **37**, 304–310

Collins, A.R., Olmedilla, B., Southon, S., Granado, F. & Duthie, S.J. (1998) Serum carotenoids and oxidative DNA damage in human lymphocytes. *Carcinogenesis*, **19**, 2159–2162

Eigen, M. (1992) *Steps Towards Life.* Oxford, Oxford University Press

Eisen, J.A. & Hanawalt, P.C. (1999) A phylogenomic study of DNA repair genes, proteins, and processes. *Mutat. Res.*, **435**, 171–213

Fenech, M. (2001) Recommended dietary allowances (RDAs) for genomic stability. *Mutat. Res.*, **480–481**, 51–54

Fretland, A.J., Devanaboyina, U.S., Nangju, N.A., Leff, M.A., Xiao, G.H., Webb, S.J., Doll, M.A. & Hein, D.W. (2001) DNA adduct levels and absence of tumors in female rapid and slow acetylator congenic hamsters administered the rat mammary carcinogen 2-amino-1-methyl-6-phenylimidaz. *J. Biochem. Mol. Toxicol.*, **15**, 26–33

Gonzalez, F.J. & Nebert, D.W. (1990) Evolution of the P450 gene superfamily: animal-plant 'warfare', molecular drive and human genetic differences in drug oxidation. *Trends Genet.*, **6**, 182–186

Goodman, M.T., Hernandez, S., Wilkens, L.R., Lee, J., Le Marchand, L., Liu, L.Q., Franke, A.A., Kukuc, O. & Hsu, T.C. (1998) Effects of beta-carotene and alpha-tocopherol on bleomycin-induced chromosomal damage. *Cancer Epidemiol. Biomarkers Prev.*, **7**, 113–117

Hemminki, K., Koskinen, M., Rajaniemi, H. & Zhao, C. (2000) DNA adducts, mutations, and cancer 2000. *Regul. Toxicol. Pharmacol.*, **32**, 264-75

Hirose, M., Takahashi, S., Ogawa, K., Futakuchi, M. & Shirai, T. (1999) Phenolics: blocking agents for heterocyclic amine-induced carcinogenesis. *Food Chem. Toxicol.*, **37**, 985–992

Hou, S.M., Yang, K., Nyberg, F., Hemminki, K., Pershagen, G. & Lambert, B. (1999) Hprt mutant frequency and aromatic DNA adduct level in non-smoking and smoking lung cancer patients and population controls. *Carcinogenesis*, **20**, 437–444

Hu, J.J., Roush, G.C., Berwick, M., Dubin, N., Mahabir, S., Chandiramani, M. & Boorstein, R. (1996) Effects of dietary supplementation of alpha-tocopherol on plasma glutathione and DNA repair activities. *Cancer Epidemiol. Biomarkers Prev.*, **5**, 263–270

Imaida, K., Ogawa, K., Takahashi, S., Ito, T., Yamaguchi, T., Totsuka, Y., Wakabayashi, K., Tanaka, K., Ito, N. & Shirai, T. (2000) Delay of DNA-adduct repair and severe toxicity in xeroderma pigmentosum group A gene (XPA) deficient mice treated with 2-amino-1-methyl-6-phenyl-imidazo [4,5-b] pyridine (PhIP). *Cancer Lett.*, **150**, 63–69

Kall, M.A., Vang, O. & Clausen, J. (1996) Effects of dietary broccoli on human in vivo drug metabolizing enzymes: evaluation of caffeine, oestrone and chlorzoxazone metabolism. *Carcinogenesis*, **17**, 791–799

Kukuc, O., Pung, A., Franke, A.A., Custer, L.J., Wilkens, L.R., Le Marchand, L., Higuchi, C.M., Cooney, R.V. & Hsu, T.C. (1995) Correlations between mutagen sensitivity and plasma nutrient levels of healthy individuals. *Cancer Epidemiol. Biomarkers Prev.*, **4**, 212–221

Li, D., Wang, M., Cheng, L., Spitz, M.R., Hittelmen, W.N. & Wei, Q. (1996) In vitro induction of benzo(a)pyrene diol epoxide-DNA adducts in peripheral lymphocytes as a susceptibility marker for human lung cancer. *Cancer Res.*, **56**, 3638–3641

Lin, H.J., Probst-Hensch, N.M., Louie, A.D., Kau, I.H., Witte, J.S., Ingles, S.A., Frankl, H.D., Lee, E.R. & Haile, R.W. (1998) Glutathione transferase null genotype, broccoli, and lower prevalence of colorectal adenomas. *Cancer Epidemiol. Biomarkers Prev.*, **7**, 647–652

London, S.J., Yuan, J.M., Chung, F.L., Gao, Y.T., Coetzee, G.A., Ross, R.K. & Yu, M.C. (2000) Isothiocyanates, glutathione S-transferase M1 and T1 polymorphisms, and lung-cancer risk: a prospective study of men in Shanghai, China. *Lancet*, **356**, 724–729

Matullo, G., Palli, D., Peluso, M., Guarrera, S., Carturan, S., Celentano, E., Krogh, V., Munnia, A., Tumino, R., Polidoro, S., Piazza, A. & Vineis, P. (2001) XRCC1, XRCC3, XPD gene polymorphisms, smoking and (32)P-DNA adducts in a sample of healthy subjects. *Carcinogenesis*, **22**, 1437–1445

Nyberg, F., Hou, S.M., Pershagen, G. & Lambert, B. (2001) Dietary fruit and vegetables, and normal but not low or high intake of carotenoids, protect against somatic mutation (at the HPRET locus) *in vivo* (abstract). ISEE Conference on Environmental and Genetic Influences on Human Health, Garmisch, September 2–8

Omenn, G.S., Goodman, G.E., Thornquist, M.D., Balmes, J., Cullen, M.R., Glass, A., Keogh, J.P., Meyskens, F.L. Jr., Valanis, B., Williams, J.H. Jr., Barnhart, S., Cherniack, M.G., Brodkin, C.A. & Hammar, S. (1996) Risk factors for lung cancer and for intervention effects in CARET, the Beta-Carotene and Retinol Efficacy Trial. *J. Natl. Cancer Inst.*, **88**, 1550–1559

Palli, D., Vineis, P., Russo, A., Berrino, F., Krogh, V., Masala, G., Munnia, A., Panico, S., Taioli, E., Tumino, S., Garte, S. & Peluso, M. (2000) Diet, DNA adducts and metabolic polymorphisms: the EPIC-Italy cross-sectional study. *Int. J. Cancer*, **87**, 444–451

Peluso, M., Airoldi, L., Magagnotti, C., Fiorini, L., Munnia, A., Hautefeuille, A., Malaveille, C. & Vineis, P. (2000) White blood cell DNA adducts and fruit and vegetable consumption in bladder cancer. *Carcinogenesis*, **21**, 183–187

Prieme, H., Loft, S., Klarlund, M., Gronbaek, K., Tonnesen, P. & Poulsen, H.E. (1998) Effect of smoking cessation on oxidative DNA modification estimated by 8-oxo-7,8-dihydro-2'-deoxyguanosine excretion. *Carcinogenesis*, **19**, 347–351

Rautalahti, M., Albanes, D., Virtamo, J., Taylor, P.R., Huttunen, J.K. & Heinonen, O.P. (1997) Beta-carotene did not work: aftermath of the ATBC study. *Cancer Lett.*, **114**, 235–236

Schut, H.A. & Yao, R. (2000) Tea as a potential chemopreventive agent in PhIP carcinogenesis: effects of green tea and black tea on PhIP-DNA adduct formation in female F-344 rats. *Nutr. Cancer*, **36**, 52–58

Tang, D., Santella, R.M., Blackwood, A.M., Young, T.L., Mayer, J., Jaretzki, A., Grantham, S., Tsai, W.Y. & Perera, F.P. (1995) A molecular epidemiological case–control study of lung cancer. *Cancer Epidemiol. Biomarkers Prev.*, **4**, 341–346

Tang, D., Phillips, D.H., Stampfer, M., Mooney, L.A., Hsu, Y., Cho, S., Tsai, W.Y., Ma, J., Cole, K.J., She, M.N. & Perera, F.P. (2001) Association between carcinogen-DNA adducts in white blood cells and lung cancer risk in the Physicians' Health Study. *Cancer Res.*, **61**, 6708–6712

Thompson, H.J., Heimendinger, J., Haegele, A., Sedlacek, S.M., Gillette, C., O'Neill, C., Wolfe, P. & Conry, C. (1999) Effect of increased vegetable and fruit consumption on markers of oxidative cellular damage. *Carcinogenesis*, **20**, 2261–2266

Van Poppel, G., Poulsen, H., Loft, S. & Verhagen, H. (1995) No influence of beta carotene on oxidative DNA damage in male smokers. *J. Natl. Cancer Inst.*, **87**, 310–311

Verhagen, H., de Vries, A., Nijhoff, W.A., Schouten, A., van Poppel, G., Peters, W.H. & van den Berg, H. (1997) Effect of Brussels sprouts on oxidative DNA damage in man. *Cancer Lett.*, **114**, 127–130

Vineis, P. & Perera, F. (2000) DNA adducts as markers of exposure to carcinogens and risk of cancer. *Int. J. Cancer.*, **88**, 325–328

Vulimiri, S.V., Wu X., Baer-Dubowska, W., de Andrade, M., Detry, M., Spitz, M.R. & DiGiovanni, J. (2000) Analysis of aromatic DNA adducts and 7,8-dihydroxy-8-oxo-2'-deoxyguanosine in lymphocyte DNA from a case–control study of lung cancer involving minority populations. *Mol. Carcinogenesis*, **27**, 34–46

Malondialdehyde-DNA adducts in relation to diet and disease risk – a brief overview of recent results

Shuker D.E.G.[1], Atkin W.[2], Bingham S.A.[3], Leuratti C.[4], Singh R.[4]

[1]Department of Chemistry, The Open University, Walton Hall, Milton Keynes MK7 6AA, UK. [2]MRC Toxicology Unit, University of Leicester, Leicester LE1 9HN, UK. [3]MRC Dunn Human Nutrition Centre, Cambridge, UK. [4]ICRF Colorectal Cancer Unit, St. Mark's Hospital, Middlesex, UK.

Introduction

Dietary fat, lipid peroxidation and arachidonic acid metabolism have all been implicated in colorectal carcinogenesis (Giovannucci & Goldin, 1997; Ozdermirler *et al.*, 1998; Hendickse *et al.*, 1994). Lipid peroxidation is initiated by free radical attack of membrane lipids, generating large amounts of reactive products, which have been implicated in tumour initiation and promotion. Since modification of DNA is believed to be an important early step in carcinogenesis, endogenous DNA adducts derived from oxidative stress, lipid peroxidation or other endogenous processes have been proposed as contributors to the etiology of human cancer (Marnett 2000).

Malondialdehyde (MDA) is a major genotoxic carbonyl compound generated by lipid peroxidation (Marnett 1999, 2000). It is also a by-product of the arachidonic acid metabolism in the synthesis of prostaglandins (Marnett 1994b). Both endogenous processes are modulated by dietary factors. For example, lipid peroxidation is stimulated by the presence of high levels of ω-6 polyunsaturated fatty acids (ω-6 PUFAs) and is inhibited by dietary antioxidants. Increased levels of MDA, together with increased levels of PUFAs and prostaglandins (e.g. PGE_2) have been reported in tumour tissues of colorectal cancer patients as compared to their normal mucosa (Hendickse *et al.*, 1994).

MDA is mutagenic in bacterial and mammalian systems (Basu & Marnett, 1983). It reacts with DNA to form adducts with deoxyguanosine, deoxyadenosine and deoxycytidine as well as cross-links (Marnett 1994a). The adduct formed upon reaction with deoxyguanosine, the highly fluorescent cyclic pyrimidopurinone, $1,N^2$ malondialdehyde-deoxyguanosine (M_1-dG), was originally detected in liver DNA from healthy individuals, at levels of 5–11 adducts per 10^7 total bases (Chaudhary *et al.*, 1994). Since then, M_1-dG has been detected in several human tissues at levels ranging from 0.02 to 21 per 10^7 normal bases (Vaca *et al.*, 1995; Rouzer *et al.*, 1997; Everett *et al.*, 2001; Kadlubar *et al.*, 1998). Very interestingly, it has been shown that M_1-dG can also be formed following direct oxidative attack on DNA (Dedon *et al.*, 1998). M_1-dG is a premutagenic lesion and can induce guanine to thymine transversions and guanine to adenine transitions in DNA (Benamira *et al.*, 1995; Fink *et al.*, 1997).

In this brief overview the use of M_1-dG as a marker of exposure to MDA in various studies is summarized. Full accounts of the methodologies and study designs are published elsewhere and can be found in the cited primary publications.

Quantitation of M_1-dG by immunoslot blot assay (ISB)

M_1-dG was quantitated in DNA using an immunoslot blot assay developed by Leuratti *et al.* (1998) with some recent modifications (Leuratti *et al.*, 2002).

The effect of dietary fat intake on M_1-dG in DNA

Fang and co-workers (1996) reported that volunteers on a diet containing high amounts of polyunsaturated fatty acids had higher levels of M_1-dG in leukocyte DNA than individuals on a diet rich in monounsaturated fatty acids. The difference between adduct levels following the two diets was greater in women than in men.

These results suggested a role of diet in modulating adduct levels. Preliminary results from our group have also suggested a dietary influence on M_1-dG levels in human leukocyte DNA (Leuratti *et al.*, 1999).

In a recent study, we have been able to make use of dietary data that had been collected in the UK arm of the EPIC study (Leuratti *et al.*, 2002). Colorectal biopsies from normal mucosa of 162 participants in both the UK Flexiscope Sigmoidoscopy Screening Trial (Atkin *et al.*, 2002) and the EPIC study (Day *et al.*, 1999) were analysed for the presence of M_1-dG, the major DNA adduct formed by reaction of MDA with DNA. The objectives of the study were to investigate whether this adduct can be regarded as a biomarker of specific dietary intake and whether it can be considered a risk factor for the presence of premalignant lesions in humans (see below).

This study showed for the first time that M_1-dG is present in the normal colorectal mucosa in humans. The levels measured had an average value, considering all participants, of 4.42 ± 2.95 per 10^7 total bases. These levels are lower than those detected in our laboratory in human gastric biopsy DNA (Everett *et al.*, 2001). It is likely that this difference in M_1-dG levels is due to tissue-specific differences in adduct formation and removal. In the present study, there was substantial inter-individual variation in adduct levels. Levels in women were slightly, but not significantly, higher than in men. Fang *et al.* (1996) reported higher levels of adducts in the white blood cells of women as compared to men. Similar findings were reported in the same leukocyte samples for etheno adducts, another product of lipid peroxidation (Nair *et al.*, 1997). Similar to our findings for colorectal biopsies, no sex differences in M_1-dG levels were reported for gastric tissue (Everett *et al.*, 2001).

In general, associations between adduct levels and anthropometric as well as environmental factors were more obvious in men than in women. Here, taller men had higher adduct levels and there was a significant inverse association with body mass index. This was an unexpected finding, which is difficult to explain since a positive association would have been predicted from the fact that cohort and prospective studies suggest that excessive body mass is positively correlated with colorectal cancer risk (Potter 1999; World Cancer Research Fund, 1997). No correlation was observed in women. Adduct levels increased with age in men, but not in women. No relationship with smoking was found, confirming other authors' findings (Everett *et al.*, 2001; Kadlubar *et al.*, 1998). A stronger dietary modulation of M_1-dG levels was observed in men, with legumes, nuts, wholemeal bread, cereals, fruits, vegetables, salads and raw tomatoes being protective. High consumption of some of these food items has been associated with protection against colon and rectum cancer.

High intake of beer, alcohol and white meat was positively correlated with adduct levels in men. Epidemiological studies have reported either an increased risk or no association between beer/alcohol consumption and colorectal cancer (Committee on Medical Aspects of Food and Nutrition Policy, COMA 1998). In studies of diet and colorectal adenomas, alcohol is usually considered to be a potential confounder, although there is little clear evidence of effects in the literature (Breuer *et al.*, 2000; Sandler *et al.*, 1998; Giovannucci *et al.*, 1992).

There were no associations between adduct levels and the recorded consumption of about 30 groups of food in women, possibly due to the smaller number of samples analysed and therefore lower statistical power. Differences between the sexes in leukocyte adduct levels in response to diet have been reported in a smaller previous study, in which mainly younger and presumably pre-menopausal women were investigated (Fang *et al.*, 1996). In the present study, all the women were aged 55–65 years and colonic adduct levels were measured. Here, there was a weak positive association between rectal biopsy M_1-dG levels and saturated fatty acid intake in women and an inverse association with the standard dietary ratio of PUFA:saturated fat.

M_1-dG levels in relation to cancer risk

One area where M_1-dG measurements have been studied extensively is in relation to cancer risk with respect to *Helicobacter* infections. *Helicobacter hepaticus* causes hepatocellular carcinoma in infected mice and *Helicobacter pylori* has been associated with increased risks of gastric cancer in humans.

The level of M_1-dG in control A/JCr mouse livers at 3, 6, 9 and 12 months averaged 37.5, 36.6, 24.8 and 30.1 adducts per 10^8 nucleotides, respectively. Higher levels of M_1-dG were detected in the liver DNA of *H. hepaticus*-infected A/JCr mice, with levels averaging 40.7, 47.0, 42.5 and 52.5 adducts per 10^8 nucleotides at 3, 6, 9 and 12 months, respectively. There was a significant age-dependent increase in the level of M_1-dG in the caudate and median lobes of the A/JCr mice relative to control mice. These results suggested that M_1-dG occurs as a result of oxidative stress associated with *H. hepaticus* infection of mice and may contribute to liver carcinogenesis in this model (Singh *et al.*, 2001).

Helicobacter pylori infection is associated with elevated gastric mucosal concentrations of MDA and reduced gastric juice vitamin C concentrations. Levels of antral mucosal M_1-dG were determined in patients

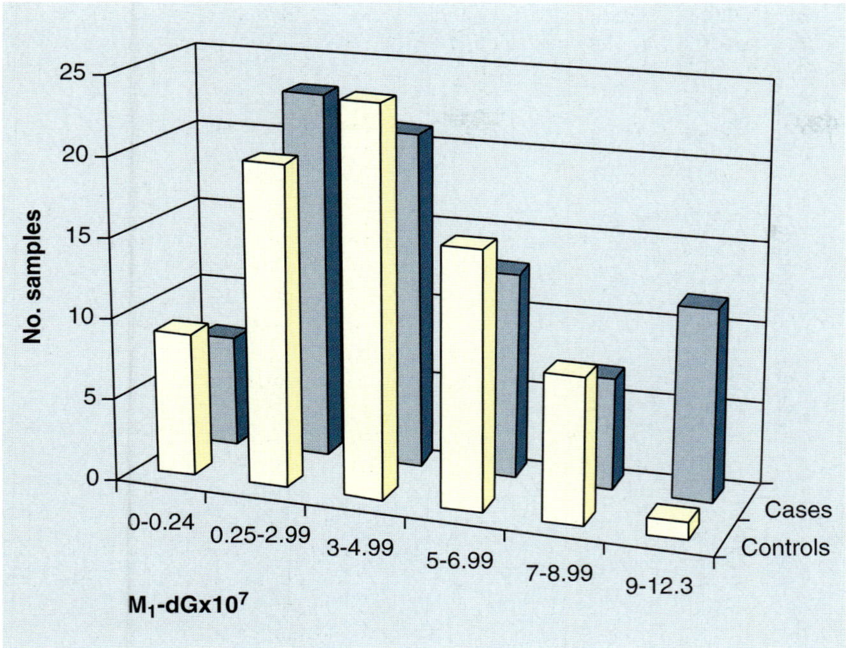

Figure 1
Distribution plot of M_1-dG levels in normal colorectal mucosa of cases and controls (men and women). M_1-dG levels ranged from undetectable (*n*=13) to 12.23 per 10^7 total bases (average, 4.42±2.95 per 10^7 bases)

(*n*=124) attending for endoscopy. Sixty-four *H. pylori*-positive patients received eradication therapy; endoscopy was repeated at 6 and 12 months. Levels of M_1-dG did not differ between subjects with *H. pylori* gastritis (*n*=85) and those with normal mucosa without *H. pylori* infection (*n*=39; 56.6 versus 60.1 adducts/108 bases) and were unaffected by age or smoking habits. Malondialdehyde levels were higher (123.7 versus 82.5 pmol/g; $P<0.001$), gastric juice ascorbic acid was lower (5.7 versus 15.0 mmol/mL; $P<0.001$), and antral mucosal ascorbic acid was unchanged (48.0 versus 42.7 mmol/g) in *H. pylori* gastritis compared with normal mucosa. Multiple regression analysis revealed that M_1-dG increased significantly with increasing levels of malondialdehyde. However, M_1-dG levels were unchanged 6 months after eradication therapy, suggesting that that the infection was not a major modulator of M_1-dG levels in the gastric mucosa. Although the clinical status of these subjects was very well characterized, there was almost no information on dietary habits (Everett *et al.*, 2001).

A recent study on the relationship between M_1-dG adducts and adenomatous polyps suggested that increased levels of DNA damage in normal mucosa were associated with increased risk of development of these precancerous lesions. Table 1 shows the characteristics and mean adduct levels in participants of the Flexiscope/EPIC study described above who were found to have adenomas, compared with adenoma-free individuals. Mean differences were not significant, although Figure 1 shows that cases tended to have higher levels. Twelve individuals with polyps had adduct levels above 9 per 10^7 bases, compared with 1 polyp-free individual. Chi squared testing of differences in adduct levels between the distributions in cases and controls failed to reach statistical significance ($P<0.065$). In females, a marginally significant (P=0.09) trend in relation to the severity of the adenomas was observed with M_1-dG levels (per 10^7 total bases) increasing from 4.06±2.0 in controls to 4.76±3.6 in low-risk and 5.40±2.6 in high-risk women. There were no differences in men (Leuratti *et al.*, 2002).

Conclusions

M_1-dG has been detected in DNA extracted from epithelial tissues from the human gastrointestinal tract as well as from white blood cells. The levels are highly variable from person to person and it is of some interest to determine whether intake of dietary fats and potential modulating factors such as intake of antioxidants contributes to this variation. Ultimately a major objective is to determine whether risk of cancer can be related to specific dietary factors or habits. Experimental models suggest that increasing M_1-dG levels are associated with increasing risk but the endogenous formation of the adduct was related to oxidative stress induced by a chronic infection and not by changes in diet. A recent study which combined collection of DNA from a likely target organ (colon) with information on dietary habits obtained through the UK EPIC study afforded a good opportunity to examine the usefulness of M_1-dG and showed that dietary habits do, to some extent, influence the levels of this mutagenic DNA adduct. Furthermore, risk of early precancerous disease (adenomatous polyps) was also related to increasing M_1-dG levels. It is likely that incorporation of biomarkers of certain types of characteristic DNA damage into studies such as EPIC will lead to an understanding of the molecular processes which link the complex exposure that is our diet to chronic diseases such as cancer.

Table 1. Anthropometric characteristics and MDA-adduct levels (M_1-dG x 10^7 total normal bases) for all participants, men and women in cases (polyps) and controls (C) in a recent study (Leuratti *et al.*, 2002)

Findings[a]	All (162)			Men (100)			Women (62)		
	C	Polyps	Correlation[b] with M_1-dG	C	Polyps	Correlation[b] with M_1-dG	C	Polyps	Correlation[b] with M_1-dG
(No.)	(79)	(83)	(*n*=162) (*P*)	(54)	(46)	(*n*=100) (*P*)	(25)	(37)	(*n*=62) (*P*)
Age (years)	57.7±2.9	58.4±3.1	0.189 ($P \leq 0.02$)	57.6±2.9	58.7±3.2	0.2586 ($P \leq 0.01$)	57.9±3.1	58.1±3.1	0.0738
Height (cm)	171.7±8.8	169.5±9.2	0.045	175.7±6.9	175.5±6.4	0.2178 ($P \leq 0.05$)	163±5.3	161.9±5.9	−0.0946
Weight (kg)	76.6±9.8	74.9±10.9	−0.046	78.4±8.0	79.8±7.7	−0.060	72.8±12.3	68.8±11.3	0.002
BMI (kg/m^2)	26.1±3.4	26.1±3.1	−0.077	25.4±2.1	25.9±2.4	−0.2506 ($P \leq 0.02$)	27.5±5.0	26.2±3.9	0.0467
M_1-dG/10^7 bases (range)	4.11±2.6 (0–11.64)	4.71±3.2 (0–12.23)		4.13±2.8 (0–11.64)	4.52±3.2 (0–12.23)		4.06±2.0 (0.23–8.54)	4.95±3.3 (0–11.56)	

[a]Values are means ± SD.
[b]Pearson's correlation test was used in the analyses.

Acknowledgements

We are extremely grateful to many colleagues, research students and technical staff, acknowledged in the cited publications, who have contributed to the development of the work described in this short overview. We gratefully acknowledge generous support from the UK Food Standards Agency. The EPIC Norfolk Study is funded by the Cancer Research Campaign, the Medical Research Council, the British Heart Foundation, the Food Standards Agency, the Department of Health, and the Europe Against Cancer Programme of the Commission of the European Communities. The UK Flexible Sigmoidoscopy Screening Trial is funded by the Medical Research Council, NHS R&D and the Imperial Cancer Research Fund.

References

Atkin, W.S., Edwards, R., Wardle, J., Northover, J.M.A., Sutton, S., Hart, A.R., Williams, C.B. & Cuzick, J. (2002) Rationale and design of a multicentre randomised trial to evaluate the suitability of flexible sigmoidoscopy as a mass population screening tool to reduce colorectal cancer morbidity and mortality. *J. Med. Screening*, in press

Basu, A.K. & Marnett, L.J. (1983) Unequivocal demonstration that malondialdehyde is a mutagen. *Carcinogenesis*, **4**, 331–333

Benamira, M., Johnson, K., Chaudhary, A., Bruner, K., Tibbetts, C. & Marnett, L.J. (1995) Induction of mutations by replication of malondialdehyde-modified $M_1$3 DNA in Escherichia coli: determination of the extent of DNA modification, genetic requirements for mutagenesis, and types of mutations induced. *Carcinogenesis*, **16**, 93–99

Breuer-Katschinski, B., Nemes, K., Marr, A., Rump, B., Leiendecker, B., Breuer, N. & Goebell H. (2000) Alcohol and cigarette smoking and the risk of colorectal adenomas. *Dig. Dis. Sci.*, **45**, 487-493

Chaudhary, A.K., Nokubo, M., Reddy, G.R., Yeola, S.N., Morrow, J.D., Blair, I.A. & Marnett, L.J. (1994) Detection of endogenous malondialdehyde-deoxyguanosine adducts in human liver. *Science*, **265**, 1580–1582

Report of the Working Group on Diet and Cancer of the Committee on Medical Aspects of Food and Nutrition Policy (COMA). Nutritional aspects of the development of cancer. Report on Health and Social Subjects No. 48. Dpt. of Health: The Stationery Office, Norwich, UK, 1998.

Day, N.E., Oakes, S., Luben, R., Khaw, K.T., Bingham, S.M., Welch, A. & Wareham, N. (1999) EPIC in Norfolk: study design and characteristics of the cohort, *Br. J. Cancer*, **80 (Suppl. 1)**, 95–103

Dedon, P.C., Plastaras, J.P., Rouzer, C.A. & Marnett, L.J. (1998) Indirect mutagenesis by oxidative DNA damage: formation of the pyrimidopurinone adduct of deoxy-guanosine by base propenal. *Proc. Natl. Acad. Sci. U. S. A.*, **95**, 11113–11116

Everett, S.M., Singh, R., Leuratti, C., White, K.L.M., Neville, P., Greenwood, D., Marnett, L.J., Schorah, C.J., Forman, D., Shuker, D.E.G. & Axon, A.T.R. (2001) Levels of malondialdehyde-deoxyguanosine in the gastric mucosa – relationship with lipid peroxidation, ascorbic acid and *Helicobacter pylori*. *Cancer Epidemiol. Biomarkers Prev.*, **10**, 369–376

Fang, J.-L., Vaca, C.E., Valsta, L.M. & Mutanen, M. (1996) Determination of DNA adducts of malondialdehyde in humans: effects of dietary fatty acid composition. *Carcinogenesis*, **17**, 1035–1040

Fink, S.P., Reddy, G.R. & Marnett, L.J. (1997) Mutagenicity in *Escherichia coli* of the major DNA adduct derived from the endogenous mutagen malondialdehyde. *Proc. Natl. Acad. Sci. U. S. A.*, **94**, 8652–8657

Giovannucci, E. & Goldin, B. (1997) The role of fat, fatty acids and total energy intake in the etiology of human colon cancer. *Am. J. Clin. Nutr.*, **66**, 1564S–1571S

Giovannucci, E., Stampfer, M., Colditz, G., Rimm, E. & Willett, W.C. (1992) Relationship of diet to colorectal adenoma in men, *J. Natl. Cancer Inst.*, **84**, 91–98

Hendickse, C.W., Kelly, R.W., Radley, S., Donovan, I.A., Keighley, M.R.B. & Neoptolemos, J.P. (1994) Lipid peroxidation and prostaglandins in colorectal cancer. *Brit. J. Surg.*, **81**, 1219–1223

Kadlubar, F.F., Anderson, K.E., Lang, N.P., Thompson, P.A., MacLeod, S.L., Chou, M.W., Mikhailova, M., Plastaras, J.P., Marnett, L.J., Haussermann, S., Nair, J., Velic, I. & Bartsch, H. (1998) Comparison of DNA adduct levels associated with oxidative stress in human pancreas. *Mutat. Res.*, **405**, 125–133

Leuratti, C., Singh, R., Lagneau, C., Farmer, P.B., Plastaras, J.P., Marnett, L.J. & Shuker, D.E.G. (1998) Determination of malondialdehyde-induced DNA damage in human tissues using an immunoslot blot assay. *Carcinogenesis*, **19**, 1919–1924

Leuratti, C., Singh, R., Deag, E.J., Griech, E., Hughes, R.M., Bingham, S.A., Plastaras, J.P., Marnett, L.J. & Shuker, D.E.G. (1999) A sensitive immunoslot-blot assay for the detection of malondialdehyde-deoxyguanosine in human DNA. In Singer, B. & Bartsch, H., eds, *Exocyclic DNA Adducts in Mutagenesis and Carcinogenesis* (IARC Scientific Publications, No. 150), Lyon, IARC, pp. 197–203

Leuratti, C., Watson, M.A., Deag, E.J., Welch, A., Singh, R., Gottschalg, E., Atkin, W., Day, N.E., Shuker, D.E.G. & Bingham, S.A. (2002) Detection of malondialdehyde-DNA adducts in human colorectal mucosa: relationship with diet and presence of adenomas. *Cancer Epidemiol. Biomarkers* Prev., in press

Marnett, L.J. (1994a) DNA adducts of α,β-unsaturated aldehydes and dicarbonyl compounds. In: Hemminki, K., Dipple, A., Shuker, D.E.G., Kadlubar, F.F., Segerback, D. & Bartsch, H., eds, *DNA Adducts: Identification and Biological Significance* (Scientific Publication, No. 125), Lyon, IARC, pp. 151–163

Marnett, L.J. (1994b) Generation of mutagens during arachidonic acid metabolism. *Cancer Metastasis Rev.*, **13**, 303–308

Marnett, L.J. (1999) Lipid peroxidation – DNA damage by malondialdehyde. *Mutat. Res.*, **424**, 83–95

Marnett, L.J. (2000) Oxyradicals and DNA damage. *Carcinogenesis*, **21**, 361–370

Nair, J., Vaca, C.E., Velic, I., Mutanen, M., Valsta, L.M. & Bartsch, H. (1997) High dietary ω-6 polyunsaturated fatty acids drastically increase the formation of etheno-DNA base adducts in white blood cells of female subjects. *Cancer Epidemiol. Biomarkers Prev.*, **6**, 597–601

Ozdemirler, G., Pabuccoglu, H., Bulut, T., Bugra, D., Uysal, M. & Toker, G. (1998) Increased lipoperoxide levels and antioxidant system in colorectal cancer. *J. Cancer Res. Clin. Oncol.*, **124**, 555–559

Potter, J.D. (1999) Colorectal cancer: molecules and populations. *J. Natl. Cancer Inst.*, **91**, 916–932

Rouzer, C.A., Chaudary, A.K., Nokubo, M., Ferguson, D.M., Reddy, G.R., Blair, I.A. & Marnett, L.J. (1997) Analysis of the malondialdehyde-2'-deoxyguanosine adduct pyrimidopurinone in human leukocyte DNA by gas chromatography/electron capture/negative chemical ionization/mass spectrometry. *Chem. Res. Toxicol.*, **10**, 181–188

Sandler, R., Lyles, C., Peipens, L., McAuliffe, C. & Woosely Kupper, L. (1998) Diet and risk of colorectal adenomas. *J. Natl. Cancer Inst.*, **85**, 884–891

Singh, R., Leuratti, C., Josyula, S., Sipowicz, M.A., Diwan, B.A., Kasprzak, K.S., Schut, H.A.J., Marnett, L.J., Anderson, L.M. & Shuker, D.E.G. (2001) Liver lobe-specific increases in malondialdehyde-DNA adduct formation in the livers of mice following infection with *Helicobacter hepaticus*. *Carcinogenesis*, **22**, 1281–1287

Vaca, C.E., Fang, J.-L., Mutanen, M. & Valsta, L. (1995) ^{32}P-postlabelling determination of DNA adducts of malondialdehyde in humans: total white blood cells and breast tissue. *Carcinogenesis*, **16**, 1847–1851

World Cancer Research Fund (1997) *Food, Nutrition and the Prevention of Cancer: A Global Perspective.* Washington, D.C., WCRF/American Institute for Cancer Research

Meat intake, metabolic genes and colorectal cancer

Le Marchand L.

Cancer Research Center of Hawaii, University of Hawaii, Honolulu, HI 96813, USA.

Recent expert reviews and meta-analyses of the epidemiological data on meat and colorectal cancer (CRC) have concluded that high red meat and processed meat intakes are probable risk factors for this disease (WCRF/AICR, 1997; Norat & Riboli, 2001; Sandhu *et al.*, 2001). These foods, especially when cooked to well-done, may be a source of exposure to chemical carcinogens, such as heterocyclic amines (HAAs), polycyclic hydrocarbons (PAHs) and other pyrolysis products. HAAs are formed when meat or fish is cooked at a high temperature for a long duration, whereas PAHs are formed when meat is cooked directly above the heat source (e.g., on a grill) (Sugimura, 1985). Exposure of the large bowel to *N*-nitroso compounds may also be increased on a high red meat diet, as these compounds are formed in the digestive tract from the reaction of amines with nitrosating agents contained in cured meat (Hecht, 1997) or generated by the colonic flora (Susuki and Mitsuoka, 1981; Bingham *et al.*, 1996). Dietary exposure to HAAs and PAHs, and endogenous formation of nitrosamines are difficult to quantify in free-living individuals.

These compounds require metabolic activation before they can bind to DNA, potentially initiating the carcinogenic process. HAAs require *N*-oxidation by cytochrome P450 1A2 (*CYP1A2*), followed by O-esterification by *N*-acetyltransferase-2 (NAT2) (Turesky *et al.*, 1991). *CYP1A1* plays a major role in metabolizing PAHs into diol-epoxides (Boyland & Sims, 1964). *CYP2E1* is also a key activating enzyme, as it catalyses the hydroxylation of many nitrosamines (Yang *et al.*, 1990). The genes encoding these metabolic enzymes often exhibit inherited sequence variations (polymorphisms), which in some instances have been shown to affect enzyme activity.

At least 10 single nucleotide polymorphisms have been identified in the *NAT2* gene, seven of them resulting in amino acid changes. Combinations of these substitutions result in alleles coding for decreased enzyme activity, five of which (**5A, *5B, *5C, *6A, *7B*) occur with significant frequency (>1%) (Cascorbi *et al.*, 1999). These polymorphisms explain most of the intraindividual variation in NAT2 activity. The *CYP1A2* gene is also thought to be polymorphic; however, no genetic variant has been clearly demonstrated to explain the interindividual variation in the activity of the enzyme. Thus, past studies have used pharmacological probes (e.g., caffeine) to characterize individuals for *CYP1A2* phenotype (Lang *et al.*, 1994). *CYP1A2* is also known to be inducible by various environmental exposures, including smoking (Lang *et al.*, 1994). It has been hypothesized that the rapid NAT2 phenotype confers an increased CRC risk, especially when combined with the rapid *CYP1A2* phenotype and consumption of well-done meat (Lang *et al.*, 1994). Recent studies, which examined the association of NAT2 alone or in combination with some measure of meat or well-done meat intake, have only been weakly supportive of the hypothesis. More striking were the results of Lang *et al.* (1994) who assessed both NAT2 and *CYP1A2* activities in their subjects and found a sixfold increased CRC risk in subjects with both the rapid NAT2 and rapid *CYP1A2* phenotypes and preference for well-done meat.

A 2455 A6G substitution polymorphism in *CYP1A1* has been shown to be associated with increased inducibility of the enzyme (Nerurkar *et al.*, 2000) and has been reported to increase risk of *in situ* CRC in a preliminary study (Sivaraman *et al.*, 1994). Recently, a 96-bp insertion polymorphism in the regulatory region of *CYP2E1* has been associated with an increased induction of the enzyme by obesity or ethanol (MacCarver *et al.*, 1998). The association of these various functional polymorphisms with CRC would provide strong evidence for a role of these classes of chemical carcinogens in the etiology of the disease.

Such associations were tested in a population-based case–control study conducted in Hawaii. We interviewed 727 CRC cases of Japanese, Caucasian or Native Hawaiian ancestry and 727 controls matched on sex, age, and ethnicity. The questionnaire inquired about cooking preference for red meat and included detailed questions on usual consumption of the main types of meat and fish for each of several cooking methods and doneness levels. Exposure to other CRC risk factors was also assessed (macro- and micronutrient intake, physical activity, smoking, aspirin use, etc.). Genotyping was performed by PCR-RFLP methods. A subgroup of 349 cases and 467 controls was also phenotyped for *CYP1A2* by caffeine challenge. *CYP1A2* activity was assessed by measuring the ratio of [1,7-dimethyluric acid (17U) + 1,7-dimethylxanthine (17X)] / caffeine (137X) by high performance liquid chromatography.

The age-, sex-, and ethnicity-adjusted odds ratios (and 95% confidence intervals) for CRC by increasing quartile of total red meat were 1.0, 1.0 (0.7–1.3), 1.3 (1.0–17) and 1.4 (1.0–1.8) (*P* for trend, 0.01). However, after adjustment for other covariates (pack-years, physical activity, aspirin use, body mass index, education, and fibre and calcium intakes), the relationship was no longer present: odds ratios of 1.0, 0.8 (0.5–1.1), 1.1 (0.8–1.5) and 1.0 (0.8–1.5), respectively. This indicates that this association was confounded by known CRC risk factors. A statistically significant association with processed meats was found for both colon and rectal cancer but the odds ratios were stronger for rectal cancer. The fully adjusted odds ratios for colon cancer by increasing quartiles of processed meats were 1.0., 1.0 (0.7–1.5), 1.2 (0.8–1.7)

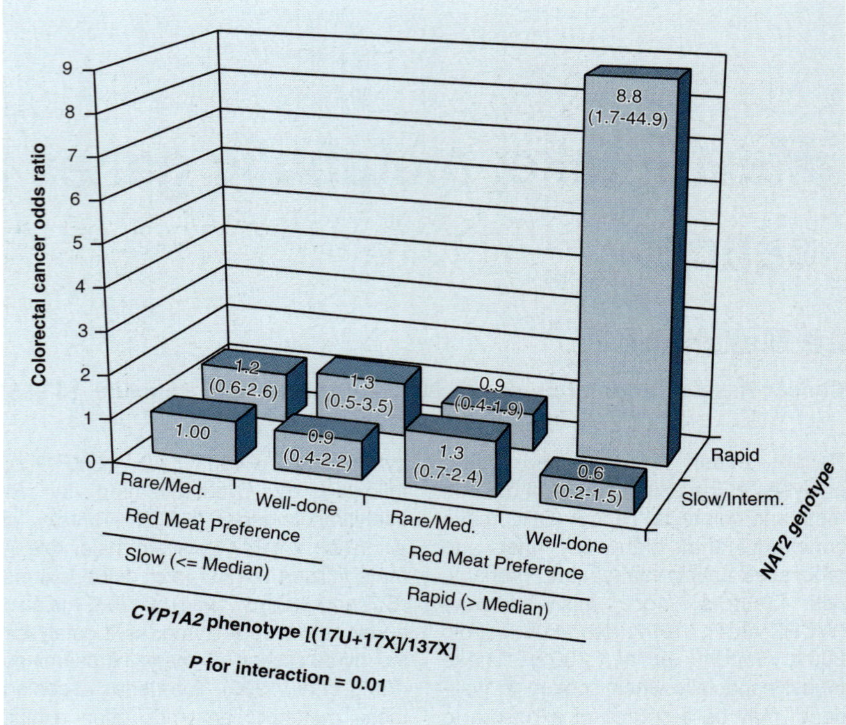

Figure 1
Odds ratios for colorectal cancer by red meat preference, *NAT2* genotype and *CYP1A2* phenotype among ever-smokers. Risk is increased only in the group of subjects with both the rapid *NAT2* and rapid *CYP1A2* phenotypes and who preferred their red meat well-done (*P* for interaction: 0.01)

and 1.4 (1.0–2.1) (*P* for trend, 0.05). The corresponding odds ratios for rectal cancer were 1.0, 1.0 (0.5–1.9), 1.9 (1.0–3.6), 2.1 (1.0–3.7) (*P* for trend, 0.03).

In this study, we also found that preference for well-done red meat was associated with an 8.8-fold increased risk of CRC (95% CI, 1.7–44.9) among ever-smokers with both the rapid NAT2 and rapid *CYP1A2* phenotypes, compared to ever-smokers with low NAT2 and *CYP1A2* activities and who preferred their red meat rare or medium (Fig. 1) (Le Marchand *et al.*, 2001). No similar association was found in never-smokers (data not shown), and there was no increased risk for well-done meat among ever-smokers with a rapid phenotype for only one of these enzymes, or for ever-smokers with both rapid phenotypes who did not prefer their red meat well-done (*P* for interaction, 0.01) (Fig. 1) (Le Marchand, *et al.*, 2001). These data are consistent with those of Lang *et al.* (1994) reviewed above in suggesting that exposure to carcinogens (presumably HAAs) through consumption of well-done meat increases the risk of CRC, particularly in individuals who are genetically susceptible (as determined by a rapid phenotype for both NAT2 and *CYP1A2*). They also suggest that smoking, probably by inducing *CYP1A2*, facilitates this effect.

In our study, the *CYP1A1* 2455G allele was also found to be associated with CRC, especially in Japanese in whom the polymorphism is relatively

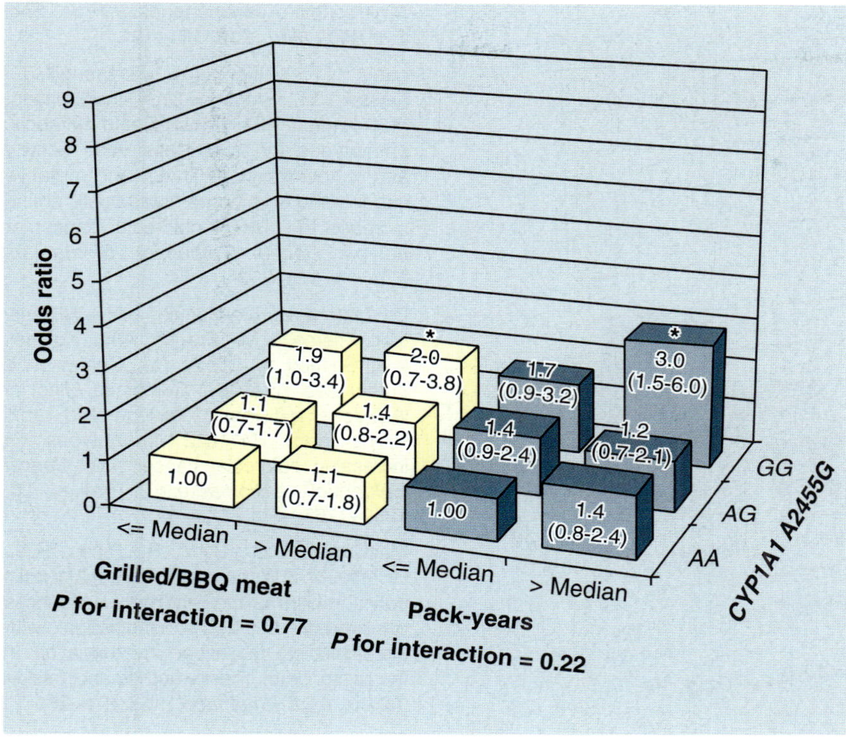

Figure 2
Odds ratios for colorectal cancer by grilled/barbecued meat intake or pack-years and *CYP1A1* A2455G genotype in Japanese. The association between the *CYP1A1* 2455G allele and colorectal cancer appears stronger among subjects with high intake levels of grilled/BBQ meat, and particularly, among heavy smokers

common. In this group, the adjusted odds ratios for the *AA, AG* and *GG* genotypes were 1.0, 1.1 (0.8–1.5) and 1.9 (1.2–2.9), respectively (*P* for gene-dosage effect, 0.02). A stronger gene-dosage effect was suggested among high consumers of grilled/barbecued meat (intake higher than the median), compared to low consumers of these meats (Fig. 2). A stronger association with the *A* allele was also observed for heavy smokers (pack-years greater than the median) compared to light smokers (Fig. 2). Although none of the interaction tests was statistically significant, the data suggest a stronger association between *CYP1A1* and CRC in individuals expected to be exposed to increased levels of PAHs through grilled meat consumption or smoking. No main effect was found for grilled/barbecued meat, whereas smoking significantly increased CRC risk. Comparable results were obtained in two recent studies of colorectal adenomas and a polymorphism in the gene for microsomal epoxide hydroxylase (*mEH*), an enzyme also involved in the metabolic activation of PAHs. In these two studies, an association was found with adenoma only in individuals who reported high levels of well-done meat intake or smoking and who carried the high activity *mEH* allele (Cortessis *et al.*, 2001; Ulrich *et al.*, 2001). Thus, exposure to PAHs appears to increase risk for CRC, especially in individuals genetically more proficient in activating these compounds.

Subjects with the insert variant at the 5' end of *CYP2E1* were found to be at a 60% increased risk (95% CI, 1.1–2.5) for rectal cancer. However, the increase in rectal cancer risk was greater (twofold to threefold) for those subjects who carry the insert and who reported a high intake of red meat or processed meat and were, thus, predicted to have been exposed to increased levels of nitrosamines (Fig. 3) (Le Marchand *et al.*, unpublished). No clear association was found for colon cancer.

Thus, our data provide additional support for the hypothesis that nitrosamines are carcinogenic to the rectum in humans and that red meat and, particularly, processed meats are significant sources of exposure for these compounds. This is consistent with the results of feeding studies conducted in Japan, which showed increased faecal excretion of *N*-nitroso compounds in subjects on a high red meat or processed meat diet. Suzuki and Mitzuoka (1981) found that volatile nitrosamines markedly increase in the faeces of traditional Japanese given a Western diet rich in bacon and beef for 8 days. Similarly, Bingham *et al.* (1996) recently showed in eight British men kept for 3 weeks in a metabolic ward that faecal levels of *N*-nitroso compounds increased fourfold on a high red meat diet (600 g/day) compared with a low red meat diet (60 g/day) or a high white meat and fish diet with similar caloric and fat contents. Faecal nitrite was also shown to increase after changing from a white to red meat diet.

In summary, the data reviewed here suggest that various pyrolysis products (particularly HAAs) that are formed when meat is cooked to well-done or directly above the heat source may increase risk of colorectal cancer, especially among subjects who are genetically more proficient in transforming these compounds into

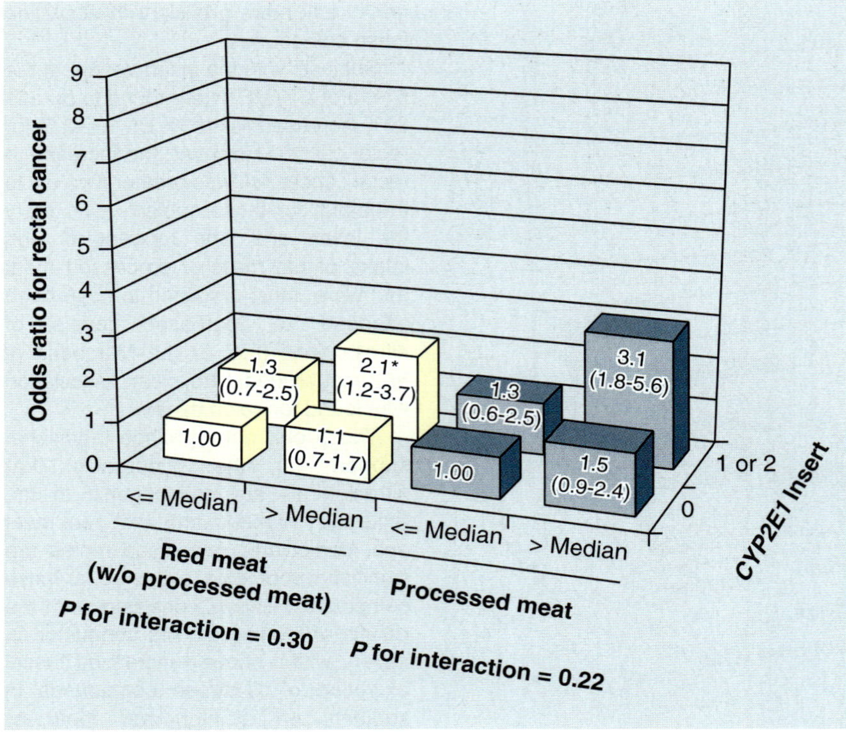

Figure 3

Odds ratios for rectal cancer by red meat intake (excluding processed meat) or processed meat intake and *CYP2E1 5'* insert genotype. The association with the insertion polymorphism is stronger among subjects expected to have had increased exposure to nitrosamines as a result of a high intake of red meat or processed meat

reactive intermediates. Similarly, overall intake of red meat and, particularly, processed meat appears to increase the risk of rectal cancer in individuals who may be genetically more apt to activate nitrosamines. These relationships need to be further explored in large studies, preferably including biomarkers of exposure or early biological effects in order to further increase the specificity of the inferences made from the data.

References

Bingham, S.A., Pignatelli, B., Pollock, J.R.A., Ellul, A., Malaveille, C., Gross, G., Runswick, S., Cummings, J.H. & O'Neill, I.K. (1996) Does increased endogenous formation of *N*-nitroso compounds in the human colon explain the association between red meat and colon cancer? *Carcinogenesis*, **17**, 515–523

Boyland, E. & Sims, P. (1964) Metabolism of polycyclic compounds: the metabolism of pyrene in rats and rabbits. *Biochem. J.*, **90**, 391–398

Cascorbi, I., Brockmoller, J., Mrozikiewicz, P.M., Muller, A. & Roots, I. (1999) Arylamine–acetyltransferase activity in man. *Drug Metab. Rev.*, **31**, 489–502

Cortessis, V., Siegmund, K., Chen, Q., Zhou, N., Diep, A., Frankl, H., Lee, E., Zhu, Q.-S., Haile, R. & Levy, D. (2001) A case–control study of microsomal epoxide hydrolase, smoking, meat consumption, glutathione S-transferase M3, and risk of colorectal adenomas. *Cancer Res.*, **61**, 2382–2385

Hecht, S.S. (1997) Approaches to cancer prevention based on an understanding of *N*-nitrosamine carcinogenesis. *Proc. Soc. Exp. Biol. Med.*, **216**, 181–191

Lang, N.P., Butler, M.A., Massengill, J., Lawson, M., Stotts, R.C., Hauer-Jensen, M. & Kadlubar F.F. (1994) Rapid metabolic phenotypes for acetyltransferase activity and cytochrome *CYP1A2* and putative exposure to food-borne heterocyclic amine increase the risk of colorectal cancer or polyps. *Cancer Epidemiol. Biomarkers Prev.*, **3**, 675–682

Le Marchand, L., Hankin, J.H., Wilkens, L.R., Pierce, L.M., Franke, A.A., Kolonel, L.N., Seifried, A., Custer, L.J., Chang, W. & Lum-Jones, A. (2001) Combined effect of well-done red meat, smoking and rapid NAT2 and *CYP1A2* phenotypes in increasing colorectal cancer risk. *Cancer Epidemiol. Biomarkers Prev.*, **10**, 1259–1266

MacCarver, D.G., Byun, R., Hines, R.N., Hichme, M. & Wegenek, W. (1998) A genetic polymorphism in the regulatory sequences of human *CYP2E1*: association with increased chlorzoxazone hydroxylation in the presence of obesity and ethanol intake. *Toxicol. Appl. Pharmacol.*, **152**, 276–281

Nerurkar, P.V., Okinaka, L., Aoki, C., Seifried, A., Lum-Jones, A., Wilkens, L.R. & Le Marchand L. (2000) *CYP1A1*, GSTM1 and GSTP1 genetic polymorphisms and urinary 1-hydroxypyrene excretion in non-occupationally exposed individuals. *Cancer Epidemiol. Biomarkers Prev.*, **9**, 1119–1122

Norat, T. & Riboli, E. (2001) Meat consumption and colorectal cancer: a review of the epidemiologic evidence. *Nutr. Rev.*, **59**, 37–47

Sandhu, M.S., White, I.R. & McPherson, K. (2001) Systematic review of the prospective cohort studies on meat consumption and colorectal cancer risk: a meta-analytical approach. *Cancer Epidemiol. Biomarkers Prev.*, **10**, 439–446

Sivaraman, L., Leatham, M.P., Yee, J., Wilkens, L.R., Lau, A.F. & Le Marchand, L. (1994) *CYP1A1* genetic polymorphisms and in-situ colorectal cancer. *Cancer Research*, **54**, 3692–3695

Sugimura T. (1985) Carcinogenicity of mutagenic heterocyclic amines formed during the cooking process. *Mut. Res.*, **150**, 33–41

Susuki, K. & Mitsuoka, T. (1981) Increase in faecal nitrosamines in Japanese individuals given a Western diet. *Nature*, **294**, 453–456

Turesky, R.J., Lang, N.P., Butler, M.A., Teitel, C.H. & Kadlubar, F.F. (1991) Metabolic activation of carcinogenic heterocyclic amines by human liver and colon. *Carcinogenesis*, **12**, 1839–1845

Ulrich, C.M., Bigler, J., Whitton, J.A., Bostick, R., Fosdick, L. & Potter, J.D. (2001) Epoxide hydrolase tyr113his polymorphism is associated with elevated risk of colorectal polyps in the presence of smoking and high meat intake. *Cancer Epidemiol. Biomarkers Prev.*, **10**, 875–882

World Cancer Research Fund/American Institute for Cancer Research. (1997) *Food Nutrition and the Prevention of Cancer: A Global Perspective*. Washington, D.C. American Institute for Cancer Research

Yang, C.S, Yoo, J.S.H., Ishizaki, H. & Hong, J. (1990) Cytochrome P450IIE1: role in nitrosamine metabolism and mechanisms of regulation. *Drug Metab. Disp.*, **22**, 147–159

Expression of cytochrome P450 enzymes in human colon

Bernauer U.[1], Ellrich R.[1], Heinrich-Hirsch B.[1], Teubner W.[2], Vieth B.[1], Gundert-Remy, U.[1]

[1]Federal Institute for Health Protection of Consumers and Veterinary Medicine (BgVV), Thielallee 88–92, D-14195 Berlin, Germany. [2]German Institute for Human Nutrition, Arthur-Scheunert-Allee 114–116, D-14558 Potsdam-Rehbrücke, Germany.

Purpose

Colon cancer is one of the most common types of cancer in developed countries. Recently, it has been estimated that environmental factors contribute to the causation of sporadic colorectal cancer by 65% (Lichtenstein *et al.*, 2000). Only about 5%–10% of colorectal tumours can be explained by inheritable susceptibilities, whose genetic basis at the DNA level is already well understood. Nevertheless, even among genetically predisposed persons, considerable variability has been observed in the clinical manifestation of colon cancer (Müller *et al.*, 2000). Therefore, further factors such as environmental impact or genetic–environmental interactions have to be considered for a better understanding of colon carcinogenesis. Formation of colon cancer may be influenced by the ability of the colon to generate reactive and toxic metabolites from orally ingested xenobiotics. Activating enzymes, among them members of the cytochrome P450 (P450) family, play an important role in the formation of reactive metabolites. Little is known about the expression of P450 enzymes in the colon and therefore it was our aim to investigate the expression pattern of xenobiotic-metabolizing P450 enzymes in the human colon. Additionally, due to the great variability in the manifestation of colorectal tumours, which might be influenced by variability in the formation of reactive toxic metabolites, it was our aim to determine P450 variability in human colon.

Methods

Human colon tissues were obtained from 23 histologically non-neoplastic surgical tissue specimens after informed consent. Colon mucosa was homogenated to yield homogenate. Microsomes were prepared and total protein contents were determined.

Western blotting

Proteins (1–30 μg) were separated and blotted as described previously (Bernauer *et al.*, 2000) and probed with commercially available antibodies recognizing the following P450 enzymes: CYP1A1, 1B1, 2A6, 2B6, 2D6, 2E1, 3A (Gentest- Woburn,MS USA), and 2C (Oxford Biomedical Research Oxford MI USA). After incubation with the appropriate second antibodies (Sigma, Saint Louis MO, USA), immunoreactive bands were visualized by the nitro blue tetrazolium method and analyzed densitometrically.

Immunoquantification

Calibration curves of known quantities of P450 standards were prepared. Integrated band densities of human colon microsomes were used to determine P450 concentrations relative to the calibration curves.

Determination of P450 activities

P450 substrates specific for CYP2E1 (chlorzoxazone), CYP2C9 (tolbutamide), CYP2C19 (mephenytoin), and CYP3A4/5 (testosterone) were incubated with pooled colon homogenate from three individuals, a NADPH-generating system, and phenacetin as the internal standard. After solid phase extraction, P450 metabolites were determined by HPLC. Effluents were monitored at 200 nm (6-hydroxy-chlorzoxazone, 6-hydroxytolbutamide, and hydroxy-mephenytoin) and at 240 nm (6β-hydroxytestosterone). Identity of P450 metabolites was confirmed by comparison of their UV spectra with those from commercially available reference compounds.

Analysis of variability

Variability is expressed in different ways: as the standard deviation of the mean value, median and range. In order to standardize the numeric value for variability, the ratios of extreme percentiles (90th/10th and 95th/5th) were calculated using Excel (Microsoft Corp.).

Results

1. After Western blot analysis of human colon microsomes, it was shown that P450 enzymes 1A1, 1B1, 2C9, 2C19, 2D6, 2E1, and 3A were present in the human colon (Fig. 1). P450 enzymes 2A6, 2B6, and 2C8 were below detectable amounts.
2. Among the 23 samples investigated, CYP2E1 and CYP3A proteins could be determined in each sample. CYP1A1, CYP1B1, CYP2C9, CYP2C19, and CYP2D6 were detectable in some samples, but not in all. CYP3A, CYP2E1, and CYP1B1 were the highest, quantitatively, of the P450 enzymes (Table 1).
3. After immunoquantification of the P450 enzymes detectable in the human colon, it was shown that their expression in the colon was low and that the P450 enzymes exhibit different and in some cases considerable variabilities, presented in Table 1.
4. The presence of catalytically active P450 enzymes in human colon was demonstrated by determining chlorzoxazone 6-hydroxylase, tolbutamide hydroxylase, and testosterone 6β-hydroxylase activities in pooled colon homogenate from three individual samples. These activities were characteristic for CYP2E1, CYP2C9, and CYP3A4/5.

Conclusions

Various xenobiotic-metabolizing P450 enzymes are expressed in the human colon, in contrast to previous studies where an absence of P450 enzymes different from CYP1A and CYP3A has been reported (de Waziers *et al.*, 1991; Massaad *et al.*, 1992).

Among the P450 enzymes expressed in human colon are those capable of metabolizing dietary carcinogens into mutagenic metabolites (e.g. CYP1A and CYP1B1, which are involved in the metabolism of food-borne heterocyclic aromatic amines).

The results also show that CYP2E1, CYP2C9 and CYP3A4/5 are expressed in their catalytically active form in the colon, which confirms the results obtained by Western blotting. Immunoquantification of P450 enzymes pointed to a high variability in the colon among different individuals. High variability of P450-dependent metabolism might be the reason for high variability in the formation of reactive metabolites from ingested xenobiotics in the colon. Therefore, variability of xenobiotic metabolizing enzymes in the colon might be a factor leading to differences in susceptibility in formation and clinical manifestation of colon cancer.

References

Bernauer, U., Vieth, B., Ellrich, R., Heinrich-Hirsch, B., Jänig, G.R., & Gundert-Remy, U. (2000) *CYP2E1*

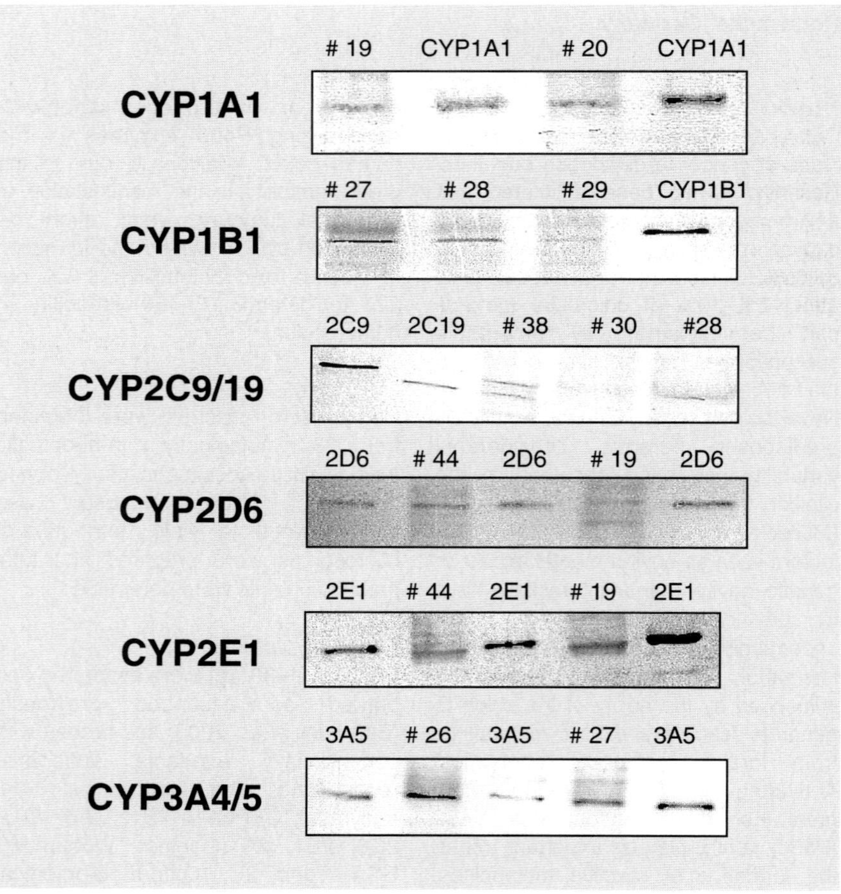

Figure 1
Western blot analysis of CYP1A1, 1B1, 2C, 2D6, 2E1 and CYP3A in selected samples of human colon microsomes (indicated by numbers) and commercially available standards

Table 1. Comparison of different xenobiotic-metabolizing P450 enzymes in human colon microsomes by results obtained after immunoquantification

P450 enzyme	Number of samples where P450 detected	Mean ± SD[a]	Median (range)[a]	P_{90}/P_{10}	P_{95}/P_{05}	Relative quantity[b]
1A1	14	0.35 ± 0.4	0.15 (0.064–1.68)	10.2	16.8	2.8
1B1	21	0.84 ± 0.72	0.54 (0.14–2.9)	7.8	17.8	10.3
2C9	19	0.35 ± 0.25	0.22 (0.07–1.1)	5.9	7.9	4.2
2C19	13	0.24 ± 0.24	0.14 (0.04–0.87)	7.5	11.8	2.7
2D6	11	0.03 ± 0.04	0.007 (0.003–0.11)	30.0	30.5	0.1
2E1	23	0.21 ± 0.1	0.198 (0.07–0.5)	3.2	4.8	3.7
3A	23	4.79 ± 3.3	4.0 (1.06–13.3)	5.8	9.9	76.1

[a]Relative quantity, pmol P450/mg protein.
[b]Percent, calculated from medians.

expression in the bone marrow and its intra- and interspecies variability: approaches for a more reliable extrapolation from one species to another in the risk assessment of chemicals. *Arch. Tox.*, **73**, 618–624

De Waziers, I., Cugnenc, P.H., Yang, C.S., Leroux, J.P., & Beaune, P.H. (1991) Drug-metabolizing enzyme expression in human normal, peritumoral and tumoral colorectal tissue samples. *Carcinogenesis*, **12**, 905–909

Lichtenstein, P., Holm, M.V., Verkasalo, P.K., Iliadou, A., Kaprio, J., Koskenvuo, M., Pukkala, E., Skythe, A., & Hemminki, K. (2000) Environmental and heritable factors in the causation of colon cancer. *N. Eng. J. Med.*, **343**, 78–85

Massaad, L., de Waziers, I., Ribrag, V., Janot, F., Beaune, P., Morizet, J., Gouyette, J., & Chabot, G. (1992) Comparison of mouse and human colon tumors with regard to phase I and phase II drug metabolizing enzyme systems. *Cancer Res.*, **52**, 6567–6575

Müller, H., Heinimann, K., & Dobbie, Z. (2000) Genetics of hereditary colon cancer – a basis for prevention? *Eur. J. Cancer*, **36**, 1215–1223

Role of *EPHX* genotype in the associations of smoking and diet with colorectal adenomas

Tiemersma E.W., Kloosterman J., Bunschoten A., Kok F.J., Kampman E.
Division of Human Nutrition and Epidemiology, Wageningen University, Wageningen, The Netherlands.

Introduction

Humans can be exposed to polycyclic aromatic hydrocarbons (PAH) via cigarette smoke and possibly via intake of foods containing PAH residues formed during production, packaging, or preparation of food. PAH are metabolized by the microsomal epoxide hydrolase enzyme, encoded by the polymorphic *EPHX* gene. Polymorphisms occur in the third and fourth exon. The exon 3 polymorphism leads to a tyrosine (Y) 113→histidine (*H*) substitution in 30%–35% of Caucasians, resulting in a markedly lower enzyme activity in *HH* homozygotes. A histidine (*H*) 139→arginine (*R*) substitution in exon 4 leads to a higher enzyme activity and is found in 15%–20% of Caucasians. As *EPHX* is involved in both activation and detoxification of PAH, genetic variation in the underlying gene may influence the rate of PAH metabolism, and through that, the effect of smoking and intake of foods potentially containing PAH residues on the risk of colorectal adenomas.

Methods

Cases (n=385) and polyp-free controls (n=396) were recruited from an ongoing study between 1997 and 2000 among those undergoing endoscopy at the outpatient clinics of eight Dutch hospitals. Eligible subjects were Dutch-speaking, of European origin, aged 18–75 years at time of endoscopy, had no hereditary colorectal cancer syndromes, chronic inflammatory bowel disease, history of colorectal cancer, or previous bowel resection. We also excluded subjects with only hyperplastic or unknown types of polyps.

Smoking and habitual consumption of foods known to possibly contain PAH residues, such as (barbecued) meat, green leafy vegetables, and fat and oil, were assessed through self-administered questionnaires, one of which was a validated semi-quantitative food frequency questionnaire described in detail elsewhere (Ocké *et al.*, 1997). Information on histology of excised polyps was obtained through medical files. Blood samples were drawn from all participants for DNA extraction. *EPHX* polymorphisms in exon 3 and 4 were determined as we described previously (Tiemersma *et al.*, 2001).

Exposure variables describing smoking habits and consumption of relevant foods were divided in quartiles based on the distribution in the control group. We considered the highest exposure category and the slow genotypes of *EPHX*, i.e. *YH* and *HH* for exon 3 and *HH* for exon 4, as high-risk categories. We calculated odds ratios adjusted for age, gender, and constipation history, and several other potential confounders, depending on the variable under study.

Results

Selected characteristics of the study population are summarized in Table 1. Exposure to cigarette smoke was higher among cases than among controls. Also, cases consumed more fat and oil and green leafy vegetables than controls. The distributions of *EPHX* exon 3 and 4 polymorphisms did not differ between cases and controls.

Table 2 shows risk estimates for colorectal adenomas for the total population and for *EPHX*-defined subgroups. Smoking increased risk of colorectal adenomas. For exon 3, this risk was confined to those with the fast (*YY*, *YH*) genotype. There was no difference in risk between carriers of fast or slow variants of exon 4. Intake of fat and oil was also positively associated with adenomas, but there were no differences between the *EPHX* variants. Total meat intake, green leafy vegetable consumption, and barbecue frequency were not associated with adenomas, and *EPHX* genotype did not influence these associations (data not shown).

Discussion

In this study, we found indications for interplay between *EPHX* genotype and smoking in the etiology of colorectal

Table 1. General characteristics of the study population.

	Cases n=385	Controls n=396
Sex (% male)	54.0[a†]	37.6
Age (years)	59.5 ± 10.5[a]	51.2 ± 13.7
BMI (kg/m^2)	26.1 ±3.8[a]	25.5 ± 4.2
History of constipation in last 3 years (%)	26.2[a]	42.9
Ever smoked cigarettes (%)	62.4[a]	53.3
Cigarette smoking, pack-years[b]	25.0 ± 20.7[a]	18.8 ± 18.9
Total energy (kJ/day)	8725 ± 2594	8652 ± 2629
Fat and oils (g/day)	27.5 ± 14.7[a]	23.8 ± 15.3
Vegetables (g/day)	127.9 ± 52.3	124.2 ± 45.5
Green leafy vegetables (g/day)	23.8 ± 17.8[a]	21.1 ± 15.7
Total meat (g/day)	109.4 ± 54.2	104.6 ± 54.7
Barbecue (frequency/year)	3.1 ± 8.0[a]	3.0 ± 5.7
EPHX exon 3 genotype (% fast, *YY*)	49.4	48.2
EPHX exon 4 genotype (% fast, *HR* or *RR*)	34.8	37.2

[a]Significantly different from controls (P<0.05).
[b]Smokers only.

adenomas. Of two recently published studies, one provided results similar to those of our study (Cortessis *et al.*, 2001), but the other presented opposite findings (Ulrich *et al.*, 2001). These conflicting results can partly be due to differences between the three studies with respect to classification of *EPHX* polymorphisms. Data on genotype–phenotype correlations *in vitro* and *in vivo* are limited, especially for the different combinations of exon 3 and 4 polymorphisms, and we therefore did not combine both. Cortessis and Ulrich both used different classifications of *EPHX*-imputed phenotypes (from fast to very slow) based on the combinations of exon 3 and 4 polymorphisms. Whereas the role of epoxide hydrolase in PAH metabolism is well established (Seidegård & DePierre, 1983), more research on the enzyme activity of combinations of exon 3 and 4 variants and on its effect on PAH-associated neoplasm is needed.

Table 2. Smoking, intake of fat and oil, EPHX-imputed phenotypes, and risk of colorectal adenomas: odds ratios (95% confidence intervals)

		EPHX			
		Exon 3		Exon 4	
	Total population	Fast (*YY*)	Slow (*YH* or *HH*)	Fast (*HR* or *RR*)	Slow (*HH*)
Smoking status[a]					
Never	1.0 (REF)	1.0 (REF)	0.9 (0.6–1.5)	1.0 (REF)	1.6 (0.98–2.8)
Former	1.2 (0.8–1.7)	1.1 (0.6–1.8)	1.2 (0.7–2.1)	1.7 (0.9–3.2)	1.6 (0.9–2.7)
Current	1.7 (1.1–2.5)	2.0 (1.1–3.5)	1.3 (0.7–2.2)	2.6 (1.3–5.0)	2.1 (1.2–3.7)
Pack-years[a]					
None	1.0 (REF)	1.0 (REF)	0.9 (0.6–1.5)	1.0 (REF)	1.7 (1.0–2.8)
≤ 10	1.1 (0.7–1.7)	0.8 (0.4–1.6)	1.3 (0.7–2.3)	2.5 (1.2–5.1)	1.1 (0.6–2.1)
10–20	1.2 (0.8–2.0)	1.5 (0.8–2.8)	0.9 (0.4–1.9)	1.5 (0.7–3.4)	1.8 (0.9–3.6)
>20	1.9 (1.2–2.9)	2.5 (1.3–4.6)	1.4 (0.8–2.6)	2.3 (1.1–4.7)	2.8 (1.5–5.2)
Intake of fat and oil (g/day)[b]					
<15	1.0 (REF)	1.0 (REF)	1.8 (0.9–3.4)	1.0 (REF)	1.6 (0.8–3.3)
15–25	1.5 (0.96–2.4)	2.7 (1.4–5.2)	1.6 (0.9–3.1)	2.1 (0.96–4.6)	2.0 (0.99–4.2)
25–35	1.5 (0.9–2.4)	2.5 (1.2–5.0)	1.5 (0.7–3.1)	1.6 (0.7–3.7)	2.3 (1.1–5.0)
≥ 35	1.8 (1.0–3.1)	2.2 (1.1–4.7)	2.5 (1.2–5.2)	2.2 (0.95–5.3)	2.5 (1.1–5.4)

[a]Adjusted for age, gender, constipation history, and alcohol consumption.
[b]Adjusted for age, gender, constipation history, total energy intake, intake of cereals, and duration of smoking.

From our study, we conclude that the *EPHX* genotype at exon 3 possibly modulates the association between smoking and colorectal adenomas, the fast variant being related to highest risk.

Acknowledgements

This study was funded by the Dutch Cancer Society, grant LUW 96-1374.

References

Cortessis, V., Siegmund, K., Chen, Q., Zhou, N., Diep, A., Frankl, H., Lee, E., Zhu, Q.S., Haile, R. & Levy, D. (2001) A case–control study of microsomal epoxide hydrolase, smoking, meat consumption, glutathione S-transferase M3, and risk of colorectal adenomas. *Cancer Res.*, **61**, 2381–2385

Ocké, M.C., Bueno-de-Mesquita, H.B., Goddijn, H.E., Jansen, A., Pols, M.A., Van Staveren, W.A. & Kromhout, D. (1997) The Dutch EPIC food frequency questionnaire. I. Description of the questionnaire, and relative validity and reproducibility for food groups. *Int. J. Epidemiol.*, **26** Suppl 1, S37–S48

Seidegård, J. & DePierre, J.W. (1983) Microsomal epoxide hydrolase. Properties, regulation and function. *Biochim. Biophys. Acta*, **695**, 251–270

Tiemersma, E.W., Omer, R.E., Bunschoten, A., Van 't Veer, P., Kok, F.J., Idris, M.O., Kadaru, A.M., Fedail, S.S. & Kampman, E. (2001) Role of genetic polymorphism of glutathione-S-transferase T1 and microsomal epoxide hydrolase in aflatoxin-associated hepatocellular carcinoma. *Cancer Epidemiol. Biomarkers Prev.*, **10**, 785–791

Ulrich, C.M., Bigler, J., Whitton, J.A., Bostick, R., Fosdick, L. & Potter, J.D. (2001) Epoxide hydrolase Tyr113His polymorphism is associated with elevated risk of colorectal polyps in the presence of smoking and high meat intake. *Cancer Epidemiol. Biomarkers Prev.*, **10**, 875–882

NQO1 and *mEH* exon 4 (*mEH4*) gene polymorphisms, smoking and colorectal cancer risk

Mitrou P.[1], Watson M.[2], Bingham S.[1], Stebbings W.S.[2], Speakman C.T.[2], Loktionov A.[1]

[1]MRC Dunn Human Nutrition Unit, Cambridge, UK. [2]Norfolk and Norwich Hospital, Norwich, UK.

Introduction

Interindividual susceptibility to colorectal cancer is attributable to environmental factors such as diet and smoking (Giovannucci & Willett, 1994). In addition, genetically inherited variations (polymorphisms) in genes involved in the detoxification of xenobiotics, thereby modulating the cell response to the genotoxic and possibly carcinogenic effects of many xenobiotic chemicals, have been implicated (Joseph & Jaiswal, 1994).

There may also be interactions between environmental and genetic factors, for example, detoxification enzymes present in the intestinal mucosa such as NQO1 and mEH (Roediger & Babidge, 1997; Lafuente *et al.*, 2000) can specifically prevent the formation of benzo(a)pyrene quinone-DNA adducts caused by cigarette smoking (Joseph & Jaiswal, 1994). In this case–control study we have examined whether a C-to-T substitution in exon 6 of *NQO1* and an A-to-G transition in exon 4 of *mEH* (*mEH4*) can confer susceptibility to colorectal cancer either causally or in linkage with environmental factors.

Methods

Study population and DNA isolation

All subjects recruited were Caucasians and included 345 healthy controls and 206 colorectal cancer (CRC) patients. The control subjects had taken part in the UK Flexible Sigmoidoscopy (FS) Screening Trial. All cancers underwent FS at the Department of Surgery of the Norwich and Norfolk Health care National Health Service (NHS) Trust and were free of cancer and polyps. Cancer cases were histopathologically confirmed and treated at the same department. All cancers were classified according to Dukes' stages (A, B, C, D) and tumour location (proximal, distal).

Polymorphism analysis

Genomic DNA was isolated from blood using standard methods and genotyped for *NQO1* and *mEH4* polymorphisms by PCR-based Restriction Fragment Length Polymorphism (RFLP) analysis. All analyses were carried out blindly on coded samples.

Statistical analysis

Data were analysed using STATA (statistical analysis software). Crude odds ratios (ORs) were calculated and logistic regression analysis was employed to test for associations between environmental factors and genetic polymorphisms in the disease groups. All participants completed a questionnaire stating their smoking habits. Subjects who reported smoking for the last 10 years prior to the time of the investigation were considered as current smokers and were used in the regression analyses.

Results

NQO1 and *mEH4* variant genotype frequencies were not significantly different between the colorectal cancer group and the control group. Logistic regression analyses did not show a significant age- and sex-adjusted risk for colorectal cancer associated with specific genotypes (OR, 0.97; 95%CI, 0.65–1.46 and OR, 0.98; 95%CI, 0.66 1.47 for *NQO1* and *mEH4* gene variants, respectively) (Table 1). There was no difference in relationship to site of colorectal cancer or Dukes' stage (data not shown). Smoking increased the risk for left-sided (distal) cancers (OR, 2.0; 95% CI, 1.04–3.84) but not for

CRC overall (Fig. 1). However, the effect of smoking status in distal CRC cancer was modulated by *NQO1* and *mEH4* genotypes. Current smokers who carried either a *NQO1* or a *mEH4* variant allele appeared to be more predisposed to colorectal cancer. This was more evident for distal cancers (OR was increased to 4.27; 95%CI, 1.92–9.51 for *NQO1* and to 3.66; 95%CI, 1.63–8.19 for *mEH4*) (Fig. 1). There was no effect in proximal cancers (data not shown).

Conclusion

This study showed that *NQO1* and *mEH4* polymorphisms influenced susceptibility to colorectal cancer in current smokers. An advantage of the present study over previous ones is that all participants underwent Flexible Sigmoidoscopy, thereby establishing a colorectal neoplasia-free control group. However, although the results for smoking status and its modulation by genotype were significant, the study is small and it is quite possible that the results may be due to the low numbers of smokers in the disease groups.

We hope to increase the statistical power of this study by expanding the genotyping studies in two further cohorts of the UK FS Screening Programme. Furthermore, considering the multifactorial nature of cancer susceptibility, stronger associations may be identified by analysis of other environmental and lifestyle variables such as diet and alcohol or by linkage with other polymorphic genes.

References

Giovannucci, E. & Willett, W.C. (1994) Dietary factors and risk of colon cancer. *Ann. Med.*, **26**, 443–452

Joseph, P. & Jaiswal, A.K. (1994) NAD(P)H:quinone oxidoreductase 1 (DT-diaphorase) specifically prevents the formation of benzo(a)pyrene quinone DNA adducts generated by cytochrome P4501A1 and P450 reductase. *Proc. Natl. Acad. Sci. U.S.A.*, **91**, 8413–8417

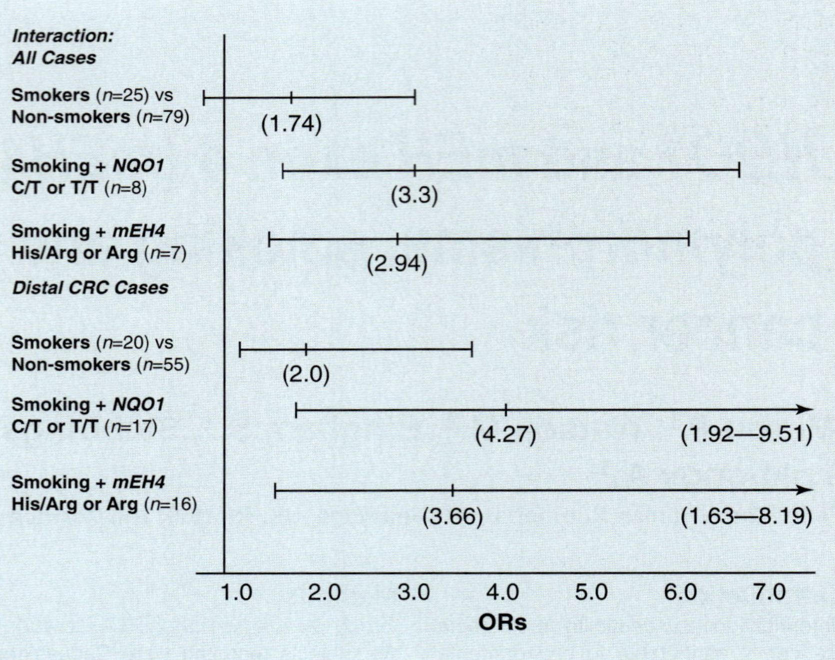

Figure 1
Forest plot of OR (95% CI) illustrating smoking–gene interactions in all CRC cases and distal CRC cases

Table 1. Distribution of *NQO1* and *mEH4* genotypes in control and CRC cases and odds ratios adjusted for age[a] and sex

	CRC Cases[b]		Controls[b]		OR (95% CI)[c]	OR (95% CI)[d]
	n	(%)	*n*	(%)		
NQO1						
C/C	131	(64)	232	(67)	e	e
C/T	72	(35)	102	(30)	0.99 (0.66–1.50)	-
T/T	3	(1)	11	(3)	0.77 (0.19–3.14)	0.97 (0.65-1.46)
mEH4						
His/His	131	(65)	221	(64)	e	e
His/Arg	64	(32)	111	(32)	0.95 (0.69–1.45)	–
Arg/Arg	8	(4)	12	(4)	1.28 (0.47–3.60)	0.98 (0.66–1.47)

[a]ORs adjusted for age: group1 ≤ 60 years of age; group 2 >60 years of age.
[b]Not every person was genotyped for each polymorphism.
[c]OR and 95% CI (any variant genotype versus wild type), adjusted for age and sex.
[d]OR and 95% CI (heterozygous and homozygous genotypes pooled together versus wild type), adjusted for age and sex.
[e]Reference group.

Lafuente, M.J., Casterad, X., Trias, M., Ascaso, C., Molina, R., Ballesta, A., Zheng, S., Wiencke, J.K., & Lafuente, A. (2000) NAD(P)H:quinone oxidoreductase-dependent risk for colorectal cancer and its association with the presence of *K*-ras mutations in tumors. *Carcinogenesis* **21**, 1813–1819

Roediger, W.E.W. & Babidge, W. (1997) Human colonocyte detoxification. *Gut*, **41**, 731–734

The role of folic acid and vitamin B_{12} in colorectal carcinogenesis in genetically different individuals – design of a study

Van den Donk M.[1], Pellis E.P.M.[1,2], Keijer J.[2], Kok F.J.[1], Nagengast F.M.[3], Kampman E.[1]

[1]Wageningen University, Division of Human Nutrition and Epidemiology, [2]State Institute for Quality Control of Agricultural Products (RIKILT), Wageningen, The Netherlands. [3]University Medical Center, Department of Gastroenterology, Nijmegen, The Netherlands.

Introduction

A high intake of fruits and vegetables may lower the risk of colorectal cancer. Folic acid may be partly responsible for this decreased risk. Low folate status and a deficiency in vitamin B_{12} may cause altered methylation of DNA and/or disturbance of DNA synthesis (Figure 1). Both DNA hypomethylation and defective DNA synthesis are important risk factors in colorectal carcinogenesis (Kim, 1999). To date, several observational and intervention studies on the role of folic acid in colorectal carcinogenesis have been published (Kim, 1999). The majority of the observational studies indicate that dietary folate intake is inversely associated with the risk of developing colorectal neoplasia. This is specifically the case among those with an inherited inefficient folate metabolism (Ulrich *et al.*, 1999). This is caused by a homozygous 677 C to T transition in the methylenetetrahydrofolate reductase (MTHFR) gene, a key enzyme in folate metabolism. Those carrying the heterozygote (CT) genotype have a 35% reduced activity, while those carrying the TT genotype have a 70% reduced activity of the MTHFR enzyme compared to people carrying the CC genotype (Frosst *et al.*, 1995).

In intervention studies, a significant effect on DNA methylation in colorectal cancer and adenoma patients was observed with a dose of 10 mg folic acid per day: a more than 50% increase of DNA methylation was seen after 6 months (Cravo *et al.*, 1994). In a more recent trial (Kim *et al.*, 2001), a folate supplementation of 5 mg per day significantly increased the DNA methylation after 6 months and after 1 year. Kim *et al.* (2001) also found that folate supplementation significantly decreased the extent of DNA-strand breaks in exons 5–8 of the *p53* gene at 6 months and 1 year. The influence of folate on the expression of genes involved in folate metabolism and folate-dependent biochemical processes in the colon has not been studied so far.

The extent to which vitamin B_{12} is related to colorectal carcinogenesis is largely unexplored. Only one intervention trial has been conducted examining the combined effect of folic acid and vitamin B_{12}: intakes of 700 μg folic acid plus 7 μg vitamin B_{12} decreased the frequency of micronucleated cells and plasma homocysteine, but was insufficient to induce alterations in DNA methylation (described in Kim, 1999). Differences in DNA synthesis and gene expression were not determined.

Objectives

The objectives of this study are to investigate:

- Whether supplementation with folic acid and vitamin B_{12} favourably alters DNA methylation and DNA synthesis processes;
- Which mechanisms are involved;
- Whether a dependency on the MTHFR C677T genotype exists.

Methods

To answer these questions, research will be conducted on three levels: the level of the cell, the individual and the population.

On the level of the cell, we will analyse the molecular effects of folic acid and vitamin B_{12}, using DNA microarray techniques. These techniques permit analysis of the expression of a large number of genes at the same time. To identify differentially expressed genes, *in vitro* experiments will be performed using human colonic cell lines. The identified genes will provide insight in the cellular effects of different concentrations of folic acid and vitamin B_{12}. To validate the *in vitro* observations, the expression of selective responsive genes will be analysed in colorectal biopsies of the participants of the intervention trial (see below).

Further, on the individual level, we will assess whether supplementation with folic acid and vitamin B_{12} alters global and gene-specific DNA methylation and DNA synthesis. Therefore, we will conduct a randomized, placebo-controlled, double-blind intervention trial in 100 subjects with a history of colorectal adenomas: 30 of them carry the MTHFR-TT genotype and 70 the MTHFR-CC genotype. Two subgroups (each including 15 TT and 35 CC) will receive folic acid (5 mg/day) and vitamin B_{12} (1.25 mg/day) or placebo for a period of 6 months. Blood samples and rectal biopsies will be collected before and at the end of the trial. In the total intervention group (n=50), an increase in DNA methylation of 30% can be detected, with a power of 90% and α=0.05 (two-sided), assuming a standard deviation of 50 (Cravo *et al.*, 1994). Within the MTHFR-TT (n=15) and MTHFR-CC (n=35) intervention groups, the detectable differences will be 60% and 40%, respectively.

On the level of the population, we will assess whether dietary intake of folic acid or vitamin B_{12} is associated with risk of adenomatous polyps and altered DNA methylation patterns in these polyps, taking into account the MTHFR-genotype. This will be evaluated in an on-going case–control study, including 600 cases and 600 polyp-free controls.

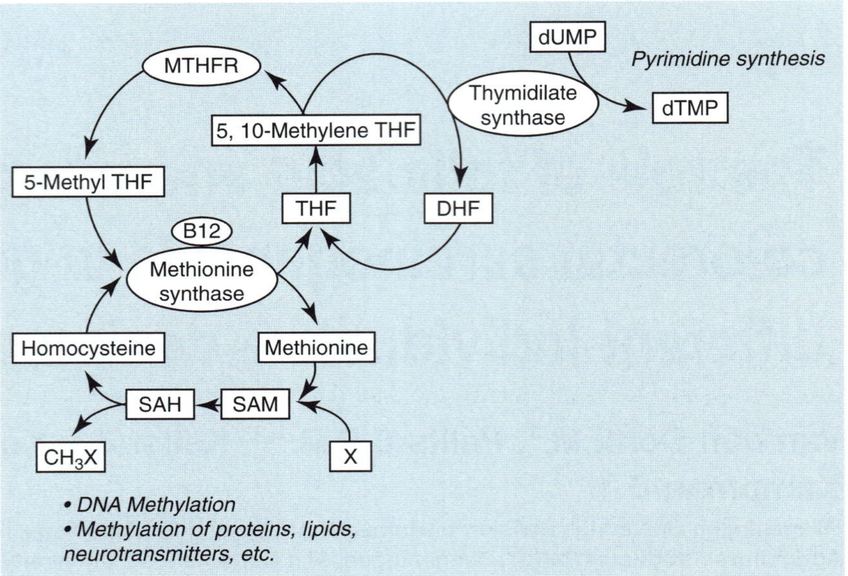

Figure 1
Folate, Vitamin B_{12}, MTHFR: links to DNA methylation and DNA synthesis.
B_{12}, vitamin B_{12}; THF, tetrahydrofolate; MTHFR, methylenetetrahydrofolate reductase; DHF, dihydrofolate; SAM, S-adenosyl methionine; SAH, S-adenosyl homocysteine; CH_3, methyl group.

This study is funded by the Netherlands Foundation of Digestive Diseases and the Netherlands Foundation of Scientific Research.

References

Cravo, M., Fidalgo, P., Pereira, A.D., Gouveia-Oliveira, A., Chaves, P., Selhub, J., Mason, J.B., Mira, F.C., & Leitao, C.N. (1994) DNA methylation as an intermediate biomarker in colorectal cancer: modulation by folic acid supplementation. *Eur. J. Cancer Prev.*, **3**, 473–479

Frosst, P., Blom, H.J., Milos, R., Goyette, P., Sheppard, C.A., Matthews, R.G., Boers, G.J.H., den Heijer, M., Kluijtmans, L.A.J., van den Heuvel, L.P., & Rozen, R. (1995) A candidate genetic risk factor for vascular disease: a common mutation in methylenetetrahydrofolate reductase. *Nat. Genet.*, **10**, 111–113

Kim, Y.-I. (1999) Folate and carcinogenesis: evidence, mechanisms, and implications. *J. Nutr. Biochem.*, **10**, 66–88

Kim, Y.-I., Baik, H.W., Fawaz, K., Knox, T., Lee, Y.M., Norton, R., Libby, E., & Mason, J.B. (2001) Effects of folate supplementation on two provisional molecular markers of colon cancer: a prospective, randomized trial. *Am. J. Gastroenterol.*, **96**, 184–195

Ulrich, C.M., Kampman, E., Bigler, J., Schwartz, S.M., Chen, C., Bostick, R., Fosdick, L., Beresford, S.A.A., Yasui, Y., & Potter, J.D. (1999) Colorectal adenomas and the C677T MTHFR polymorphism: evidence for gene–environment interaction? *Cancer Epidemiol. Biomarkers Prev.*, **8**, 659–668

Diet and *K-ras* mutations in colorectal cancer

Moreno V.[1], Guinó E.[1], Bosch F.X.[1], Peinado M.[2], Capellà G.[1], Navarro M.[1], Martí J.[3], Cambray M.[1], Lloberas B.[1] and the Bellvitge Colorectal Cancer Study Group

[1]Catalan Institute of Oncology (ICO), Barcelona, Spain. [2]Cancer Research Institute (IRO), Barcelona, Spain. [3]CSUB, L'Hospitalet, Barcelona, Spain.

Introduction

It is currently believed that colorectal cancer (CCR) develops after a series of genetic alterations accumulate in the cells that confer the ability to avoid normal cell-growth control, either promoting proliferation or inhibiting apoptosis. Some key genes in this process have been identified whose expression may be modified by mutations or epigenetic changes. Among them, mutations in *K-ras* are frequently seen in about 40% of CCR and have previously been found to interact with diet (Bautista *et al.*, 1997; Slattery *et al.*, 2000).

Purpose

To assess the relationship between diet and *K-ras* mutations of colorectal tumours.

Methods

A hospital-based case–control study was conducted from January 1996 to December 1998. All cases had confirmation of their diagnosis by tumour histology typification. Controls without colorectal cancer were recruited among patients of the same hospital admitted for a newly diagnosed disease. Approval from Ethics Committee was granted and written consent was obtained for all participating subjects. All data were handled according to Good Clinical Practices. Cases and controls were personally interviewed by trained personnel for demographic characteristics, personal and familial antecedents of cancer, reproductive and metabolic variables, physical activity, diet, alcohol, smoking and drug habits, including chronic use of medications. Diet was assessed with a structured dietary history questionnaire that had been validated previously (The EPIC group of Spain, 1997). The focus was on average past diet, relating at least 1 year prior to development of symptoms for current disease. We report here the analysis for selected food groups. For patients who underwent operation, samples of tumour tissue were screened for mutations in *K-ras* oncogene (codons 12 and 13) by PCR amplification and SSCP separation. Dubious cases were sequenced. Cases were classified according to wild type or mutated *K-ras* status. To test the hypothesis of the association between dietary risk factors and genetic alterations, multivariate methods based on logistic regression analyses were used. When cases were subdivided into groups, polytomous logistic regression was used, comparing each group of cases to the entire set of controls. Quantitative measures of exposure were categorized into quintiles to avoid the effect of extreme values. Odds ratios (OR) and 95% confidence intervals (CI) were calculated for quintiles 2 to 5 compared to the first one. Tests for a linear trend on the ORs were calculated using the categorized variable as a quantitative variable. All analyses were adjusted for age, sex, body weight and total caloric intake. *P* values were derived from likelihood ratio tests.

Results

From 501 cases and 461 controls identified, 424 cases and 401 controls could be interviewed and 419 cases provided tumour samples. Mutations in *K-ras* were found in 39% of cases. Table 1 shows the odds ratios for highest versus lowest quintile of intake, 95% confidence intervals and trend test *P* values for all cases compared to controls and for the subgroups of cases with wild type *K-ras* and mutated *K-ras*. For all cases, protective factors were vegetables, fruits and potatoes, though this latter food was not significant. Risk was increased for pastry, alcoholic beverages and beef, but not significantly for all meat or other varieties of meat. Similar findings were found for colon

Table 1. Odds ratios for colorectal cancer associated with high intake of selected food groups

	All		*K-ras* WT		*K-ras* MUT	
	OR[a] (95% CI)	P[b]	OR[a] (95% CI)	P[b]	OR[a] (95% CI)	P[b]
Potatoes	0.79 (0.50–1.28)	0.21	0.78 (0.44–1.36)	0.26	0.87 (0.45–1.67)	0.59
Green vegetables	0.56 (0.35–0.88)	0.01	0.51 (0.30–0.87)	0.01	0.69 (0.36–1.30)	0.21
Fruits	0.69 (0.44–1.08)	0.05	0.58 (0.35–0.98)	0.03	0.96 (0.51–1.80)	0.53
Legumes	1.09 (0.62–1.86)	0.99	1.57 (0.91–2.71)	0.60	0.98 (0.51–1.89)	0.52
Dairy	0.94 (0.60–1.47)	0.26	0.75 (0.44–1.26)	0.19	1.00 (0.53–1.91)	0.23
Cereals	1.32 (0.81–2.14)	0.28	1.20 (0.67–2.14)	0.50	1.39 (0.73–2.66)	0.37
Meat	0.95 (0.56–1.55)	0.66	0.98 (0.54–1.78)	0.46	0.87 (0.44–1.75)	0.65
Beef	2.81 (1.09–7.26)	0.02	2.80 (1.00–7.85)	0.05	3.22 (1.03–10.0)	0.04
Fish	1.38 (0.87–2.19)	0.32	1.20 (0.69–2.08)	0.71	1.61 (0.87–2.99)	0.17
Eggs	1.17 (0.74–1.84)	0.62	1.53 (0.88–2.65)	0.21	0.85 (0.45–1.61)	0.62
Pastry	1.58 (1.09–2.30)	0.02	1.39 (0.89–2.17)	0.19	1.88 (1.15–3.07)	0.01
Alcohol	1.63 (1.08–2.46)	0.02	1.51 (0.93–2.45)	0.05	1.82 (1.05–3.15)	0.04

[a]OR for 5th versus 1st quintile.
[b]*P* value for trend test.

and rectum tumours (data not shown). The protective effect of fruits was only seen for tumours with wild type *K-ras*. For vegetables, the protective effect was smaller and nonsignificant in *K-ras* mutated cases. No differences according to *K-ras* status were observed for the increase in risk for alcohol or beef. However, for pastry, the increase in risk was higher in cases with mutated *K-ras* than in cases with wild type *K-ras*.

Discussion

Our data show an interaction between diet and *K-ras* mutations. The protective effect of high fruit and vegetable consumption is stronger in cases with wild type *K-ras* than in cases with mutated *K-ras*. One possible interpretation of this observation is that high consumption of fruits and vegetables leads to the selection of tumours without mutation in the *K-ras* oncogene. Another possibility is that tumours with this mutation are resistant to the protective effect of these foods, irrespective of the amount of intake. We did not find an interaction of *K-ras* mutations with meat consumption. In our study only beef was associated with an increase in risk, but this was similar both for tumours with wild type or mutated *K-ras*. Similar results were observed by O'Brien *et al.* (2000). Other studies like this one have explored interactions between *K-ras* mutations and diet and found some associations (Bautista *et al.*, 1997; Slattery *et al.*, 2000). All these studies, including ours, provide preliminary knowledge in the field and generate different hypotheses that should be confirmed by replication.

References

Bautista, D., Obrador, A., Moreno, V., Cabeza, E., Canet, R., Benito, E., Bosch, X., & Costa, J. (1997) KI-RAS mutation modifies the protective effect of dietary monounsaturated fat and calcium on sporadic colorectal cancer. *Cancer Epidemiol. Biomarkers Prev.*, **6**, 57–61

The EPIC group of Spain (1997) Validity and reproducibility of a diet history questionnaire in Spain. I. Foods. *Int. J. Epidemiol.*, **26** (Suppl. 1), S91–S99

O'Brien, H., Matthew, J.A., Gee, J.M., Watson, M., Rhodes, M., Speakman, C.T., Stebbings, W.S., Kennedy, H.J. & Johnson, I.T. (2000). *K-ras* mutations, rectal crypt cell proliferation, and meat consumption in patients with left-sided colorectal carcinoma. *Eur. J. Cancer Prev.*, **9**, 41–47

Slattery, M.L., Curtin, K., Anderson, K., Ma, K.N., Edwards, S., Leppert, M., Potter, J., Schaffe, D. & Samowitz, W.S. (2000) Associations between dietary intake and Ki-ras mutations in colon tumors: a population-based study. *Cancer Res.*, **60**, 6935–6941

Dietary factors, genetic susceptibility and somatic mutations in colorectal cancer: a prospective study

Weijenberg M.P.[1], Brink M.[1], Lüchtenborg M.[1], Wark P.A.[2], de Goeij A.F.P.M.[3], de Bruïne A.P.[3], van't Veer P.[2], Kampman E.[2], van Muijen G.N.P.[4], Goldbohm R.A.[5], van den Brandt P.A.[1]

[1]Department of Epidemiology, Maastricht University, The Netherlands. [2]Division of Human Nutrition and Epidemiology, Wageningen University, The Netherlands. [3]Department of Pathology, Maastricht University, The Netherlands. [4]Department of Pathology, University Medical Centre Nijmegen, The Netherlands. [5]Consumer Research and Epidemiology, TNO, Zeist, The Netherlands.

Introduction

A diet rich in red meat and saturated fat and low in fruits, vegetables, folate and dietary fibre is thought to increase the risk of colorectal cancer, but associations tend to be weak or inconsistent (Potter, 1996). Taking into account individual variations in susceptibility (i.e. polymorphisms in genes coding for metabolic enzymes), the molecular pathways of carcinogenesis and the nature of the impaired gene function may improve etiological insight into the disease.

A high intake of meat, especially when cooked at high temperatures or smoked, may increase exposure to heterocyclic aromatic amines and polycyclic aromatic hydrocarbons, respectively. These compounds might be mutagenic, especially among individuals who are fast acetelators due to polymorphisms in N-acetyltransferase 1 and 2 (*NAT1* and *NAT2*) genes (Chen *et al.*, 1998).

The protective effect of vegetables has been attributed to nutrients (e.g. folate by influencing methylation, antioxidants by scavenging free radicals) as well as specific subgroups such as cruciferous vegetables. Cruciferous vegetables, namely the *Brassica oleracea* (broccoli), are potentially able to induce the phase II enzyme glutathione S-transferase (GST). Thus, one would expect that the protective effect is more apparent in those carrying the GST plus genotype compared to the null genotype (Cotton *et al.*, 2000). However, GST may also conjugate isothiocyanates and thereby enhance its excretion. Hence, broccoli consumption in combination with the *GSTM1* null genotype may be associated with a lower prevalence of colorectal adenomas or cancer because of higher isothiocyanate levels. This hypothesis was supported in a study by Lin *et al.* (in Cotton *et al.* 2000). A high consumption of fruits and vegetables may also decrease the number of aberrations in colorectal cancer genes. The strength of this association may depend on *GSTM1* genotype.

Based on the adenoma-carcinoma sequence, Fearon & Vogelstein (1990) proposed a gradual accumulation of genetic alterations in sporadic colorectal carcinogenesis, with different genes subsequently involved in adenoma formation (the adenomatosis polyposis coli (*APC*) and *β-catenin* genes) and the transition to carcinomas (the *K-ras* gene). Microsatellite instability, as a result of aberrations in DNA mismatch repair genes (*MMR*), is also of importance in colorectal carcinogenesis. Heterocyclic aromatic amines, polycyclic aromatic hydrocarbons and arylamines, which can be formed during high-temperature cooking, smoking and processing of meat, respectively, have all been shown to induce specific patterns of mutations. Heterocyclic aromatic amines can give rise to G deletions at 5'-GGGA-3' sites in *APC* and are thought to induce point mutations. Polycyclic aromatic hydrocarbons are associated with an increased prevalence of G to T transversions in *K-ras*. Nitrosamines are related to G to A transitions. Folate, abundant in green leafy vegetables, is a main methyl donor in the diet. A lack of folate is associated with global hypomethylation of the genome and hypermethylation of the promotor region of many genes, including *APC* and the *MMR* gene *hMLH1*.

Most of the evidence relating dietary factors to somatic mutations in the key genes involved in colorectal cancer is based on *in-vitro* studies and animal experiments; there is very limited epidemiological and pathological evidence from humans. No studies have yet incorporated information on genetic susceptibility in studying these relationships. Therefore, we will evaluate the following hypotheses:

1. A high consumption of red meat and meat products is related to an increased frequency of aberrations in *APC/β-catenin*, *K-ras* and *MMR* genes, depending on *NAT* genotypes.

2. A high consumption of fruits and vegetables is related to lower frequency of aberrations in *APC/β-catenin*, *K-ras* and *MMR* genes, depending on the *GSTM1* genotype.

Methods

The Netherlands Cohort Study on Diet and Cancer (NCLS) was initiated in 1986 and included 58 279 men and 62 573 women aged 55–69 years (Van den Brandt *et al.*, 1990). Participants completed a self-administered questionnaire on dietary habits and other risk factors for cancer. A semi-quantitative food frequency questionnaire was used containing questions on the average consumption of 150 food items over the past year. Follow-up for cancer was established by an annual computerized record linkage with the Netherlands Cancer Registry and with a nationwide pathology registry. After 7.3 years of follow-up and exclusion of the first 2 years of follow-up, 819 cases with colorectal cancer have been detected. Paraffin-embedded tissue of the cases has been collected from all pathology labs in the country. Molecular analyses are currently being performed. These include direct sequencing of relevant parts of *APC/β-catenin* and *K-ras* genes, immunohistochemistry for microsatellite instability, and PCR/RFLP techniques for polymorphisms in *NAT1*, *NAT2* and *GSTM1* genes. For statistical analysis, case–case comparisons as well as case–cohort analyses will be performed. A subcohort of 3500 subjects was randomly selected at baseline and is being followed-up biannually to estimate the person-years at risk for the entire cohort.

Results

The first results with respect to dietary factors are expected by 2002.

References

Chen, J., Stampfer, M.J., Hough, H.L., Garcia-Closas, M., Willett, W.C., Hennekens, C.H., Kelsey, K.T. & Hunter, D.J. (1998) A prospective study of N-acetyltransferase genotype, red meat intake, and risk of colorectal cancer. *Cancer Res.*, **58**, 3307–3311

Cotton, S.C., Sharp, L., Little, J. & Brockton, N. (2000) Glutathione S-transferase polymorphisms and colorectal cancer: a HuGE review. *Am. J. Epidemiol.*, **151**, 7–32

Fearon, E.R. & Vogelstein, B. (1990) A genetic model for colorectal tumorigenesis. *Cell*, **61**, 759–767

Potter, J.D. (1996) Nutrition and colorectal cancer. *Cancer Causes Control*, **7**, 127–146

Van den Brandt, P.A., Goldbohm, R.A., van 't Veer, P., Volovics, A., Hermus, R.J. & Sturmans, F. (1990) A large-scale prospective cohort study on diet and cancer in The Netherlands. *J. Clin. Epidemiol.*, **43**, 285–295

Diet and truncating *APC* mutations in sporadic colon tumours

Diergaarde B.[1], van Geloof W.L.[2], van Muijen G.N.P.[2], Kok F.J.[1], Kampman E.[1]

[1]Division of Human Nutrition & Epidemiology, Wageningen University, Wageningen, The Netherlands.
[2]Department of Pathology, UMC St Radboud, Nijmegen, The Netherlands.

Introduction

The etiology of colon cancer is complex, involving both environmental and genetic factors. Known dietary risk factors for colon cancer include meat and alcohol consumption, fat intake, and possibly smoking. Inverse associations are found with vegetable consumption, use of nonsteroidal anti-inflammatory drugs, and, although less consistent, with fruit consumption (WCRF, 1997). Though much is known about the genetic events involved, the relationship between dietary factors and the (epi)genetic mutations that drive colon carcinogenesis is less clear. Mutations in the adenomatous polyposis coli (*APC*) gene are believed to be a critical initiating event in familial and sporadic colon cancer. Nearly all *APC* mutations identified predict truncation of the protein product and loss of function. The occurrence of somatic truncating *APC* mutations in colon carcinomas may well be influenced by specific dietary factors associated with colon cancer. We investigated this in a Dutch population-based case–control study on diet and sporadic colon cancer.

Materials and Methods

Participants were recruited between 1989 and 1993. Details were described previously (Kampman *et al.*, 1994). In short, cases (n=184) were women and men diagnosed with a first primary incident colon carcinoma. Controls (n=259) were randomly recruited by the general practitioners of the cases. All participants were Caucasian, up to 75 years old, and without known previous cancer, familial adenomatous polyposis, hereditary nonpolyposis colorectal cancer, ulcerative colitis, and Crohn's disease.

Usual dietary habits were assessed by an interview-based questionnaire. Paraffin-embedded tumour tissue was available for all 184 cases. Single-strand conformation polymorphism analysis and DNA sequencing (see Voskuil *et al.*, 1999) were used to screen codons 1286–1585 of the *APC* gene for mutations. This region includes the mutation cluster region (codon 1286–1513) in which the majority of somatic mutations are located.

Cases were classified as APC$^+$ (containing a truncating *APC* mutation) or APC$^-$ (without a truncating *APC* mutation). Case–case comparisons were conducted to evaluate differences in dietary risk factors for the two carcinoma subsets. case–control comparisons were conducted to estimate the relative risk of developing carcinomas with and without truncating *APC* mutation.

Results

In 63 (34%) of the 184 colon carcinomas, a truncating APC mutation

Table 1. Dietary factors and colon tumours with (APC$^+$) and without (APC$^-$) truncating *APC* mutation

	APC$^+$ vs APC^{-a}	APC$^+$ vs controls[a]	APC$^-$ vs controls[a]
Vegetables	2.3 (1.0–5.3)	0.6 (0.3–1.3)	0.3 (0.2–0.5)
Red meat	1.7 (0.7–3.8)	1.7 (0.8–3.6)	0.9 (0.5–1.7)
Fish	1.6 (0.7–3.4)	1.4 (0.7–2.8)	0.9 (0.5–1.6)
Alcohol	0.3 (0.2–0.7)	0.5 (0.3–1.1)	1.7 (1.0–3.0)

[a]Odds ratios (95% confidence intervals). Highest versus lowest tertile. Adjusted for age, sex and total energy intake. Alcohol also adjusted for smoking.

was identified. Table 1 presents results of case–case and case–control comparisons conducted to assess associations between several dietary factors and APC$^+$ and APC$^-$ tumours. Vegetable and alcohol intake were significantly associated with APC$^+$ compared to APC$^-$ tumours, but in a different way. case–control comparisons showed that vegetable intake was inversely associated with both tumour subsets, more pronounced with APC$^-$ tumours. Alcohol was found positively associated with APC$^-$ tumours only. Red meat and fish were more notably, although not significantly, associated with APC$^+$ than with APC$^-$ tumours (*P* trend, respectively, 0.18 and 0.26).

Conclusions

Our data suggest that vegetables play a protective role in the etiology of APC$^+$ as well as APC$^-$ tumours, though the protective effect of vegetables appears to be less influential in the APC$^+$ subset. Alcohol seems to promote the development of APC$^-$ tumours in our population while red meat and fish appear to enhance the development of APC$^+$ tumours.

Acknowledgements

This study was funded by the Dutch Cancer Society grant LUW 98-1687.

References

Kampman, E., Van't Veer, P., Hiddink, G.J., Van Aken-Schneijder, P., Kok, F.J. & Hermus, R.J.J. (1994) Fermented dairy products, dietary calcium and colon cancer: a case–control study in the Netherlands. *Int. J. Cancer*, **59**, 170–176

Voskuil, D.W., Kampman, E., Van Kraats, A.A., Balder, H.F., Van Muijen, G.N.P., Goldbohm, R.A. & Van 't Veer, P. (1999) *P53* overexpression and *p53* mutations in colon carcinomas: relation to dietary risk factors. *Int. J. Cancer*, **81**, 675–681

World Cancer Research Fund Panel (Potter, J.D. Chair) (1997) *Diet, Nutrition and the Prevention of Cancer: A Global Perspective.* WCRF/American Institute for Cancer Research, Washington, D.C.

Cruciferous vegetable intake, *GSTM1* genotype and lung cancer risk in a non-smoking population

Lewis S.[1], Brennan P.[1], Nyberg F.[2], Ahrens W.[3], Constantinescu V.[4], Mukeria A.[5], Benhamou S.[6], Batura-Gabryel H.[7], Bruske-Hohlfeld I.[8], Simonato L.[9], Menezes A.[10], Boffetta P.[1]

[1]International Agency for Research on Cancer, Lyon, France. [2]Institute of Environmental Medicine, Karolinska Institute, Stockholm, Sweden. [3]Bremen Institute for Preventative Research, Bremen, Germany. [4]Institute of Public Health, Bucharest, Romania. [5]Institute of Carcinogenesis, Cancer Research Center, Moscow, Russia. [6]INSERM, Villejuif, France. [7]Pneumological Hospital, Poznan, Poland. [8]GSF Institute for Epidemiology, Munich, Germany. [9]University of Padua, Padua, Italy. [10]Federal University of Rio Grande do Sul, Pelotas, Brazil.

Isothiocyanates, which have been shown to inhibit tumorigenesis in animal models, are non-nutrient compounds found in cruciferous vegetables. Glutathione-S-transferase (GST)-catalysed conjugation of glutathione with isothiocyanates promotes the elimination of these compounds (Koln *et al.*, 1995). Among individuals who are genetically deficient with respect to the GST enzymes, elimination of isothiocyanates is likely to be less rapid, which may enhance their chemopreventive effect. In support of this hypothesis, Spitz *et al.* (2000) described a greater protective effect of high cruciferous vegetable intake for lung cancer risk among individuals who were null for both *GSTM1* and *GSTT1* genotypes compared with those who had positive alleles for both genes, and London *et al.* (2000) found a greater protective effect of isothiocyanates among *GSTM1* null compared with *GSTM1* wild-type individuals. This may represent an important example of a gene–environment interaction in human carcinogenesis.

Using data from a multicentre study of lung cancer among non-smokers (Malats *et al.*, 2000), we examined associations between *GSTM1* genotypes, cruciferous vegetable intake and lung cancer risk. GST genotyping data was available for 122 lung cancer cases and 123 controls. Subjects recruited at nine different centres throughout Europe and South America were included in the analysis. The majority of both lung cancer cases and controls were female (Table 1). Among cases, age ranged from 18 to 92 years with a mean of 64.0 years, while in controls these figures were 23 to 85 years and 59.0 years, respectively. Age, sex and centre were adjusted for in the analysis. Cruciferous vegetable intake (including broccoli, cabbage and cauliflower) was measured using a food frequency questionnaire and consumption was classified as follows: low, less than one portion per month (n=105); medium, between one portion per month and one portion per week (n=90); and high, greater than one portion per week (n=50).

In this population, *GSTM1* null was found to be a risk factor for lung cancer (OR, 1.53; 95% CI, 0.87–2.71), which is in agreement with previous findings (Houlsten *et al.*, 1999). Overall, a high consumption of cruciferous vegetables was associated with a decrease in lung cancer risk in this population (OR, 0.64; 95% CI, 0.25–1.67, Table 1). The protective effect of cruciferous vegetable consumption was observed in both *GSTM1*-positive and -null individuals although a weak dose–response relationship was apparent only in *GSTM1*-null individuals (Table 2).

Isothiocyanates appeared to reduce lung cancer risk in this population. However, whereas Spitz *et al.* found a protective effect among current smokers

Table 1. Characteristics of the study population

Characteristics	Cases n=122	Controls n=123
Sex		
Male	17 (13.9)	35 (28.5)
Female	105 (86.1)	88 (71.5)
Age		
Minimum to 49	19 (15.6)	26 (21.1)
50–59	25 (20.5)	36 (29.3)
60–69	26 (21.3)	36 (29.3)
70 to maximum	52 (42.6)	25 (20.3)
Centre		
1	60 (49.2)	28 (22.8)
2	4 (3.3)	28 (22.8)
3	5 (4.1)	4 (3.2)
4	8 (6.6)	11 (8.9)
5	3 (2.5)	8 (6.5)
6	14 (11.5)	13 (10.6)
7	15 (12.2)	15 (12.2)
8	3 (2.5)	6 (4.9)
9	10 (8.2)	10 (8.1)
Cruciferous vegetables		
Low	54 (44.3)	51 (41.5)
Medium	37 (30.3)	53 (43.1)
High	31 (25.4)	19 (15.5)
GSTM1		
+	57 (46.7)	70 (56.9)
–	65 (53.3)	53 (43.1)

Table 2. Cruciferous vegetable intake and lung cancer risk stratified by *GSTM1* genotype

		Cruciferous vegetable consumption[a]			
	Cases/controls	Low	Medium	High	*P* for trend
All individuals	122/123	1	0.58 (0.26, 1.32)	0.64 (0.25, 1.67)	0.35
GSTM1-positive	57/67	1	0.28 (0.08, 1.04)	0.65 (0.16, 2.66)	0.57
GSTM1-null	62/53	1	0.68 (0.20, 2.29)	0.27 (0.06, 1.33)	0.12

[a]Odds ratios and 95% confidence intervals were adjusted for age (4 categories), sex and centre.

only, we found this among non-smokers. The fact that we found a dose–response relationship between cruciferous vegetable intake and lung cancer risk among *GSTM1*-null individuals only supports the hypothesis that isothiocyanates may be more important in lung cancer prevention among those individuals who can eliminate these compounds less rapidly. However, the strength of our findings is limited by the sample size of the study and much larger studies will be required to accurately measure the modest effects of genes such as *GSTM1* and identify the extent of gene–environment interactions.

References

Houlsten, R.S. (1999) Glutathione S-transferase M1 status and lung cancer risk: a meta-analysis. *Cancer Epidemiol. Biomarkers Prev.*, **8**, 675–682

Koln, R.H., Danielson, U.H., Zhang, Y., Talay, P. & Mannervik, B. (1995) Isothiocyanates as substrates for human glutathione transferases: structure-activity studies. *Biochem. J.*, **311**, 453–459

London, S.J., Yuan, J.M., Chung, F.L., Gao, Y.T., Coetzee, G.A., Ross, R.K. & Yu, M.C. (2000) Isothiocyanates, glutathione S-transferase M1 and T1 polymorphisms, and lung cancer risk: a prospective study of men in Shanghai, China. *Lancet*, **356**, 724–729

Malats, N., Camus-Radon, A.M., Nyberg, F., Ahrens, W., Constantinescu, V., Mukeria, A., Benhamou, S., Batura-Gabryel, H., Bruske-Hohlfeld, I., Simonato, L., Menezes, A., Lea, S., Lang, M. & Boffetta, P. (2000) Lung cancer risk in nonsmokers and *GSTM1* and *GSTT1* genetic polymorphism. *Cancer Epidemiol. Biomarkers Prev.*, **9**, 827–833

Spitz, M.R., Duphorne, C.M., Detry, M.A., Pillow, P.C., Amos, C.I., Lei, L., de Andrade, M., Gu, X., Hong, W.K. & Wu, X. (2000) Dietary intake of isothiocyanates: evidence of a joint effect with glutathione-S-transferase polymorphisms in lung cancer risk. *Cancer Epidemiol. Biomarkers Prev.*, **9**, 1017–1020

Risk factors, genetic predisposition and mutations in the *VHL* gene in sporadic renal cell carcinoma: The Netherlands Cohort Study

Van Dijk B.A.C.[1], Schouten L.J.[1], Hulsbergen-van de Kaa C.A.[2], van Houwelingen K.P.[3], Schalken J.A.[3], Kiemeney L.A.L.M.[3], Geurts van Kessel A.H.M.[4], Bausch-Goldbohm R.A.[5], van den Brandt P.A[1]

[1]Epidemiology, Maastricht University. PO Box 616, 6200 MD Maastricht, The Netherlands. [2]Pathology, University Medical Centre Nijmegen, The Netherlands. [3]Urology, University Medical Centre Nijmegen, The Netherlands. [4]Department of Antropogenetics, University Medical Centre Nijmegen, The Netherlands. [5]Consumer Research and Epidemiology, TNO, Zeist, The Netherlands.

Kidney cancer is the ninth most common tumour in the European Union. It comprises different types of kidney cancer, the most frequent being clear-cell renal cell carcinoma (CC-RCC). The estimated incidence of kidney cancer in the European Union in 1996 was 10 per 100 000 persons at risk (Age Standardized Rate, European standard population); the estimated mortality is 4.5 per 100 000 persons at risk (ASR(E)). Both the incidence and mortality rates are about twice as high for males as for females (Ferlay *et al.*, 1999). Associations between risk factors such as hypertension and/or hypertension medication, obesity, dietary components and CC-RCC are weak or inconsistent (Wolk *et al.*, 1996; McLaughlin & Lipworth, 2000).

In 1993, the Von Hippel Lindau (*VHL*) tumour suppressor gene was identified as a causative gene for Von Hippel Lindau disease, a rare inherited disorder characterized by various outcomes, one being clear-cell renal cancer. Since then, it has been recognized that approximately 75% of all CC-RCCs, not associated with VHL disease, also show *VHL* defects (Cohen 1999). Polymorphisms in xenobiotic-metabolizing enzymes are under investigation because they may modulate cancer susceptibility (Taningher *et al.*, 1999). The presence of (specific) mutations in the *VHL* gene and/or polymorphisms in xenobiotic-metabolizing enzymes may explain the weak and inconsistent associations between risk factors and CC-RCC.

The aim of the present study is to investigate associations between risk factors and CC-RCC. Associations between risk factors and mutations in the *VHL* gene, as a specific endpoint, will also be investigated. For certain risk factors, the role of polymorphisms in certain xenobiotic-metabolizing enzymes in the relationship between this risk factor and CC-RCC will be investigated.

In 1986, a population-based cohort of 120 852 men and women, aged 55–69 was recruited. A self-administered food frequency and lifestyle questionnaire was administered. A subcohort of 3500 men and women was formed by drawing a random sample from the cohort. The subcohort was followed up to estimate person-time for the complete cohort and to investigate the stability of dietary habits. Cases were identified through annual computerized record linkage with The Netherlands Cancer Registry and PALGA, a nationwide pathology register. In 1997, after 11 years of follow-up, 305 cases of RCC have been identified. At the moment, paraffin blocks from cases are being collected in the pathology laboratories in The Netherlands. From these paraffin blocks DNA from malignant and healthy tissue will be isolated. DNA from malignant tissue will be sequenced to map mutations in the *VHL* gene. PCR/RFLP techniques will be used on DNA isolated from healthy tissue to determine polymorphisms in xenobiotic-metabolizing enzymes.

The risk factors that will be investigated are smoking, hypertension and hypertension medication, obesity and possible mediation by energy intake, the intake of certain kinds of vegetables (e.g. cruciferous vegetables), and the intake of fruit. Furthermore, cases will be subdivided according to the presence of (specific) mutations in the *VHL* gene, and for these subgroups risk ratios will be computed. Moreover, the role of some xenobiotic-metabolizing enzymes will be investigated (e.g. the role of cytochrome P450 1A1 in the relation of smoking and CC-RCC).

The first results are expected in the year 2004.

References

Cohen, H.T. (1999) Advances in the molecular basis of renal neoplasia. *Cur. Opin. Nephrol. Hyperten.*, **8**, 325–331

Ferlay, J., Bray, F., Sankila, R. & Parkin, D.M. (1999) *EUCAN: Cancer Incidence, Mortality and Prevalence in the European Union 1996*, version 3.1. Lyon, IARC Press

McLaughlin, J.K. & Lipworth, L. (2000) Epidemiologic aspects of renal cell cancer. *Sem. Oncol.*, **27**, 115–123

Taningher, M., Malacarne, D., Izzotti, A., Ugolini, D. & Parodi, S. (1999) Drug metabolism polymorphisms as modulators of cancer susceptibility. *Mut. Res.*, **436**, 227–261

Wolk, A., Lindblad, P. & Adami, H.O., (1996) Nutrition and renal cell cancer. *Cancer Causes Control*, **7**, 5–18

Chapter 10

Cancer prevention: global implications of new European evidence

Trends in foods available for consumption: Europe, 1961–1999

Burlingame B.

Nutrition Impact, Assessment and Evaluation Group, The Food and Agriculture Organization of the United Nations, Rome, Italy.

Introduction

The Food and Agriculture Organization of the United Nations, as part of its mandate, compiles information and data on various aspects of food from all its member countries. The data are analysed and interpreted to support the FAO's programmes and activities and, in accordance with the basic functions of the Organization, they are widely disseminated as CD-ROMs (FAO, 2001a) and via the Internet (FAO, 2001b).

The databases can be broadly classified into three groups: (a) country-level data referring to items such as agricultural production and trade, producer prices, land use, means of production, etc., (b) data referring to items such as population and labour force that are derived by, or in collaboration with, other international agencies and (c) derived data such as agricultural production, food supply and nutrition data. The data of direct relevance to nutrition include dietary energy supply (DES) (kcal/person/day), dietary protein supply (g/person/day) and dietary fat supply (g/person/day), as well as food supply (kg/person/year) in a time series from 1961 to the present period of data acquisition and validation (there is a 2-year lag period, e.g. the 1999 data are released in 2001).

These data are widely used, most commonly to analyse a population's food availability and eating habits (Kowrygo *et al.*, 1999; Sekula, 1997; USDA, 2001). However, they have been used in a variety of ways including prediction of famine (Atwood, 1991), estimations of nutrient losses from irradiation (Narvaiz & Ladomery, 1998) and exposure assessments for lead (Tahvonen, 1997). Much of the elucidation of the Mediterranean diet came from analysis of data from FAOSTAT (Ferro-Luzzi *et al.*, 1994; Helsing, 1995), as have earlier analyses of the relationship between dietary patterns and cancer (Kesteloot *et al.*, 1994).

Methods

FAOSTAT 2001 (FAO, 2001a) data sets provide time series food supply information from 1961 to 1999 for 130 food commodities or aggregations of commodities, and 363 countries and aggregations of countries.

Country aggregations

The aggregations for European countries include the following: the political-economic aggregations of EU12 (Belgium-Luxemburg, Denmark, France, Germany, Greece, Ireland, Italy, Luxembourg, Netherlands, Portugal, Spain, UK) and EU15 (EU12 + Austria, Finland, Sweden); and the geopolitical aggregations of Europe (51 countries), Western Europe (30 countries), Europe + Baltic (47 countries); Eastern Europe (14 countries); USSR Europe (7 countries). Data are preserved for countries even when they cease to exist, for continuity and the least disruption to the time series data. For example, Czechoslovakia data end in 1992, and Czech Republic and Slovak Republic data begin in 1993.

European countries are also included in other groupings: the Moldova Republic and the Ukraine part of Europe and are on the list of Low Income Countries (LIC), a World Bank per caput income classification, which for 1999 was US$755. All or most European countries are among the aggregations of Developed, OECD, Industrialized, World, and Former World countries.

Foods and Data

All data are expressed as the primary commodity equivalents. FAOSTAT accommodates the fact that commodities are often not consumed in the primary form – cereals enter the household mainly in processed form such as flour, meal, bread, husked or milled rice – by applying the appropriate food composition factors to the quantities of the processed commodities and not by multiplying the quantities shown in the commodity balance with the food composition factors relating to primary commodities. These factors were recently reviewed and updated (FAO, 2001c). Export and non-food uses are accounted for and are excluded from the calculations. Data are presented as food availability in kg/cap/year, dietary energy supply (DES) in kcal/cap/day, dietary protein supply (DPS) in g/cap/day, dietary fat supply (DFS) in g/cap/day. Other macro- and micronutrient data sets are available within the FAO, but are not available for external use at this time.

Per caput supply figures shown in the commodity balances represent the average supply available for the population as a whole and do not indicate what is actually consumed. Notwithstanding certain well-documented weaknesses (FAO 2001d; FAO 2001e), they are used as proxies for per caput consumption. Overestimation is likely to be a problem; it is linked to perishable foods, food-chain losses, household waste and other factors. Vegetable and fruit data are prone to overestimation; starchy staples are less prone. Underestimation is linked to home/community gardens, gathered foods and some other foods outside formal economic systems.

Results

Europe

In Europe, plants provide 72.5% of the energy from the food supply, against 27.5% from animal products. In contrast, animal products supply 54% of total protein, and plants only 46%. The same situation is found with regard to dietary fats, where animal and plant products provide, respectively, 54% and 46%.

Within plant foods, wheat is the main source of energy and protein, supplying almost 37% and 57%, respectively, of total plant intake. Other important sources of energy are sweeteners (sugar cane and sugar beet mainly), potato, sunflower, barley and maize, while low levels of protein are provided by potato, maize, rye, barley, beans and rice. Lipids are mainly supplied by sunflower and olive, followed by rape, soybean, wheat, maize, peanut and cacao.

Energy

In 1961, the DES range was approximately 2500 kcal/cap/day in Portugal to nearly 3400 kcal/cap/day in Ireland. By 1999, all European countries exceeded 3200 kcal/cap/day, with Portugal having the highest DES, at nearly 3700 kcal/cap/day (see Fig. 1).

The distribution of energy between plant and animal sources has changed little over time. In 1961 and in 1999, the average for Europe was about 70% of the DES from plant products against 30% from animal products. A country-by-country analysis for the recent 3-year period shows that animal sources contributed just over 20% of the energy to the diet in Greece, and nearly 40% in France (see Fig. 2).

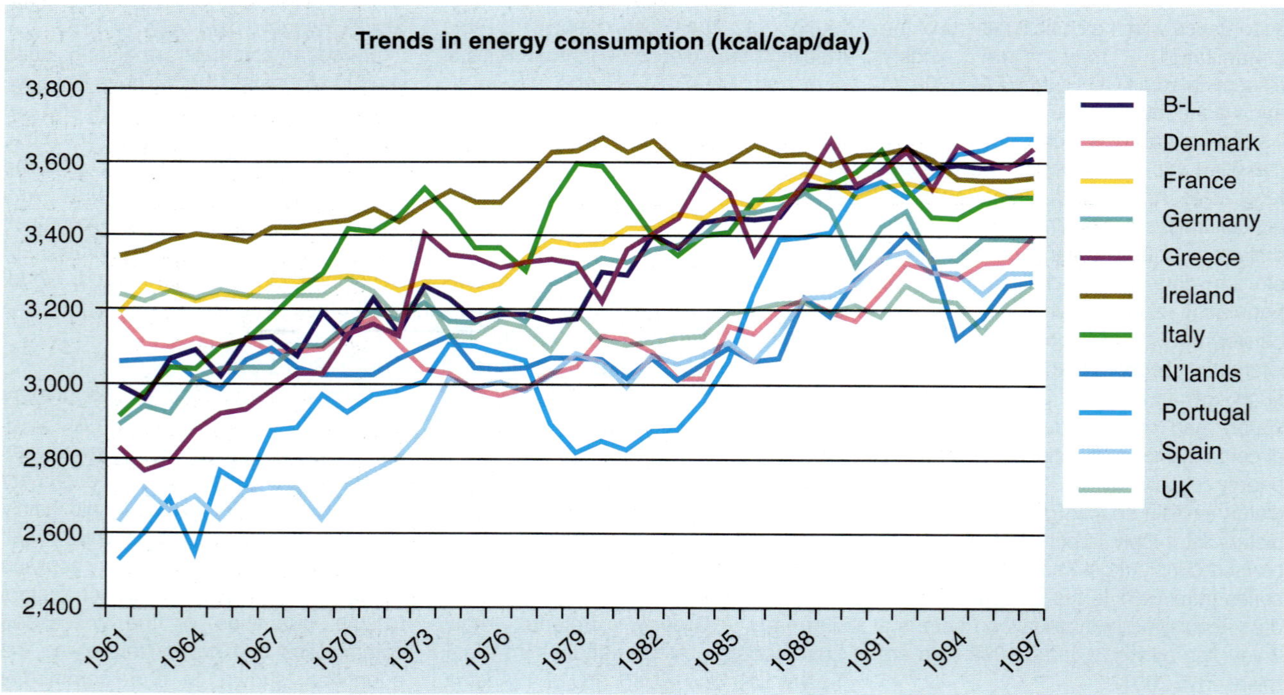

Figure 1
Trends in energy consumption in selected European countries

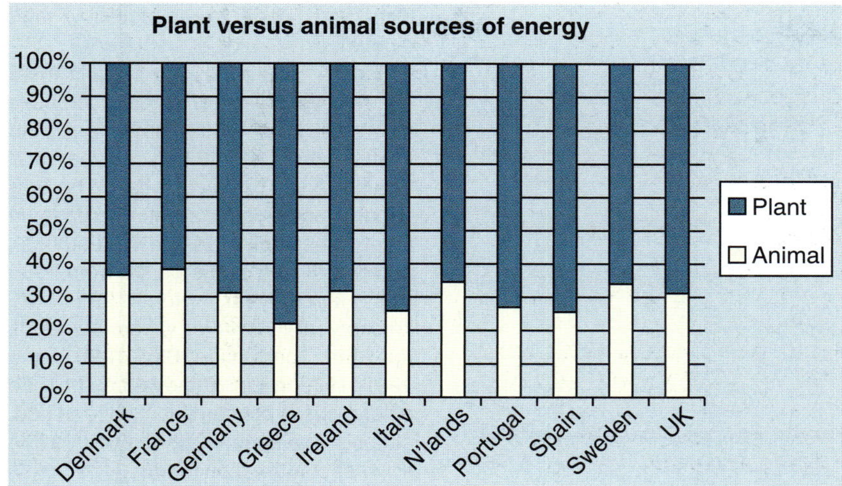

Figure 2
Percentages of energy from plants and animals (3-year averages, 1997–1999)

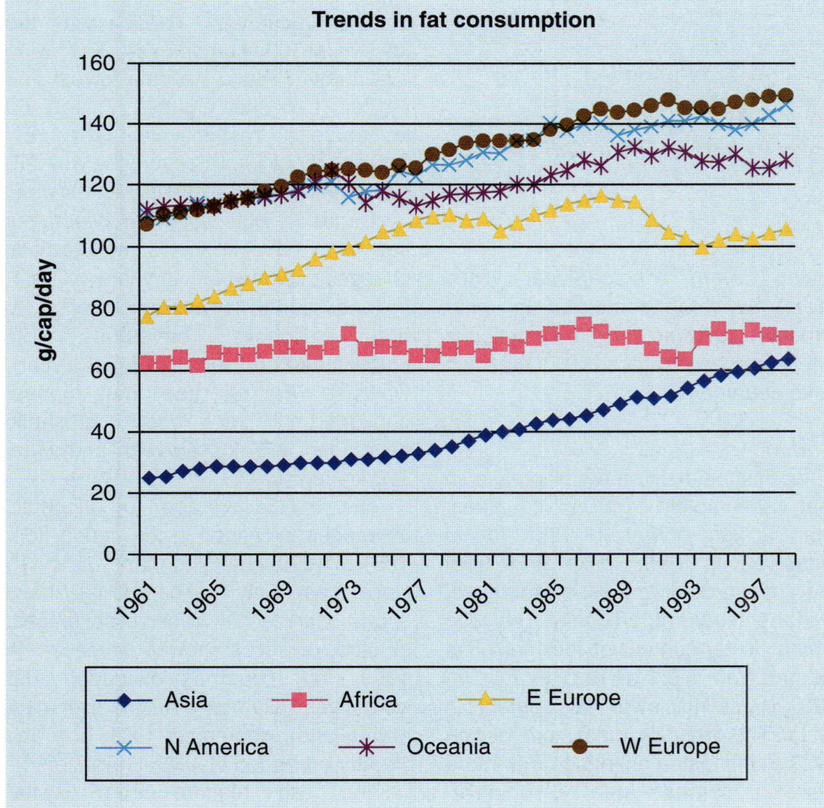

Figure 3
Worldwide trends in fat consumption, by region

Fat

Developed country aggregations by region show that DFS over time has increased everywhere.

In 1961, the developed countries in the regions Western Europe, North America and Oceania had a DFS of approximately 110 g/cap/day. By 1999, every region (except Africa) had added 20–40 g fat/cap/day (see Fig. 3).

The fat comes from a variety of sources and this too has changed over time. In 1997, Sweden had the highest DFS from fish, at 3.8 g/cap/day, and also the lowest DFS from meat, at 21.6 g/cap/day. France had the highest DFS from meat, at nearly 43 g/cap/day. Four countries had 30 g/cap/day fat from meat (Ireland, Netherlands, Spain and UK), and all countries except Denmark, Portugal and Sweden had DFS from fish of less than 2 g/cap/day.

Dairy

In 1999 fat/cap/day from milk, including all dairy except butter, averaged 16.2 g for Eastern Europe and 19.4 for Western Europe. There is a cluster of Eastern European countries on the low end of the scale, with fat from dairy under 15 g/cap/day, and a cluster of Western European countries on the high end, with fat from dairy above 25 g/cap/day. The exceptions are Denmark, with the countries lowest in dairy fat intake, Albania topping the chart with the highest intake and the Netherlands only slightly lower.

Analysis of trends in dairy product supply, again expressed in fat, between the highest and lowest of the Western European countries shows that they were nearly equivalent in 1961. Converging a few times through the late 1980s and then separating dramatically from about 1989. The inclusion of butter increases the fat from milk and milk products by another 4 g/cap/day in Denmark, and another 5 g/cap/day in the Netherlands for the latest time period.

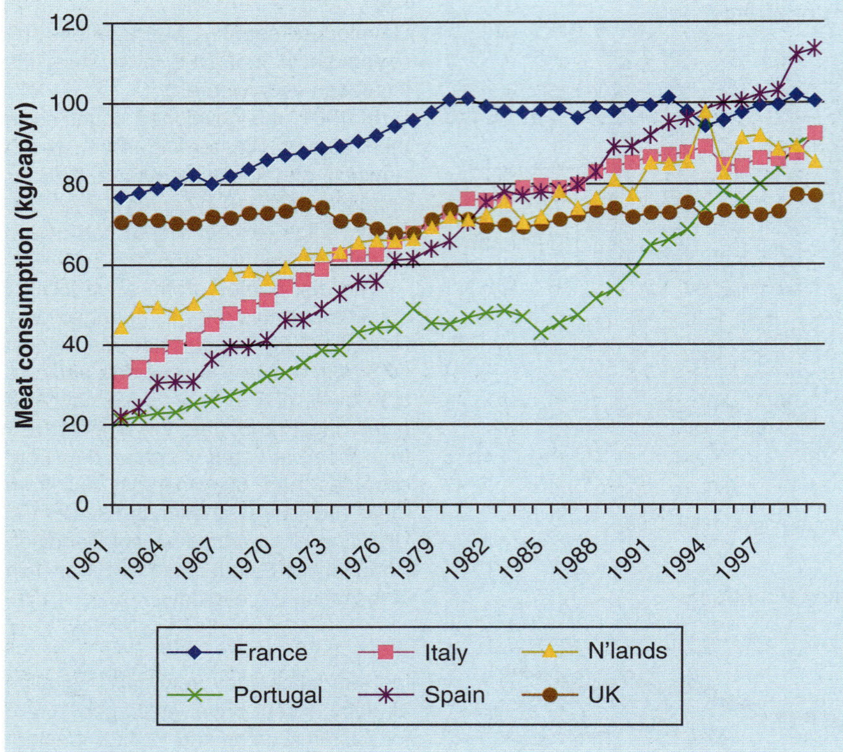

Figure 4
Trends in meat consumption in selected European countries

Sugar

Sugar consumption patterns show increases and decreases over the past 40 years. Denmark, Ireland and the UK have all decreased their apparent consumption of sugar. Denmark and the Netherlands have the highest supply, currently around 50 kg/cap/year.

Soybeans

In 1999, Asia led the world in consumption of soybeans, with 3.5 kg/cap/year, Europe averaged around 0.1 kg/cap/year.

Through the late 1980s, all European countries registered zero for soybeans and most still did in 1999. However, there are three countries with a measurable supply for human consumption: Hungary, since 1995, and Germany and Austria. All three are moving toward 1 kg/cap/year. While noteworthy when compared to other European countries, this consumption is negligible when compared to the high intake countries of Asia.

Meat

There has been a steady increase in meat consumption in EU15 countries, from 53 kg/cap/year in 1961 to 90 kg/cap/year in 1999. Intake of fat from meat (g/cap/day) has also increased, but not entirely proportionally. The ratio of meat to fat content of the meat has changed from 6.9:1 in 1961 to 7.5:1 in 1999, indicating lower fat content in meats. This trend in meat composition needs continual monitoring and more data on carcass quality, point-of-purchase fat trimming and household food waste (e.g. fat trimmed and discarded) need to be collected and evaluated.

Figure 4 illustrates the trend in meat consumption. The sharpest increases from 1961 to 1999 have been in Portugal (from 21 to 93 kg/cap/year) and Spain (22 to 113 kg/cap/year). The only country showing a slight decrease in meat consumption is the Netherlands, and it is for the single period from 1998 (90 kg/cap/year) to 1999 (86 kg/cap/year). However, 3-year averages for the periods 1994–1996 and 1997–1999 in the Netherlands show no differences in consumption in the period, although the suggestion of a decreasing trend should be monitored.

Wine and alcoholic beverages

In 1999, Ireland showed the highest per capita availability of alcoholic beverages, at 159 kg/cap/year. Greece was the lowest at 63 kg/cap/year. For wine availability, Finland had the lowest and France had the highest, 7 and 60 kg/cap/year respectively. The EU average for alcoholic beverages was 115 kg/cap/year, and 34 kg/cap/year for wine.

Trends in both alcoholic beverages and wine have shown some dramatic changes over the past 40 years. In 1961, Finland had the lowest consumption for both alcoholic beverages (27 kg/cap/year) and wine (<1 kg/cap/year), whereas France had the highest consumption for both: alcoholic beverages, 177 kg/cap/year, and wine, 120 kg/cap/year.

The EU15 average for alcoholic beverages increased in the period from 1961 to 1999, changing from 105 to 115 kg/cap/year. Only France and Italy have shown decreases in alcoholic beverages; all other countries showed increases. In 1999, four countries exceeded 150 kg/cap/year (Germany, Austria, Denmark and Ireland), whereas in 1961, only one country exceeded that level (France).

The two highest EU15 wine-consuming countries in 1961, France and Italy, were also the two highest in 1999.

However, total wine supply has decreased by half for both countries. France decreased from 120 to 60 kg/cap/year and Italy, from 108 to 55 kg/cap/year over the 1961–1999 period. Other decreases in wine supply from 1961 to 1999 were seen in Greece (34 to 22 kg), Portugal (from 65 to 51 kg) and Spain (from 60 to 39 kg). Wine supply increased for all the other EU15 countries, with Denmark increasing by a factor of 10 over the period, from 3 to 30kg. The EU15 average decreased from 46 kg in 1961 to 34 kg in 1999.

Fish

There has been substantial stability in the consumption of fish and seafood in most European countries over the time series of these data. Portugal has, for most of the time series, achieved the highest levels of consumption. Aside from the period from 1975 to 1983, the consumption of fish and seafood has exceeded 50 kg/cap/year. From the early 1960s through the mid-1980s, Austria achieved a per capita consumption of less than 10 kg/cap/year and continues to have the lowest consumption of the EU15 countries, at approximately 14 kg/cap/year. Ireland, in spite of its coastal resources, also appears on the low end of the consumption scale, with a gradual increase over the time series from less than 9 to approximately 15.5 kg/cap/year. The other low-consuming countries for fish and seafood, both currently and over the time series, are Germany, the Netherlands and Belgium.

Conclusions

The food supplies and dietary patterns in Europe are changing markedly. FAO Statistical Databases provide a tool for making useful assessments of these changes. Although other survey methodologies may give differing pictures of dietary patterns at the community, household and individual levels, and at different time periods, FAOSTAT provides a unique resource for national and global level standardized assessments over a 40-year period. These data, in combination with other data sets, are necessary for monitoring changes in food supplies and dietary patterns, currently and retrospectively, against the changing morbidity and mortality from cancer and other diseases.

References

Atwood, D.A. (1991) Aggregate food supply and famine early warning. *Food Policy*, **16**, 245–251

FAO (2001a) *FAOSTAT 2001 CD-ROM.* Rome, FAO Statistical Databases

FAO (2001b) FAOSTAT On-Line. http://www.apps.fao.org/

FAO (2001c) Inter-temporal changes of conversion factors, extraction rates, and productivity of crops and livestock and related matters: 1963–67 to 1993–97. http://www.fao.org/WAICENT/FAOINFO/ECONOMIC/ESS/totdoc.htm

FAO (2001d) Supply utilization accounts and food balance sheets in the context of a national statistical system. http://www.fao.org/WAICENT/FAOINFO/ECONOMIC/ESS/suafbs.htm

FAO (2001e) Problems of compiling internationally comparable agricultural statistics and estimation of missing data. http://www.fao.org/WAICENT/FAOINFO/ECONOMIC/ESS/prob.htm

Ferro-Luzzi, A., Cialfa, E., Leclercq, C. & Toti, E. (1994) The Mediterranean diet revisited. Focus on fruit and vegetables. *Int. J. Food Sci. Nutr.*, **45**, 291–300

Helsing, E. (1995) Traditional diets and disease patterns of the Mediterranean, circa 1960. *Am. J. Clin. Nutr.*, **61**, 1329S–1337S

Kesteloot, H., Sasaki, S., Verbeke, G. & Joossens, J.V. (1994) Cancer mortality and age: relationship with dietary fat. *Nutr. Cancer*, **22**, 85–98

Kowrygo, B., Gorska-Warsewicz, H. & Berger, S. (1999) Evaluation of eating patterns with different methods: the Polish experience. *Appetite*, **32**, 86–92

Narvaiz, P. & Ladomery, L.G. (1998) Estimation of the effect of food irradiation on total dietary vitamin availability as compared with dietary allowances: study for Argentina. *J. Sci. Food Agric.*, **76**, 250–256

Sekula, W. (1997) Recent developments in the dietary pattern and health status in Poland. *BNF Nutr. Bull.* **22**, 123–126

Tahvonen, R. (1997) Contents of lead in foods and diet in Finland in the early 1990s. *Food Rev. Int.*, **13**, 77–90

USDA (2001) Changing structure of global food consumption and trade. *Agriculture and Trade Reports*, WRS 01-1. Washington, D.C., USA, United States Dpt of Agriculture, Economic Research Service.

WHO's strategy on nutrition and noncommunicable diseases prevention

Puska P.

Noncommunicable Diseases Prevention and Health Promotion, World Health Organization, Geneva, Switzerland.

WHO's mission is to improve global public health through effective, evidence-based measures to reduce the burden of diseases and to promote health. Assessment of burdens caused by different diseases and of their major determinants is vital to this mission.

During the last few years, important information has been obtained on the global burden of diseases. It shows how the world's health situation is rapidly changing. The relative role of infectious diseases is diminishing and that of some major noncommunicable diseases (NCD) increasing. Of major importance is the fact that NCDs are so rapidly increasing in the developing world.

According to WHO's latest estimates, some 60% of all deaths in the world are now caused by noncommunicable diseases, together with injuries and violence. Every third death is cardiovascular and coronary heart disease is the number one killer in the world. In all regions of the world, except in Sub-Saharan Africa, NCDs are the leading cause of death and the majority of the world's NCD deaths occur in the economically developing countries.

NCDs were once referred to as diseases of affluence. This is wrong; these diseases are rapidly increasing also in poor countries and in most populations these diseases and their risk factors tend to accumulate in lower socioeconomic groups. This changing picture of global public health is due to successes in infectious disease control, to rapidly changing lifestyles, notably in urban areas, and to rapid demographic shifts. This development and the predicted further increase in the NCD burden form a great threat to the national economies and are a vast new public health challenge.

Nutrition – a major determinant

Noncommunicable diseases are not inevitable consequences of ageing. Research has clearly identified a few powerful causal factors. Although an individual's risk is influenced by genetic predisposition, the disease development is closely linked to a few risk factors that are closely related to lifestyle-related factors that can be changed, notably nutrition, tobacco use and physical inactivity – factors that have their roots in social and physical environments.

This solid evidence forms a strong basis for prevention. Although improvement in treatment of diseases is important, the public health potential in control of NCDs lies in prevention. Strong evidence shows that prevention is possible. NCD rates can change markedly and in a relatively short time as a consequence of changes in lifestyles. Such changes can take place in response to major social, economic or political actions, whether intended for public health consequences or not.

Nutrition is one of the major lifestyle factors related to development of NCDs. Numerous international expert reviews, including those of WHO, have identified the close links between certain nutritional factors and risks of major cardiovascular diseases (CVD). Important nutritional risk factors are blood LDL cholesterol, elevated blood pressure, elevated blood glucose tolerance and obesity. Research has also convincingly shown major links between dietary or nutritional factors and many forms of cancer, diabetes and dental caries. Alzheimer's disease, musculoskeletal problems and other conditions have also been associated with nutritional factors.

During the last few years, great progress has been achieved in the drugs used to reduce nutrition-related risk factors (such as serum cholesterol or blood pressure). While these products have an important place in treatment of high-risk patients, dietary changes have a great potential in reducing the need for drugs and will remain the main method, from a public health point of view, in reducing the NCD rates in the population.

Global trends, nutrition in transition

The emerging epidemics of NCDs are associated with changing dietary patterns, which lead to increased risks of NCDs. Worldwide, we can see trends in reduced intake of fruit and vegetables and dietary fibre, and in increased intake of fats (especially saturated fats), sugar and alcohol. Together with reduced physical activity, this leads to increasing weight and the growing problem of obesity. Salt consumption is high in many populations, greatly contributing to elevated blood pressure values and risk of cerebrovascular strokes.

Although undernutrition remains a problem in many developing countries, even in the same countries we see growing rates of overweight and obesity. It should be pointed out that nutritional issues underlying NCDs are not limited to obesity. Many nutrition-related problems, e.g. elevated blood cholesterol or elevated blood pressure, can be seen in people with normal weight – but with unbalanced nutrition.

The changing and unhealthy patterns of nutrition in the world are often linked with so-called globalization. While globalization can clearly bring benefits in alleviating global poverty and in infection disease control – and is seen by many as inevitable – there are obvious negative consequences for NCD-related risk factors. For example, it gives transnational industry powerful means to promote tobacco products as well as foods and drinks that replace healthier traditional food habits.

Although increases in NCDs often relate to economic development in countries in transition, NCDs are not inevitable consequences of economic growth. Instead, with successful health promotion and policies, economic development can be linked with healthier lifestyles and nutrition, and consequently with reduced NCD rates.

Policy framework for nutrition in NCD prevention

The science base for nutrition in NCD prevention is strong. This is, however, not enough for effective prevention in real life. Dietary habits and nutrition can be deeply rooted in cultural, economic and political structures.

Substantial changes in national diets can take place as a consequence of major crisis or political changes. However, attempts to influence diets for health reasons usually have to employ more elaborate interventions. Basically it is a question of communicating the healthy information and skills to people, persuading people to implement healthy changes and providing social and environmental support for such changes. From a health policy point of view, this calls for a sound policy framework that is based on careful analysis of the local situation and on relevant, evidence-based theoretical approaches, and leads to appropriate policy decisions.

Although dietary changes for prevention are needed for high-risk people (e.g. with hypercholesterolaemia or hypertension), major changes in national NCD rates can only be based on a population approach, that is, on influencing the general nutrition in the population. This is the case because risks often concern a great proportion of the population and lifestyle changes cannot be isolated for only a fraction of the population. Thus, generally healthy diets should be promoted – diets needed for prevention of a range of NCDs are safe and in many ways promote health generally (the integrated approach).

Intervention activities

Practical activities within a national policy framework for healthy nutrition and NCD prevention are multiple. Particularly the following sectors/areas should be involved:

- Health services (especially primary health care).
- Schools: curricula, school lunches and school health.
- Mass communication, media.
- Civil society organisations (health-related and others)
- Restaurants, catering, etc.
- Supermarkets, food industry.
- Legislation and policy.
- Monitoring and research.

Strategies to prevent NCDs should be organized at the national level. Ministries of Health should have the political leadership, but effective national strategies require intersectoral collaboration. To implement national policies and strategies, a technical focal point linked with the government is essential, as is collaboration with relevant expert institutes. National guidelines are needed, as well as surveillance on different levels: rapid and simple monitoring of key dietary habits should be supplemented by less frequent but more comprehensive surveys on nutrition and nutritional risk factors.

As far as policy and legislation are concerned, the aim should be to remove obstacles and to enhance people's possibilities to enjoy healthy diets. Practical areas concern taxation and pricing, agriculture, food labelling and nutritional claims, institutional nutrition and support to healthy nutrition programmes.

Healthy changes in national diets do not occur with policy plans and programme protocols alone, however good they are. Policies and plans need to be implemented well and enough resources should be allocated for effective implementation. Financial resources are needed for dietary interventions, although the investments are tiny compared with the costs of treatment of nutrition-related diseases. Such investments are certainly a cost-effective way to improve a nation's health.

WHO's role

WHO's traditional role is to provide technical expertise and support to Member States. To help tackle global health challenges, WHO's strong leadership is needed, but at the same time partnerships with national governments and other international agencies and organisations are vital.

WHO is now building a strong structure to respond effectively to the growing burden of NCDs at its headquarters. Within the cluster of Noncommunicable Diseases and Mental Health, the department of NCD Prevention and Health Promotion has started its work, a major area being Nutrition in NCD Prevention. This area of work contributes to many other activities of the cluster. The aim is to build up a core team that, in close collaboration with international collaborating centres, other agencies and organizations, can carry out work that can meaningfully contribute to global nutritional changes for NCD prevention.

The work will involve the three levels:

1. Technical support and advocacy (science-based, evidence-based for interventions and policies).
2. Support to national programmes (particularly through regional networks such as CINDI, CARMEN, etc.).
3. Global initiatives and activities.

Working at the global level is essential because of the increasingly global background of dietary trends. The work of the food industry, international trade agreements and supranational communication (Internet, satellite channels, etc.) all mean that the scope of individual nations to intervene to promote healthy nutrition is increasingly limited.

Thus national programmes should be strongly supplemented by global initiatives to put health and healthy nutrition effectively on the global agenda. This calls for WHO leadership that we are prepared to take, but only in broad collaboration and partnerships. Success in these actions is measured in such improvements in global health that can be matched by very few other possible measures.

The World Cancer Research Fund Expert Report: the next steps

Wiseman M.J.

World Cancer Research Fund International, 19 Harley Street, London W1G 9QJ, UK.

Introduction

It is now generally accepted that nutrition status, dietary patterns and other lifestyle factors are important determinants of the risk of a number of cancers. However, until relatively recently, this was not the case. While the link between smoking and lung cancer has been accepted since the 1950s, it was 1982 before the first authoritative statement on the issue was made. The US National Academy of Sciences report on Diet, Nutrition and Cancer (NAS, 1982) heralded an increasing worldwide interest in the role that diet and nutrition could play in the development – and prevention – of cancer.

Serious consideration of the influence of diet on cancer risk was stimulated by the seminal paper by Doll and Peto (1981), in which they estimated that around 35% of cancers in the United States might be related to dietary exposures. Though confidence intervals around their estimate were wide – between 10% and 70% – it nevertheless highlighted the potential for prevention across a wide range of cancer sites. Subsequent estimates by other workers have come to similar conclusions and confidence in the estimates is increasing (Riboli, 1992; Willett, 1995).

By the early 1990s, an impressive literature surrounding diet, nutrition and cancer had developed. This diverse database comprised epidemiological studies, clinical studies and laboratory data in animals and humans. In all areas, the quality of studies was varied and in particular, data on diet itself was often unsatisfactory. In spite of this diversity of quality and study type, some patterns of association became apparent, such as the link between higher consumption of fruit and vegetables and lower risks of a number of cancers (Block *et al.*, 1992). Nevertheless considerable heterogeneity in the data remained and a number of individuals and groups considered it timely for a further review of the topic.

WCRF/AICR Expert Report

The World Cancer Research Fund/American Institute for Cancer Research (WCRF/AICR) Expert Report *Food, Nutrition and the Prevention of Cancer: a Global Perspective* was published in 1997 (WCRF/AICR, 1997). The result of 5 years and an exhaustive review by a panel of independent experts from around the world, this Report changed the landscape of how people perceive not only the links between diet, nutrition and cancer, but also the potential for prevention through dietary and other lifestyle changes. It provided in one volume a comprehensive analysis of the status of the evidence base up to 1995, incorporating assessments of epidemiological, clinical and laboratory data.

Four years on, there has been a substantial accumulation of new evidence. Just as in the original evidence base for the Expert Report, not all studies come to identical conclusions and their quality is variable. Clearly the new data will impact on the overall body of evidence, which must form the basis of any comprehensive interpretation.

Technical developments

Over the last few years there has been an explosion of interest in the methods used to synthesize research evidence. There have been major developments in both qualitative and quantitative aspects, including systematic reviews and meta-analysis. However, the principal focus for this activity has been in relation to healthcare interventions to inform clinical decisions. Relatively little attention has been given to applying these principles to questions surrounding the causation and prevention of disease.

One consequence of this approach has been that a hierarchy of evidence developed in the context of healthcare interventions has become regarded as universally applicable. However, this may not always be so (Harbour & Miller 2001). For many questions, particularly those related to the factors involved in the development of chronic disease, this hierarchy has problems. At the root of the problems lies a reliance on randomized controlled trials (RCTs). RCTs are often the best way of testing whether a particular intervention impacts on the progress of a disease – and therefore are conducted in relatively small numbers on groups at relatively high risk of developing an end-point. In contrast, etiological studies need to be carried on for decades in large numbers at low risk. The practical problems of conducting RCTs in such circumstances are insurmountable and the vast majority of studies addressing such questions are epidemiological. In addition, the few direct intervention studies and the voluminous laboratory data often offer only indirect insights into the questions of relevance.

The outcome is a misperception by health professionals and policy makers that the studies necessary to help develop rational strategies for primary prevention, by understanding the causation of disease, are not of adequate quality to underpin decisions. However, if prevention is to be part of the approach to managing cancer in the community, as it must, such decisions do need to be made on the best evidence available. The question therefore arises as to what constitutes the best evidence in relation to the development of chronic disease over decades.

The perception that RCTs offer a universally better approach bears examination. Well-conducted RCTs are the best way of avoiding various biases. However, experimental constraints may mitigate this advantage. For instance, the intervention applied may not be directly related to the question of relevance, the application of the intervention may be unrepresentative of usual practice, and the population studied may differ from the eventual target group.

In some healthcare situations, it has been possible to examine whether well-conducted observational studies produce more biased results than randomized clinical trials. Concato *et al.* (2000) compared the results of randomized intervention studies with observational evidence relating to a number of clinical situations in a systematic way. They concluded that, at least for the situations they studied, observational data from well-conducted studies did not appear to produce biased results as compared to randomized interventions. Possible reasons for this disparity from a long-standing perception include better control for confounding factors and definition of inclusion and exclusion criteria. While it may be difficult to extrapolate widely from the few situations Concato *et al.* studied, in situations where randomized interventions can only bear indirectly on the etiological question of relevance, it appears reasonable to use the existing data to draw conclusions.

World Cancer Research Fund International – the next steps

However, if observational data are to be used to underpin important educational, policy and clinical decisions, it is essential that the data are analysed in the most rigorous way. While true objectivity is an impossible goal, it is possible to minimize the effects of subjectivity in a number of ways. Firstly, it is necessary to separate the processes of collating and displaying the data from that of interpreting the evidence, drawing conclusions and deriving recommendations. Secondly, it is important to collate the evidence in a systematic way. Thirdly, it is necessary for the process to be transparent so that it is open to external scrutiny and any necessary judgements are overt. Finally, it is helpful to have the evidence displayed in a systematic and common format.

From the outset, WCRF International has made clear its commitment to keeping the Report and the recommendations derived from it up to date. WCRF International, as a start to revisiting and updating the Report, has convened a Methodology Task Force to address the question of how best to assimilate the evidence relating to the causation and development of cancer. We expect this to become a widely accepted convention when reviewing such data and to impact on the perception of clinicians and policy makers with regard to the evidence for a role of diet in the development and prevention of cancer.

References

Block, G., Patterson, B. & Subar, A. (1992) Fruit, vegetables, and cancer prevention: a review of the epidemiological evidence. *Nutr. Cancer*, **18**, 1–29

Concato, J., Shah, N. & Horwitz, R.I. (2000) Randomized, controlled trials, observational studies, and the hierarchy of research designs. *N. Engl. J. Med.*, **342**, 1887–1892

Doll, R. & Peto, R. (1981) The causes of cancer: quantitative estimates of avoidable risks of cancer in the United States today. *J. Natl. Cancer Inst.*, **66**, 1191–1308

Harbour, R. & Miller, J. (2001) A new system for grading recommendations in evidence-based guidelines. *Br. Med. J.*, **323**, 334–336

National Academy of Sciences (1982) *Diet, Nutrition and Cancer.* Washington, National Academy Press

Riboli, E. (1992) Background and rationale of EPIC. *Ann. Oncol.*, **3**, 783–791

Willett, W. (1995) Diet, nutrition, and avoidable cancer. *Environ. Health Perspect.*, **103** (Suppl. 8), 165–170

World Cancer Research Fund/American Institute for Cancer Research (1997) *Food, Nutrition and the Prevention of Cancer: A Global Perspective.* London, UK/Washington, D.C., World Cancer Research Fund/American Institute for Cancer Research

A global perspective on food, environment and health, with particular reference to diet and cancer

McMichael A.J.

National Centre for Epidemiology and Population Health, Australian National University, Canberra, ACT 0200, Australia.

Introduction

The world population will reach an estimated 8–9 billion by 2050. Meanwhile, consumer expectations are rising. Hence, we can anticipate an approximately two- to threefold increase in total food requirements over the coming half-century (Cohen, 1996). Yet, even as new technologies emerge, we face newly occurring global environmental changes such as climate change that are likely to impair food production. Other incipient large-scale environmental changes likely to affect food production include stratospheric ozone depletion, the accelerating loss of biodiversity (with knock-on effects on crop and livestock pest species), and the perturbation of several of the great elemental cycles of nitrogen and sulfur. Indeed, modern agricultural practices, worldwide, are themselves a source of increasingly severe environmental damage, jeopardizing the productivity of agroecosystems and contributing to large-scale environmental changes.

Against this background of environmental change, epidemiologists are tackling an array of intriguing questions about the relationship between diet and cancer in the foreground. The research imperative drives us to seek to elucidate the mechanisms underlying these observed relationships. Consistency of findings allows confident application in the policy realm, modulating individual and community behaviours, and perhaps influencing patterns of food production and processing. Meanwhile, there are large, historically based and often environmentally determined differences in regional diets. Further, as environmental conditions alter, as technologies (molecular and otherwise) evolve, and as consumer preferences change, so the configuration of dietary risks of cancer (and many other diseases) changes. There is both a need and opportunity to marry the results of epidemiological findings with the discourses on biologically desirable and ecologically sustainable food production.

Compared to potent genotoxic chemicals, the human diet might appear to be a rather mundane cause of cancer. Further, it presents as a methodological morass that has challenged, and sometimes thwarted, many good epidemiological studies and good epidemiologists. Yet it is hardly surprising that many components of the diet – themselves not genotoxic – may influence the probabilities of cancer occurrence, given the important role of diverse factors such as hormones, other chemokines and viruses in affecting rates of cellular proliferation and, hence, the occurrence of cancer. We also recognize that various micronutrients can reduce oxidative damage to cells, a role that those same micronutrients play in the natural world within the plant species from which they predominantly derive. Thus, our ideas about the dietary influences on cancer have widened beyond those of the more molecular-mechanistic chemical carcinogenesis, which prevailed 3–4 decades ago.

Now that we have begun to think in more life-course and human ecological terms about dietary influences on disease, we are recognizing that diets can also act over time via influences on, for example, early life (including perhaps fetal life, especially in the case of breast cancer) programming of metabolic or physiological phenomena, and the metabolic and hormonal consequences of obesity.

Again, it may seem mundane that, alongside laboratory carcinogens such as aflatoxin and the *N*-nitrosamines, one of the clearest diet-related risk-factor complexes is physical inactivity and elevated relative weight. Yet, in 2001, the IARC concluded that: "Taken together, excess body weight and physical inactivity account for approximately one-fourth to one-third of breast cancer, and cancers of the colon, endometrium, and kidney and oesophagus." And: "Limiting weight gain during adult life, thereby avoiding overweight and obesity, reduces the risk of postmenopausal breast cancer, and cancer of the colon, uterus (endometrium), kidney (renal cell) and oesophagus (adenocarcinoma)."

The recent epidemiological research on diet and cancer has revealed a spectrum of results and has suggested some new insights and emphases. At the risk of oversimplification, one might summarize the main results as follows:

- Alcohol and breast cancer risk shows a consistent, moderate, mostly linear increase. EPIC studies show a relatively weak association.
- EPIC studies confirm well-documented effects of alcohol on upper aerodigestive system cancers (and not attributable to fruit and vegetables which display an independent protective effect).
- Findings on fruit and vegetables are suggestive but uneven.
- Meta-analysis indicates a differential effect of types of meat/fish on colon cancer. Processed meats appear to confer the greatest risk increase.
- Modes of cooking meat may also have a real – but minor – contribution to colon cancer.
- Postmenopausal estrogens (estradiol) increase breast cancer risk.
- Consistent evidence is available supporting an increase in risk with raised BMI and physical inactivity.
- Dietary influences on prostate cancer remain unclear, although there is clear population-level evidence of a protective effect of plant food diets.
- Factors influencing cell proliferation appear to play a central role – hormonal (sex, insulin, IGF1), inflammatory processes, and perhaps body size.

Our ideas in the realm of diet and cancer have thus broadened over the past two decades. Indeed, we are interested in thinking about dietary influences on human disease risks at several levels. Certainly, mainstream epidemiological research will continue to pursue essentially reductionist questions about the cancer risks associated with specific aspects of the human diet. But we are also interested in how these exposures arise and change within the larger ecological context, since the environmental and social context influences the types and amounts of foods available to local populations. In macroscopic terms, that wider context can be summarized thus:

- The world population is increasing, especially in developing countries (South Asia and sub-Saharan Africa).
- Urban consumers, worldwide, are becoming more affluent.
- Global corporations are increasingly shaping food preferences and availability.
- The prevalence of obesity is rising, alongside urbanization and diminished physical activity levels.
- Macro-pressures on the natural environment are causing land degradation, biodiversity losses, climate change, and increases in some infectious diseases. This is leading to some reconsideration of industrial farming and intensive livestock production.
- The world cannot, with foreseeable technologies, feed a population of 8–9 billion a current Western diet.

Let us stand back from the conditions of the present and review the longer history of food, environment, and human health and disease.

An historical perspective on food, environment and health

Historically, food availability has been the most fundamental constraint on human population size. Over time, humans have found ways to expand food supplies and hence the environmental carrying capacity. Having gradually replaced foraging and hunting over the past 10 000 years, farming has become both more extensive and intensive, such that the expansion of local environmental carrying capacity has tended to become less sustainable. There are many celebrated historical examples (Diamond, 1997). The fratricide in Rwanda in 1994 is deemed by some commentators to have reflected the land pressures, and food shortages, in a rapidly growing population of 8 million living in a tiny country with an environmental carrying capacity estimated at only 6–7 million.

In his apocalyptic vision, 1900 years ago, St. John the Divine saw a world continuously ravaged by the Four Horseman: conquest, warfare, famine and pestilence (McMichael, 2001a). The terrible Third Horseman rode on a black steed. Indeed, subsistence crises, with famine and starvation, have long been part of the human story. However, over the past two centuries, modernization, extended trading networks, other forms of interconnectedness and an emerging ethos of international aid have reduced the occurrence and impact of local famines.

Today, however, we face the unprecedented macro-Malthusian prospect of population size exceeding food supplies at a global level. World population size appears set to undergo a sixfold increase, from 1.5 billion in 1900 to around 8–9 billion in 2050, after which it may level off at something not much higher than that. Meanwhile, the modern agricultural revolution, with its beginnings in the late eighteenth century, has intensified, the Green Revolution has boosted grain yields during the latter half of the twentieth century, and we stand now on the brink of applying genetic biotechnologies and precision farming techniques to the future expansion of world food production. The classic Malthusian tension between increasing numbers and the expansion of environmental carrying capacity persists (Malthus, 1798).

Nevertheless, malnutrition remains a serious international public health, social and economic problem. Although the proportion of persons who are malnourished has declined gradually over recent decades, the absolute numbers are not yet obviously declining. The estimated total number, in the year 2000, is 830 million, of which 790 million are within the less developed countries (FAO, 1999). In the Global Burden of Disease assessment made by the World Health Organization (Murray & Lopez, 1996), malnutrition accounts for 16% of the world's total burden of disabling illness and premature death, measured in DALYs (disability-adjusted life-years).

Environmental stresses and food production

An understanding of the emerging world food situation requires more than simple arithmetic and linear extrapolations. There are qualitative shifts occurring to the ecological infrastructure that underpins the world's food-producing systems. Indeed, some scientists now argue that, worldwide, agriculture is set to cause more global environmental damage than the better-known examples such as global climate change. Land degradation has occurred widely, with, now, approximately one-third of fertile soil moderately or severely damaged via erosion, salination, water-logging, chemicalization, loss of organic material and physical compaction (Greenland *et al.*, 1998; McMichael, 2001a).

The spread of irrigation has caused salination and water-logging in many locations. Ground-water supplies have been widely depleted as aquifers have been overexploited – now a critical problem in northern China, the American Midwest and north-west India. The chemicalization of soil and waterways will increase as the use of nitrogenous fertilizer increases. Already the past half-century's combination of huge increases in nitrogenous fertilizer use, in livestock production, and in the combustion of fossil fuels has added greatly to the level of biologically active (fixed) nitrogen within the biosphere. This has contributed to the acidification of soils and has resulted in increasingly high nitrate levels in ground water.

Against this background, questions arise about how, in future, other great changes in global environmental systems and processes might affect food production. Global climate change is an acknowledged major source of likely future stress on both terrestrial and marine food production, and is attracting much of the scientific and policy debate (Conroy *et al.*, 1994; Rosenzweig & Iglesias, 1998). However, the world is, as ever, multivariate: there are other incipient large-scale environmental changes that will affect food production, including stratospheric ozone depletion, the accelerating loss of biodiversity (with knock-on effects on crop and livestock pest species), and the perturbation of several of the great elemental cycles (nitrogen, sulfur and phosphorus). Further, the impacts will not be simply additive: many of these processes will interact with one another. For example, the probability of crop infestations by pests may be influenced multiplicatively by changes in climatic conditions, the weakening of photosynthesis and plant biology by both increased ultraviolet irradiance and micronutrient deficiencies, the depletion of predator species, and water shortages.

In the latter half of the twentieth century, population growth rates accelerated; indeed, the world passed through its highest-ever annual growth rates, over 2%. The pressures to boost food production were therefore increased. The Green Revolution relieved the situation during the 1960s–1980s. However, in the final decade or so of the last century, the rate of increase in the production of cereal grain – which accounts for around two-thirds of world food energy – fell below the (gradually declining) rate of increase in world population. Per-person production of cereal grains peaked in 1985 (King, 1999), but to perhaps a large extent, the subsequent decline reflected political decisions and realities in several regions of the world rather than an impairment of agroecosystem yields (Dyson, 1999a).

Will world production of cereal grains keep pace with the increased population growth and the increased consumer demand (as more grain is diverted into livestock production)? Forecasts by most international agencies remain optimistic: they foresee future food production matching increased population size and rising consumer demand at the global level over the next 2–3 decades. At the regional level, however, the prospect is for worsening food security in sub-Saharan Africa and for only marginal improvement in South Asia. Whatever else, it seems clear that cereal grain exports from North America, Europe, Australia and Argentina will have to rise to meet the increased demand in many developing countries as their populations continue to grow (Dyson, 1999b). The answer to the above question will depend on the balance achieved between the positive and negative influences. Global environmental changes loom as a major source of potentially negative influences.

Global climate change and food production

From long human experience, we know that climatic fluctuations can disrupt food production, leading to famine, deaths and social unrest. The climate is less irregular in Europe and North America than in most other regions of the world, particularly tropical and subtropical regions. Floods and famines in China and famines in India have been notorious killers over the centuries (Bryson & Murray, 1997; Fagan, 1999). In China, where vegetables and rice have long accounted for nearly all of the caloric intake by the toiling peasantry, famines have been recorded (by China's long-centralized bureaucracy) in one or more provinces in over 90% of all years between 108 BC and 1910 AD. Great famines have occurred once or twice every century in India over the past 1000 years, causing hundreds of thousands, sometimes millions, of deaths (Fagan, 1999).

Today, we face the prospect of human-induced climate change (IPCC, 2001). The anticipated globally averaged warming is on the order of 2–3 °C over the coming century. The warming would be greater at higher latitudes than at low latitudes, greater on land than at sea, and greater in winter than in summer. Overall, rainfall would increase because of the intensification of the hydrological cycle at higher temperatures, with increased evaporation. There would, nevertheless, be considerable regional variation in patterns of change in temperature and rainfall. This has potentially great implications for future food production. Further, climate change will entail not just shifts in mean temperatures and seasonal rainfall levels; climatologists also foresee an increase in climatic variability. This would result in an increase in extreme weather events in many regions of the world.

Food yields, especially of agricultural crops, are likely to be affected by shifts in mean climatic conditions (Rosenzweig & Iglesias, 1998; Winters *et al.*, 1999; IPCC, 2001). Those shifts would entail warmer temperatures, changes in growing seasons, altered patterns of precipitation, and, in many rain-dependent regions, reduced soil moisture. The impacts of a change in mean climatic conditions may not all be adverse. Regions with a temperate or cold climate might undergo increased yields in response to increased temperature. However, many mid-continental and semi-arid regions would be vulnerable to crop failures caused by small increases in warming and soil drying. Irrigation-dependent agriculture would be vulnerable to reduced rainfall, exacerbated by heightened evaporative losses. Less predictably, climatic changes would influence the ecology of plant pests and pathogens. Further, a less quantifiable risk arises from the likely increase in extreme weather events under a climate change regime. Floods, droughts, storms and fires all pose episodic, sometimes severe, risks to regional food production.

Scientists have used dynamic crop growth models to simulate the effects of climate change, in conjunction with increased atmospheric carbon dioxide on cereal crop yields (Rosenzweig & Iglesias, 1998; McMichael, 2001b). These models represent the important physiological processes responsible for plant growth and development. They also include other major factors that affect yields: climatic conditions, soil characteristics, management practices and genotypic features. The models can be used to predict both rain-fed and irrigated crop yields. Note, however, that none of the models yet in use include consideration of the climatic modulation of pest or pathogen activity. The estimated impact of standard scenarios of global climate change is for an approximately 70 million additional hungry people by the 2080s (equivalent to around a 40% increase on the background expectation for that decade) (Parry *et al.*, 1999). Regionally, most of this nutritional adversity would occur in sub-Saharan Africa. The resultant additional hunger and malnutrition would increase the risk of infant and child mortality and cause physical and intellectual stunting. In adults, energy levels, work capacity and health status would be compromised.

Water is an essential input to agriculture and animal husbandry: for example, currently four-fifths of water usage in India is for agriculture. In many regions, water supplies may be adversely affected by climate change. Reductions in rainfall are most likely in South Asia, the Middle East, North Africa and Central America. Tensions over freshwater shortages would be exacerbated by climate-related changes in rainfall where adjoining countries share river basins, particularly in North Africa, the Middle East, South Asia and South-east Asia. Conflict and a public health crisis might then result (McMichael, 2001a).

The rise in the sea level is another environmental consequence of global warming. A half-metre rise (at today's population) would approximately double the number who experience flooding annually from around 50 million to 100 million. Some of the world's coastal arable land and fish-nurturing mangroves would be damaged by a rise in sea level. Rising seas would also salinate coastal freshwater aquifers, particularly those beneath small islands.

Dietary heterogeneity, and change, around the world

It is evident that there are current and impending stresses on the world's food producing systems, on land and at sea. Meanwhile, as is well known, there are major differences in the types of foods and the nutrient profile consumed by populations in different parts of the world. Much of this variation reflects the particularities of local environments and their associated repertoire of natural and introduced species of plants and animals. The following diagram displays the differences in nutrient composition of regional diets. This, of course, is merely a snapshot of an evolving global profile of human diets. As societies modernize and grow wealthier, social diets change. Classic micronutrient deficiencies and food contaminants are replaced by the

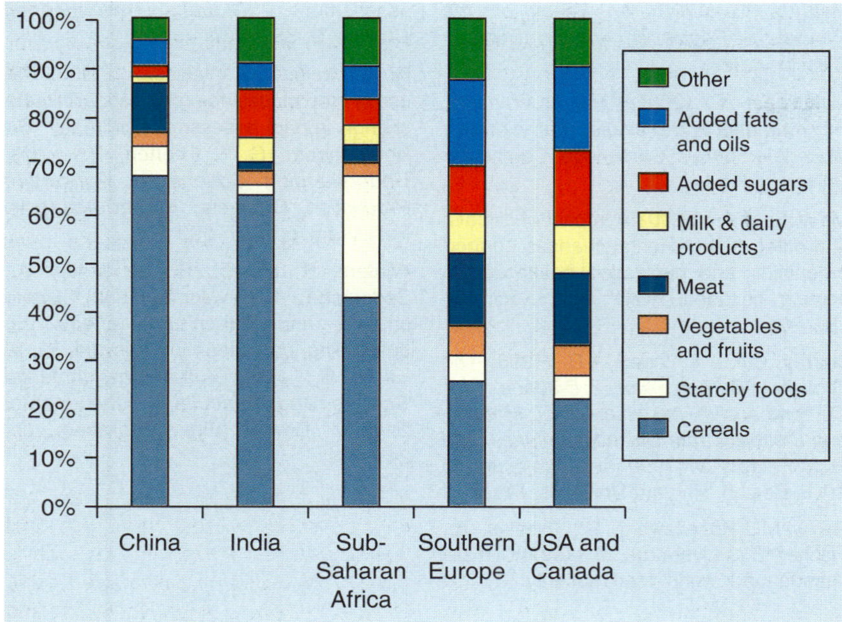

Figure 1
Geographical regional differences in dietary profile

imbalances of affluence, compounded by physical inactivity. This process has been referred to as the nutrition transition.

These differences between regional populations have many implications for the anticipation of diet-related risks of cancer. Much of the epidemiological research has been done in developed countries, eating a Western-type of diet. Yet much of the interest lies in estimating risks for the much larger number of people living in other countries, where dietary changes are spreading as urbanization grows and as consumer preferences and buying power change.

We therefore need to enquire about the likelihood of nutrient–nutrient interactions occurring. For example, might fruits and vegetables have a stronger cancer-protective effect in (poorer) developing countries characterized by micronutrient-deficient populations? There may also be some gene–nutrient interactions that have significant influences on diet-related risks of cancer. For example, many of the metabolic polymorphic active alleles are more prevalent in Asian than in African and European populations. And we must also remember that the shape of the dose-response function is often not known outside the range of Western observations.

Finally, it should be stressed that the public health goal is a food-and-nutrition policy that optimizes the population's health outcome. Avoiding cancer is not our only task. Reassuringly, the main findings in relation to dietary protective effects are convergent across major disease outcomes: cardiovascular disease, diabetes and cancer. This applies, for example, to obesity, physical inactivity, fruit and vegetable intake, red meat versus fish intake, and antioxidants in food. It also appears that reducing the consumption of saturated fats (thus affecting either their direct metabolic action or their role as an obesity promoter) confers general health benefits. This convergence is probably not coincidental, but reflects the long play of underlying biological evolutionary forces.

Conclusions

Environmental influences on the production of food – crops and livestock on land, wild and cultivated fisheries – are diverse, complex and interactive. So, as ever, are cultural influences. These, and the prospects for molecular genetics (GM foods), comprise the main background conditions that will influence future patterns of human diets. Those diets, in turn, will influence the probabilities of cancer occurrence.

In light of the various uncertainties pertaining to future world food yields and the possibility that climatic and other environmental changes could adversely affect world food production, there is a clear need to apply the precautionary principle. There are finite, and increasingly evident, limits to agroecosystems and to wild fisheries. Our capacity to maintain food supplies for an increasingly large and increasingly expectant world population will depend on maximizing the efficiency and sustainability of production methods, incorporating socially beneficial genetic biotechnologies, and taking preemptive action to minimize the future course of detrimental, ecologically damaging, global environmental changes.

References

Bryson, R.A. & Murray, T.J. (1997) *Climates of Hunger: Mankind and the World's Changing Weather*, Madison, University of Wisconsin

Cohen J.E. (1996) *How Many People Can the Earth Support*? New York, Norton

Conroy J.P., Seneweera, S., Basra, A.S., Rogers, G. & Nissenwoller, B. (1994) Influence of rising atmospheric CO_2 concentrations and temperature on growth, yield and grain quality of cereal crops. *Aust. J. Plant Physiol.*, **21**, 741–758

Diamond, J. (1997) *Guns, Germs and Steel*, London, Jonathan Cape

Dyson, T. (1999a) World food trends and prospects to 2025. *Proc. Natl. Acad. Sci. U.S.A.*, **96**, 5929–5936

Dyson, T. (1999b) Prospects for feeding the world. *Br. Med. J.*, **319**, 988–990

Fagan, B. (1999) *Floods, Famines and Emperors. El Nino and the Fate of Civilisations*, New York, Basic Books

Food and Agricultural Organization (1999) *Food Insecurity Report.* 2000. Rome, Food and Agricultural Organization

Greenland, D.J., Gregory, P.J. & Nye, P.H. (1998) Land resources and constraints to crop production. In: Waterlow, J.C., Armstrong D.G., Fowden L., Riley R., eds, *Feeding a World Population of More Than Eight Billion*, Oxford, Oxford University Press, pp. 39–55

Intergovernmental Panel on Climate Change (IPCC) (2001) *Climate Change 2000. Third Assessment Report*, Cambridge, Cambridge University Press

King, M. (1999) Commentary: bread for the world – another view. *Br. Med. J.*, **319**, 991

Malthus, T. (1798) *An Essay on the Principle of Population*, London (Penguin Classics, 1985)

McMichael, A.J. (2001a) *Human Frontiers, Environments and Disease: Past patterns, Uncertain Futures*. Cambridge: Cambridge University Press

McMichael, A.J. (2001b) Impact of climatic and other environmental changes on food production and population health in the coming decades. *Proc. Nutr. Soc.*, **60**, 195–201

Murray, C.J.L. & Lopez, A.D. (1996) *The Global Burden of Disease. A Comprehensive Assessment of Mortality and Disability from Diseases, Injuries, and Risk Factors in 1990 and Projected to 2020.* Boston, Harvard University Press

Parry, M., Rosenzweig, C., Iglesias, A., Fischer, G. & Livermore, M. (1999) Climate change and world food security: a new assessment. *Global Environmental Change*, **9**, S51–S67

Rosenzweig, C. & Iglesias, A. (1998) The use of crop models for international climate change impact assessment. In: Tsuji, G., Hoogrnboom, G. & Thorton, P.K., eds, *Understanding Options for Agriculture Production*, Dortrecht, Kluwer Academic Publishers, pp. 267–292

Winters, P., Murgai, R., de Janvry, A., Sadoulet, E. & Frisvold, G. (1999) Climate change and agriculture: effects on developing countries. In: Frisvold, G. & Kuhn, B., eds, *Global Environmental Change and Agriculture*, Cheltenham, England, Edward Elgar Publishers, pp. 241–264

The dietary prevention of ischaemic heart disease

Saracci R.

Division of Epidemiology, IFC-National Research Council, Pisa, Italy. Nutrition and Cancer Unit, International Agency for Research on Cancer, Lyon, France

Introduction

Links between nutritional factors and cardiovascular diseases have been foreseen for more than a century: early anatomical recognition of fatty degeneration in major arteries goes back to the nineteenth century and seminal experiments showing coronary atheromas in rabbits fed diets high in cholesterol have been carried out since the beginning of the twentieth century (Leibowitz, 1970). Based on clinical observations, recommendations had also been issued on dietary approaches to heart disease. In 1894, one classic medical textbook (Strumpell, 1894) advised that treatment for "coronary sclerosis' should be based . . . on dietary and general hygiene measures. In adipose subjects simple and moderate eating is prescribed reducing to a minimum or eliminating alcoholic drinks, and allowing no more than two to three cigars daily. Regular exercise . . . is not only useful but necessary . . . avoiding violent efforts." For obesity it firmly stated: "All slimming methods, however numerous, stand on the same principle: reduction of intake and increase in consumption. This principle can be applied in several different ways." More than a century later, a vast amount of experimental and epidemiological research has validated, qualified and extended the broadly correct foresight of this advice.

The current evidence

Currently available evidence establishes three factors as causally related to ischaemic heart disease (IHD): energy imbalance, dietary fats and alcoholic drinks.

The evidence for a causal role of *energy imbalance* (Willett, 1998; Willett *et al.*, 1995; Larsson, 1994) derives from three sources. First the Nurse Health Study, among other large observational cohort studies, shows that the risk of symptomatic non-fatal myocardial infarction and of fatal IHD rises steadily with the rise in BMI above 21; no excess for other causes of death is apparent below a BMI of 21 once the data have been adjusted for confounders. Weight gain since age 18 also shows a clear relation to IHD incidence. Second, several prospective cohort studies show an increase in incidence of IHD, independently of BMI, with an increase in intraabdominal fat, measured directly by CAT scan or indirectly through body anthropometric indices. Third, randomized clinical trials demonstrate that weight loss over the medium term lowers blood pressure, glucose, total cholesterol, LDL cholesterol and raises HDL cholesterol. These variables, pathogenetically connected to IHD, appear to be mediators of most if not all of the relationship between overweight and IHD, as indicated in observational data by the weakening of the association between overweight and IHD risk, once the variables have been controlled for confounders.

In the second half of the century, a large number of investigations, including direct studies in humans, have established the role of *dietary fats* in IHD occurrence. In contrast, the specific role of total fats, individual fats as well as of the balance between them and with other energy-providing nutrients, in particular carbohydrates, is still open to discussion. Support for the fats–IHD causal link comes from the interconnected evidence of six kinds of studies in humans (Willet *et al.*, 1995). First, striking mortality differences for IHD have been observed between populations with different fat intakes: in the classic seven-country study (Menotti *et al.*, 1989) IHD mortality rates spanned over a 50-fold range between Crete (Greece) and East Finland. Second, more than 20 prospective cohort studies show a relation between fat intake and IHD occurrence rates. Third, metabolic studies under controlled conditions demonstrate that total blood cholesterol (TC) and its fractions are responsive to the qualitative and quantitative fat composition of diet, allowing calculation of predictive equations. Fourth, multiple prospective cohort studies show a smooth, continuous increase in IHD risk with increasing TC levels: the MRFIT study reported a fourfold rise in risk for TC levels above 264 mg/dL compared to levels below 167 mg/dL. An even sharper dose–response relationship is observed with respect to the TC/HDL-cholesterol ratio, HDL cholesterol being itself inversely related to IHD risk. Fifth, a primary prevention randomized trial in healthy hypercholesterolemic men (Shepherd *et al.*, 1995) using pravastatin, a cholesterol-lowering drug, has shown a near 30% reduction in cardiac deaths; another randomized trial (Gotto *et al.*, 2000) using lovastatin has shown a more substantial effect on the occurrence of first major coronary events in healthy subjects extending beyond those with a high-risk lipid profile. Finally, there is evidence, more from secondary than from primary prevention trials, of a reduced IHD risk when saturated fats are replaced by polyunsaturated fats, in particular those of the n-3 category.

Evidence from large prospective cohort studies (Doll, 1997) shows that moderate *alcohol* drinkers, up to about 30 g/day, incur, regardless of the type of drinks, a myocardial infarction risk 30% lower compared to nondrinkers. Higher consumptions steadily increase, among other conditions, the risk of hypertension and haemorrhagic stroke.

Besides these now established causal factors *other dietary components*, including foods, macronutrients and micronutrients, have been studied in relation to IHD (Willett, 1998). The evidence supporting, to a varying degree, their etiological or protective role leaves room for doubt. They include the potentially adverse effects of high salt intake, saturated fats, trans-fatty acids; the potentially protective effects of monounsaturated fats, n-3 polyunsaturated fats, fruit, vegetables and fibre, and folic acid; and the uncertain role of n-6 polyunsaturated fats. Pragmatically, the knowledge available today on these foods and nutrients is generally given some weight for recommendation purposes.

Recommendations

In the light of present knowledge, recommendations have been issued (for example in Krauss *et al.*, 2000 and (National Heart, Lung and Blood Institute, 2000), which should be regarded as approximate and bound to change, particularly as to the quantitative aspects.

The *primary recommendation* is for Mediterranean-style diets, which are not harmful and highly likely beneficial, calorically matched to individual requirements. The dietary pattern is based on vegetables, fruits, legumes, whole grains, fish and poultry, with a balance between caloric intake and physical activity expenditure. General recommendations to eat moderately do not make sense if the energy expenditure of an individual is not known: in fact, large dietary intake often derives from a high-energy requirement for physical activity. Hence overweight needs to be individually screened by measuring weight and height, and dietary counseling tailored to keep BMI around or below 25. To obtain and maintain this target, moderate and regular physical exercise (as can be comfortably sustained for at least 1 hour, e.g. walking or cycling) is an indispensable complement of dietary control.

Additional quantitative specifications, more open to uncertainty and liable to modification, involve the following:

- Salt: reduce added salt to keep the total daily amount to less than 6 g;
- Fats: total intake contributing less than 30% of energy, with less than 10% from saturated fat, 10%–15% from monounsaturated fats, and 5%–10% of polyunsaturated fats with an approximate 4:1 ratio of n-6 to n-3 fats;
- Alcohol: a maximum of 30 g per day for men and even less (or none) for women because of the risk of breast cancer, particularly in high-incidence families or populations and the usually smaller benefit for IHD prevention.

The EPIC-Heart project

Firmer quantitative recommendations depend on clarifying the role of factors which remain in doubt, by the possible identification of additional dietary determinants of IHD and by a better definition of specific protective dietary patterns. For these purposes, a primary source of information will derive from ongoing large prospective studies such as the EPIC-Heart project, which represents the cardiovascular disease component of EPIC. There is an obvious advantage to investigating diseases other than cancers within EPIC. From a research point of view, EPIC offers the excellent infrastructure consisting of a large array of exposure variables collected with uniform or close procedures, the availability of stored biological samples and follow-up facilities. From a public health point of view, results will be obtained in the same European populations both for cancers and cardiovascular diseases, thus placing on a common basis whatever dietary recommendations may derive from the study. Twenty-one centres in ten countries are taking part in EPIC-Heart. The first step of the project is an investigation of dietary factors in relation to fatal myocardial infarction. More than 1000 deaths from IHD have already been accumulated. Initially, the relation of food groups and alcohol consumption to these deaths will be explored, followed by analyses by key nutrients as soon as data on nutrients become available: a nested case–control investigation is then planned focusing on blood lipid and fatty acid profiles, with the particular aim of examining the potential protective role of the n-3 alfa-linolenic acid (Leaf, 1999). This first step of the project will also be of value to identify possible needs to make the EPIC resource, primarily designed for cancer studies, an optimal resource for investigating other diseases as well.

References

Doll, R. (1997) One for the heart. *BMJ*, **315**, 1664–1668

Gotto, A.M. Jr., Whitney, E., Stein, E.A., Shapiro, D.R., Clearfield, M., Weis, S., Jou, J.Y., Langendorfer, A., Beere, P.A., Watson, D.J., Downs, J.R. & de Cani, J.S. (2000) Application of the National Cholesterol Education Program and joint European treatment criteria and clinical benefit in the Air Force/Texas Coronary Atherosclerosis Prevention Study (AFCAPS/TexCAPS). *Eur. Heart J.*, **21**, 1627–1633

Krauss, R.M., Eckel, R.H., Howard, B., Appel, L.J., Daniels, S.R., Deckelbaum, R.J., Erdman, J.W. Jr., Kris-Etherton, P., Goldberg, I.J., Kotchen, T.A., Lichtenstein, A.H., Mitch, W.E., Mullis, R., Robinson, K., Wylie-Rosett, J., St Jeor, S., Suttie, J., Tribble, D.L. & Bazzarre, T.L. (2000) AHA dietary guidelines. *Circulation*, **102**, 2284–2299

Larsson, B. (1994) Obesity and body fat distribution as predictors of coronary heart disease, In: Marmot, M. & Elliott, P., eds, *Coronary Heart Disease Epidemiology*, Oxford, Oxford University Press

Leaf, A. (1999) Dietary prevention of coronary heart disease: the Lyon diet heart study. *Circulation*, **99**, 733–735

Leibowitz, J.O. (1970) The History of Coronary Heart Disease, London, *Wellcome Institute of the History of Medicine*

Menotti, A., Keys, A., Arvanis, C., Blackburn, H., Dontas, A., *et al.* (1989) Seven Countries Study. First 20-year mortality data in 12 cohorts of six countries. *Ann. Med.*, **21**, 175–9

National Heart, Lung and Blood Institute. (2000) *Clinical Guidelines on the Identification, Evaluation and Treatment of Overweight and Obesity in Adults*, (NIH Publication no. 00-4084), Washington, D.C., National Institutes of Health

Shepherd, J., Cobbe, S.M., Ford, I., Isles, C.G., Lorimer, A.R., MacFarlane, P.W., McKillop, J.H. & Packard, C.J. (1995) Prevention of coronary heart disease with pravastatin in men with hypercholesterolemia. West of Scotland Coronary Prevention Study. *N. Engl. J. Med.*, **333**, 1301–1307

Strumpell, A. (1894) *Treatise of Medical Pathology and Therapeutics*, 8th ed. Erlangen, Germany

Willett, W.C., Manson, J.E., Stampfer, M.J., Colditz, G.A., Rosner, B., Speizer, F.E. & Hennekens, C.H. (1995) Weight, weight change, and coronary heart disease in women. *J.A.M.A.*, **273**, 461–465

Willett, W. (1998) *Nutritional Epidemiology, 2nd ed.* New York, Oxford University Press, ch.17

Malignant tumour follow-up in Italy, 1993–1998

Evangelista A.[1], Tagliabue G.[2], Del Sette D.[1], Tittarelli A.[2], Contiero P.[2], Krogh V.[1], Crosignani P.[2], Berrino F.[1]
(The EPIC cohort in Varese)

[1]Epidemiology Unit, [2]Lombardy Cancer Registry Unit, Istituto Nazionale per lo Studio e la Cura dei Tumori, Milan, Italy.

Aim of study

EPIC is a multicentre prospective cohort study investigating the relation between diet, nutrition, and lifestyle and cancer risk (Riboli & Kaaks, 1997). This study reports on follow-up in the EPIC cohort of Varese, in northern Italy.

Materials and methods

Cohort

12 079 volunteers were enrolled (9525 women and 2554 men) from 31 August 1993 to 17 December 1997. Mean age at recruitment was 51.6 years: 51.2 in women and 53.2 in men. Eight subjects were younger than 35 and 199 were over 70 at recruitment. All completed food frequency and lifestyle questionnaires, provided blood samples and were actively followed.

Lombardy Cancer Registry

The Lombardy Cancer Registry (LCR) collects all cases of malignant disease incident in the province. Malignant neoplasms are those defined by ICD-9 classification (World Health Organisation, 1977).

Follow-up

To identify EPIC cohort members in the Lombardy Regional Population Database and to verify vital status, we used semiprobabilistic linkage software (EPILINK) developed by the LCR. Once identified, each EPIC participant was assigned, within the EPIC anagraphic database, the official code that identified that individual within the Lombardy Region Files. This made it possible to speed up the subsequent phase of the follow-up.

We then used this code to link EPIC participants to several official databases made available by the LCR:

- Regional Population Health Database of Lombardy, which includes approximately 11 million subjects, 1 million of these in Varese Province.
- Admission and discharge reports for hospital patients, which accumulate about 26 000 oncological records per year.
- Lombardy Cancer Registry, which has data on 91 000 cancer patients and 102 000 cancers, registered from 1976.

The linked subjects were then compared with records in another database containing records from the three main pathology laboratories in Varese Province in order to check the histological or cytological diagnoses of the tumours.

Results

The vital status of the cohort at 31 December 1998 is shown in Table 1.

The most frequent cancer sites were breast (108 tumours), skin (15), ovary (13), stomach (10), corpus uteri (9) and kidney (9) for women, whereas skin cancer (6) and non-Hodgkin's lymphoma (4) were the most frequent cancers in the (few) men of the cohort.

Of these neoplasms, 95.3% were confirmed histologically, 4.3% were confirmed cytologically and 0.4% were verified medically or by imaging.

With regard to causes of death in the Varese EPIC cohort, the main underlying causes were cancer (65.7%) followed by cardiovascular disease (22.9%) and other causes (11.4%).

Observed/expected cases

We used the ECIDC computer program to calculate expected cancer cases at 31 December 1998 in a dynamic cohort (Micheli & Krogh, 1994). The observed/expected ratio for women is shown in Table 2.

For most cancers – the exceptions being kidney, breast and ovary cancer – the actual incidence was lower than expected.

Table 1. Varese EPIC cohort: vital status on December 31, 1998

VS Code	Description		No. of subjects
1	Alive		11 728
2	Dead		70
7	Emigrated to another region of Italy		87
8	Emigrated to another country		0
9	Unknown	Lost to follow up	4
		To be followed actively because not covered by the National Health Service	
	Total		12 079

Median length of follow-up was 3.68 years: 3.98 in women and 2.04 in men.

Table 2. Varese EPIC cohort: observed/expected case ratio for malignant cancers in women at 31 December 1998

IDC-9 site	Description	Obs/exp	95% CI
151	Stomach	1.17	0.45–1.90
153	Colon	0.49	0.15–0.82
154	Rectum	0.57	0.01–1.13
162	Lung	0.87	0.22–1.51
172	Melanoma	1.09	0.14–2.05
173	Skin	0.74	0.37–1.11
174	Breast	1.28	1.03–1.53
182	Corpus uteri	0.66	0.23–1.09
183	Ovary	1.23	0.56–1.89
189	Kidney	1.82	0.63–3.00
202	Non-Hodgkin lymphoma	0.57	0.07–1.08

Obs, observed; exp, expected; CI, confidence interval.

The observed/expected ratios for men are unlikely to be meaningful in view of the small number of enrolled males (2554) and the correspondingly low length of follow-up (2.04 years) and person-years (7065). It is important to note, however, that the expected cases of lung cancer in men were 13.83, whereas we observed only three.

Conclusions

The incidence relative to the general population was significantly low for colon cancers in women and also for lung cancer in men (Obs/exp, 0.22). This suggests that the enrolled population is self-selected on the basis of dietary or other lifestyle factors (Faggiano *et al.*, 1997).

The number of breast cancer cases was significantly higher than expected, suggesting that women at high risk were more motivated to participate.

The results on incidence are remarkably complete, mainly due to the use of multiple follow-up methods by this experienced cancer registry. Only 281 persons (2.3%) were lost or had emigrated. Furthermore, the percentage of death certificate-only cases in the LCR database was low at 2.4% (Zanetti *et al.*, eds, 1997).

Acknowledgements

The EPIC study is being financed by the Europe Against Cancer Programme, the Italian Ministry of Health and the Italian Association for Cancer Research (AIRC).

We are indebted to Mrs. Manuela Bellegotti and Mr. Donald C. Ward for technical support.

References

Faggiano, F., Partanen, T., Kogevinas, M. & Boffetta, P. (1997) *Socioeconomic Differences in Cancer Incidence and Mortality*, (IARC Scientific Publications No. 138). Lyon, IARC, pp. 65–177

Micheli, A. & Krogh, V. (1994) A computer program to calculate expected cases in a dynamic cohort. *Epidemiol. Prev.*, **18**, 164–169

Riboli, E. & Kaaks, R. (1997) The EPIC project: rationale and study design. *Int. J. Epidemiol.*, **26** (Suppl 1), S6–S14

World Health Organisation (1977) *International Classification of Diseases, 9th Revision, Vol. 1*, Geneva, World Health Organisation

Zanetti, R., Crosignani, P. & Rosso, S., eds, (1997) Il Cancro in Italia. I dati di incidenza dei registri tumori 1988–1992, Vol. 2, Roma, Il Pensiero Scientifico Editore

Benign neoplasms: a follow-up study in Italy, 1993–1998

Contiero P.[2], Evangelista A.[1], Tittarelli A.[2], Del Sette D.[1], Krogh V.[1], Berrino F.[1], Tagliabue G.[2]
(the EPIC cohort in Varese)

[1]Epidemiology Unit, [2]Lombardy Cancer Registry Unit, Istituto Nazionale per lo Studio e la Cura dei Tumori, Milan, Italy.

Aim of study

Few population-based data are available on the frequency of benign compared to malignant neoplasms. However, pathological data indicate that certain histotypes of benign tumours are relatively common (Marshall *et al.*, 1997) in the population. The etiologies of these tumours are largely unknown and very few studies have been published (Faerstein *et al.*, 2001; Sharara *et al.*, 1995). In the present study we analysed the various types of benign tumours present within the Varese EPIC cohort for subjects requiring hospitalization or biopsy.

Methods

Cohort

The Varese, Italy EPIC cohort consists of 9525 women and 2554 men, all resident in the Province of Varese, who enrolled voluntarily in the study during the period 1993–1997. The Province of Varese (800 000 inhabitants) is covered by the Lombardy Cancer Registry and is part of the Region of Lombardy (9 000 000 inhabitants). Anagraphic, anthropometric, professional, and educational information was collected from the volunteers at enrolment. Blood samples were also taken and stored in liquid nitrogen. In addition, detailed dietary and lifestyle questionnaires were compiled for each volunteer and transferred to a database.

Follow-up

From 31 August 1993 to 31 December 1998 all neoplasms, including benign types, that arose in the cohort were registered firstly by accessing the files in the Lombardy Cancer Registry, and secondly by active searches in admission and discharge files in all hospitals and clinics of the Lombardy Region. Additional data were obtained by accessing the files of several pathology laboratories. The median length of follow-up was 3.68 years: 3.98 years for women and 2.04 years for men (enrolment for men began in 1995).

Definition of benign neoplasms

Histotypes with morphological behaviour 0 (ICD-0, WHO, 1990) or topography code between 210 and 229 (ICD-9, WHO, 1977) were considered benign. Benign transitional papilloma of the bladder was not included.

Results

Of the 296 cases of benign tumour found, 59.8% were confirmed histologically, 31.8% were confirmed medically, 5.7% were confirmed by imaging and 2.7% were diagnosed by other means.

The most common benign neoplasm in women was uterine leiomyoma (124 cases) followed by lipoma (22 cases), benign breast neoplasms (22 cases), and benign nervous system neoplasms (18 cases). In men, lipoma (6 cases) followed by neoplasms of other parts of the digestive system (5 cases), central nervous system (4 cases), skin (4 cases) and oral cavity (4 cases) were the most common (Table 1).

Associations between malignant and benign tumours in females are shown in Table 2. Leiomyoma was associated with breast and ovarian malignancy in two cases each. Leiomyoma was most frequently associated with benign neoplasms of the ovary (5 cases) and the breast (2 cases).

Conclusions

Leiomyoma, probably a hormone-dependent tumour (Marshall *et al.*, 1998), was the most common benign

Table 1. Varese EPIC cohort: vital status on December 31, 1998

Women ICD-9 site	Description	No. of cases
218	Uterine leiomyoma	124
216	Skin	24
214	Lipoma	22
217	Breast	22
225	Brain and other parts of nervous system	18
228	Haemangioma and lymphangioma	14
220	Ovary	11
227	Other endocrine glands and related structures	10
210	Lip, oral cavity and pharynx	6
211	Other parts of digestive system	5
226	Thyroid gland	3
215	Connective and other soft tissues	3
219	Other uterus	3
213	Bone and articular cartilage	1
221	Other female genital organs	1
223	Kidney and other urinary organs	1
Men		
214	Lipoma	6
211	Other parts of digestive system	5
225	Brain and other parts of nervous system	4
216	Skin	4
210	Lip, oral cavity and pharynx	4
213	Bone and articular cartilage	2
228	Haemangioma and lymphangioma	1
227	Other endocrine glands and related structures	1
223	Kidney and other urinary organs	1

The cohort has many more females than males because males began to be recruited later.

Table 2. Associations between benign and malignant tumours in individual patients

Benign	Malignant	No. of cases
Leiomyoma	Breast	2
Leiomyoma	Ovary	2
Breast	Breast	2
Lipoma	Ovary	1
Skin	Breast	1
Breast	Endometrium	1
Leiomyoma	Thymus	1
Leiomyoma	Endometrium	1
Other Uterus	Endometrium	1
Ovary	Endometrium	1
Brain	Pleura	1
Thyroid	Colon	1
Haemangioma	Colon	1
Haemangioma	Breast	1

All the reported associations were found in women only.

tumour in women. The high frequency of this tumour suggests that the EPIC study will be able to analyse the relation of this tumour to hormone levels and dietary factors, and possibly other tumours with longer follow-up. The epidemiological association between benign meningiomas and tumours of the female reproductive tract has recently been shown to be related to receptor-mediated hormone sensitivity in the affected cell types (Carrol *et al.*, 1999).

Leiomyoma may also be considered a marker of hormonal exposure, which may contribute to our understanding of the etiology of hormone-dependent malignant tumours of other organs (e.g. breast, endometrium and ovary).

Whereas most malignant tumours mainly affect epithelia (88.0% of malignant cases in our cohort), benign neoplasms mainly (86.9%) affect mesenchyme.

Acknowledgement

The EPIC study is being financed by the Europe Against Cancer Programme, the Italian Ministry of Health and the Italian Association for Cancer Research (AIRC). We are indebted to Manuela Bellegotti and Donald Ward for technical support.

References

Carroll, R.S., Zhang, J. & Black, P.M. (1999) Expression of estrogen receptors alpha and beta in human meningiomas *J. Neurooncol.*, **42**, 109–116

Faerstein, E., Szklo, M. & Rosenshein, N. (2001) Risk factors for uterine leiomyoma: a practice-based case–control study. *Am. J. Epidemiol.*, **153**, 1–10

International Classification of Diseases (ICD-9), 1977, World Health Organization, Geneva

International Classification of Diseases for Oncology (ICD-O), 1990, World Health Organization, Geneva

Marshall, L.M., Spiegelman, D., Barbieri, R.L., Goldman, M.B., Manson, J.E., Colditz, G.A., Willett, W.C. & Hunter, D.J.

(1997) Variation in incidence of uterine leiomyoma among premenopausal women by age and race. *Obstet. Gynecol.*, **90**, 967–973

Marshall, L.M., Spiegelman, D. & Goldman, M.B. (1998) A prospective study of reproductive factors and oral contraceptive use in relation to the risk of uterine leiomyomata. *Fertil. Steril.*, **70**, 432–439

Sharara, F.I. & Nieman, L.K., (1995) Growth hormone receptor messenger ribonucleic acid expression in leiomyoma and surrounding myometrium. *Am. J. Obstet. Gynecol.*, **13**, 198–202

Age at exposure to the Dutch famine of 1944–1945 has opposing effects on adult mammographic density (DY); a study in the DOM cohort

Van Noord P.A.H., Haars G., Peeters P.H.M.

Julius Center for General Practice and Patient-Oriented Research, University Medical Center Utrecht, Utrecht, The Netherlands.

Purpose

Caloric restriction in rodents is known to extend their life span, in part due to a reduction in hormone-dependent tumours. Our group studies whether similar protective effects can be found for humans. This is being done among a cohort of women, unfortunately exposed to a historical "experiment" known as the Dutch famine of 1944–1945.

Radio-density, first described by Wolfe in 1976 and at that time called dysplasia (DY), is a clear breast cancer risk indicator, now considered an intermediate endpoint in the study of breast cancer. DY tends to decline with age, an early first childbirth, a higher parity, while it may increase when women start taking hormone replacement therapy (HRT).

After our earlier demonstration that famine exposure at well-defined age categories of development can affect, already before puberty, reproductive maturation (menarche) (van Noord & Kaaks, 1991) and (long) bone growth (van Noord & Arias-Careaga, 1995), both of which are breast cancer risk factors, we studied the impact of exposure to famine early in life on DY later in life.

Methods

Mammograms and famine exposure data were available for about 20 000 women born between 1911 and 1943, so between 2 and 34 years of age at the peak of the famine. The women volunteered in the DOM cohort, a population-based breast cancer screening study, and lived in the famine-exposed area of The Netherlands.

Analyses were performed by four different, biologically relevant age-at-exposure categories: age 2–9, representing prepubertal development; 10–12, the age covering the peak growth spurt in girls; 13–18, the age from menarche to first childbirth; and the ages over 18 (18–34 years), the age when most women have a first child. All screening mammograms had been classified as yes or no for DY. Based on individual recollections, women had reported their exposure to hunger, cold and/or weight loss during the famine.

Results

For women exposed after the age of 18, significant effects were found for having DY as adults, effects that were independent of parity, body weight and adult height.

Conclusions

The youngest age window that we could study in this cohort (2–9 years) showed a decrease in DY later in life, although nonsignificant. This is, however, also the age category most vulnerable to an increase in breast cancer in the Japanese women exposed to nuclear fall-out in Hiroshima and Nagasaki (Boice *et al.*, 1979).

The finding of higher DY levels in women exposed to the famine after age 18 seems contradictory. These effects seemed stronger in women that had

Table 1. Risk of having DY breast patterns when exposed to the famine, stratified to age categories when famine occurred and parity

Age at exposure	*n*	Women without children *n*=2757 OR (95% CI)	Women with children *n*=16 973 OR (95% CI)	All women *n*=19 730 OR (95% CI)
2–9 years	6560	0.69 (0.36–1.33)	0.84 (0.64–1.09)	0.83 (0.65–1.06)
10–12 years	2560	0.55 (0.20–1.51)	1.11 (0.78–1.63)	1.02 (0.72–1.44)
13–18 years	3586	0.53 (0.27–1.01)	1.05 (0.76–1.43)	0.96 (0.72–1.27)
>18 years	7024	1.20 (0.85–1.70)	1.37 (1.17–1.62)	1.32 (1.14–1.53)
Total	19 730	0.90 (0.70–1.17)	1.19 (1.06–1.34)	1.16 (1.04–1.29)

given birth to a child. Exposure, however, after age 18 and a first childbirth, could have nullified a known DY, reducing the effect of (first) pregnancy. This could be due to a breast gland stimulating growth effect due to a gonadotrophin and/or insulin-like growth-factor surge, induced by the abrupt refeeding after the famine (Thissen *et al.*, 1994). Such effects may only occur in postpubertal adult women who have an already fully developed, mature reproductive system. Such a rebound phenomenon would be similar to the temporary (glandular) gynaecomastia observed among male prisoners of war upon refeeding after liberation, related to higher production and availability of endogenous hormones. Also, women starting HRT can show a return of DY. Immediately after birth is another period in life when gonadotrophins and reproductive hormones can be even higher than in adult women, showing rapid changes that can also cause gynaecomasty and even the production of 'witches' milk or abnormal nipple discharge (Neele *et al.*, 1995).

This study indicates that possible effects of caloric deprivation on cancer risk may be entirely dependent on the age at exposure. These caloric effects, either direct or indirect, may not necessarily have a cancer risk-reducing impact.

The time window before age 10 may be specifically vulnerable for breast cancer risk modification. This is the age category in Western countries where now the greatest impact of caloric abundance, causing overweight, is seen. Abruptness and/or fluctuations in caloric intake later in life may have deleterious effects on (breast) cancer risk factors, though by different mechanisms.

Acknowledgements

This study was supported by WCRF GRANT 9969.

References

Boice, J.D., Land, C.E., Shore, R.E., Norman, J.E. & Tokunaga, M. (1979) Risk of breast cancer following low-dose radiation exposure. *Radiology*, **131**, 589--597

Neely, E.K., Hintz, R.L., Wilson, D.M., Lee, P.A., Gautier, T., Argente, J. & Stene, M. (1995) Normal ranges for immunochemiluminometric gonadotropin assays. *J. Pediatr.*, **127**, 40–46

Thissen, J.P., Ketelslegers, J.M. & Underwood, L.E. (1994) Nutritional regulation of the insulin-like growth factors. *Endocr. Rev.*, **15**, 80–101

Van Noord, P.A.H. & Kaaks, R. (1991) The effect of wartime conditions and the 1944–45 'Dutch Famine' on recalled menarcheal age in participants of the DOM breast cancer screening cohort. *Ann. Hum. Biol.*, **18**, 57–70

Van Noord, P.A.H. & Arias-Careaga, S. (1995) The Dutch Famine 1944–45: lasting effects on adult height. *Am. J. Epidemiol.*, **141**, S11–S44

Diet, energy intake and breast cancer risk in an Asian country

Rattanamongkolgul S.[1], Muir K.[1], Armstrong S.[2], Sriamporn S.[3], Vatanasapt V.[3]

[1]Division of Public Health Sciences, University of Nottingham, UK. [2]Trent Institute for Health Services Research, University of Nottingham, UK. [3]Faculty of Medicine, Khon Kean University, Thailand.

Background

Geographical variations, migration studies and worldwide increased incidence rates of breast cancer point to influences of environmental factors on breast cancer risk, in particular lifestyle and diet. Recent prospective studies do not support the association between breast cancer and fat intake as suggested by geographical correlation and animal studies (Willett *et al.*, 1987). In addition, the link between specific nutrients and breast cancer has not been consistently observed. As a result, the hypothesis of excess total energy intake in relation to elevated breast cancer risk has emerged. The imbalance of total energy intake and energy expenditure can lead to changes in body composition and consequently endogenous hormone metabolism. The hypothesis of this association is supported by evidence that calorie restriction is associated with decreased incidence and mortality of mammary carcinoma in rats and mice. Furthermore, rapid growth and early menarche, which are the risk factors of breast cancer, were suggested to be associated with excess energy intake in childhood (World Cancer Research Fund & American Institute for Cancer Research, 1997). However, most of the evidence was derived from affluent populations where breast cancer incidence rates have been high and excess energy intake and sedentary lifestyle are prevalent. Consistent evidence from low-risk countries would strengthen the association. To investigate this association, we conducted a case–control study in a rural area of Thailand where the age-standardized incidence rate of breast cancer is only 13 per 100 000, about five times lower than the European and the US rates (Parkin *et al.*, 1997).

Methods

A hospital-based case–control study was conducted in rural areas of Thailand, in 1999–2000 after receiving ethics committee approval. All subjects identified through the seven hospitals were women, aged 70 years or less, who had lived in north-east Thailand for at least 1 year. We recruited 405 pathologically confirmed new breast cancer patients diagnosed from 1 November 1998 to 30 June 2000; 811 control patients randomly selected from the same hospitals as the indicator cases were matched for age and residence area. Patients with pregnancy-related conditions, critical illnesses, malignancy and mental disorders were excluded. Face-to-face interviews were conducted using structured questionnaires requesting demographic information, reproductive history, physical activity and family history of breast cancer, including food frequency questionnaires asking for diet in the past year. Body weight, height, and waist and hip circumference were measured at the interviews. Unconditional logistic regression analyses were performed to calculate odd ratios for pre- and postmenopausal women using the statistical package SPSS.

Results

In Table 1, women with a high income or education level tended to have a decreased risk of breast cancer. It was also found that parity and family history of breast cancer were significantly associated. From Tables 2 and 3, it can be seen that height was not associated with breast cancer regardless of menopausal status. High present body weight, body mass index and waist-to-hip ratio were significantly associated with an elevated risk of postmenopausal breast cancer while in postmenopausal women, the results showed a significant reduction

Table 1. Distribution for selected characteristics and breast cancer risk among 405 cases and 811 controls.

Characteristics	Categories	Cases: no. (%)	Controls: no. (%)	Odds ratio (95% CI)	*P* trend[a]
Total annual income (Baht)	1000–16 700	110 (28)	185 (24)		
	16 701–36 000	115 (29)	214 (27)	0.90 (0.65–1.25)	
	36 001–97 200	85 (21)	181 (23)	0.78 (0.55–1.10)	
	97 200–552 600	87 (22)	207 (26)	0.69 (0.49– 0.98)	0.03
Highest education	Pre-primary school	38 (9)	71 (9)	1.00	
	Primary school	271 (67)	497 (61)	0.98 (0.64–1.50)	
	Secondary school	38 (9)	110 (14)	0.55 (0.31–0.98)	
	College or higher	56 (14)	132 (16)	0.71 (0.42–2.00)	0.04
Age at menarche	10–14 years	108 (27)	215 (27)	1.00	
	15–16 years	156 (39)	348 (43)	0.90 (0.66–1.22)	
	17–24 years	140 (35)	244 (30)	1.16 (0.84–1.56)	0.32

[a]*P* Trend calculated across categories.

Table 2. Adjusted[a] odd ratios of body mass index, weight, height and waist-to-hip ratio in relation to breast cancer risk in pre- and postmenopausal women

Risk factors	Categories	Premenopausal women (*n*=224/409)		Postmenopausal women (*n*=172/371)	
		Cases/controls: no. (%)	OR (95% CI)	Cases/controls: no. (%)	OR (95% CI)
Height (cm)	132–50	64/101 (29/24)	1.00	68/141 (40/37)	1.00
	150.1– 155	68/133 (30/32)	0.84 (0.54–1.31)	52/140 (30/37)	0.72 (0.46–1.12)
	155.1–173	92/179 (41/43)	0.82 (0.53–1.25)	52/96 (30/25)	1.04 (0.65–1.67)
			P trend[b] = 0.37		*P* trend[b] = 1.00
Weight (kg)	24–49.5	57/116 (25/28)	1.00	49/146 (28/39)	1.00
	49.6–59	90/152 (40/37)	1.15 (0.75–1.77)	60/133 (34/35)	1.44 (0.90–2.31)
	59.1–110	80/146 (35/35)	1.02 (0.65–1.59)	68/99 (38/26)	2.31 (1.43–3.73)
			P trend[b] = 0.99		*P* trend[b] = 0.001
Body mass index (kg/m^2)	<21.0	64/119 (29/29)	1.00	54/136 (31/37)	1.00
	21.0–24.9	86/176 (38/43)	0.84 (0.56–1.28)	47/140 (27/38)	0.94 (0.58–1.52)
	25.0–29.9	58/87 (26/21)	1.19 (0.74–1.93)	55/74 (32/20)	1.92 (1.16–3.18)
	≥ 30	16/27 (7/7)	1.04 (0.50–2.17)	16/21 (9/6)	2.50 (1.15–5.40)
			P trend[b] = 0.54		*P* trend[b] = 0.002
Waist-to-hip ratio	0.36–0.78	83/159 (38/39)	1.00	34/101 (20/27)	1.00
	0.79–0.83	60/128 (27/31)	0.80 (0.52–1.22)	56/111 (32/30)	1.51 (0.89–2.56)
	0.84–1.41	78/125 (35/30)	1.07 (0.71–1.62)	83/159 (48/43)	1.96 (1.18–3.25)
			P trend[b] = 0.77		*P* trend[b] = 0.001

[a]Adjusted for age, parity, lactation, income and family history of breast cancer.
[b]*P* trend calculated across categories.

Table 3. Adjusted[a] odd ratios of energy intake and physical activity in relation to breast cancer risk in pre- and postmenopausal women

Risk factors	Categories	Premenopausal women (*n*=224/409) Cases/controls: no. (%)	OR (95% CI)	Postmenopausal women (*n*=172/371) Cases/controls: no. (%)	OR (95% CI)
Energy intake	Restricted	126/258 (56/62)	1.00	101/245 (57/64)	1.00
	<15% excess	43/60 (19/15)	1.60 (0.99–2.58)	39/63 (22/17)	1.40 (0.84–2.36)
	≥ 15% excess	58/98 (26/24)	1.55 (1.00–2.39)	38/73 (21/19)	1.24 (0.74–2.09)
			P trend[b] = 0.030		*P* trend[b] = 0.30
Physical activity	Light	53/68 (23/16)	1.00	34/68 (19/23)	1.00
	Medium	89/185 (39/44)	0.42 (0.26–0.70)	89/185 (40/44)	1.15 (0.68–1.95)
	High	85/163 (37/39)	0.39 (0.23–0.68)	85/163 (40/33)	1.52 (0.86–2.69)
			P trend[b] = 0.003		*P* trend[b] = 0.13

[a]Adjusted for age, parity, lactation, income, family history of breast cancer and BMI.
[b]*P* trend calculated across categories.

of breast cancer risk for self-reported physical activity and an increase in the risk for excess energy intake.

Discussion

Although the findings are somewhat consistent with studies from Western populations, they reflect Asian population characteristics. In contrast to a report of a small increased risk of breast cancer with increased height (Hunter & Willett, 1993), body height did not appear to be associated with breast cancer risk in pre- or postmenopausal women. The lack of an association here may be due to the generally short stature in this population as a result of restricted nutrition. The failure to observe a reduced risk of breast cancer in obese premenopausal women may be due to the low prevalence of obesity and therefore the suggested mechanism of anovulation was not likely to influence the risk. The lack of an observed influence of physical activity on postmenopausal breast cancer can be explained by the high prevalence in the population of women with a high level of physical activity and lean body mass. The pattern of excess energy intake associated with breast cancer in pre- but not postmenopausal women was similar to the pattern of association between breast cancer risk and insulin-like growth factor-I, which is suggested to be associated with high energy intake and breast cancer risk (Kaaks, 1996).

However, the limitations of the study should be considered. Physical activity data was self-reported and reflected day-to-day activity rather than exercise, since exercise is not a common practice. Thus exercise is likely to provide a minor contribution to total energy expenditure. In addition, if misclassification occurred because of the self-reported data, it could lead to attenuation of the associations. Body measurements were considered to be accurate as these were measured by the interviewers.

In summary, despite a few differences with data from affluent communities, indicators of excess energy intake from this low-incidence population were associated with increased breast cancer risk in premenopausal women in particular. These factors may possibly partly explain the low incidence of breast cancer in this nation. Provided that these are modifiable factors and obesity is prevalent in particular in Western populations and potentially in Asian populations, modifications of these lifestyle factors could considerably reduce the incidence of cancer.

References

Hunter, D.J. & Willett, W.C. (1993) Diet, body size, and breast cancer. *Epidemiol. Rev.*, **15**, 110–132

Kaaks, R. (1996) Nutrition, hormones, and breast cancer: is insulin the missing link? *Cancer Causes Control*, **7**, 605–625

Parkin, D.M., Wheland, S.L., Ferlay, J., Raymond, L. & Yong, J. (1997) *Cancer Incidence in Five Continents Vol. VII.* (IARC Scientific Publications No. 143) Lyon, International Agency for Research on Cancer, France

Willett, W.C., Stampfer, M.J., Colditz, G.A., Rosner, B.A., Hennekens, C.H. & Speizer, F.E. (1987) Dietary fat and the risk of breast cancer. *N. Engl. J. Med.*, **316**, 22–28

World Cancer Research Fund & American Institute for Cancer Research. (1997) *Food, Nutrition and the Prevention of Cancer: A Global Perspective.* Washington, D.C., American Institute for Cancer Research

Epidemiological characteristics of colorectal cancer in Vojvodina

Miladinov-Mikov M., Lukic N., Petrovic T.

Institute of Oncology-Cancer Registry of Vojvodina-Sremska Kamenica, Yugoslavia

The epidemiological characteristics of colorectal cancer were analysed for the 25-year period from 1973 to 1997. The analysis is based on the official data of the Cancer Registry of Vojvodina, which covers about 2 000 000 inhabitants. It is a population-based registry, the oldest of this type in the entire country, which routinely collects and analyses data on all cancer patients in the province (Mikov *et al.*, 1994).

Using a descriptive epidemiological method, basic characteristics of colorectal cancer in Vojvodina are presented.

Excluding nonmelanotic skin cancer, colorectal cancer was the second most commonly diagnosed cancer in Vojvodina, accounting for more than 12% in both sexes in 1997. It was also the second most common cancer death in males (11.4%) and females (12%).

Over a period from 1973 to 1997, the total of 15 920 cases of colorectal cancers were registered, on average 637 per year, in the territory of Vojvodina. Just over half of these (52.5%) occurred in males. Colon cancer was slightly less frequent than rectal cancer, comprising 48.8% of all malignancies of the large bowel. At the same time, a total of 11 434 cases died from colorectal cancer, on average 457 cases per year. This indicates an overall case fatality rate of 71.7%.

Vojvodina has relatively low incidence rates of colon cancer compared with other regions in the world (Parkin *et al.*, 1997). Nevertheless, rates in Vojvodina have increased, particularly in males. The crude incidence rate of colon cancer varied from 7.8/100 000 in 1973 to 24.2/100 000 in 1997 in males, while in females it varied from 8.8/100 000 in 1973 to 23.1/100 000 in 1990. The crude mortality rate varied from 5.4/100 000 in 1973 to 18.8/100 000 in 1997 for males and for the females from 7/100 000 in 1973 to 15.5/100 000 in 1996 (Fig. 1 and 2). The overall linear time trends for both genders in incidence and mortality of colon cancer increased steadily and significantly over the observed period, with a greater increase, however, in incidence rates than in mortality rates (Miladinov-Mikov *et al.*, 1999). A similar tendency is noted worldwide (Coleman *et al.*, 1993).

The crude incidence rate of rectal cancer varied from 11.3/100 000 in 1976

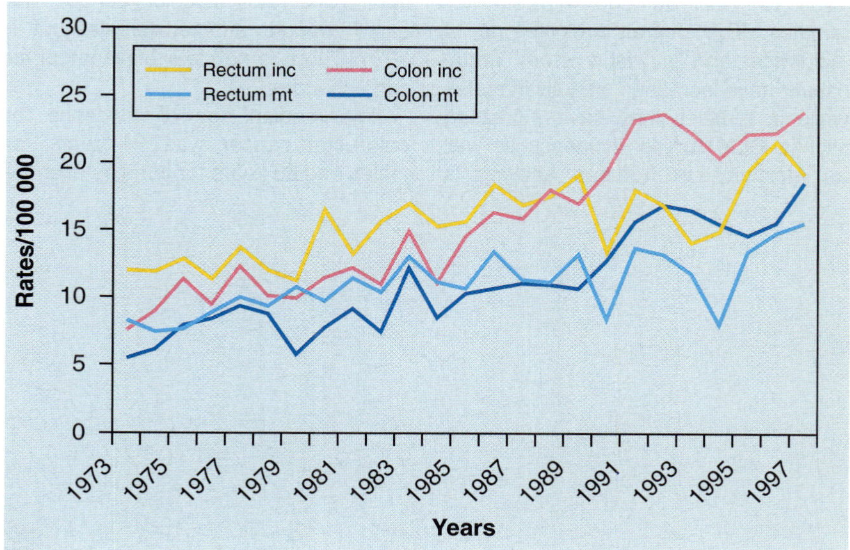

Figure 1
Incidence (inc) and mortality (mt) rates of colon and rectal cancer, Vojvodina, males, 1973–1997

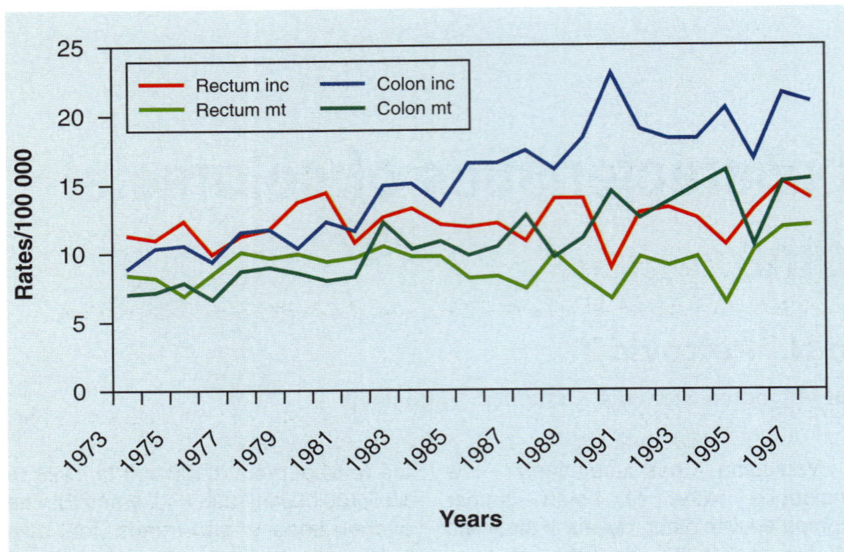

Figure 2
Incidence and mortality rates of colon and rectal cancer, Vojvodina, females, 1973–1997

to 21.7/100 000 in 1996 for males, while in females it varied from 8.9/100 000 in 1990 to 15.3/100 000 in 1996. Mortality rates from rectal cancer varied from 7.7/100 000 in 1974 to 15.7/100 000 in 1997 for males and from 6/100 000 in 1994 to 11.9/100 000 in 1997 for females. The overall time trends of incidence and mortality from rectal cancer have increased steadily in males while in females they have increased slightly. Both curves, incidence as well as mortality, in females showed a fluctuating pattern.

Incidence and mortality rates of rectal cancer in males fell in 1989 and were exceeded by the rates of colon cancer. Although the rates of rectal cancer increased afterwards, they remained behind the rates of colon cancer. The same changes affected females but in 1981. There is no clear explanation for such changes.

The median age of incidence for colorectal cancer was 64 years for males and 65 years for females over the observed period. At the same time, the median age for mortality was 64 and 67 years, respectively.

The age-specific incidence and mortality rate patterns showed a large increase starting with the age group 40–45 years, reaching the highest values in the age group 65–75 years.

The epidemiological situation in regard to colorectal cancer in Vojvodina is unsatisfactory, especially in view of increasing incidence and mortality over time and the absence of organized primary and secondary prevention in our society.

References

Coleman, M.P., Esteve, J., Demiecki, P., Arsland, A. & Rendar, H. (1993) *Trends in Cancer Incidence and Mortality* (IARC Scientific Publication No. 121), Lyon, IARC

Mikov, M., Burany, B. & Popovic, S. (1994) Koncepcija kompjuterske obrade podataka u Registru za maligne neoplazme u Vojvodini. *Arh. Celok. Lek.*, **122**, 302–304

Miladinov-Mikov, M., Lukic, N. & Petrovic, T. (1999) Epidemiology of colon cancer in Vojvodina. *Arch. Oncol.*, **7**, 109–112

Parkin, D.M., Whelan, S.L, Ferlay, J., Raymond, L. & Young, J. (1997) *Cancer Incidence in Five Continents, Vol VII* (IARC Scientific Publication No. 143), Lyon, IARC

Diet and colorectal cancer in Portugal

Amaral T.[1], de Almeida M.D.V.[1], Barros H.[2]

[1]Faculty of Nutrition and Food Sciences, Porto University, Rua Dr. Roberto Frias, 4200-465 Porto, Portugal.
[2]Faculty of Medicine, Porto University, Portugal.

Purpose

In Portugal, a southern European country with several particular food consumption characteristics, the association between diet and colorectal cancer (CRC) has never been studied. The identification of which foods and nutrients are associated with the risk of CRC could give etiological clues and provide preventive strategies.

The aim of the present study was to evaluate the effect of diet – food habits, food and nutrient intake – independently of the contribution of tobacco, alcohol intake and other lifestyle factors, in the risk of CRC in the Portuguese population.

Methods

We conducted a hospital-based case–control study in Porto between 1993 and 1996. Colorectal cancer cases were Portuguese Caucasian males and females, aged 40 or over, with incident colon/rectum histologically confirmed adenocarcinomas, admitted consecutively for treatment in the major central hospital in Porto. This group included 184 participants: 104 men (mean age of 65.4 years; standard deviation, 9.1) and 80 women (65.9 years; SD, 9.3).

The control group included 435 participants, 241 men (mean age of 58.3 years; SD, 10.8) and 194 women (58.4 years; SD, 10.4) admitted to the same hospital, during the same period and from the same residence area as cases, for non-tumoral pathology (minor general or osteoarticular surgery).

Data was collected using a questionnaire for sociodemographic characteristics, physical activity, smoking, self and family history of cancer, prescribed drugs, anthropometry, medical, gynaecological and reproductive history, alcohol intake and other food habits.

A food frequency questionnaire (180 foods and recipes) was developed to measure food intake during the previous year and to classify the participants according to quartiles of daily intakes. Relative validity was assessed in a sample of university students and in a sample of the control group. Results showed that this food frequency questionnaire could be regarded as a reliable source of information for most nutrients (Amaral, 1998).

Trained nutritionists collected data by direct interview. We considered information on food portion sizes, obtained with visual aids, and on culinary methods and seasonal variation in data analysis. The conversion of foods to nutrients was done by the software package Microdiet® completed with Portuguese data. Cases and controls were distributed in quartiles according the distribution of each variable of total sample in the study. Food groups, foods and nutrients were adjusted for total energy intake that was made by the residual method.

The association between the disease and possible risk factors was calculated by the means of odds ratios (OR) and 95% confidence intervals (CI), in univariate analysis and adjusted using non-conditional logistic regression (OR for the highest category versus the lowest).

Results

As an interaction between total energy intake and sex was found, different models were calculated (Table 1).

Both for men and for women (Table 2), high intakes of calcium, fibre (soluble or insoluble), vitamin C and vegetables, including cruciferous vegetables (for men OR, 0.37; CI, 0.16–0.82 and for women OR, 0.28; CI, 0.12–0.66), decreased the risk of CRC.

High consumption of folate, carotene and fruits, coffee, low intake of CHO-rich foods and a high ratio alfa-tocopherol/PUFA (>0.4) were also associated with decreased CRC risk in women. For men, high intake of fatty red meat, white fish and the habit of non-removal of visible fat in meat, increased the risk of CRC.

Cases consumed more energy, protein, total fat and cholesterol than controls, although without reaching the level of statistical significance. In men, long-term smoking and low physical activity were also associated with an increased risk of CRC.

Table 1. Colorectal cancer risk – separate models in multivariate analysis for men and woman						
	Men OR	95% CI	*P*	Women OR	95% CI	*P*
Age (years)	1.1	1.05–1.11	<0.001	1.10	1.06–1.14	<0.001
Education (years)						
0	1.0			1.0		
1–4	1.6	0.8–3.5	0.213	1.4a	0.9–2.3	0.173
≥ 5	1.1	0.4–2.7	0.913			
Positive family history of CRC (yes vs no)	6.5	1.9–22.7	0.003	8.8	2.8–27.8	<0.001
Total physical activity (hours x intensity x years)						
>111 vs <70	0.3	0.1–0.7	0.003	0.7	0.3–1.6	0.407
Energy intake (100 kcal)	1.05	0.99–1.11	0.089	1.03	0.97–1.09	0.393
Tobacco (packs/year)						
0.0				1.0		
0.1–20.1	1.8	0.8–3.8	0.140			
20.2–40.1	2.3	1.0–5.4	0.051			
≥ 40.2	2.5	1.3–5.0	0.008			
Non-removal of visible fat in meat						
Never vs ever	1.9	1.0–3.6	0.040			
Ethanol (g/day)						
0.06–1.6	1.0					
23.8–56.2	1.7	0.7–4.0	0.260			
56.3–326.3	1.5	0.6–3.9	0.442			

[a]≥ 1 vs 0.

Discussion and conclusions

The results of this study suggest an inverse independent association of CRC for both men and women with vegetables and fruits and some of their components, such as vitamin C, fibre, carotenes and folate, as already described for other countries (WCRF/AICR, 1997).

In this sample with a wide range of exposure, high calcium intake, but not high dairy product consumption, decreased the risk of CRC, suggesting that total calcium or calcium from other sources, such as vegetables, could be more relevant in reducing CRC risk (Janneke *et al.*, 1996).

In women, the high ratio alfa-tocopherol eq/g PUFA (>0.4 mg) (Dupont *et al.*, 1996) was associated with a lower risk of CRC and the intake of more than one cup of coffee/day independently decreased the risk of CRC.

As recently described (Ekbom *et al.*, 2001), we found an increased risk with long-term tobacco smoking in men. We were not able to study the role of tobacco in CRC risk in women, because only 5% of cases and 3% of controls were exposed.

The role of energy, protein, total lipids and cholesterol needs to be further confirmed. Other nutrient or dietary patterns were not associated with CRC.

Table 2. Nutrients and foods and colorectal cancer risk: multivariate analysis

	Men[a] Cases/controls *n*	OR	95% CI	Women[b] Cases/controls *n*	OR	95% CI
Protein (g/day)						
30.4–68.0	29/69	1.00	–	16/40	1.00	–
68.1–78.4	24/61	1.01	0.47–2.18	19/51	0.80	0.31–2.06
78.5–89.9	21/62	1.37	0.61–3.07	18/53	1.44	0.54–3.84
90.0–162.9	30/49	2.02	0.88–4.56	27/50	1.40	0.55–3.53
Total lipids (g/day)						
12.4–37.6	33/80	1.00	–	10/32	1.00	–
37.7–45.7	27/72	0.95	0.47–1.65	19/36	1.53	0.57–4.11
45.8–81.5	20/50	1.07	0.48–2.40	24/61	1.40	0.56–3.50
81.6–98.8	24/39	2.18	0.96–4.97	27/65	1.21	0.48–3.09
Cholesterol (mg/day)						
9.1–162.4	29/60	1.00	–	18/47	1.00	–
162.5–217.2	23/67	0.74	0.35–1.54	18/47	1.19	0.48–2.99
217.3–272.6	26/70	0.88	0.41–1.87	12/46	0.78	0.28–2.16
272.7–585.0	26/44	1.87	0.81–4.29	32/54	1.90	0.75–4.81
Calcium (mg/day)						
198.5–538.7	36/58	1.00	–	23/37	1.00	–
538.8–743.3	25/72	0.62	0.30–1.28	17/41	0.55	0.23–1.32
743.4–1024.4	32/51	0.87	0.42–1.79	18/53	0.47	0.20–1.10
1025.5–3094.5	11/60	0.29	0.12–0.71	22/63	0.38	0.17–0.87
Vitamin C (mg/day)						
13.4–71.3	41/57	1.00	–	31/25	1.00	–
71.4–107.7	27/66	0.60	0.30–1.21	18/43	0.52	0.22–1.25
107.8–153.8	21/65	0.39	0.18–0.83	13/56	0.22	0.01–0.55
153.9–622.6	15/53	0.39	0.17–0.89	18/70	0.28	0.12–0.63
Fibre (g/day)						
4.6–16.0	42/58	1.00	–	24/31	1.00	–
16.1–19.6	26/55	0.73	0.34–1.55	24/49	0.75	0.33–1.70
19.7–23.8	19/76	0.37	0.18–0.78	16/43	0.56	0.23–1.36
23.9–39.8	17/52	0.49	0.20–1.16	16/71	0.32	0.14–0.76
Folate (μg/day)						
132.4–302.5	35/52	1.00	–	23/23	1.00	–
302.6–383.4	31/65	0.76	0.36–1.59	22/58	0.45	0.19–1.09
383.5–455.1	19/65	0.50	0.23–1.12	18/52	0.30	0.12–0.74
455.2–919.4	19/59	0.49	0.21–1.12	17/61	0.26	0.11–0.63
Carotene (μg/day)						
24.3–1728.3	35/64	1.00	–	29/26	1.00	–
1728.4–2812.6	34/54	0.76	0.36–1.59	17/49	0.29	0.12–0.70
2812.7–4362.9	19/68	0.50	0.23–1.12	16/52	0.22	0.01–0.55
4363.0–21396.4	16/55	0.49	0.21–1.12	18/67	0.21	0.01–0.48

Table 2 (cont). Nutrients and foods and colorectal cancer risk: multivariate analysis

	Men[a] Cases/controls n	OR	95% CI	Women[b] Cases/controls n	OR	95% CI
Vegetables (g/day)						
8.2–124.9	39/56	1.00	–	30/29	1.00	–
125.0–183.3	29/57	0.67	0.33–1.36	14/55	0.25	0.10–0.61
183.4–287.4	24/66	0.63	0.30–1.31	21/44	0.54	0.24–1.22
287.5–761.1	12/62	0.32	0.14–0.76	15/66	0.23	0.01–0.54
Fatty red meat (g/day)						
0.0–0.01	25/95	1.00	–	9/24	1.00	–
0.2–2.1	28/57	1.71	0.74–3.97	19/52	1.24	0.36–4.29
2.2–5.4	9/30	0.81	0.24–2.72	33/82	1.71	0.41–7.14
5.5–286.0	42/59	2.28	1.12–4.62	19/36	2.98	0.72–10.01
White fish (g/day)						
0.0–3.4	21/73	1.00	–	15/44	1.00	–
3.5–11.4	34/76	1.24	0.58–2.63	15/31	2.06	0.76–5.59
11.5–23.0	25/58	1.76	0.80–3.87	23/48	1.77	0.75–4.22a
23.1–227.9	24/34	3.25	1.33–7.98	27/71	1.64	0.70–3.85
Alfa-tocopherol (eq)/PUFA (g)<0.4			0.69	0.38–1.24		0.45 0.24–0.83
Coffee (≥ 50 ml vs 0)		0.65	0.32–1.34		0.36	0.47–0.93

[a]Adjusted for age, education, family history of CRC, total physical activity, tobacco, ethanol and total energy.
[b]Adjusted for age, education, family history of CRC, physical activity at work and total energy.

Acknowledgements

The first author was funded by the "Junta Nacional de Investigação Científica e Tecnológica – Program Ciência (BD/2223/92) and Program Praxis XXI (BD/5481/95)".

References

Amaral, T. (1998) *Nutritional risk in the epidemiology of breast and colo-rectal cancer*. Ph D Thesis. Faculty of Nutrition and Food Sciences, Porto University, Portugal

Dupont, J., Holub, B.J., Knapp, H.R. & Meydani, M. (1996) Fatty acid-related function. *Am. J. Clin. Nutr.*, **63**, 991S–993S

Terry, P., Ekbom, A., Lichtenstein, P., Feychting, M. & Wolk, A. (2001) Long-term tobacco smoking and colorectal cancer in a prospective cohort study. *Int. J. Cancer*, **91**, 585–587

Bergsma Kadijk, J.A., Van't Veer, P., Kampman, E. & Burema, J. (1996) Calcium does not protect against colorectal neoplasia. *Epidemiology*, **7**, 590–597

World Cancer Research Fund/American Institute for Cancer Research (1997) *Food, Nutrition and the Prevention of Cancer: A Global Perspective*, Washington, D.C., American Institute for Cancer Research

Calorie restriction reduces the incidence of radiation-induced myeloid leukaemia

Yoshida K.[1], Hirabayashi Y.[2], Inoue T.[2]

[1]Radiation Hazard Research Group, National Institute of Radiological Sciences, Chiba 263-8555, Japan.
[2]Division of Cellular & Molecular Toxicology, National Institute of Health Sciences, Tokyo 158-8501, Japan.

Introduction

Dietary restriction, especially caloric restriction, is a major carcinogenic modifier in experimental carcinogenesis, and is known to decrease significantly not only spontaneous, but also induced cancers by chemicals. In view of the potential importance in the contribution of dietary calories on radiation-induced cancers in animals as well as in man, we attempted to examine the effects of caloric restriction on the radiation-induced myeloid leukaemia (MyL) as an experimental model, because the incidence of MyL is known to have increased significantly among the survivors of atomic bombs in Hiroshima and Nagasaki.

Materials and methods

Mice and irradiation

C3H/HeNirMs male mice, 6 weeks old and bred in our institute, were used. Mice were exposed to 3 Gy of whole-body X irradiation, by a 200KV 20 mA through a therapeutic X-ray irradiator (Shimadzu, Tokyo, Japan). All the mice in the irradiated groups were given 3 Gy at the age of 10 weeks.

Diets

Detailed methods of caloric restriction and diets used are reported elsewhere (Yoshida *et al.*, 1997). Briefly, the diets consisted of four different calorie controlled regimens, i.e. 60, 65, 70 and 95 kcal per week per mouse (Table 1). The calorie intake was adjusted weekly by varying the amount of carbohydrate and dextrose with the four regimens, under the constant amount of other nutrients, such as protein, lipid, vitamins and minerals.

Experimental groups and procedures

Caloric restriction was designed so as to distinguish the group restricted from the age of 6 weeks until irradiation at 10 weeks (RC) from the other restricted groups: after irradiation (RB), the other groups restricted throughout the life span from 6 weeks of age (RA) and the group without restriction (NR) (Table 2). According to the theory of multi-step

Table 1. Composition of diet (g per mouse per week)

Diets[a]: kcal/ mouse/week	Cornstarch	Dextrose	Milk casein	Corn oil	Fibre	Alpha starch	Vitamin mixture	Mineral mixture
95	1.3	2.7	6.3	0.8	1.4	0.3	0.3	1.9
75	9.18	1.82	6.3	0.8	1.4	0.3	0.3	1.9
70	8.5	1.8	6.0	0.8	1.3	0.3	0.3	1.9
65	7.4	1.4	6.0	0.8	1.3	0.3	0.3	1.9
60	5.9	1.2	6.3	0.8	1.4	0.3	0.3	1.9

[a]Diets consisted of five different calorie-controlled regimens. The calorie intake was adjusted by controlling the amount of carbohydrate and dextrose, while keeping intake amount of other nutrients, such as protein, lipid, vitamins and minerals, constant.

Table 2. Experimental groups

Groups	No. of mice	Diet 6 weeks ~10 weeks	Kcal per mouse per week Weeks ~ throughout the life span	Radiation (3 Gy) At the age of 10 weeks
CNR	262	95 kcal	95 kcal	No
3NR	272	95 kcal	95 kcal	Yes
CRAa	70	65 kcal	60~95 kcal (Average 75 kcal)	No
3RAa	76	65 kcal	60~95 kcal (Average 75 kcal)	Yes
CRBa	135	95 kcal	60~95 kcal (Average 75 kcal)	No
3RBa	131	95 kcal	60~95 kcal (Average 75 kcal)	Yes
CRC	95	65 kcal	95 kcal	No
3RC	99	65 kcal	95 kcal	Yes

[a]The body weight of mice was measured weekly, and then mice in the groups were controlled to keep their body weight between 25 and 27g. The average caloric intake from the age of 10 weeks and thereafter was about 75 kcal per mouse per week.

carcinogenesis, the experiment was designed so that the RC group would predict an initiation effect and the RB group, a promotion effect.

Cell cycle analysis on haematopoietic stem cells

Cell cycle analysis on the haematopoietic stem cells (HSC) was made on mice at age 40 weeks. Incorporation of bromodeoxyuridine followed by ultraviolet exposure (BUUV) cytocide assay (Hirabayashi *et al.*, 1998) was performed to evaluate the size of the cycling stem cell compartment for both restricted (CRB) and control (CNR) groups.

Results

Incidence of myeloid leukemia

The incidence of MyL decreased with caloric restriction. Incidence of MyL in non-irradiated groups, CNR, CRA, CRB and CRC, were 1.1, 1, 0 and 2.1%, respectively. When irradiated, the incidences increased up to 21.6% in 3NR, 7.9% in 3RA, 10.7% in 3RB and 16.2% in 3RC. Therefore, a significant decrease from 3NR to 3RA and 3RB was observed. A decrease was also observed from the 3RC to the 3NR; however, the difference was not statistically significant.

Number of haematopoietic stem cells at irradiation

When the number of HSC, the possible target cells for radiation-induced leukemogenesis, was evaluated in both restricted and non-restricted groups at the time immediately before the irradiation (10 weeks old), the number of CFU-S in the spleen decreased from 38 per 10^6 cells in the non-restricted group to 10 per 10^6 cells in the restricted group. The total number of CFU-S per spleen in the restricted group (0.93×10^3 per spleen) decreased to 10% in the non-restricted group (9.1×10^3 per spleen), whereas the number of CFU-S in the bone marrow was less significant in the restricted group compared with the non-restricted group.

Size of cycling fraction of the stem cells

A statistically significant decrease was observed in the size of CFU-S in the cell cycle in the femur, dropping from 46% in the group for NR to 26% in the RA and RB. In the spleen, the size of CFU-S also decreased from 31.4% in the NR to 17.7% in the RA and RB.

Conclusions

The incidence of MyL decreased with caloric restriction, which may have contributed to reduce the incidence of leukaemia the initiation stage of leukaemogenesis, but more significantly to reduce the effect in the promotion process of leukaemogenesis after irradiation.

The number of haematopoietic stem cells was significantly decreased in the restriction groups, RC and RA, especially in the spleen, at the time of radiation exposure. Since the incidence of leukaemia was greatly decreased in the RB group in which the number of stem cells was naturally similar to the NR group, and further the suppression of leukaemia in RC was less significant, the decrease in stem cell number at irradiation did not seem to be a major reason for the reduction of leukaemia incidence by caloric restriction.

The cycling fraction of the HSC in the restricted group was smaller than the non-restriction group, implying that the haematopoietic stem cells in the restriction groups proliferate at a rate much slower than those in NR mice do, and the proliferation rate after irradiation may also contribute the reduction seen in groups, RA and RB.

Acknowledgements

The authors thank Ms. F. Watanabe, S. Wada, K. Nojima, M. Terada for their technical assistance. This work was supported by a special project grant for experimental studies on the radiation health detriment and its modifying factors from the Japan Science and Technology Agency.

References

Hirabayashi, Y., Matsumura, T., Matsuda, M., Kuramoto, K., Motoyoshi, K., Yoshida, K., Sasaki, H. & Inoue, T. (1998) Cell kinetics of hematopoietic colony-forming units in spleen (CFU-S) in young and old mice. *Mech. Ageing Dev.*, **101**, 221–223

Yoshida, K., Inoue, T., Nojima, K., Hirabayashi, Y. & Sado, T. (1997) Calorie restriction reduces the incidence of myeloid leukemia induced by a single whole-body radiation in C3H/He mice. *Proc. Natl. Acad. Sci. U.S.A.*, **94**, 2615–2619

Dietary factors and brain tumours in adults: pilot study results of a case–control investigation in Rio de Janeiro, Brazil

Pereira R.A.[1], Monteiro G.T.R.[2], Koifman S.[2]

[1]Institute of Nutrition, Federal University of Rio de Janeiro, Brazil. [2]Department of Epidemiology, National School of Public Health, Rio de Janeiro, Brazil.

Background

Brain tumours are important because of apparent increases in incidence and mortality rates and the low survival rates observed. Legler *et al.* (1999) consider that the rise in brain cancer rates is probably due to the introduction of more precise and less invasive diagnosis procedures such as computerized tomography and magnetic resonance imaging. However, Schechter (1999) maintains that the increasing brain tumour rates could be related to the introduction of unidentified neurocarcinogens into the environment. In Brazil, brain cancer mortality rates have been increasing since 1980, particularly in elderly people and women.

Purpose

This work presents preliminary results on diet profiles obtained in the pilot study of a hospital-based case–control study in progress in the Rio de Janeiro metropolitan area since 1999.

Methods

Cases were identified among selected hospitals' in-patients with primary brain tumour and included 30- to 65-year-old patients living in the study area. Controls were selected among in-patients of the same hospitals; they were matched for frequency, age and sex, lived in the same area, and had a diagnosis of other than cancer or diet-related diseases.

A food frequency questionnaire was used in 64 cases and 77 controls to assess food intake during adolescence and in the year before hospitalization. The patients were asked about changes in their diet between adolescence and the year before diagnosis.

The contribution of food groups to brain cancer risk was ascertained by stratified analysis and by unconditional logistic regression procedures.

Results

Changes in diet between adolescence and the year before diagnosis were more often reported among controls than cases: 54.5% and 32.8%, respectively. Changing diet showed a protective effect against brain cancer: odds ratio (OR), 0.42; 95% confidence interval (95% CI), 0.21–0.85, even after stratification in individuals with and without familial history of cancer (OR, 0.56; 95% CI, 0.26–1.22).

Industrialized-food intake during adolescence (OR, 2.07; 95% CI, 0.69–6.39) and a high intake level of cholesterol in the year before diagnosis (OR, 3.60; 95% CI, 1.22–10.63) were associated with increased brain cancer risk, even after adjustment for total energy intake and familial history of cancer (Table 1).

Discussion and conclusion

The category "industrialized products" could be a marker of the dietary habits pattern, possibly indicating intensive intake of *N*-nitroso compound precursors and a reduced fruit and vegetable intake.

Boeing *et al.* (1993) mentioned that the heating of plant oils could be relevant to the development of brain tumours. Giles *et al.* (1994) observed an increased risk of brain cancer with a high intake of eggs and oils and Blowers *et al.* (1997) also observed an increase in the risk of brain tumours in association with intake of eggs and fried potatoes.

The limitation imposed by the data of a pilot study does not allow more complex analysis to evaluate the

Table 1. Brain cancer and dietary intake in adolescence and in the year previous to diagnosis, Rio de Janeiro, Brazil, 1998–2000

Models and variables	βa	OR[b]	CI[c]
1 Frequency of industrialized food intake during adolescence	0.253	1.29	0.52–3.17
Cholesterol intake in the year before diagnosis	0.893	2.44	1.09–5.49
2 Frequency of industrialized food intake during adolescence	0.725	2.07	0.69–6.39
Cholesterol intake in the year before diagnosis	1.281	3.60	1.22–10.63
Familial history of cancer	–0.038	0.96	0.40–2.29
Energy intake in adolescence (100 kcal variation)	–0.074	0.93	0.76–1.13
Energy intake in the year before diagnosis (100 kcal variation)	0.012	1.01	0.83–1.23

[a]β, regression coefficient.
[b]OR, odds ratio.
[c]CI, 95% confidence interval.

modifier effect of other variables or the specific effect for the different histological types of brain tumours.

The results support previous reports that some dietary factors could act by modulating brain carcinogenesis. Following new case enrolment, evaluation of such associations will be further carried out taking into account specific histological strata.

References

Blowers, L., Preston-Martin, S. & Mack, W.J. (1997) Dietary and other lifestyle factors of women with brain gliomas in Los Angeles County (California, USA). *Cancer Causes Control.* **8**, 5–12

Boeing, H., Schlehofer, B., Blettner, M. & Wahrendorf, J. (1993) Dietary carcinogens and the risk for glioma and meningioma in Germany. *Int. J. Cancer,* **53**, 561–565

Giles, G.G., McNeil, J.J., Donnan, G., Webley, C., Staples, M.P., Ireland, P.D., Hurley, S.F. & Salzberg, M. (1994) Dietary factors and the risk of glioma in adults: results of a case–control study in Melbourne, Australia. *Int. J. Cancer,* **59**, 357–362

Legler, J.M., Gloecker, R., Smith, M.A., Warren, J.L,. Heineman, E.F., Kaplan, R.S. & Linet, M.S. (1999) Brain and other central nervous system cancer: recent trends in incidence and mortality. *J. Natl. Cancer Inst.*, **91**, 1382–1390

Schechter, C.B. (1999) Re: brain and other central nervous system cancer: recent trends in incidence and mortality. *J. Natl. Cancer Inst.*, **91**, 2050

Diet and cancer of oral cavity and pharynx: a case–control study in São Paulo, Brazil

Marchioni D.L., Fisberg R.M., do Rosário M., Latorre D.O., Wunsch V.

University of São Paulo, São Paulo, Brazil.

Introduction

Cancer of the oral cavity and the pharynx is the fifth incidence of cancer worldwide and presents great geographical variability (La Vecchia *et al.*, 1997). Data from the report of the Sao Paulo cancer registries presents one of the highest incidences for cancer of the oral cavity and pharynx in Latin America (Wunsch & Camargo, 2001).

Tobacco and alcohol, recognized risk factors for oral cancer in general, are also important risk factors in Latin America and the Caribbean (La Vecchia *et al.*, 1997; Wunsch & Camargo, 2001). Diet and eating habits could have important implications in the causality of oral cavity and pharynx cancer, considering the particular dietary cultures in different regions. The objective of this study was to investigate the role played by dietary factors in oral cavity and pharynx cancer in the city of São Paulo.

Material and methods

Data referred to in this paper is part of a Latin American multicentre hospital-based case–control study coordinated by the International Agency for Research on Cancer (Boffetta *et al.*, 1998). Between November 1998 and March 2001, 260 cases of oral cavity, oropharynx and hypopharynx cancer, including 36 women (median age, 55.5 years; range, 30–90 years) were identified in seven hospitals in São Paulo City. All interviews were performed before any cancer treatment began. Controls were 257 subjects, including 68 women (median age, 57 years; range, 23–85 years) who had been admitted to the same hospitals of the study for conditions unrelated with diseases that are negatively or positively associated with known or suspected risk factors for cancer of the oral cavity and pharynx. Control subjects were frequency matched with cases by sex and quinquennia of age.

Written consent to participate in the study was obtained from cases and controls. All interviews were conducted by trained interviewers using a structured questionnaire, which included information on age, education and other socio-economic factors such as detailed occupational histories, smoking and drinking habits and history of cancer in first-degree relatives. Information about diet included questions on the weekly frequency of consumption of 27 food items before the appearance of any symptoms of the disease. The answers were open and consumption was converted into times per day. The food items were regrouped into dairy (milk, yogurt, cheese), cereals (bread, pasta or rice and corn), meat (beef, poultry, fish, pork or any other meat), sausages

Table 1. Mean intake of portions per day of selected food groups. São Paulo, 1998–2001

Food group portions per day	Controls (n=257) Mean (SD)	Cases (n=260) Mean (SD)	P (t test)
Dairy	1.25 (0.95)	1.35 (1.54)	0.376
Pulses	1.56 (0.89)	1.40 (0.75)	0.023
Cereals	2.96 (1.25)	2.90 (1.23)	0.614
Meat	1.15 (0.63)	1.18 (0.74)	0.761
Sausage	0.16 (0.25)	0.19 (0.31)	0.163
Vegetables	1.55 (0.94)	1.52 (1.07)	0.741
Fruits	1.86 (1.50)	1.57 (1.23)	0.016
Desserts	0.30 (0.38)	0.27 (0.40)	0.349

(sausages, ham or salami), vegetables (raw, cruciferous, tomato or carrot), pulses, fruits (juice, banana, apple or pear) and desserts. The total frequency of intake per day was divided into tertiles.

Data analysis

Student's *t* test was performed to compare means of intake of food groups among cases and controls. The associations were assessed by chi-square test. Odds ratios (OR) for oral and pharynx cancer and the corresponding 95% confidence interval for tertiles of each food group were estimated using unconditional logistic regression. The final model was adjusted for age, sex, tobacco and alcohol consumption.

In the unconditional logistic regression analyses, a statistically significant inverse association emerged for the highest intake for pulses and cereals compared with the lowest. A protective but nonsignificant effect was also observed for fruits and for the highest tertile of intake of vegetables. The intake of desserts showed a linear

Table 2. Odds ratio of oral cancer and pharyngeal cancer (with 95% confidence intervals), according to approximate tertiles of food groups, São Paulo, 1998–2001

Food group	Tertiles of intake[a]	Control	Case	$P(\chi^2)$	OR (95% CI)[b]	Linear trend
Dairy	0.714	71	92	0.099	1.00	0.258
	1.429	93	75		0.69 (0.44–1.11)	
	14.14	93	93		1.08 (0.68–1.74)	
Pulses	1.00	98	112	0.000	1.00	0.007
	2.00	4	37		4.73 (1.58–14.14)	
	9.14	155	111		0.48 (0.32–0.73)	
Cereals	2.43	76	91	0.305	1.00	0.132
	3.14	91	80		0.63 (0.39–1.03)	
	10	103	89		0.56 (0.35–0.90)	
Meat	0.86	73	78	0.918	1.00	0.777
	1.28	91	89		1.02 (0.64–1.65)	
	5.00	93	93		1.01 (0.63–1.62)	
Sausage	0.00	116	114	0.027	1.00	0.143
	0.14	84	64		0.77 (0.49–1.22)	
	2.86	57	82		1.30 (0.82–2.07)	
Vegetables	1.00	74	87	0.225	1.00	0.099
	1.71	89	96		1.05 (0.66–1.66)	
	6.00	94	77		0.86 (0.54–1.39)	
Fruits	0.85	81	106	0.056	1.00	0.144
	2.00	85	66		0.71 (0.45–1.15)	
	8.00	91	88		0.87 (0.55–1.37)	
Desserts	0.00	71	107	0.003	1.00	0.021
	0.28	115	87		0.45 (0.29–0.71)	
	2.14	71	66		0.63 (0.38–1.04)	

[a]Upper limit, portions per day.
[b]Estimates from multiple logistic regression equations adjusting for age, gender, smoking and alcohol consumption. OR, odds ratio; CI, confidence interval.

trend protective risk. There was nonsignificant risk associated with oral cancer for dairy, meat and sausage.

Discussion

In our study, preliminary analyses showed that cases had significantly smaller mean intake of pulses and fruits. High intake of cereal and pulses were associated with significant decrease of risk. Grains and legumes were reported as protective in an earlier study conducted in Uruguay (De Stefani *et al.*, 1999). Increased nonsignificant risk was detected in the highest tertile sausage intake. An unexpected protective effect of desserts with a significant trend was observed. Fruits and vegetables, factors recognized as protective against these kinds of cancer by numerous studies (La Vecchia, 1997; De Stefani *et al.*, 1999; Franceschi, 1999), were also protective in our study.

A limitation of this study is the small number of food items. The recall of the past diet may also be affected by early symptoms of cancer, psychosocial issues and current diet. Such biases should weaken the associations observed.

In conclusion, the results are suggestive that diets rich in cereals and pulses, such as the Brazilian diet composed basically of rice and beans, plus high intakes of vegetables and fruits could be protective for oral and pharynx cancer.

References

Boffetta, P., Brennan, P. & Herrero, R. (1998) *International study on environment, viruses and cancer of oral cavity and larynx study protocol.* Lyon, International Agency for Research on Cancer (IARC)

De Stefani, E., Deneo-Pellegrini, H., Mendilaharsu, M. & Ronco, A. (1999) Diet and risk of cancer of the upper aerodigestive tract: 1 – foods. *Oral Oncol.*, **35**, 17–21

Franceschi, S., Favero, A., Conti, E., Talamini, R., Volpe, R., Negri, E., Barzan, L. & La Vecchia, C. (1999) Food groups, oil and butter, and cancer of oral cavity and pharynx. *Br. J. Cancer*, **80**, 614–620

La Vecchia, C., Tavani, A., Franceschi, S., Levi, F., Corrao, G. & Negri, E. (1997) Epidemiology and prevention of oral cancer. *Oral Oncol.*, **33**, 302–312

Wunsch, V. & Camargo, E.A. (2001) The burden of mouth cancer in Latin America and the Caribbean: epidemiological issues. *Semin. Oncol.*, **28**, 158–168

Achevé d'imprimer sur les presses
de l'Imprimerie Darantiere à Dijon-Quetigny
en août 2002

Dépôt légal : août 2002
N° d'impression : 22-1002

Imprimé en France